Digital Dentistry

Antigoni Delantoni • Kaan Orhan
Editors

Digital Dentistry

An Overview and Future Prospects

Springer

Editors
Antigoni Delantoni
Faculty of Dentistry
Aristotle University of Thessaloniki
Thessaloniki, Greece

Kaan Orhan
Faculty of Dentistry
Ankara University
Ankara, Turkey

Ankara University Medical Design
Application and Research Center
(MEDITAM)
Ankara, Turkey

Department of Oral Diagnostics
Faculty of Dentistry
Semmelweis University
Budapest, Hungary

ISBN 978-3-031-52825-5 ISBN 978-3-031-52826-2 (eBook)
https://doi.org/10.1007/978-3-031-52826-2

This Springer imprint is published by the registered company Springer Nature Switzerland AG
The registered company address is: Gewerbestrasse 11, 6330 Cham, Switzerland

Paper in this product is recyclable.

To my family for always loving and supporting me.
They always inspire me and make me a better person.
Without your continuous support this project would not have been possible.

—Antigoni Delantoni

To my family: In gratitude for the unwavering support, encouragement, and inspiration that fueled the journey of bringing these pages to life. Your love has been a guiding light, turning mere words into a heartfelt narrative. This book is dedicated to you, with heartfelt appreciation for the role you've played in making this dream a reality.

—Kaan Orhan

Contents

Part I

Basic Digital Systems in Dentistry

Introduction to Digital Dentistry

1

Kaan Orhan and Antigoni Delantoni

1.1 Introduction

Digital dentistry refers to any dental technology or device that incorporates digital or computer-controlled components. The introduction of digital imaging led to the development of three-dimensional (3D) models and the manufacturing of dental prosthesis. 3D medical modelling began in almost two decades ago and has now exploded using different 3D software. The introduction of digital technology saves time and also provides clinical control of the design, which is very specific to each patient.

Today, the digital revolution is changing the workflow and consequently changing operating procedures. In modern digital dentistry, the four basic phases of work are image acquisition, data preparation/processing, the production and the clinical application on patients. One of the most significant changes is the introduction of 'digital dentistry'—when real teeth and gums are scanned and converted into three-dimensional models on a computer. These models can be used together with computer-aided design to help plan and facilitate more predictable outcomes for dental treatment.

There are different applications for various digital dentistry using digital radiographs. Some of the technologies involved in digital dentistry include CAD/CAM restorations, digitally designed implants, crowns and bridges, digital radiography, digital impressions, digitally based surgical guides, imaging for implant placement, electronic prescriptions.

There are several benefits for utilizing digital dentistry for both the patient and the dentist. The primary benefit is its improved accuracy. The traditional approach to creating dental moulds for crowns and other restorations can sometimes be inaccurate. This can often lead to poorly fitting restorations, not to mention discomfort for the patient. The precision that comes along with the practices involved in digital dentist techniques provides a more up to date solution to these issues.

Digital dentistry allows for streamlined, less invasive and accurate treatments and processes. Furthermore, these innovations allow for greater predictability in the outcome of treatments.

Besides, an additional benefit is the improved comfort patients experience in contrast to traditional dentistry. There is no need to utilize an impression tray as well as the added benefit of digital treatments being far less time-consuming. This is because this technology makes it possible to design, create and place restorations in one

K. Orhan
Faculty of Dentistry, Ankara University, Ankara, Turkey

Ankara University Medical Design Application and Research Center (MEDITAM), Ankara, Turkey

Department of Oral Diagnostics, Faculty of Dentistry, Semmelweis University, Budapest, Hungary

A. Delantoni (✉)
Faculty of Dentistry, Aristotle University of Thessaloniki, Thessaloniki, Greece
e-mail: andelant@dent.auth.gr

A. Delantoni, K. Orhan (eds.), *Digital Dentistry*, https://doi.org/10.1007/978-3-031-52826-2_1

visit, allowing the patient to experience ultimate convenience. The precision achieved through digital dentistry comes in the form of laser technology that creates and reconstructs the image of the patient's tooth with great accuracy. This also has a direct effect on the aesthetics of the tooth as natural colours and contours can also be achieved.

Besides, clinical advancement, the studies as well as new workflow and materials are being advancing. Today, technology is playing an important role in driving innovation and shaping student experience in dentistry education. As learning methods and tools continue to advance understanding educational methodologies is crucial to optimizing educational effectiveness,

Figure 1.1 shows the analysis of search from the www.scopus.com for 'Digital Dentistry' on 21.03.2024. The results show that the papers published increasing eventually and the works including Digital Dentistry are increasing. Figure 1.2 shows the distribution of subjects found in Scopus until March 2024. The vast majority in dentistry scope papers and following medicine.

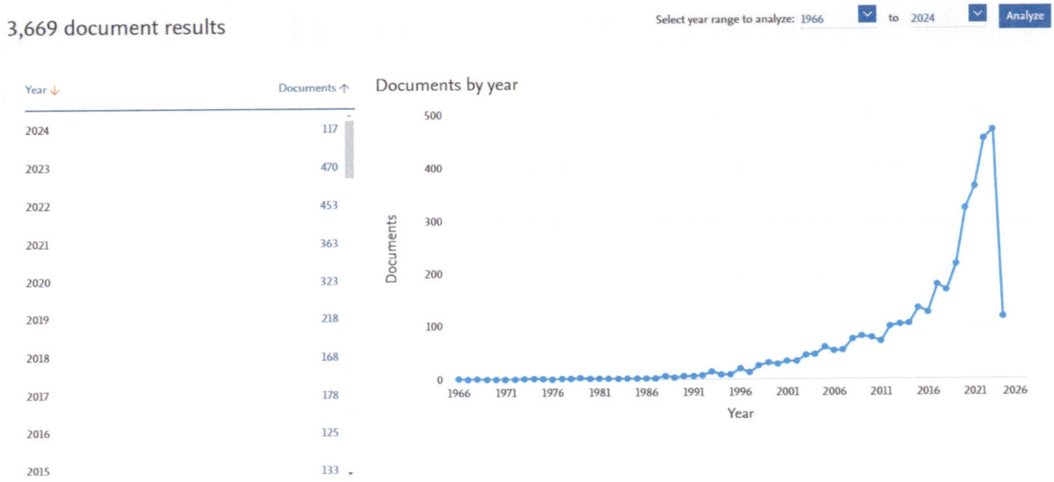

Fig. 1.1 Analysis of search from the www.scopus.com for 'Digital Dentistry' on 21.03.2024

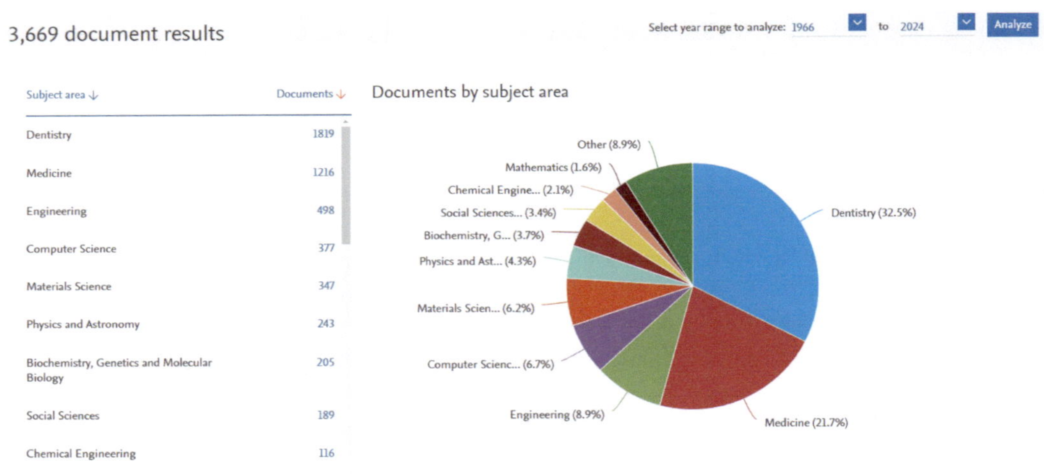

Fig. 1.2 The distribution of subjects found in Scopus until 2023

1.2 What Does the Life Sciences Profession Need in Terms of Digital Dentistry?

The scientific studies, an objective diagnosis using imaging techniques must be reproducible. Although there are criteria and conventional as well as contemporary evaluation methods in life sciences, there are still an unclear correlation often exists between clinical relevance and symptoms and the imaging findings in diseases.

Digital dental technologies available for dental clinics or labs have a wide range of purposes. Imaging, scanning, digital design and 3D printing or milling are technologies developed on their own but complement each other for treatment planning, design and delivery of the final product. Research done by David Guichet shows us how digital dental processes and scanning technologies help to improve strength and aesthetic qualities of restorations, as well as decrease costs and improve practice efficiency. Digital scanners in dentistry can be classified into different types depending on where and how they are used: in dental clinics, facing the patient, or in dental laboratories, not facing the patient. Dental scanning equipment for clinics can be categorized into CBCT or intraoral scanners. Dental cone beam CT (CBCT) scanners are used for taking X-rays of the mouth area, and intraoral scanners or dental 3D scanners replace the conventional impression method, where patients are asked to sit with gooey impression material in their mouth in order to get an accurate impression. The two scan types can be combined, for example, when full denture treatment is needed.

Intraoral scans are built up by polygons and can be combined with an image taken by an intraoral camera which allows the dentist to see even the smallest problems and defects of teeth, and other parts of the cavity. Some scanners can even detect caries in the very early stages.

In today's dentistry education, digital microscopes, virtual pathology slides, digital radiography and chairside applications of restorative and prosthetic procedures have strengthened their position, while virtual reality, haptic-enhanced VR simulations and robot patients used in preclinical laboratory education systems are still in the initial stage and increasing interest in their future development is apparent. Many research questions still need to be answered to accept these technological advancements more broadly in dentistry education. Expansion of software to increase the number of dental procedures available would also be advantageous. Many research questions have yet to be answered both to direct these technological developments and to establish a wider acceptance of simulation in dental education [1–6].

Moreover, in the age of big data and analytics, perhaps students will need more computer programming knowledge to support evidence-based decision making and to fully discover the information needed, and therefore will need to take computer courses. In this way, digital technology can become an educational goal and desired competence that will replace other parts of the curriculum.

With the advent of diagnosis, patient and case documentation, treatment planning, novel treatment techniques and more recently throughout the workflow in oral rehabilitation, digital dentistry is a reality with a promising future. However, much more is yet to come and other fields such as artificial intelligence (AI) will play a major and currently unimaginable role in overcoming all known boundaries. Already considered a rising field, AI technology in dentistry has been the focus of serious research. Software with deep learning capabilities is already helping to improve orthodontic treatment outcomes, caries diagnosis, diagnosis and prediction of periodontal diseases, risk assessment of oral cancer, treatment plan suggestions, patient data analysis, and smile design, among others.

This book will discuss all the terms and definitions that the dental professional needs to know to understand the procedures discussed in the following chapters. Such definitions include abbreviations and general concepts of digital imaging and digital workflow. This chapter also presents a history of the use of CAD-CAM in dentistry in the last two decades, and the basic knowledge required plus ideas and alternatives to start with digital dentistry.

The chapters that follow fall into three categories: Basic Digital Systems in Dentistry which will be discussed in Chaps. 1–5. Chapters 2–4 briefly reviews the fundamentals of digital dentistry and Basic principles of systems and techniques in Dentistry. Chaps. 6–15 will be reviewing Novelties and advances in digital dentistry. The rest of the book will focus both medical applications are covered as the future of digital dentistry and applications in Chaps. 16–21.

References

1. Schweiger BJ, Edelhoff D. Digital dentistry: an overview of recent developments for CAD/CAM generated restorations. Br Dent J. 2008;204:505–11.
2. Gonulol N, Kaalyancuoglu E. Education and learning in digital dentistry. J Exp Clin Med. 2021;38:163–7.
3. Cooper LF. Digital technology: Impact and opportunities in dental education. J Dent Educ. 2019;83:379–80.
4. Jackson TH, Zhong J, Phillips C, Koroluk LD. Selfdirected digital learning: when do dental students' study? J Dent Educ. 2018;82:373–8.
5. da Silva RLB, Kim JH, Markarian RA, Falacho R, Cortes DN, Costa AJM, Cortes ARG. Introduction to digital dentistry. In: Cortes ARG, editor. Digital dentistry. Hoboken: Wiley; 2022. https://doi.org/10.1002/9781119852025.ch1.
6. Chatham C, Spencer M, Wood D, et al. The introduction of digital dental technology into BDS curricula. Br Dent J. 2014;217:639–42. https://doi.org/10.1038/sj.bdj.2014.1049.

2 General Considerations Basic Principles and History Overview of Digital Applications in Dentistry

Kaan Orhan, Antigoni Delantoni, and Seçil Aksoy

2.1 Digital Applications in Dentistry

Digital technology revolution is changing the way many industries, and dentistry is no exception. In recent years, digital applications have been developed to reduce the patient radiation dose and to improve the quality and accuracy of dental procedures, as well as to enhance the patient experience. This chapter will explore the various technologies in which digital application is being used in dentistry, including digital radiography, digital impressions, cone beam computed tomography (CBCT), and virtual consultations.

K. Orhan (✉)
Faculty of Dentistry, Ankara University, Ankara, Turkey

Ankara University Medical Design Application and Research Center (MEDITAM), Ankara, Turkey

Department of Oral Diagnostics, Faculty of Dentistry, Semmelweis University, Budapest, Hungary

A. Delantoni
Faculty of Dentistry, Aristotle University of Thessaloniki, Thessaloniki, Greece
e-mail: andelant@dent.auth.gr

S. Aksoy
Faculty of Dentistry, Department of Dentomaxillofacial Radiology, Near University, Nicosia, Cyprus

2.2 Digital Imaging

Digital imaging technology has transformed the field of dentistry in recent years. This technology allows dentists to obtain high-resolution images of a patients teeth and surrounding maxillary and mandibular bones, which can then be used to diagnose and treat a wide variety of dental disease.

For over a century, radiographs have been obtained using direct exposure X-ray films. However, traditional radiography is now being replaced by digital imaging in dental offices, which is widely considered to be one of the most significant innovations in the field of dentistry in recent times. A number of factors have contributed to the transition from film to digital systems. The negative impact of inadequate film processing on diagnostic accuracy and the difficulties in maintaining high-quality chemical processing are well-entrenched. Digital imaging, on the other hand, eliminates the need for chemical processing, thereby reducing the environmental impact through the reduction of hazardous waste. Additionally, digital images can be easily transmitted to other healthcare providers without compromising image quality. Furthermore, the use of digital intraoral receptors results in lower radiation exposure to patients compared to film-based systems. Finally, digital imaging affords greater flexibility in terms of modifications, measurements, and corrections, which are not possible with film-based systems [1].

Digital radiography (DR) systems are composed of a standard X-ray machine, a digital sen-

A. Delantoni, K. Orhan (eds.), *Digital Dentistry*, https://doi.org/10.1007/978-3-031-52826-2_2

sor or screen in place of film, and a computer with appropriate software, all of which are enhanced by a high-resolution monitor [2]. The advent of DR in dentistry began in the mid-1980s with the launch of the first digital radiography system, known as RadioVisioGraphy (RVG), in Europe by the French company Trophy Radiologie [3–5]. The inventor of this system, Dr. Francis Mouyen, developed a method of using fiber optics to reduce a large X-ray image to a smaller size that could be captured by a charge-coupled device (CCD) image sensor chip. Trophy Radiologie then sought the aid of Fairchild CCD Imaging Company in Silicon Valley, California, where a Finnish physicist and CCD image sensor design engineer named Paul Suni helped in creating the necessary CCD image sensor technology [4].

At present, there are two different types of DR technologies which do not require an analog precursor. Direct digital imaging are achieved using a solid state sensors utilizing charge-coupled device (CCD) or complementary metal oxide semiconductor (CMOS). Other method, referred to as semi direct digital imaging, involves the use of a phosphor plate system (PSP) [1, 6].

Another type of digital imaging technology that is commonly used in dentistry is cone beam computed tomography (CBCT). This technology was first implemented in the field of vascular imaging in the 1980s and has undergone many improvements [7]. The first dental and maxillofacial CBCT units were made available for commercial use in the late 1990s and early 2000s [8]. This technology uses a cone shaped beam of X-rays to capture three dimensional images of a patients' teeth and hard tissue [7]. These images can be used to plan and perform dental procedures such as implant placement and root canal therapy, with a high level of accuracy.

Digital imaging technology is also used in patient education. Dentists can use digital imaging software to show patients a virtual simulation of the current status of teeth that need treatments. In addition, digital images can be used to create a digital model and customized treatment plan of a patient.

Overall, digital imaging technology has a significant impact on the dentistry. It allows dentists to diagnose and to do treatment planning for dental conditions with greater accuracy and efficiency, while also reducing the amount of radiation exposure for patients.

2.3 Digital Planning

The integration of digital tools such as computer-aided design (CAD) and computer-aided manufacturing (CAM) into the practice of dentistry has led to a change toward digital planning. Digital planning in dentistry involves to create virtual accurate and precise models of a patient using digital imaging technology and to simulate various treatment options. These virtual models are used to position dental implants and design custom made restorations and prosthesis. Surgical guides, copings, abutments, bars, copings, etc. are different types of 3D models which can then be exported to 3D printers or milling machines.

Computer-aided design and manufacturing, or CAD/CAM, were first developed in the 1960s for use in the aircraft and automotive industries and were later applied to dentistry in the 1970s [9]. Notable figures in the development of dental CAD/CAM include Drs. Francois Duret, Werner Mormann, Dianne Rekow, and Matts Andersson. Dr. Duret was the first person to develop a dental CAD/CAM device, creating crowns based on an optical impression of the abutment tooth in 1971 and later developed the Sopha system [10]. Dr. Mormann, in collaboration with Dr. Marco Brandestini, developed the first commercial CAD/CAM system called CEREC, which was capable of performing chair side inlays using an intraoral scanner and milling device by 1985 [11]. CAD/CAM is also used in orthodontics, like Invisalign, a treatment that uses multiple clear, removable appliances designed and manufactured via CAD/CAM to straighten teeth [10].

CAD and CAM software are used to design and manufacture a variety of dental restorations such as crowns, bridges, and veneers. CAD software allows for the creation of digital models of the restoration that can be modified and adjusted on a computer screen for a perfect fit for the patient. CAM software then converts these digital models into physical restorations through milling machines or 3D printers, leading to greater precision and efficiency in the treatment process [12].

Intraoral scanners are an integral part of the digital planning, as they improve the efficiency of the practice and enhance the patient experience when compared to traditional impression methods. An intraoral scanner consists of a handheld camera, a computer, and software that is used to record the 3D geometry of an object [13].

The use of digital tools and digital planning decreases the need for multiple appointments and reduces chair time for patients, making the process more efficient and less time-consuming. Digital planning also improves communication between dentists, dental technicians, and patients. Patients can see a virtual simulation of the potential outcome of a procedure before starting treatment, allowing them to make more informed decisions.

2.4 Digital Communication

Digital communication channels represents an essential part of modern dentistry, thanks to the incorporation of digital technology such as teleconferencing or teledentistry. These technologies have enabled dental practitioners to connect with patients and other healthcare providers in a more efficient and convenient way.

The idea of teledentistry originated as a component of dental informatics, a discipline that combines computer science, information technology, engineering, and oral health. This concept was first presented at a 1989 conference in Baltimore [14].

The integration of digital technology in dentistry has an impact on patient management and communication. The implementation of mobile applications offers new prospects for both patients and dental practitioners. Prior to the digitalization of healthcare, there was no mechanism for maintaining active communication with patients after they left the dental practice. With the utilization of mobile applications, dental practices now have the ability to employ online scheduling systems, send recall and news messages to patients, and provide standardized or personalized applications for a more comprehensive understanding of the patient's health status. The ongoing coronavirus pandemic has resulted in a marked increase in interaction between patients and dental clinics through digital video software such as Zoom, Skype, and Microsoft Teams. This is particularly useful for patients who live in remote areas or have mobility issues, making it easier for them to access dental care. The pandemic has provided an opportunity to implement innovative technologies and it is expected that this form of communication will become established with patients in the future. This is due to the increased acceptance of this mode of communication resulting from experiences with remote work and video conferencing [15].

Telemedicine services are another option for dental practices in the future. Although there will always be a need for in-person visits for procedures such as drilling, cutting, filling, or fixing, telemedicine apps offer the potential for multidisciplinary communication between dentists, general physicians, pharmacies, and even insurance companies on a common platform. These systems can be AI-driven and connected to a cloud, but legal barriers and the risk of cyberattacks present challenges for implementation. Telemedicine apps also bring new dimensions to the dentist-patient interaction, such as the potential to motivate patients to take better care of their oral health through gamification. This could help prevent caries, periodontitis, and periimplantitis, and would be a long-term strategy. The impact of chronic periodontitis on widespread diseases such as diabetes highlights the need for an app that can collect health care and additional data. Such an app would be especially valuable for doctors of internal medicine as they could get information and motivate patients with diabetes to use dental hygiene services to avoid further risks to their health. Overall, telemedicine apps that connect all health data could bring added value to patients and be part of a long-term prevention strategy, which would ultimately lead to reduced costs in the healthcare system [15].

The incorporation of digital technology also facilitates communication among healthcare providers. Dental practitioners can share patient records and treatment plans with other healthcare providers through secure, online platforms, improving coordination of care, and reducing the risk of errors.

2.5 Digital Education

Digital education in dentistry refers to the use of technology to enhance learning and training in oral healthcare. This encompasses the utilization of digital mediums such as e-learning platforms, webinars, virtual reality simulations, and interactive videos which complement the traditional classroom-based education. The incorporation of digital education in dentistry has several advantages, including the expansion of the reach of education, improved access for remote and underserved populations, and increased adaptability for learners. Additionally, digital education can provide real-time feedback and personalized learning experiences, which can enhance the retention and transfer of knowledge in a more efficient and convenient way. Furthermore, digital education in dentistry can also provide a cost-effective alternative to traditional method. Moreover, digital education can bridge the gap between theoretical knowledge and practical skills by providing hands-on training using virtual reality simulators, which can increase the readiness of students to enter the workforce.

Online courses are an increasingly popular way for dental students to access educational content. The use of various technological advancements, such as the internet, digital satellite technology, and virtual reality applications, has significantly impacted the way learning is conducted at all levels. Online learning environments, such as virtual classrooms or virtual learning environments (VLE), can be accessed through the web, and provide electronic materials for learning. These environments also have the capability for interactions between students, hands on learning and collaborative tasks. Examples of VLE software include Moodle™, Blackboard™, and WebCT (Web Course Tools). To maximize the effectiveness of these tools, active learning strategies should be incorporated, which go beyond simply downloading materials. Additionally, web based learning tools can enhance the educational experience by providing students with challenging tasks and resources that promote higher level thinking and collaboration [16].

The use of multimedia, such as visual images and audio prompts, can enhance the learning and teaching process of practical skills in dental education. This is particularly effective for millennial learners, who are known to be technologically savvy and thrive on immediate and continual feedback [17]. Videos provide a hands-on learning experience by demonstrating procedures and communicating facts. The ability to stop, start, and rewind videos also allows students to review complex procedures and improve their understanding. Additionally, the use of instructional videos in addition to traditional classroom instructions has been shown to be effective in developing cognitive skills, enhancing psychomotor skills, and improving knowledge retention [18, 19].

The use of virtual patients (VPs) in dental education is a new strategy that allows students to learn and practice in an environment that closely resembles live patient encounters. This can include using simulated patient records, computer-aided and/or virtual reality-based simulations, and self-paced methods with immediate feedback. Virtual patients can also provide students with the opportunity to develop overall decision-making skills that will increase confidence and consistency. The latest technology trends involve creating a more immersive simulation experience by establishing connections between the learner and VP, and by creating realistic personalities and backstories for the VPs [20]. This may include the use of social media and decision tree technology to enhance problem-solving, critical thinking, and reflective learning [21].

In conclusion, the use of digital resources such as online courses, virtual patients, and instructional videos has greatly improved dental education and training. This advancements made it more efficient and convenient for dental students and practitioners to access educational content and training materials. As technology continues to advance, digital education is likely to become an even more integral aspect of dental education and training.

2.6 Digital Workflow

Digital technology has greatly affected the way dental practices operate by streamlining and optimizing the dental workflow. The integration of digital tools and systems has made it possible for dental practices throughout the entire dental treatment process, from appointment scheduling to treatment planning and follow-up.

Digital workflow in dentistry can also include the use of practice management software and electronic health records (EHRs) to manage patient data and appointments, as well as digital communication tools such as telehealth and virtual consultations. The appointment scheduling process can be streamlined using digital tools such as online appointment booking systems, which allow patients to book appointments at their convenience without the need for phone calls or in-person visits [22]. This can also help to reduce administrative tasks for the dental practice.

Treatment planning is another area that can benefit from digital technology. Digital tools such as 3D imaging and virtual reality simulations can be used to plan and communicate treatment options to patients, helping them to understand and make informed decisions about their dental care.

During the treatment process, digital tools such as intraoral scanners, CAD/CAM systems, and digital impression systems can be used to improve the accuracy and efficiency of procedures. This can lead to better outcomes for patients and increased productivity for the dental practice.

After the treatment, digital tools such as patient portals, text and email reminders, and telehealth consultations can be used to improve communication and follow-up care. These tools can help to keep patients informed and engaged in their own dental care, and can also help to reduce the risk of complications or treatment failure.

Overall, the use of digital workflow in dentistry can provide a number of benefits, such as improved accuracy and efficiency in diagnosis and treatment planning, increased communication and collaboration between dental professionals, and enhanced patient education and engagement. Additionally, digital workflow can also help to reduce the need for multiple appointments, minimize the use of traditional analog materials, and improve the speed and precision of dental procedures. However, it is important to note that the implementation of digital workflow in dentistry requires both technical and clinical expertise and should be performed by trained and qualified dental professionals.

References

1. Mol A. Digital imaging. In: Mallya SM, Lam EWN, editors. White and Pharoah's oral radiology: principles and interpretation. 8th ed. St. Louis, Missouri: Elsevier; 2019.
2. Wenzel A, Gröndahl HG. Direct digital radiography in the dental office. Int Dent J. 1995;45(1):27–34.
3. Farman AG. Image-guidance...The revolution in dental treatment facilitated by digital radiology. Oral Surg Oral Med Oral Pathol Oral Radiol Endod. 2006;101(3):273–5.
4. Dhir P, David CM, Keerthi G, Sharma V, Girdhar V. Digital imaging in dentistry: an overview. IJDMS. 2011;23(6):62–8.
5. van der Stelt PF. Filmless imaging: the uses of digital radiography in dental practice. J Am Dent Assoc. 2005;136(10):1379–87.
6. Serindere G, Gündüz K. Digital imaging and dental record. J Exp Clin Med. 2021;38:113–8.
7. Angelopoulos C, Scarfe WC, Farman AG. A comparison of maxillofacial CBCT and medical CT. Atlas Oral Maxillofac Surg Clin North Am. 2012;20(1):1–17.
8. Mozzo P, Procacci C, Tacconi A, Martini PT, Andreis IA. A new volumetric CT machine for dental imaging based on the cone-beam technique: preliminary results. Eur Radiol. 1998;8(9):1558–64.
9. Duret F, Preston JD. CAD/CAM imaging in dentistry. Curr Opin Dent. 1991;1(2):150–4.
10. Davidowitz G, Kotick PG. The use of CAD/CAM in dentistry. Dent Clin N Am. 2011;55(3):559–70.
11. Mörmann WH. The evolution of the CEREC system. J Am Dent Assoc. 2006;137:7S–13S.

12. Vasques MT, Urbano GS, Gialain IO, et al. Computer-aided manufacturing (CAM). In: Cortes ARG, editor. Digital dentistry a step-by-step guide and case atlas. 1st ed. West Sussex: Wiley; 2022.
13. Richert R, Goujat A, Venet L, et al. Intraoral scanner technologies: a review to make a successful impression. J Healthc Eng. 2017;2017:8427595.
14. Kiser AL. Dental informatics and the evolution of computers—the roles of organized dentistry. In: Abbey LM, Zimmerman JL, editors. Dental informatics: integrating technology into the dental environment. 1st ed. New York: Springer; 1992.
15. Plugmann P. Digitalization in dentistry. In: Glauner P, Plugmann P, Lerzynski G, editors. Digitalization in healthcare. Cham: Springer; 2021.
16. Feeney L, Reynolds PA, Eaton KA, Harper J. A description of the new technologies used in transforming dental education. Br Dent J. 2008;204(1):19–28.
17. Monaco M, Martin M. The millennial student: a new generation of learners. Athl Train Educ J. 2007;2(2):42–6.
18. Fakhry A, Dehkordi-Vakil FH. Video-assisted clinical instruction in dentistry (VACID) enhances real-time visualisation of clinical procedures. Eur J Dent Educ. 2007;11(4):238–44.
19. Wong G, Apthorpe HC, Ruiz K, Nanayakkara S. An innovative educational approach in using instructional videos to teach dental local anaesthetic skills. Eur J Dent Educ. 2019;23(1):28–34.
20. Cederberg RA, Bentley DA, Halpin R, Valenza JA. Use of virtual patients in dental education: a survey of U.S. and Canadian Dental Schools. J Dent Educ. 2012;76(10):1358–64.
21. Barrows HS. Problem-based learning in medicine and beyond: a brief overview. New Dir Teach Learn. 1996;68:3–12.
22. Tang PC, Ash JS, Bates DW, Overhage JM, Sands DZ. Personal health records: definitions, benefits, and strategies for overcoming barriers to adoption. J Am Med Inform Assoc. 2006;13(2):121–6.

3 Digital Radiographic Systems

Antigoni Delantoni, Alexandros Sapountzis, and Kaan Orhan

3.1 Introduction

X-rays were discovered in December of 1895 by W.C. Röntgen who studied for several months the properties of a new kind of "invisible rays," and shortly after presented his findings in the proceedings of the WürzburgPhysico-Medical Society (Fig. 3.1).

In a very short amount of time, the value of X-rays and radiographs was recognized by the medical community. In February of 1896 in the USA the first radiograph for "purely medical" reasons was taken for investigating a wrist fracture on a patient. In the following years, radiography became the leading diagnostic method in medicine and found an ever-growing field of use.

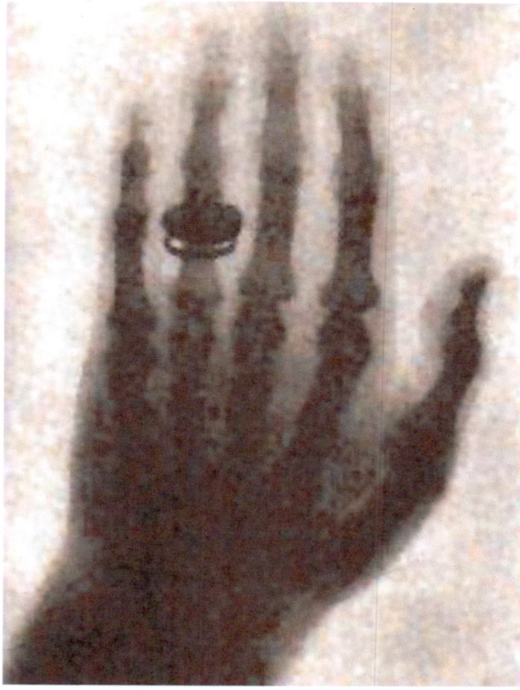

Fig 3.1 A film of Röntgen's wife's hand with a ring, produced on Friday, November 8, 1895, is one of the first radiographs ever produced

From the early "X-ray" machines to the latest state of art tomographs, X-rays are still one of the leading tools in our diagnostic arsenal.

Although the first documented "dental X-ray" was produced in 1896 by DrWalkhoff after a 25-min exposure as shown in Fig. 3.2 the use of dental X-ray machines became widely-used

A. Delantoni (✉)
Faculty of Dentistry, Aristotle University of Thessaloniki, Thessaloniki, Greece
e-mail: andelant@dent.auth.gr

A. Sapountzis
Oral Radiology Faculty of Dentistry, Department of Dentoalveolar Surgery, Implant Surgery and Radiology, Thessaloniki, Greece

K. Orhan
Faculty of Dentistry, Ankara University, Ankara, Turkey

Ankara University Medical Design Application and Research Center (MEDITAM), Ankara, Turkey

Department of Oral Diagnostics, Faculty of Dentistry, Semmelweis University, Budapest, Hungary

A. Delantoni, K. Orhan (eds.), *Digital Dentistry*, https://doi.org/10.1007/978-3-031-52826-2_3

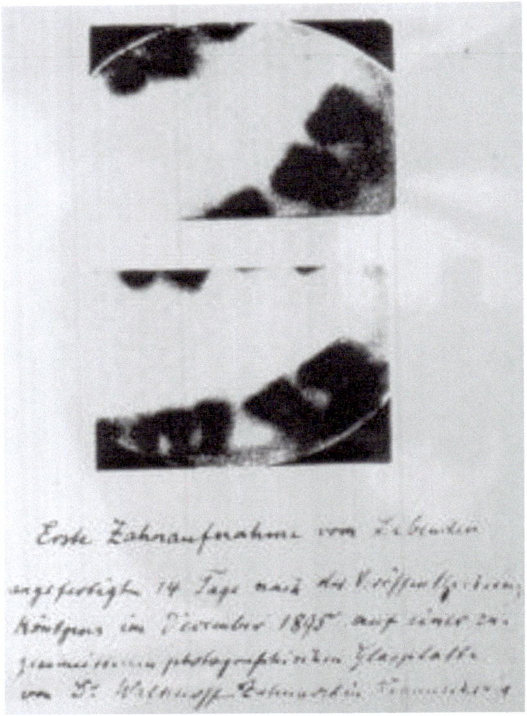

Fig. 3.2 The first dental radiograph known taken by Dr. Walkhoff

around 1950 when X-rays became a routine part of the dental exam. From the early years of radiography, concerns were raised about the potentially harmful effects of X-rays on patients and operators.

Around 1901 William Herbert Rollins a dentist and a physician who suffered radiation burns during the usage of X-rays published over 200 articles detailing the shielding of both the operators and the X-ray machines with lead, ways to expose only the areas of interest to the beam, and shielding the other areas of patients body from radiation. He also raised safety considerations regarding the dosage of X-rays for the average patient.

As modern dentistry evolved over the years, the need for improving the amount of information and details from the various modalities grew in proportion with the needs of the patients and the more complicated treatment plans. Thus the use of X-rays in dentistry increased in both quantity and intensity, especially with the introduction of exams like the panoramic X-ray and later the various CT scans. It was becoming apparent that the film as a radiation detector was an inefficient medium that while producing images of good quality still required relatively high radiation exposure, and offered very few options for post-exposure image processing and enhancement.

In the late 1980s and mid-1990s, dentistry entered the digital era, starting to shift from conventional film to CCD sensors. In 1987 a French dentist Dr. Francis Moyen using a charge-coupled device (CCD) image sensor designed by engineer Paul Suni created and patented the first digital dental radiographic intraoral technic which he named Radiovisiography (RVG). The first RVG system called DRS—short for digital radiography system did not interface with a computer and so although the radiographic images could be seen on a video screen, the operator did not have the option to store them.

Later in 1991 Philips Dental Systems launched Visualix—the first computer-coupled RVG system that consisted of an intraoral CCD sensor coupled with a Gd_2O_2S scintillator. Visualix was the world's first RVG system that in conjunction with a personal computer could store and export the produced radiographs in a standard file format such as Tiff, Jpeg, etc.

While at the time most of the digital radiographic systems were developed and produced in Europe using the technology of charge-coupled devices, or CCDs for image acquisition, around 1996 in the US David Schick, founder of Schick Technologies acquired a license from Jet Propulsion Labs for CMOS technology—a metal-oxide semiconductor chip that was both easier to make and more cost-effective in comparison to the CCD sensors—and started on working to implement it on X-ray sensors. Two years later in 1998, the first CMOS X-ray sensor was introduced to the dental world.

Today in modern dentistry film radiology is almost nonexistent due to the superiority that digital radiography has offered in terms of X-dosage for the patient and image quality, processing storage, and sharing capabilities.

3.2 Digital Dental Radiographic Systems

3.2.1 Part I Intraoral Systems

3.2.1.1 How the Digital Image Is Produced

Digital images are made up of digits and are essentially distinct in terms of the resolution of the image elements (pixels) and terms of the different shades of gray of each element (pixels) of the image. Essentially a digital image consists of horizontal and vertical pixel arrays. Each pixel has a column and row mapping in the image that marks its position in the image and represents a shade of gray.

The production of the digital image requires certain steps that start with the conversion of the image from analog to digital (analog-to-digital conversion) with the amount of radiation received. This value is specific and is stored on the computer and one could say that it represents the image. This defines the parameters and monitors the images during their production. The difference in this absorption is detected and recorded by special detectors, which are located directly opposite the X-ray tube.

3.2.2 Types of Dental Digital X-Ray Systems

Different types of receptors form the digital image. These are

- PSP (Photostimulable Phosphor) and SPS (Storage Phosphor Systems) where the image must be "scanned" and there is a small time-lapse from receiving the image and presenting it on the screen (closer as a technique to conventional intraoral x-ray) [1, 4, 5, 7, 8].
- Fixed CCD (charge-coupled device) and CMOS (complementary metal-oxide semiconductors) sensors where the sensor is connected to the computer and there is a direct image obtained [23, 24].

As for the first receptors, CMOS technology is a newer technology than CCD and both have been around since 1967, although CMOS was introduced into dental X-rays only in recent years by Trophy and Schick [2, 3, 17].

CCD receptors are generally considered better for dental radiology while CMOS is still under research.

3.2.2.1 Photostimulable Phosphor Plates (PSP)

Although in PSP technology conventional film is not used, most of the literature refers to it as "computed radiography" and does not classify it as a digital radiographic technique.

The first PSP was introduced by Fuji corporation in 1981 and the first commercial PSP dental scanner was introduced later by Soredex in 1994. The system which was called Digora used intraoral PSP plates of various sizes covered with disposable plastic pouches which prevented the ambient light to interact with the plate after the exposure and avoided cross-infection.

PSP technology is based on the effect of Photostimulated luminescence which is the release of energy stored in a phosphor plate after stimulating it with a form of visible light.

In PSP technology the radiograph is created in a two-stage process and thus it is classified as an indirect radiographic technic. First, the X-rays are absorbed from a photostimulable phosphor plate which consists of a crystalline halide emulsion on a polyester base and a latent image is "stored" on it. The emulsion is made of a europium-barium fluorohalide compound (BaFBrEu). In the second stage, the stored energy is released in the form of a blue-violet 400 nm luminescence when exposed to helium-neon laser energy within the scanner. The produced "luminescence" is captured by a photomultiplier tube which converts the incident photons to an amplified electrical signal which in turn is quantized by an analog-to-digital converter or ADC. The digital values produced for each pixel by the ADC are used to produce the final radiographic image which is projected on a computer screen.

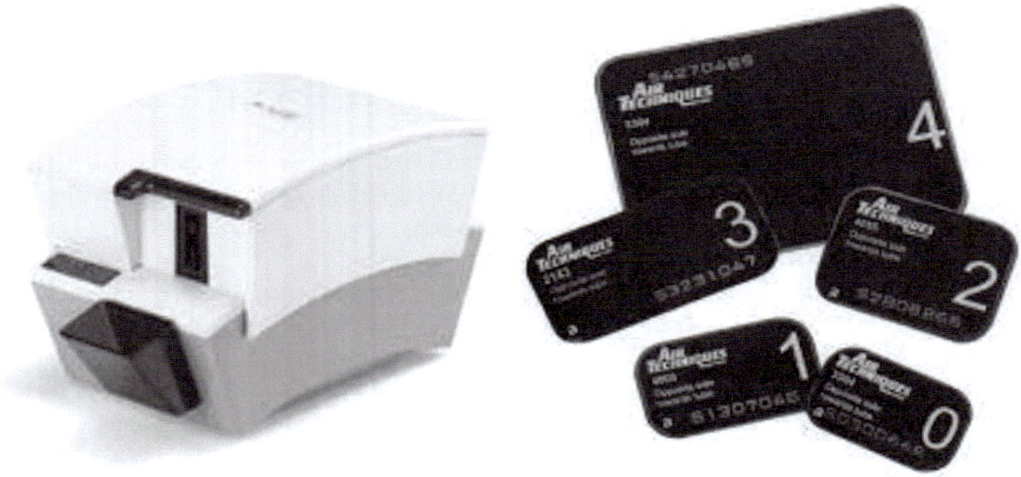

Fig. 3.3 An example of a PSP scanner. Also, various sizes of plates give us corresponding size images

After the scanning is finished, the plate gets erased usually with exposure to red light from LEDs within the scanner. The plate is then ready to be used again for a new radiograph (Fig. 3.3).

According to manufacturer specifications and modern literature each plate can be used several hundreds of times in a clinical environment with fading (when the PSP plate is exposed to ambient light before scanning), bitemarks, image size reduction, scratches, and delayed scanning being the most common problems.

Many articles evaluate PSP technology and the literature shows that in terms of the total time required for the imaging procedure (preparation, placement, exposure, and image production), patient comfort, and subjective image quality in real clinical settings they fall short from their CMOS/CCD counterparts. That being said the wireless nature of the plates, the availability in several sizes with relatively low cost, and the acceptable imaged quality make them an acceptable alternative for X-ray examination in modern dentistry.

3.2.2.2 CCD and CMOS Sensors

These sensors are often referred to as direct digital sensors. Generally CMOS and CCD sensors convert images (light) into electronic signals. CCD sensors are slightly cheaper and are the older, more mature technology. CCD and CMOS sensors are susceptible to different problems. CCD sensors are more susceptible to vertical smear from bright light sources, while CMOS sensors are susceptible to skewing, wobbling, and partial exposure. However, neither technology is a clear winner over the other in overall image quality.

One can say that CCD receptors have a better light response with the X-ray photons used for this, thus they are considered more efficient than CMOS. However, CMOS receptors have a better "optical" package (microfiches and scintillators) with similar efficiencies, although this makes them more expensive.

The key features of digital sensors are as follows:

- Contrast analysis.
- Spatial resolution.
- Detector latitude.
- Detector sensitivity.

Contrast analysis is the ability to distinguish different optical frequencies in the radiographic image.

It is a function of the following factors:

- The effect of tissue weakening characteristics is depicted.
- The ability of the receptor to distinguish differences in the number of X-ray protons coming from different parts of the object being irradiated.
- The ability of the computer screen to show differences in density.
- The ability of the observer to recognize the differences presented on the screen by the system.

Spatial resolution is the ability to discern detail (resolution). A theoretical limitation in digital imaging is the function of the pixel size of the image measured in line pairs per millimeter [9, 10]. In theory this analysis is determined by the manufacturers and is dependent on the size of the pixels while it does not take into account the loss due to diffusion from the scintillator, and the electronic systems of the receptor. At the highest CCD resolution, over 20 microns per pixel have been measured corresponding to a ratio of 8 microns Ag grain. At these 20 microns per pixel, a theoretical resolution of 25 pairs of lines per millimeter can be obtained [10]. Therefore, because the human eye can distinguish 6 pairs of lines per millimeter most digital systems perform very well (more than 7 pairs of lines per millimeter).

Receptor amplitude is the ability of a receptor to receive a range of random photon energy, which clinically varies from the gums to the enamel and allows slight variations in radius permeability to be apparent in the image.

Receptor sensitivity is the ability to respond to small amounts of radiation. It is how the receptor responds and reacts to small amounts of radiation exposure.

3.2.2.3 Advantages of Digital Radiography

Digital radiography requires over 80% lesser dose compared to classic dental radiographic film. In digital imaging, the quality may be manipulated after image acquisition to improve the final image result and even provide more information to the examiner, i.e., contrast, blur, and noise alterations. The diagnostic accuracy of the detection of carious lesions is increased by digital contrast enhancement and additional filtering. The dentist can perform measurements of length, angle, and area on a digital image. Smoothing of the image can reduce the image noise but at the same time, it decreases image resolution. Hardening of the image enhances edges to create a crisper image, but with more noise. In digital radiography, the same image can be used for various diagnostic purposes with the use of different filters. With the CCD system, the image is displayed immediately after radiation exposure. Although there is a lag time between scanning and the appearance of an image exists with the PSP sensors, it is faster than the conventional method. Digital Imaging and Communications in Medicine (DICOM) standards encompass primary and secondary diagnostic images acquired digitally that provide a basis for interoperability of the digital system's output. DICOM-compliant system utilizes common file formats that are universally recognized.

The advantages of digital radiographic systems can be summed up to the following

- Immediacy in image production, resulting in better ergonomics (for CCD and CMOS sensors).
- The presentation of the image on the computer helps the patient to understand the disease.
- Ease of storing images and archiving them.
- Ease of making copies where necessary.
- The simplification of the measurements is required mainly for endodontics.
- There are no chemicals or other materials in the doctor's office.
- Ability to communicate with colleagues and discuss the diagnosis.
- The low radiation dose.

3.2.2.4 Disadvantages of Digital Radiography

Though there are very few disadvantages to digital radiographic dental systems and one cannot argue that they ease our lives, the main disadvantages of intraoral digital radiography are as follows:

- The unfamiliarity of the staff with the sensors results in multiple repetitions in the production of the images.
- The technique of digital radiography has low sensitivity in cases where the patient is irradiated more than he should be (although it is not easy since many radiological machines now have a choice of digital or non-digital image) [6].
- when the image is printed on plain paper diagnostically there may be a loss of original image info,
- It is possible to modify and edit the image so that digital images are not accepted as evidence.
- This in the future can be solved as a problem with techniques such as in medical radiological files where after the image is entered into the program it is not possible to process the image.

Conclusions In conclusion, one can argue that technology is evolving rapidly, and the dentist must monitor it.

Sensors are capable of producing high-resolution X-rays with radiation doses much lower than conventional radiographic images, the time required to produce the image is less than that required with conventional files, and the images can be stored in formats. That have no data loss. Dentists must emphasize not only the purely radiological part of the machine but also the image of the image taken and the screen on which it is projected.

3.3 Part II

3.3.1 Digital Panoramic Systems

The dental panoramic X-ray or orthopantomogram is an X-ray imaging modality in which a single curved tomographic slice of the face, jaws, teeth, and supporting anatomical structures of the area is produced. The panoramic X-ray image is formed by the simultaneous and opposite movement of an X-ray source and the X-ray receptor both of which are mounted on a rotating gantry. To avoid the radiation exposure of the patient in places that are not of interest and are not opposed to the thin X-ray beam, metal barriers are used, which allow the generated rays to fall only on a limited and desired small area. As in intraoral radiographic techniques, panoramic radiography, mostly due to the distance between the source of the rays and the anatomical structures under examination, results in a magnification in radiographic image which can be noted and varies between 10 and 30% depending on the characteristics of the orthopantomograph and can increase more in case of incorrect positioning of the patient during the exam. The magnification is different in the horizontal and vertical planes of the radiographic image and is balanced within a curved region known as the focal plane. All structures contained within the focal plane of a radiograph show the same degree of magnification and optimal sharpness, while anatomical structures located outside the focal plane are distorted and show various degrees of magnification depending on their distance from it [11–16].

Initially in panoramic radiography, the film was used as the X-ray receptor. In most cases to reduce the number of X-rays needed to form the image on the film, a technique was used in which the film was encased in a specially build cassette between two fluorescent intensifying screens. The screens were 10–60 times more sensitive than the film itself and as the X-rays fell on them they fluoresced thus forming the panoramic image on the film while reducing the dose of radiation needed.

Regarding digital systems, they were initially presented in 1995 when a company called Signed presented at the IDS in Germany the first digital panoramic sensor called DXIS. The system consisted of a CCD sensor and an acquisition program that run on a computer with MS-DOS. Axis could be retrofitted on an existing orthopantomograph and although it had several issues like the fact that it required an adaptation of the hosting machine which in most cases would cancel the warranty of the manufacturer, it was greeted with positive reactions from the dental community.

Around 1997 Siemens offered the first digital-Ortophos Plus panoramic unit and Trophy offered digipan an upgrade for several panoramic machines on the market like OP100 made by the Finnish Instrumentarium, Orthoralix made by Genedex, etc.

At the same time, Genedex released Denoptix the first dental Photo Stimulated Phosphor Plate (PSP) scanner which could scan both panoramic/cephalometric and intraoral plates (Fig. 3.4).

In 2001 a new technology called laminographic tomosynthesis reconstruction was patented by AJAT a Finnish company founded by Konstantinos Spartiotis. In this technique, an addon kit is used that combines a single-crystal Cadmium Telluride (CdTe) semiconductor detector with a CMOS array sensor. The method uses a large number of raw images that are processed by a sophisticated algorithm that creates the image after the acquisition allowing the user to select any panoramic plane to be reconstructed after the acquisition of the raw data.

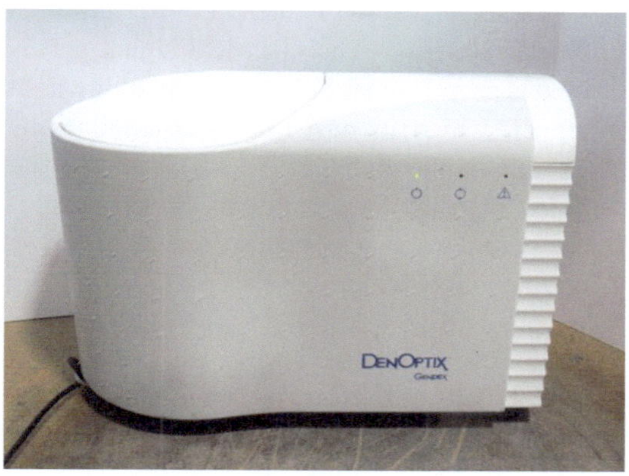

Fig. 3.4 The first Digital PSP scanner for Panoramic and cephalometric radiographs by Gendex

3.4 Part III

3.4.1 Cone Beam Computer Tomography

Cone beam computed tomography is an evolution of computed tomography. While it originally was used in angiography, radiotherapy, and mammography, it found many uses in dental science. The first cone beam scanner for use in dental science was installed in Europe in 1998 (NewTom −9000) and later in the United States of America the CommCat (previous to the iCat model). Cone beam computed tomography or Cbctis an imaging modality that uses a rotating X-ray tube attached to an X-ray detector. As the system rotates similarly to the rotation that a panoramic machine, multiple and successive radiographic images of the patient are created and collected by the detection system. This is achieved by giving the X-rays a characteristic cone shape and by using a detection system e that can capture almost all of the attenuated beams from the patient's tissues thus resulting in a more efficient use of the X-ray beam when compared to a fan beam computed tomography [18–22].

There are four basic stages of image production in cone beam tomography:

(a) Beam generation.
(b) X-ray detection system.
(c) Image reconstruction.
(d) Image display.

3.4.2 Beam Production-Scanning

Most cone beam tomographs use a fixed-anode tube not different from those used in panoramic machines. The main difference lies in the use of several beam confinement components that give the X-ray beam the characteristic cone shape, the base of which will correspond to the surface of the X-ray detector. During the scan, hundreds of images are produced corresponding to projections of the area under examination from each angle. Because the X-ray detection system is unable to collect the beam signal continuously due to technical limitations, the X-ray tube produces a pulsed beam. The frequency of the pulsed beam coincides with the periodicity of the scanning system, in terms of the time it requires to collect the data of each projection. The short time interval between the X-ray projections is used by the detection system to process the data of each projection. As a result, the actual patient exposure time to radiation is significantly shorter than the time taken for the scan. Furthermore, the beam confinement system allows only the area of interest to be irradiated.

As mentioned before during the scan, the X-rays produce a series of single exposures that correspond to each position of the tube during its rotational movement around the area of interest. These produce simple view images called basic or structural images. The number of these images per scan is constant for most tomographs. The amount of information collected by the scanning system is in direct proportion to the number of basic images produced, which will later be used to reconstruct the tomographic images. However, increasing the number of structural images leads to increased scan time and therefore increased patient irradiation.

3.4.3 Detection of the Beam

The purpose of the detection system is to collect the radiation attenuated by the patient's tissues and convert it into images on the tomographs computer.

The main types of the detection system in cone beam tomographs fall into two categories: image intensifier tubes and flat panel detectors.

1. Image intensifier tubes usually consist of an array of scintillation screens, two cesium iodide intensifier plates, corrective lenses, and a charge-coupled device (CCD) sensor array. The beam of X-rays, after entering the tube, is converted into light utilizing an amplifying plate called an input phosphor. The light signal is in turn converted into an electron beam in the photocathode of the tube. The resulting electron beam is accelerated by an electric field inside the tube and is re-converted into light by a second amplifying plate called an output phosphor. The intensity of the signal is modified by a series of lenses. The final light signal is converted into an electrical signal by an array of CCD-type sensors. The final electrical signal produced is proportional to the intensity of the light signal, which in turn is proportional to the energy of the radiation incident on the amplifier tube. The image produced after this process suffers geometric distortion as well as a relative loss in image sharpness due to the shape of the amplifier tube and the existence of multiple stages in the image production. Therefore, several algorithms are applied to correct the distortion and limit the artifacts created by the tube.
2. In flat panel detectors, the sensors that capture the X-rays are contained within a thin layer of amorphous silicon (a-si). Therefore, there is no restriction on their size. The intensifying screen converts incident radiation into light (light signal) which is then converted into an electrical signal. The electrical signal generated is proportional to the intensity of the light signal, which in turn is proportional to the energy of the radiation incident on the flat panel display. These systems do not exhibit the geometric distortion that can be found in an image intensifier tube.

In both types of detectors, the dimensions and number of cells collecting the signal play a major role in the analytical capability of the detection system. As the area of the sensitive cells is reduced, the analytical capability (resolution in space) of the detection system increases but at the same time, the signal-to-noise ratio (SNR) decreases.

In cone beam computed tomography, voxel size is determined by the size of the pixels (sensitive cells) of the detection system and not by the thickness of the slice as in CT (axial) computed tomography.

3.4.4 Reconstruction of the Images

The reconstruction of the tomographic images is a complex process performed by the scanner's computer which converts the electrical signal into a tomographic image. This process involves several steps. First, a pre-correction of the inhomogeneity of the structural images produced is performed. This inhomogeneity is the result of the variation of the sensitivity of the cells of the detection system in different parts of its surface and the inhomogeneity of the efficiency of the intensifying plate. Next, the data collected from each voxel will be sorted by radiation attenuation, filtered to smooth out any residual inhomogeneities, and finally projected with diametrically opposite pixel brightness from the one they originally had by a complex algorithm. The best-known and most widely-used algorithm for processing cone beam computed tomography data is the Feldkamp algorithm (FDK).

3.4.5 Display of Tomographic Images

Most of the available tomographic systems display the tomographic images to the user as a package of secondary reconstructed images in the three main planes (axial, frontal, and ocular). The user can select the thickness of the slice in each reconstruction, enhance the resulting images with several tools available in the scanner software, as well as perform various measurements.

Finally, as in conventional computed tomography, by using specific algorithms, the scanner's computer creates shadows by illuminating the projected volumes in such a way as to give a three-dimensional appearance to the resulting image.

3.4.6 Advantages of Cone Beam Tomography

Cone beam computed tomography has several advantages compared to other imaging modalities. The scanning and data acquisition time is short (5–40 s), thus reducing the possibility of image distortion due to the physical or respiratory movements of the patient. In modern cone beam scanners, the isotropic voxel size ranges from 80 to 400 microns and thus they manage to visualize the structures of the maxillofacial region with sufficient resolution, allowing the operator to obtain measurements accurately. Compared to conventional computed tomography, cone beam computed tomography shows significantly fewer artifacts due to metallic structures in the region of interest, and the radiation dose to the patient, depending always on the scanner, protocol, and field size is lower. An important advantage is also the interactivity, i.e., the ability of modern systems to allow the transfer of tomographic data and their study in other computer systems. Finally, the size but also the cost of acquiring a cone beam computed tomography scanner is significantly reduced compared to conventional computed tomography scanners.

There are different type of machines, others working with the patient seated and the rotation like a panoramic system, others with the patient standing like a panoramic system and few with the patient laying down like in a medical CT. Examples of the types of machines are given in the following image (Fig. 3.5).

The ability to reconstruct the tomographic images in each plane (beyond the three main planes mentioned above) is the main advantage of cone beam computed tomography over conventional dental imaging methods. This property is called multi-planar reformatting and is made possible because since all the initial scan data are stored in the scanner's computer, rearranging these data will lead to the creation of new images according to the diagnostic needs.

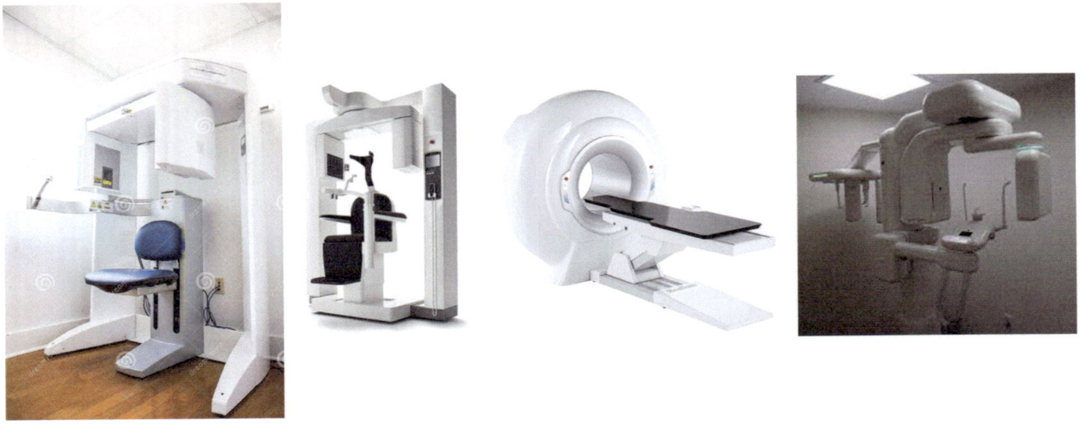

Fig. 3.5 Example of various CBCT systems with the patient in different positions either standing, sitting or laying down

3.4.7 Limitations

Cone beam computed tomography has some limitations related to the beam geometry, the sensitivity of the detection system, and the contrast resolution compared to fan beam computed tomography. In addition, various artifacts, noise, and low soft tissue contrast can affect the sharpness of the tomographic images.

Due to the conical shape of the X-ray beam, a relatively large part of the patient's head is irradiated during the acquisition of each of the structural images during the scan. This increases the probability of scattering of photons involved in attenuation interactions. The scattered rays deviate from the position of the object or tissue that attenuated them and therefore when captured by the detector, they are recorded as information at a spatially different position on the detector (noise). This reduces the sharpness of the tomographic image and degrades its overall quality. In conventional CT scanners, the fan-shaped beam produced improves the secondary (scatter radiation) to primary radiation ratio (SPR), compared to cone beam scanners. Finally, increasing the angular range of the cone beam leads to a larger area of the cone base, a larger imaging field, and consequently increased secondary radiation and noise generation.

References

1. Mehralizadeh S, Anaraki SN, Orshesh M. Comparison of CMOS and PSP intraoral digital sensors in the diagnosis of secondary caries adjacent to amalgam restorations. J Res Dent Maxillofac Sci. 2017;2(4):44–9.
2. Körner M, Weber CH, Wirth S, Pfeifer KJ, Reiser MF, Treitl M. Advances in digital radiography: physical principles and system overview. Radiographics. 2007;27:675–86.
3. Bushong SC. Radiologic science for technologists: physics, biology, and protection. 5th ed. St. Louis: Mosby; 1993. p. 325–35.
4. Jayachandran S. Digital imaging in dentistry: a review. Contemp Clin Dent. 2017;8:193–4.
5. Kamburoğlu K, Samunahmetoğlu E, Eratam N, Sönmez G. Sevilay Karahan· clinical comparison of intraoral CMOS and PSP detectors in terms of time efficiency, patient comfort, and subjective image quality. Imaging Sci Dent. 2022;52(1):93–101.
6. Elkhateeb SM, Aloyouny AY, Omer MMS, Mansour SM. Analysis of photostimulable phosphor image plate artifacts and their prevalence. World J Clin Cases. 2022;10(2):437–47.
7. Mann J, Hacking C, Bell D, et al. Photostimulable phosphors. Reference article, Radiopaedia.org. Accessed 12 Dec 2022.
8. Ponce AZ, McDavid WD, Langland OE. The use of added erbium filtration in intraoral radiography. Oral Surg Oral Med Oral Pathol. 1988 Oct;66(4):513–7.
9. White SC, Pharoah M. Oral radiology: principles and interpretation. 6th ed. St Louis: Mosby; 2008. p. 79–99, 207–224.
10. Molteni R. The way we were (and how we got here): fifty years of technology changes in dental and

maxillofacial radiology. Dentomaxillofac Radiol. 2021;50(1):2020.
11. Ogawa K, Langlais RP, McDavid WD, Noujeim M, Seki K, Okano T, et al. Development of a new dental panoramic radiographic system based on a tomosynthesis method. Dentomaxillofac Radiol. 2010;39:47–53.
12. Noujeim M, Prihoda T, McDavid WD, Ogawa K, Yamakawa T, Seki K, Okano T, et al. Pre-clinical evaluation of a new dental panoramic radiographic system based on the tomosynthesis method. Dentomaxillofac Radiol. 2011;40:42–6.
13. Dental Reach—Leading Dental Magazine—Dentistry Journal, News & Events. 2022. The journey of panoramic radiography—a review.
14. Beckmann EC. CT scanning in the early days. Br J Radiol. 2006;79(937):5–8.
15. Bushong SC. Radiologic science for technologists: physics, biology, and protection. 5th St. Louis: Mosby, 1993, pg 325–335.
16. Rustemeyer P, Sireubühr U, Suttmoeller J. Low-dose dental computed tomography: significant dose reduction without loss of image quality. Acta Radiol. 2004;45(8):847–53.
17. Robb RA. The dynamic spatial Reconstructor: an X-ray video-fluoroscopic CT scanner for dynamic volume imaging of moving organs. IEEE Trans Med Imaging. 1982;1(1):22–33.
18. Chen B, Ning R. Cone-beam volume CT breast imaging: a feasibility study. Med Phys. 2002;29(5):755–70.
19. Cho PS, Johnson RH, Griffin TW. Cone-beam CT for radiotherapy applications. Phys Med Biol. 1995;40(11):1863–83. Detection PU. 154/Pulmonary Disease. 2007;154–5.
20. Araki K, Maki K, Seki K, Sakamaki K, Harata Y, Sakaino R, et al. Characteristics of a newly developed dentomaxillofacial X-ray cone beam CT scanner (CB MercuRayTM): system configuration and physical properties. Dentomaxillofacial Radiol. 2004;33(1):51–9.
21. Venkatesh E, Elluru SV. CBCT: basics and applications in dentistry. J Istanbul Univ Fac Dent. 2017;51:102–21.
22. Yamamoto K, Ueno K, Seo K, Shinohara D. Development of beam X-ray computed tomography system. Orthod Craniofac Res. 2003;6:160–2.
23. Scarfe WC, Farman AG. What is cone-beam CT and how does it work? Dent Clin N Am. 2008;52(4):707–30.
24. Scarfe WC, Farman AG, Sukovic P. Clinical applications of cone-beam computed tomography in dental practice. J Can Dent Assoc (Tor). 2006;72(1):75–80.

4 Digital Impressions

Konstantinos Michalakis, Lea Hajjar, Luis Del Castillo, and Hiroshi Hirayama

4.1 History and Introductory Data

Preliminary and definitive (final) impressions are a vital part of the restorative process, as the former are used for the fabrication of the diagnostic casts and treatment planning, while the latter are employed for the fabrication of the master casts, on which the definitive prostheses of the patients are made [1]. Irreversible hydrocolloids (alginates) and non-aqueous elastomeric materials are traditionally used for preliminary impressions, depending on the clinician's preferences regarding accuracy, existence of laboratory support within the dental practice, as well as the need to re-pour the impression or not. On the contrary, until quite recently the definitive impressions were made only with non-aqueous elastomeric materials, which included condensation silicones, polyvinylsiloxanes, polyether, vinylsiloxanethers, and polysulfides [2]. An accurate impression of prepared teeth is a prerequisite for restorations which will maintain tooth integrity and periodontal health, through accurate marginal fitting and establishment of correct emergence profile. Some inelastic materials, such as plaster, zinc-oxide eugenol, and impression compounds have also been employed as impression materials in the past, especially for the construction of removable complete dentures.

To fulfill their purpose, the impression materials should have some ideal characteristics. They should: (1) be easy to handle, (2) be hydrophilic before and after setting, (3) be accurate in reproduction, (4) have resistance to tear, (5) provide reasonable working and setting times, (6) be biocompatible and hypoallergenic, (7) have dimensional stability, (8) provide elastic recovery, (9) be compatible with dental stone and other pouring materials (e.g., epoxy resins), (10) have pleasant odor and taste [2]. Although all impression materials in the dental market satisfy ADA's nos. 18 (alginate) and 19 (non-aqueous elastomeric) specifications for impression materials, there is no material which possesses all the aforementioned ideal characteristics. Each one of the aforementioned impression materials has certain

K. Michalakis (✉)
Department of Restorative Sciences and Biomaterials, Boston University Henry M. Goldman School of Dental Medicine, Boston, MA, USA

Boston University Center for Multiscale and Translational Mechanobiology, Boston, MA, USA
e-mail: kmich@bu.edu

L. Hajjar
Department of Prosthodontics, Tufts University School of Dental Medicine, Boston, MA, USA

L. Del Castillo · H. Hirayama
Department of Restorative Sciences and Biomaterials, Advanced Education Program in Prosthodontics, Boston University Henry M. Goldman School of Dental Medicine, Boston, MA, USA

A. Delantoni, K. Orhan (eds.), *Digital Dentistry*, https://doi.org/10.1007/978-3-031-52826-2_4

indications, as well as advantages and disadvantages, which are beyond the scope of this chapter, and can be found in Dental Materials books. Two of the biggest disadvantages of the impressions, especially when these are made for the fabrication of definitive prostheses and they involve a large number of prepared teeth, is that quite often one or more of the teeth may not be adequately impressed. In these cases, especially when the impression is made for fixed partial dentures, the whole procedure has to be repeated. This procedure, which involves retraction cord packing in the sulci of the prepared teeth, is usually time-consuming for the dentist and annoying for the patient, especially if it involves multiple teeth. It can also result, depending on patient's biotype (i.e., patients with thin biotype) to soft tissue recession, with adverse effects in the final restorative esthetic result [3, 4]. Moreover, there are many patients who have a strong pharyngeal (gag) reflex and the impression procedure is extremely unpleasant for them.

It should be mentioned that the accuracy of the definitive restorations does not rely only on the properties of the impression material used, but also on the characteristics of other materials used during the laboratory procedures. These inaccuracies result from the setting expansion (0.1–0.3%) of the dental stone; shrinkage distortion (0.4%) of the casting wax; setting (0.23–0.50%), hygroscopic (0.35–1.20%) and thermal (1.33–1.58%) expansion of the investment material; and thermal contraction (1.42–1.56%) of dental alloys [2].

With the advent of digital technologies in dentistry impressions can be made by using an intraoral scanner (IOS), which eliminates the need for an impression material. Moreover, computer-aided design/computer-aided manufacturing (CAD/CAM), which includes digital restoration design on virtual casts, as well as milling, printing, or sintering of restorations, has minimized all errors associated with laboratory procedures. The introduction of this concept into the dental field was first made by Dr. Francois Duret, in his 1974 thesis "Empreinte Optique" ("Optical Impression") which was submitted at the faculty of dentistry of Université Claude Bernard, in Lyon, France [5]. This thesis was based on the knowledge gained by Dr. Duret's studies in physics and dentistry. His knowledge of these two different fields gave him the opportunity to think about the thermodynamics of quantum systems and the need for digitization of information in dentistry. In 1980, along with Hennequin, Déchelet and Blouin, he developed the first handheld optical probe (IOS), which consisted of a laser diode source and a charge-coupled-device (CCD) photoreceptor. As the probe was passing over the teeth the laser light was reflected by the teeth to the CCD, converted then to a digital signal and transmitted to the personal computer. For each tooth, the process had to be repeated 4 times to ensure acceptable images could be collected. The system had a resolution of 20 μm and it was theoretically based on Moire fringe techniques [6]. As during the procedure unwanted reflections could be produced, a non-reflective substance (powder) was needed, in order to eliminate those reflections. The CAD/CAM system used was the Euclid (Matra Datavision, Woburn, MA), and it was capable of creating solid models of the surfaces, on which the restorations would be placed [7, 8]. It was in 1985 at the ADF congress in Paris that the first crown was made for Dr. Duret's wife, by using this technology [9]. Between 1986 and 1993 the company Hennson/Sopha financed, developed, and produced 80 CAD/CAM devices, of which 61 were sold. In 1989, at the Chicago Midwinter Meeting, Dr. Duret presented his CAD/CAM technology from the Northwestern University School of Dentistry through a live closed-circuit television session. The attendees of that meeting witnessed the fabrication of a crown in a few hours. This was a breakthrough event in fabrication of a crown, which had a tolerance of <80 μm.

In the early 1980s, a Swiss Professor of dentistry, Werner Mörmann, and an Italian electrical engineer, Marco Brandestini, presented their concept of chairside CAD/CAM technology for the fabrication of ceramic restorations, intended to substitute composite fillings, which presented several disadvantages [10–12]. This technology was branded as CEREC (computer-assisted CERamic REConstruction) (Brains, Brandestini

Instruments, Zollikan, Switzerland), and the prototype unit (CEREC 1) was presented on May 1, 1986 [13]. That system was using an optical topographical scanning process along with an electronically controlled milling unit [14]. The system was complemented by a 3-dimensional IOS, specially designed for that purpose, which was providing data to an interactive CAD unit. The IOS had a light-emitting diode, joined by a lens system which was capable of illuminating the cavity prepared by the dentist. The system had also a set of mirrors, so as the light rays could be reflected and reach the tooth easier. The emitted rays were passing through a set of ruled lines and a lens system. In this way a pattern of light and dark areas, in the form of stripes, was created on the prepared tooth cavity. The light was reflected back to the head of the scanner and was sensed by a CCD sensor, at a different angle from that which was emitted. The CCD sensor had a resolution of 256 × 256 pixels, and the intensity of the light was converted to voltage values, which were then sent to the personal computer for analysis. The computer was programmed to transform the voltage values, which—as previously mentioned—represented different light intensities depending on the depth of the cavity. The complexity of the preparation was determined by shift differences between the reflected and incident light, as shallow areas exhibited less apparent shift than deeper areas [15]. The system was quite accurate, and it was determined that its accuracy could be further enhanced by the use of a powder (CAVISON, Svedia Dental industry, Enkoeping, Sweden), which could eliminate undesired reflections, due to saliva, well-polished tooth surfaces, metallic restorations, etc. The whole scanning process could be seen in the monitor of the computer, as the dentist was progressing with image acquisition. The IOS was complemented by a 3-axes milling machine, which possessed three translatory platforms mounted on a frame, providing position control for the x, y, z axes. The machining of the prefabricated rod-shaped blocks of feldspathic porcelain (Vitadur 353 N; VITA Zahnfabrik, Bad Sackingen, Germany) was taking place by a diamond bur rigidly connected to the y-axis which was powered by a high-speed turbine [16, 17].

At that time the first patient was treated, using Vita Mark I feldspathic porcelain (VITA Zahnfabrik). However, it was not until the early 1990s that the first clinical results were published. Until 2000 the software had only a two-dimensional imaging capability, while from 2003 three-dimensional image capturing was made feasible. The founders of the CEREC system named the whole process as "optical impression" [17, 18]. The basic principles of imaging have not changed since then (Table 4.1). With the advancement of the hardware and the software the need for an anti-glare white TiO_2 powder was made obsolete and in 2012 the company marketed CEREC Omnicam, which also produced colored images. It should be mentioned however that there are still IOS devices requiring the teeth to be powder-coated before the scanning procedures, as this method has been shown to be very accurate for partial impressions [19]. This powder coating has a thickness of 20–40 μm, or even more, depending on the operator. To overcome this problem the systems which still require anti-reflection powder have incorporated in their software an average thickness, for compensation reasons [20]. However, use of the powder presents some drawbacks, including patient's relative discomfort and additional scanning time, especially when the powder is moistened with saliva and necessitates cleaning and reapplication [21]. As maintenance of a dry field for full mouth scanning is difficult, systems which do not require powder application are recommended for cross-arch digital acquisition procedures [22].

At about the same time, a third group at the University of Minnesota, in the United States, was also working on the digital impression concept. Their approach however was different from the ones previously described. It required data acquisition with a 35 mm camera through a 10 mm diameter single-rod lens laryngo-pharyngoscope (Richard Wolf Medical Instruments, Rosemont, IL), which could be attached to a standard 55 mm lens, surrounded by fiber optics for illumination purposes [23]. An attached prism system at the end of the sin-

Table 4.1 The evolution of CEREC system

Year	Hardware (brand name)	Software capability	Restorations	Producer
1980	Initial concept (no brand name)	2-dimensional	Inlays	Mörmann & Brandestini
1985	CEREC 1	2-dimensional	Inlays	Mörmann & Brandestini
1988	CEREC 1	2-dimensional	Inlays (I), Onlays (O), veneers (V)	Mörmann & Brandestini
1994	CEREC 2	2-dimensional	I, O, V, partial crowns (PC), full crowns (FC), copings (C)	Siemens
2000	CEREC 3 (Redcam)	2-dimensional	I, O, V, PC, FC, C, 3-unit FPD	Sirona
2003	CEREC 3 (Redcam)	3-dimensional	I, O, V, PC, FC, C, 4-unit FPD	Sirona
2005	CEREC 3 (Redcam)	3-dimensional	I, O, V, PC, FC, C, 4-unit FPD, with automatic virtual occlusal adjustment	Sirona
2009	CEREC 4 (Bluecam)	3-dimensional	I, O, V, PC, FC, C, 4-unit FPD, with automatic virtual occlusal adjustment	Sirona
2012	CEREC 5 (Omnicam)	3-dimensional	I, O, V, PC, FC, C, 4-unit FPD, with automatic virtual occlusal adjustment	Sirona
2019	CEREC (Primescan)	3-dimensional	I, O, V, PC, FC, C, 4-unit FPD, with automatic virtual occlusal adjustment	Sirona

gle-rod lens was providing a 90° view with an infinite depth of field, so as to be able to capture with great accuracy the preparation along with the margins, from a distance of 25 mm above the occlusal surface of the tooth. Obviously, a number of images were needed to capture every detail of the prepared teeth and minimize the risk of unclear images due to patient movement. A drawback of the system—which was done for keeping the cost low for the dentists—was that it needed image recording on a standard film. The slides were then digitized by an Eikonix system (Eikonix Corp., Bedford, MA) with a resolution of 4096 × 4096 pixels. The prepared tooth's three-dimensional reconstruction from the acquired images was then performed by applying either a direct linear transformation or by using the theory of human stereo vision proposed by Grimson [24, 25]. The system had also a library with ideal tooth forms and it could machine a full coverage restoration with a five axis CAD/CAM system (Integrated Computer-Aided Engineering and Machining-Design, Drafting and Numerical Control, Control Data Corp., Minneapolis, MN). It should be mentioned that while the Minnesota and the Duret systems were designed to be able to produce full coverage restorations, the CEREC system was initially developed for inlays. Nevertheless, the fact that an immediate digitization was not feasible with the Minnesota system made its use impractical. This approach was selected by the inventors to keep the cost for the dentist in the region of $5000, which was much lower than the $35,000 to $90,000 cost of the other two systems [17].

4.2 Digital Impression Modalities

There are basically two ways of digitizing the tooth preparations in order to proceed with the CAD/CAM manufacturing process of a restoration. The first method (*direct*) utilizes an intraoral scanner (IOS), while the second one (*indirect*) requires making of an analog impression with a non-aqueous elastomeric material, fabrication of a definitive stone cast, and scanning of this cast with a laboratory scanning unit. Both the direct and the indirect methods have as an endpoint the digitization of the prepared teeth and their antagonists through the generation of datasets called Standard Tessellation Language (STL) files in order to be able to:

- Design single or multiple fixed provisional or definitive restorations
- Design partial or complete removable dentures
- Design surgical stents for implant placement
- Design occlusal appliances

4.3 Scanning Technologies and Related Concepts

The ultimate purpose of every scanning method (direct or indirect) is to record with high precision the three-dimensional geometries of the teeth and/or the soft tissues by generating STL files, as previously mentioned. These files which, depending on the system, can be either open or closed (locked), have been used for rapid prototyping, three-dimensional printing, as well as for CAM purposes in several industrial areas, and they were first released in 1987, by 3D systems [26, 27]. In simple words it can be said that the STL file is nothing more than the "translation of a three-dimensional object." The STL file encodes an object's surface geometry. These files define the geometrical surfaces of three-dimensional objects, without however providing any texture or color representation. Most often, Polygon File Formats (PLY) are being employed for transparency, color, and texture representations. These formats are also known as Stanford Triangle Formats (STF) [28]. The geometry of the model in STL files is reproduced by a series of linked triangles in the three-dimensional Cartesian coordinate system. This file encodes an object's surface geometry, and the applied concept is termed tessellation. Therefore, *tessellation* is the action of construction of a surface with geometric shapes, which are most often triangles. Thus, the whole procedure involves the concept of triangulation, where 3D objects are subdivided into tetrahedral elements joined together. These triangles are most often met in an edge-to-edge and vertex-to vertex fashion. As the number of triangles increases so does the resolution of the triangulated object (Fig. 4.1). These triangles (or other geometrical entities) can be saved in two different ways: (a) by *binary* encoding, and (b) by ASCII encoding. Both ways of encoding store the components of the unit normal vector of each triangle, as well as the vertices' coordinates.

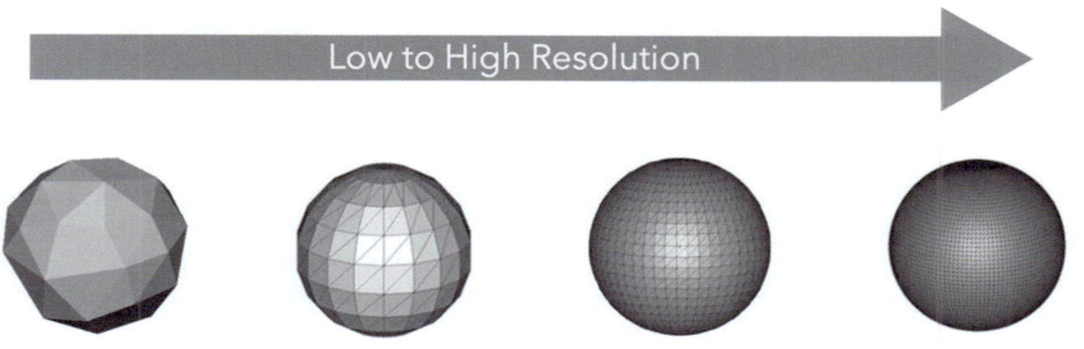

Fig. 4.1 As the number of geometrical entities (triangles) increases so does the resolution of the object (sphere)

4.4 Direct Method

The direct method, which utilizes the use of an IOS, has many advantages, and it has gained great popularity worldwide in the last fifteen years. It requires an initial moderate to high investment, which is however much cheaper than what it used to be when the IOSs became readily available in the dental market (Fig. 4.2).

The direct method presents many benefits for the patients, who avoid the unpleasant procedure of analog impressions, and for the dentists, who don't have to spend a significant amount of money for purchasing non-aqueous elastomeric impression materials, stock trays, and impression disinfection solutions. In addition, the fact that all impression data are stored in computers eliminates the need for physical space for stone cast storage. Furthermore, the communication with the lab becomes easier and the need of couriers or mail is eliminated. In this way the paperwork for both the dental office and the laboratory is reduced too. Other significant advantages include the reduction of turnaround times, reduction of waste which would end in landfills, immediate evaluation of the digital impression on the screen, and repetition of the procedure if the digital impression is considered inadequate. Another major advantage of the direct method is the critical evaluation of the preparation features under magnification, which can be up to 20 times the actual size. Even minute details of tooth's prepared surfaces as well as the continuity of the margin can be immediately assessed and corrected, if needed. This immediate feedback is a great advantage for the restorative dentist, especially for the inexperienced one. It should be mentioned however that certain procedures which are needed for a good analog impression are also required for the intraoral digital impression too. These include gingival retraction for sufficient exposure of subgingivally placed margins and tooth isolation from moisture contamination, i.e., from blood and saliva. These are prerequisites for the acquisition of an accurate digital impression, and they are also limitations of this technology. Obviously, these shortcomings could be eliminated if the digital impression was performed via high-frequency ultrasound technology, which is an area of current research [29, 30]. New data comparing conventional optical intraoral (Lava COS; 3 M/ESPE, St. Paul, MN, USA) and laboratory (CARES Scan CS2, Straumann, Basel, Switzerland) scanners with a high-frequency ultrasound prototype developed at the Department of Medical Engineering, Helmholtz Institute, RWTH Aachen University, Germany, have demonstrated that there was no statistical difference between the methods examined. The mean deviation error was 75 ± 41.43 μm for the laboratory scanner, 57.40 ± 17.44 μm for the high-frequency ultrasound, and 38.55 ± 24.34 μm for the intraoral one. Furthermore, the ultrasound scanner demonstrated a similar trueness, with those exhibited by the two optical scanners examined [31]. Nevertheless, the thickness of the gingiva has still an effect on the quality of the image. Thin gingival layers demonstrated better image quality than thick layers [30]. The positive results of the latest research demonstrate that soon there

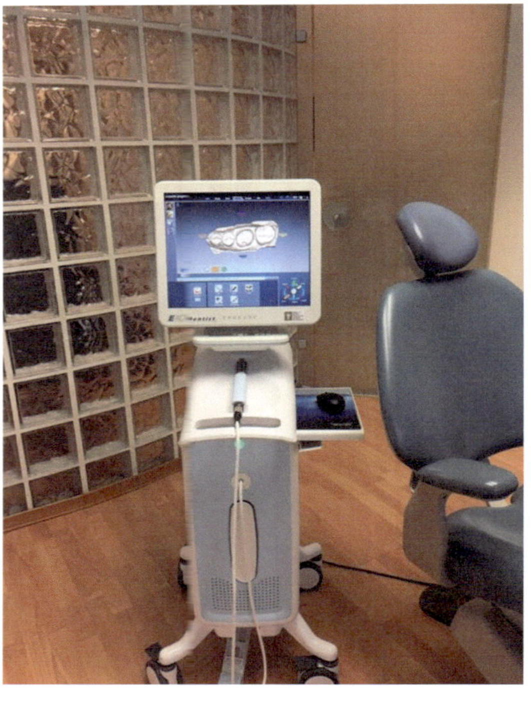

Fig. 4.2 One of the most popular intraoral scanners in the late 2000s-early 2010s was the E4D® system

will be some changes in this field. It can be understood that the development of high-frequency ultrasound impression could be a very big step towards a simplified digital impression procedure, as neither gingival retraction nor tooth isolation would be needed, with a positive impact on patient comfort, soft tissue response, and dentist's efforts.

Until this technology becomes readily available, optical IOSs are considered the gold standards for this purpose. Although the original concepts of Drs. Duret and Mörmann have been highly improved, a handheld optical scanner, a computer, and a software developed for this purpose are still needed.

Today there are several different ways of imaging technologies adopted by companies manufacturing IOS and/or lab scanners. Two basic techniques are used: (1) the *passive*, which relies on ambient lighting for teeth and tissue illumination, and (2) the *active*, which requires blue, red, or white light emission. The passive technique relies on the texture of the object being recorded, while the active technique does not need to rely on that as much [32, 33]. The light which is emitted from the scanner head onto the object is used for distance calculation. This can also be done by a projection of either multiple points or of a mesh on the object, which is going to be registered, and the surfaces of the object are reconstructed by a compilation of multiple images [34, 35]. Several ways have been employed for calculation of the distance between the anatomical structure recorded and the lens. These include:

1. *Active Wavefront Sampling (AWS),* which is a three-dimensional surface imaging technique, utilizing one camera and an AWS module, which is an off-axis aperture. The optical wavefront traversing a lens is sampled at ≥2 off-axis locations, and as a result the motion of each target feature can be accurately measured. The advantage of this method is that only a single optical train and a sensor are needed for depth information, and thus the size of the equipment and its cost are decreased. In intraoral scanning, the image reflected from an intraoral anatomical structure (e.g. tooth) is led to a sensor through a lens system. If the image of the tooth is in focus, then the distance of that tooth corresponds to the focal length of the lens. If it is out of focus, the distance is calculated from the software, based on the size of the blurred image [36–39] (Fig. 4.3).
2. *Confocal* imaging is one of the most precise methods used in today's scanning technologies and is based on three-dimensional scanning of the intraoral structures by employment

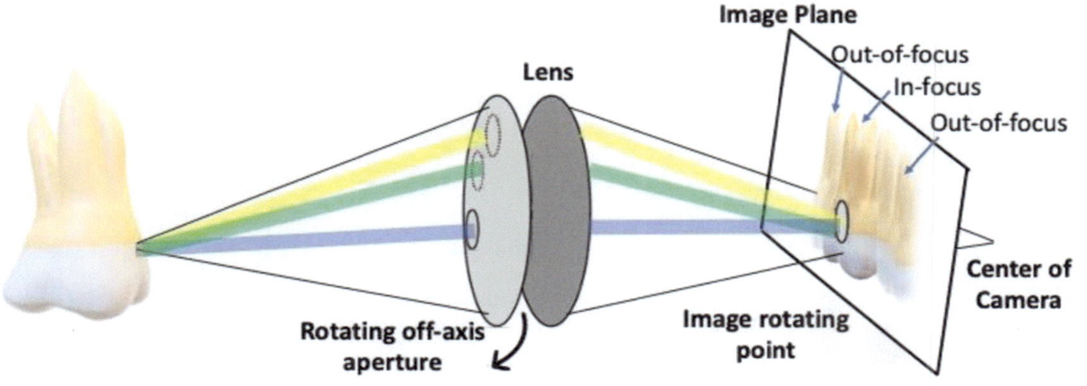

Fig. 4.3 Active Wavefront Sampling (AWS) requires a camera with an off-axis aperture which revolves around the optical axis and produces a rotation of points of interest

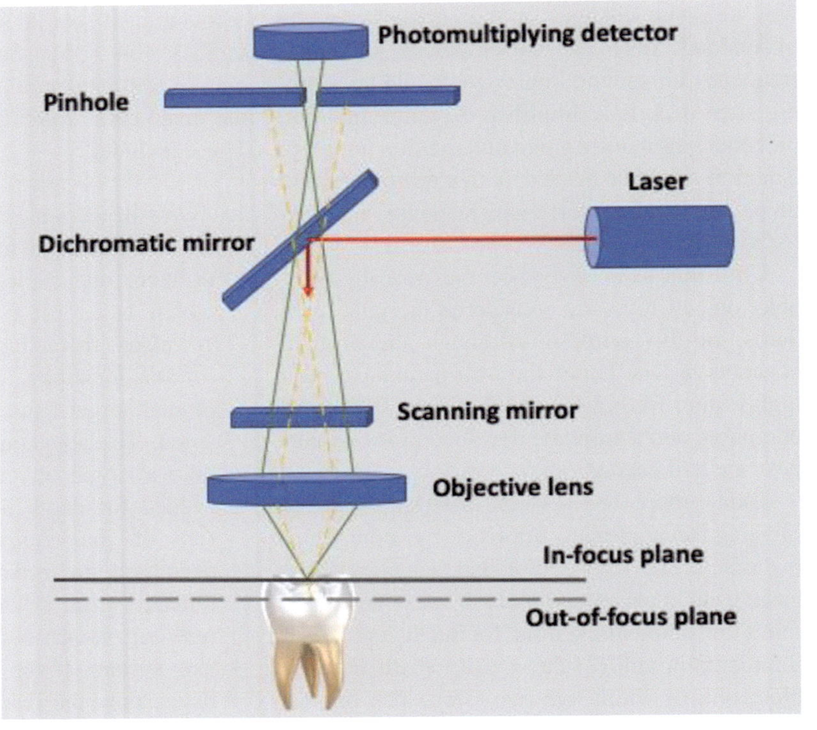

Fig. 4.4 Basic configuration of a confocal scanning device. Only the rays (green) from the in-focus plane reach the photomultiplying detector. The dotted yellow rays originating from an out-of-focus plane do not reach the detector

of a focused laser probe and spatial filtering through a pinhole in the image plane. The purpose of the pinhole is to reduce the laser light intensity when this comes from out-of-focus areas. This results in the confocal signal on the detector. This concept was developed and patented by Marvin Minsky in the late 1950s [40, 41]. In Minsky's configuration, a pinhole was in front of a zirconium (Zr) arc light source, in order to provide to the object a point of focused light by an objective lens. The system required also an additional objective lens, which focused the object onto a second pinhole, which was in front of the detector. The idea was to provide a double focusing system, which would reject all out-of-focus light rays emanating from the object, thus they do not reach the low-noise photomultiplying detector. This technology is both very accurate and advantageous, as it allows data acquisition from regions with difficult access, such as the interproximal areas [42, 43] (Figs. 4.4 and 4.5).

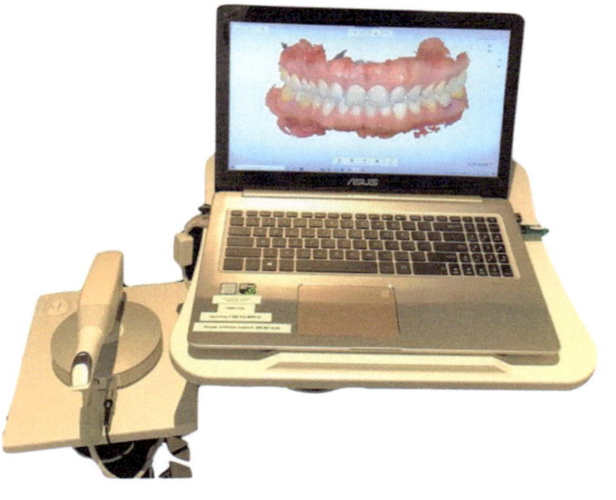

Fig. 4.5 The Trios/3shape® intraoral digital scanner, which uses confocal imaging technology (courtesy Dr. Andre Hashem)

3. *Stereophotogrammetry* represents a relatively cheaper approach to the digital imaging issue. It requires a small high-resolution camera which can estimate the x, y, z coordinates of the object, via multiple images analysis, with

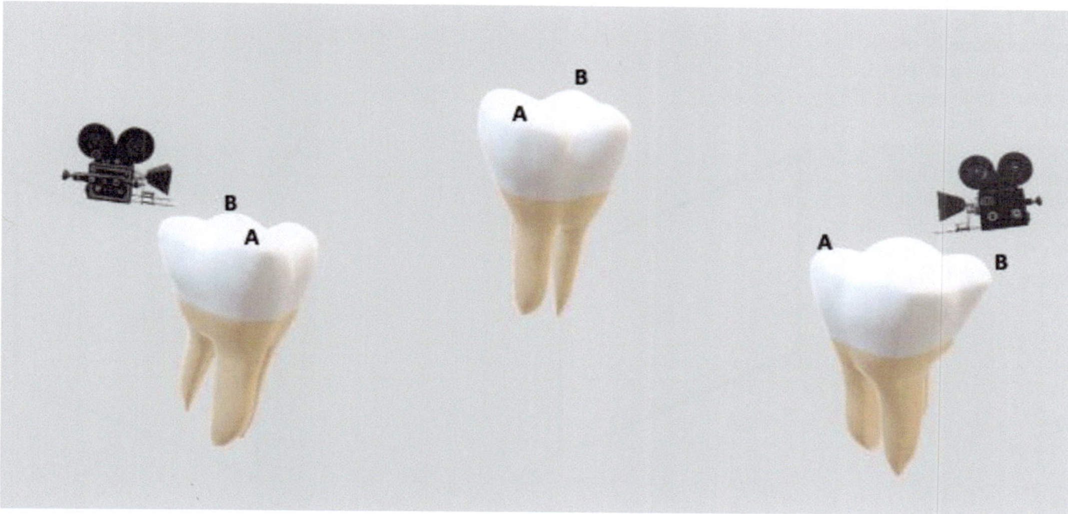

Fig. 4.6 In stereophotogrammetry the three-dimensional coordinates of several points are registered in multiple images, and these are merged in one final image

appropriate algorithms. These images are taken in milliseconds from different positions, generating a collection of points acquired along the three-dimensional coordinate system which are interrelated to each other and cannot be separated. The resulting images are overlapped and merged into one final image, which can be viewed, turned in all possible directions, and analyzed. As a method, stereophotogrammetry depends on passive light projection [44] (Fig. 4.6).

4. *Triangulation* represents a method of determining the exact location of a point in three-dimensional space, by knowing the angles and the positions either of two cameras, or of a single camera moving and capturing images at different points of time. This is considered to be a simple problem to solve, as each point in an image corresponds to a line in the three-dimensional space. Therefore, every point on that line in the three-dimensional space is actually projected to that point in the image. Thus, if two corresponding points can be found in more than one image, it can be assumed that they represent the projection of a common three-dimensional point x. There are several ways to calculate the coordinates of point x, as the set of lines produced by the image points should intersect at point x. Although the geometric solution of the triangulation problem is considered simple, there are some factors which create inaccuracies in this process. These factors include various types of noise, like the geometric noise, which results from detection errors or from lens distortion. As a consequence, the computed coordinates of the image are not accurate, since the lines which correspond to the points of interest do not intersect in the three-dimensional space. Several ways of optimization have been proposed for the solution of this problem [45] (Figs. 4.7, 4.8, and 4.9).

Several IOS systems have been developed during the last few years, incorporating the principles and the methods previously described. These devices have been thoroughly evaluated for their ease of handling, speed, scanning technique, and accuracy by different research groups worldwide [39, 46–53] (Table 4.2).

When it comes to implant dentistry, conventionally, the position of the implant is transferred to the physical model with the use of components known as impression copings and implant replicas. Digitally, the position of the implant is transferred with the aid of a scan body, which is a

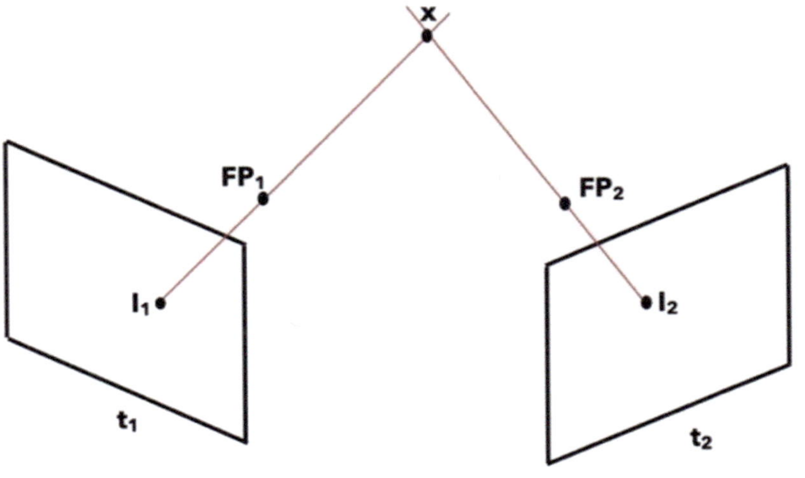

Fig. 4.7 The two planes represent images of a single camera at two different time points t_1 and t_2. Point x is projected on the images through the two lines, which intersect at the two focal points FP_1 and FP_2. These result in the image points I_1 and I_2

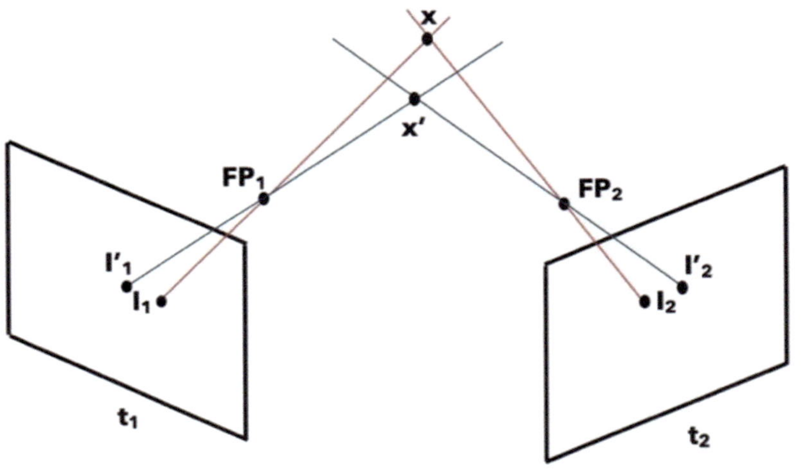

Fig. 4.8 In reality, due to geometric noise or lens distortion, points I_1 and I_2 cannot be accurately measured. Points I'_1 and I'_2 are the ones which are actually detected and used. The lines which connect I'_1 and FP_1, and I_2 and FP_2, intersect at point x', but not at the point of interest x

component with a specific geometric shape that will be scanned and recognized by a virtual library incorporated in the CAD software to identify the location of an implant. A virtual analog is then generated from the overlap of the scanned scan body STL with the virtual library of the same scan body, and a digital design of the prosthesis is then made on it (Fig. 4.10).

The concept of photogrammetry, which relies on the stereophotogrammetry method previously described, has been strictly reserved for the registration of implant position in dentistry, and so far does not apply to the registration of soft tissues intraorally. Thus, the STL file obtained from this technology only contains information about the implant position and would therefore require a second STL file of a soft tissue registration to be overlapped to it. It would be reasonable to say that this extra step may present a drawback to the use of this technology. Since photogrammetry is also based on the interrelation of points to each other in space to construct an image, it would be considered unbeneficial to use this technology for the registration of a single implant only.

Photogrammetry has been widely employed in the areas of naval engineering, automobile, and topography since the early 1980s and was only recently integrated to the field of dentistry for the registration of implants in cases of edentulous patients with full-arch implant-supported prostheses. The photogrammetry systems currently available in the market contain 2–4 cameras (Fig. 4.11), which present a larger scanning range and a faster scanning speed compared to intraoral scanning devices. The implant positions are acquired from an extraoral standpoint as the cameras are positioned outside the patient's mouth for the registration, reducing the influence that the oral cavity environment has on the accuracy of the device (Table 4.3).

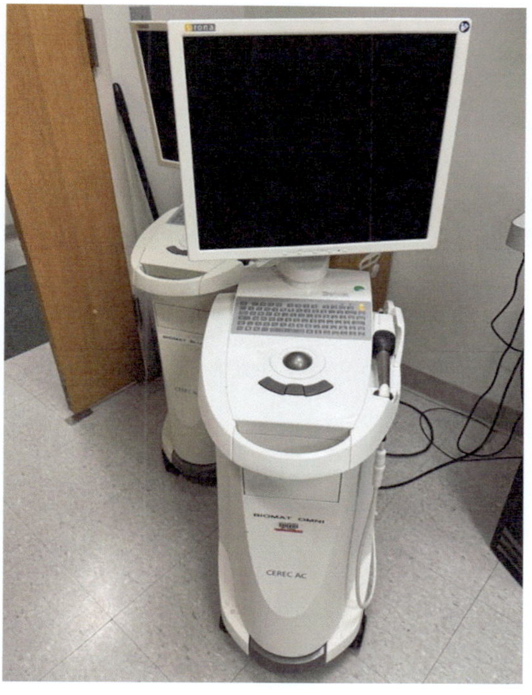

Fig. 4.9 The Sirona Omnicam® intraoral scanner, which uses the triangulation method

Since the technology behind photogrammetry allows the data to be generated by vectors of the exact position of the scan bodies in relation to one another, it does not rely on the superimposition of images also known as the "stitching effect," which is inevitable with intraoral scanning technology. That being said, scanners and photogrammetry work in different ways when it comes to capturing information from the scan body over the implant. Photogrammetry uses a scan body that presents white markers called "targets" which are precisely positioned on the scan bodies and are specific to each metric system (Fig. 4.12).

Another difference between the two technologies lies in the design and registration method of a photogrammetry scan body versus that of an IOS system: the former only needs 3 target points from two surfaces to capture the 3D position of implants whereas the latter needs to cover at least 180 degrees of the surface (Fig. 4.13).

The ICam4D from Imetric is firstly calibrated using the specific calibration plate immediately prior to the scan body measurement procedure. The optimum distance that should be maintained between the photogrammetry device and the scan bodies placed intraorally is monitored on the screen and is indicated on the left side by a green circle. In order to improve the "triangulation angle," the scanning protocol recommended by the manufacturers is to start at one side of the model and to slowly move to the other side until the ICamBodies turn green, which means the software considers the measurement precise enough (Fig. 4.14).

Table 4.2 Characteristics of different IOS systems

Intraoral scanner (IOS)	Recording method	Coating powder	Accuracy (μm)	Color
Carestream	Color-coded fringe projection pulsed light	No	24.8–65.5 [50]	Yes
Cerec Primescan	Triangulation/color-coded fringe projection	No	23.25–26.75 [52, 53]	Yes
iTero	Parallel confocal	No	45–87.25 [39]	Yes
Lava C.O.S.	Active wavefront sampling	No	12.7–14.2 [39]	Yes
Planmeca Emerald	Projected pattern triangulation	No	64–76 [52, 53]	Yes
3shape/Trios	Confocal	No	39–42 [52, 53]	Yes
True Definition	Monochrome fringe projection/disparity	Yes	19.5–75.3 [50]	No
Zfx Intrascan	Confocal/moire effect	No	112.4–126.2 [54]	No

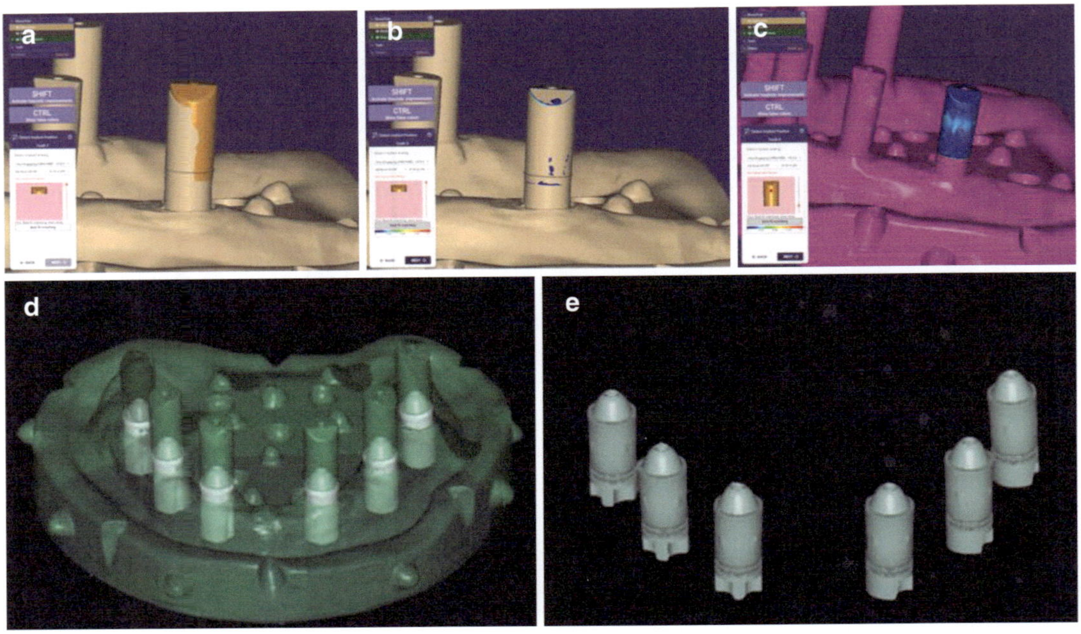

Fig. 4.10 Scan body from the scanned STL merged with the scan body from the virtual library on a CAD software (Exocad® DentalCAD; Darmstadt, Germany). (**a**) Initial alignment done between the virtual and scanned scan body; (**b**) Verification of initial merge using a colorimetric map; (**c**) Second alignment done for best fit. (**d**) Full view of the STL file with scan body and virtual analogs generated; (**e**) View of virtual analogs only

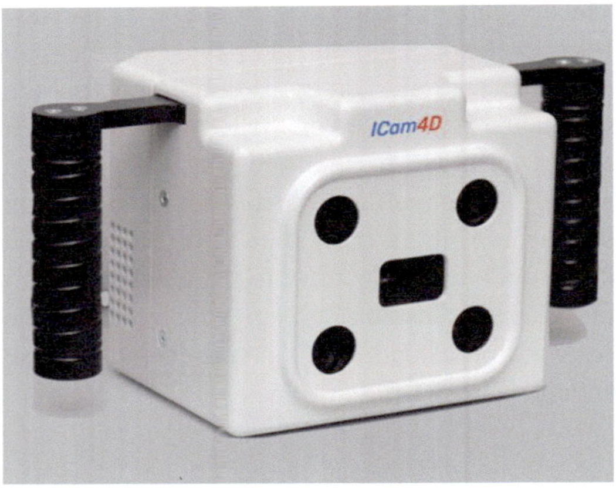

Fig. 4.11 Photogrammetry system with 4 cameras (ICam4D®, Imetric, Switzerland)

Table 4.3 Characteristics of different photogrammetry systems

Photogrammetry system	Number of cameras	Scan body shape	Coating powder	Color
PIC Camera by PIC Dental	2 cameras	Flag—1 visible surface to the cameras	No	no
ICam 4D by Imetric	4 cameras	Cuboid—2 visible surfaces to the cameras	No	No

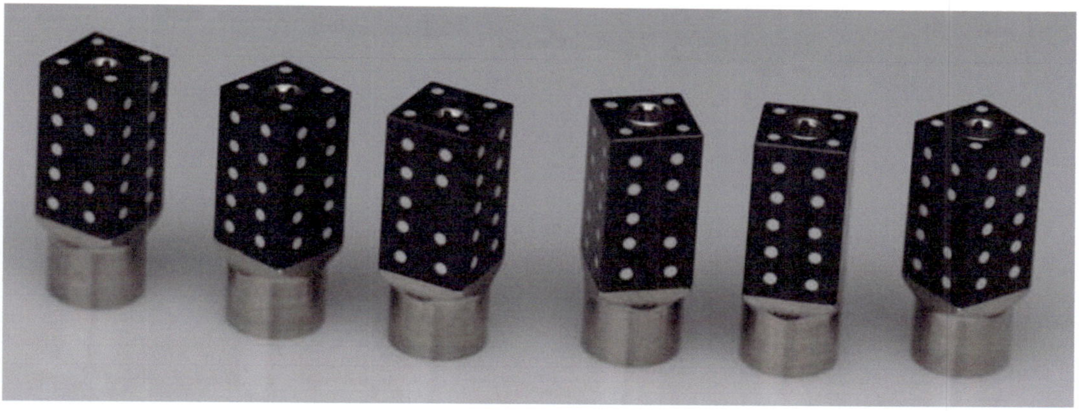

Fig. 4.12 The ICam4D® Scan bodies from Imetric (also known as ICamBodies) which presents targets on each of its cuboid surfaces

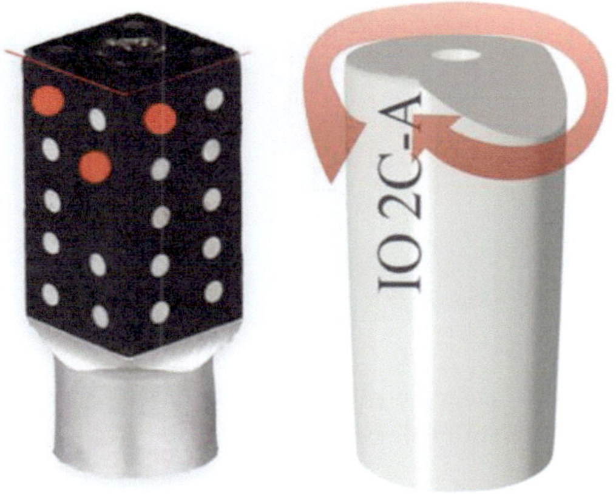

Fig. 4.13 Scan bodies represented in red by scanning surface that is necessary for registration: on the left, a photogrammetry scan body (ICam Body used for the Imetric's ICam 4D) versus an intraoral scan body on the right (ELOS Accurate scan body used for a multi-unit abutment)

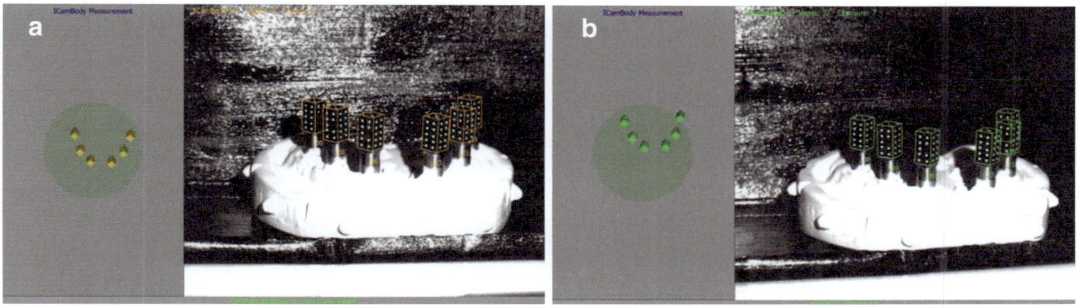

Fig. 4.14 Screen during measurement of ICamBodies showing on the left green circle indicating optimum distance and on the right the view from the camera during measurement. (**a**) ICamBodies are yellow at this stage of capture because there are not enough captures; (**b**) ICamBodies are green at this stage indicating an optimal number of captures have been taken

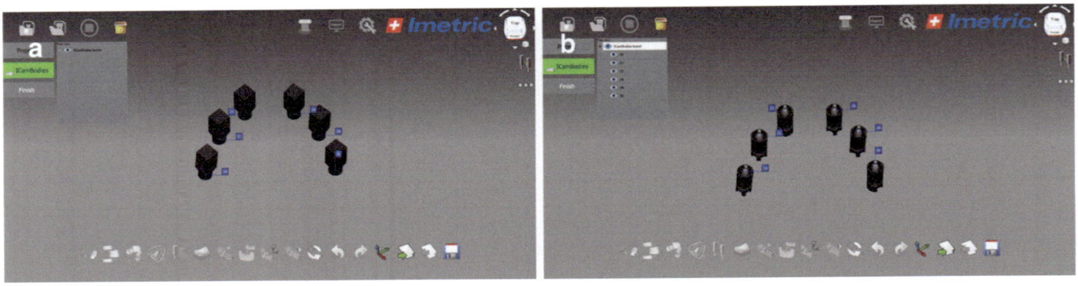

Fig. 4.15 Virtual conversion of ICamBodies into implant abutment analogs (**a**) ICamBodies measurement obtained from capture; (**b**) ICamBodies converted to Multi-unit implant abutment analogs, using the "change geometryu" feature of the software

Once the capture is completed, the ICamBodies geometry is converted into the corresponding virtual implant abutment analogs, without a need to merge any scan bodies, by simply using a "change geometry" feature incorporated in the software (Fig. 4.15).

4.5 Indirect Method

Digitization of tooth preparations and of residual alveolar ridges of complete and/or partially edentulous patients can be also completed indirectly by employing laboratory scanning equipment, which can digitize either conventional (analog) impressions, or definitive stone casts (Figs. 4.16 and 4.17). This approach is preferred many times from clinicians, especially older ones, who feel comfortable with the analog impression procedures, and they are reluctant in investing money and time for purchasing IOSs and being trained in intraoral scanning procedures. Therefore, analog impressions still represent the dominant method for impression taking in clinical settings, although this trend is expected to change in the next few years as the prices of IOSs will become lower. There are many manufacturers of laboratory scanners, and their prices are usually considerably lower than those of the IOSs.

There are several disadvantages of the indirect method, including the need for purchasing non-aqueous elastomeric materials, stock trays, dental stone, as well as the need for using additional storage space and mail/couriers for sending the impressions and/or the casts to the laboratory. Moreover, some additional errors can be introduced in the definitive restorations fabrication process, resulting from the dimensional stability and elastic recovery properties of the non-aqueous elastomeric materials and from the expansion of the dental stone. These parameters may negatively affect the marginal adaptation of the definitive restoration on the tooth, which has been considered to be one of the most important factors for the longevity of the prosthesis, as it can lead to cement dissolution, microleakage, secondary caries, endodontic inflammation, and plaque accumulation which can result in gingival inflammation if the restorative margin has been placed subgingivally [55–59].

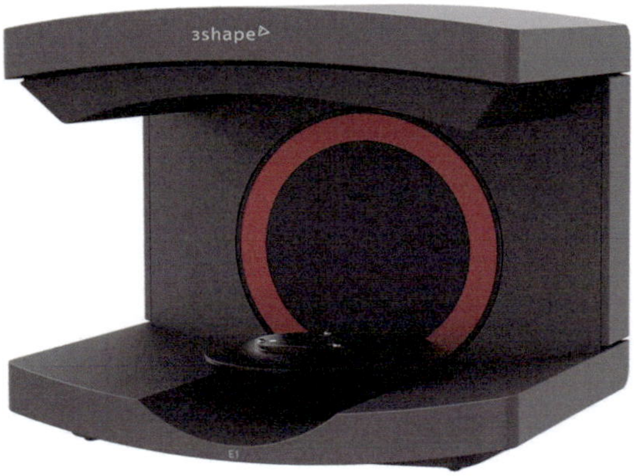

Fig. 4.16 Indirect digitization system (3shape®) used in a laboratory environment

Although there is a lot of research regarding IOSs, there is limited research on laboratory scanners. Nevertheless, the available literature suggests that the definitive restorations which were made based on intraoral digital impressions demonstrated significantly smaller marginal

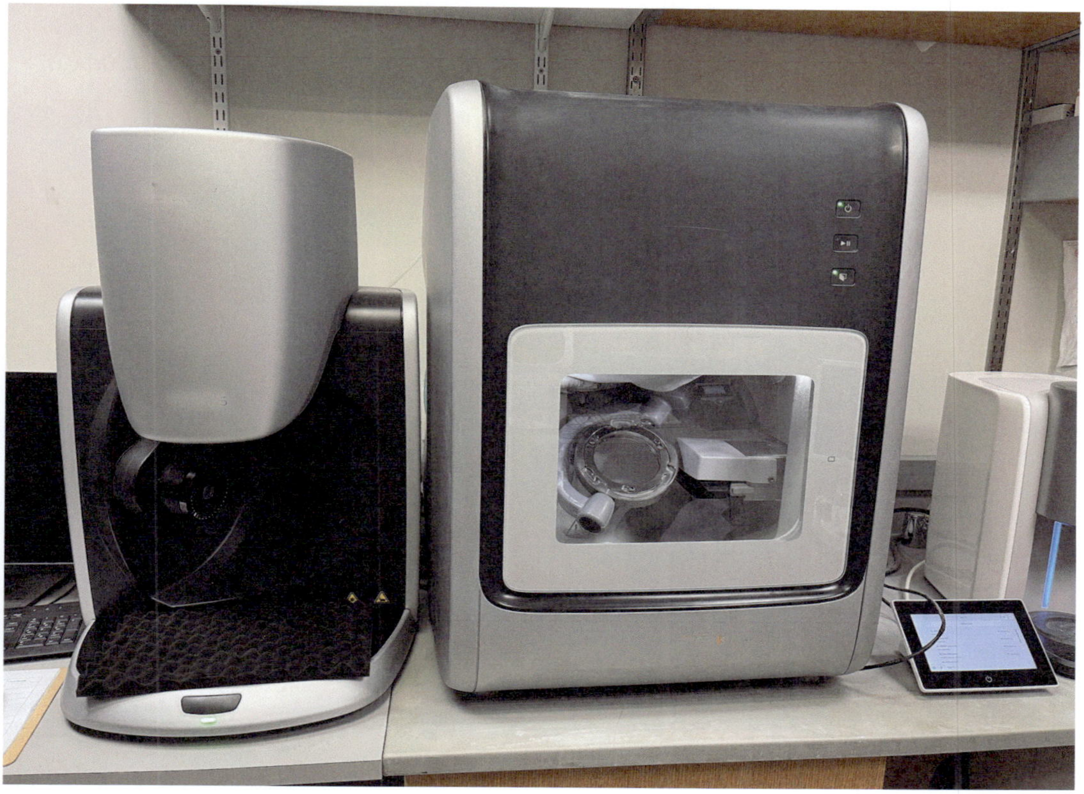

Fig. 4.17 Indirect digitization system and 5-axis milling unit (Sirona®) used in a laboratory environment

openings (from 86.09 μm ± 61.46 μm to 88.95 μm ± 54.46 μm) than those which were fabricated based on laboratory scanning procedures (143.29 μm ± 100.71 μm) [60]. The research of Güth et al. has shown that if the laboratory procedure is going to be implemented, then it is preferable to digitize the analog (conventional) definitive impression than the definitive stone model [61]. This may be attributed to the fact that one more laboratory step is added in the workflow when a stone model is fabricated, and to the expansion of high strength dental stone, which ranges between 0.08% and 0.1% [62]. Other research however has demonstrated that scanning of the stone model results in smaller discrepancies than the digitization of the definitive impression [63]. Moreover, there seems to be a difference in the marginal openings of restorations made for different teeth groups. Greater marginal gaps are usually demonstrated for incisors and canines, which have bigger axial walls and are more angulated, when compared to premolars and molars. The digitization process seems to show inefficiency in capturing deep hollow spaces, as those met in definitive impressions of anterior teeth [63].

4.6 Accuracy of Digital Impression

IOSs are mainly used to digitally impress prepared teeth and assist in the CAD/CAM process of definitive or provisional restorations. Therefore, the accuracy of the impression method is of paramount importance for the longevity of these restorations. According to the International Organization for Standardization (ISO) 5725-1, the term *accuracy* refers to the combination of *trueness* and *precision* [64]. The term *trueness* refers to the closeness between the arithmetic mean of a big number of test results and the true or accepted reference value. *Precision* is another term which is used widely for optical impres-

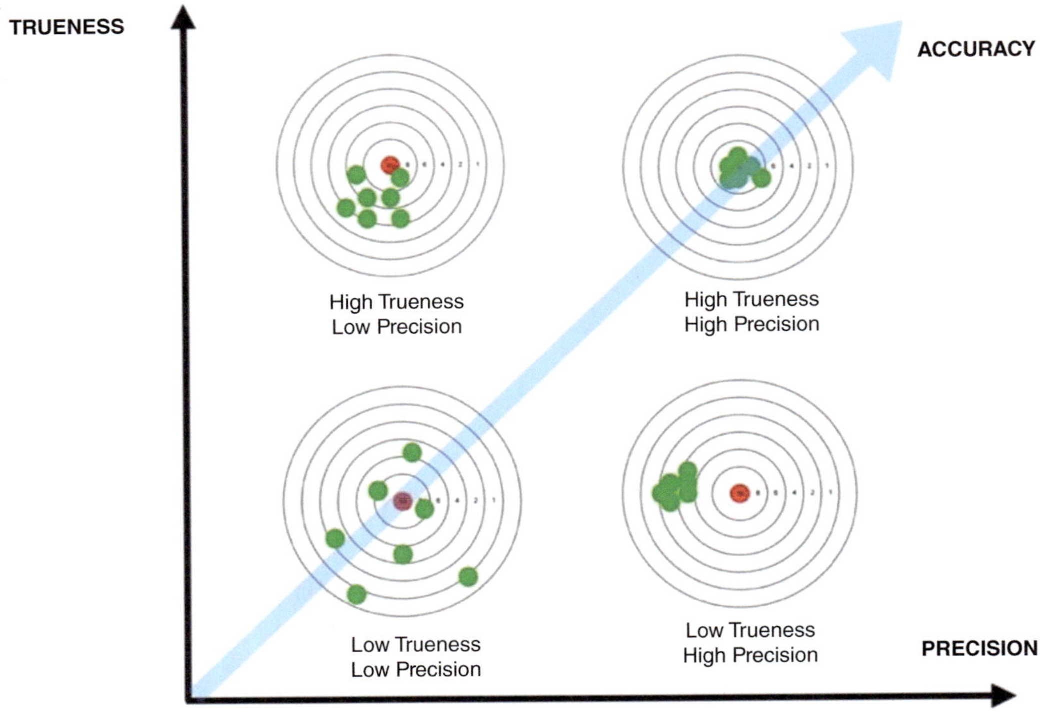

Fig. 4.18 Accuracy is the combination of trueness and precision

sions. This term refers to how close several measurements of the same quantity are close to each other. It can be understood that both trueness and precision are extremely important in digital impression procedures, and therefore an ideal IOS should have both high trueness and high precision (Fig. 4.18) [64, 65].

Trueness and precision values are used to check the accuracy of a digital scanning system. The first thing to do with a system is to verify if it is precise. If a system is precise, it can then be made to be accurate through calibration. Usually a high-resolution desktop scanner or an industrial scanner (e.g., Artec Space Spider, ATOS Core 80, etc.) is used for a reference scan. This is considered essential in determining both trueness and precision [66]. It should be mentioned however that the use of industrial scanners presents certain difficulties, as they cannot be used for intraoral scanning, and their use may require application of a powder to overcome problems with shiny and reflecting objects. Repeated scans by an IOS can give an indication regarding the precision, but not about trueness [67]. The *trueness* values of IOSs are obtained by superimposing the STL files from the IOSs in question, with the STL files from the/a reference scan chosen from a high accuracy source. Nevertheless, it should be noted that there is still no way to obtain an ideal reference or exact coordinates to evaluate the trueness of a system, and it is even more challenging to evaluate in clinical studies as the "gold standard" is yet to be determined in those settings [68]. The *precision* values of the IOS are examined by overlapping the STL files from subsequent scans of the same IOS. The final overlapping of the meshes of the different STL files is determined by an algorithm (e.g., iterative closest point algorithm) checking the best fit through an inspection or a reverse engineering software [69] (Fig. 4.19).

A color map is then used to evaluate differences between the overlapping analyzed meshes, and different colors indicate inward displacement, outward displacement, or absence of changes

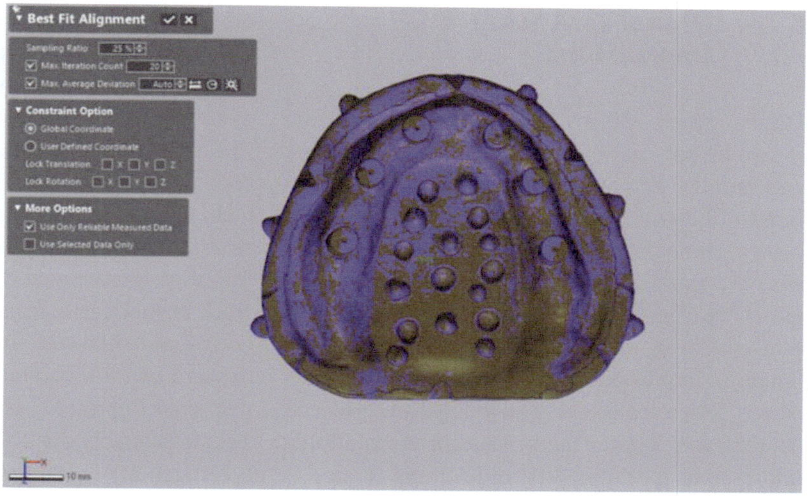

Fig. 4.19 Best-fit alignment between the test STL file and the reference file done on an inspection software (Geomagic Control X) to compare the two files

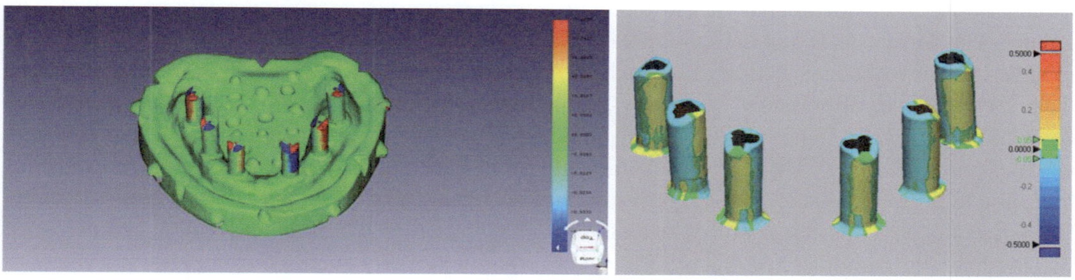

Fig. 4.20 Colorimetric map generated for visual inspection of existing deviations between a reference STL file and a test file

between the examined STL file and that of the reference scanner [70] (Fig. 4.20). A root mean square value, also known as the "RMS" value, is a measure of the magnitude of all deviation values and is obtained throughout those analyses.

As technology advances very fast, all, or nearly all, IOSs demonstrate high accuracy. This can be also demonstrated by the fact that the precision of the older intraoral scanning systems is lower than those of the newer systems [71]. Today, different scanners may vary slightly at precision values, but these differences are within the acceptable clinical criteria set. Differences between scanners exist more frequently when the full arch is digitally impressed. Since the scanning path is longer, more stitching is required due to the superimposition of the images captured, amounting to more errors, especially if the arch is edentulous and lacks distinct anatomical landmarks or distinguishing features [72, 73]. These differences are anticipated to extinct soon, as the continuous research will improve both the hardware and the software employed in intraoral imaging [74]. Almost every scanner in the dental market performs adequately when scanning is limited to a quadrant.

4.7 Digital Vs. Analog Impressions

Digital impressions are considered efficient regarding preparation, working time, rescan time, and number of rescan times. This is especially true for the younger generation of dentists, predoctoral students, and graduate program residents who are familiar with modern digital technologies [75] (Fig. 4.21). For these people, preparation, working, and making of a conventional (analog) impression are more demanding processes. As mentioned previously, experienced dentists who master the process of conventional impressions have less difficulties in this area.

The accuracy of digital impressions for single tooth restorations or for fixed partial dentures of a quadrant has been documented in the dental literature. The consensus is that digital impressions in these cases are of equal accuracy or even better than conventional impressions made by non-aqueous elastomeric materials (i.e., polyether and polyvinylsiloxanes) [76]. A recent clinical trial on a total of 38 patients requiring 45 monolithic zirconia fixed partial dentures retained on two implants has demonstrated that the clinical fit of FPDs made from digital impressions was comparable to the ones made from conventional impressions. Furthermore, this research has shown that there are no statistically significant differences between the FPDs made with the two different impression approaches, while the complication rates were very low within the first year of service [77]. However, there is not enough data to support that the same applies in cases of full-arch impressions. This is an important question that needs to be answered, as an accurate impression is of paramount importance for one piece full-arch fixed prostheses in which the framework is fabricated from materials which cannot be cut and soldered, like zirconia. The available dental literature cannot answer clearly if a conventional impression is better than a digital one. This is probably due to the fact that there is a big heterogeneity in published studies. Furthermore, most of the research is taking place in vitro, as these studies are simpler to perform, and the influencing factors can be easily controlled. The up-to-date research, however, indicates that there are not substantial differences between the two modes of impression taking. Most of the research has been done on dental casts with implants, and they have shown that conventional impressions do not differ statistically from digital scanning. On the other hand, there is published evidence that in partially edentulous impressions, the conventional approach presents better results than the digital one [78]. The accuracy of full-arch digital scans can be affected by several factors, including inter-implant distance and angulation, operator experience, scan body and design, scanning strategy, shape of the arch, as well as ambient scanning light conditions [48, 79–84]. The latter has been shown to influence both the precision and the trueness of different IOSs. An interesting fact is that an ideal lighting condition does not seem to exist, as three of the leading IOSs in the dental market perform better in different lighting conditions, which range from natural lighting (500 lux) to room lighting (1000 lux), to operating chair lighting (10,000 lux) [85]. These scanning accuracy differences are probably due to the different recording technologies adopted by the companies. As mentioned earlier, most of the published data come from in vitro studies and therefore they must be interpreted very cautiously. There are many factors in a clinical setting which may influence the outcome.

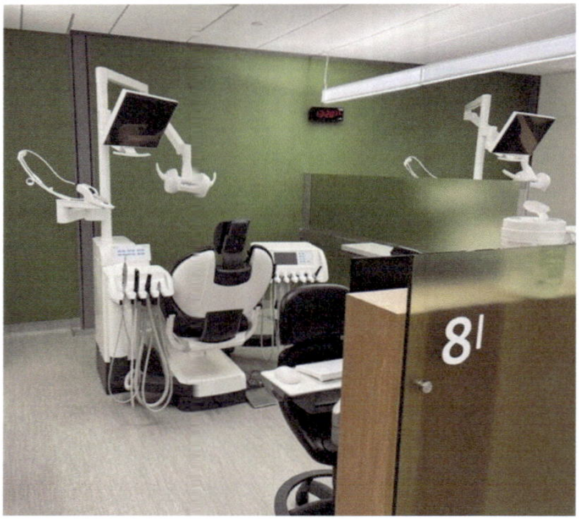

Fig. 4.21 The Omnicam® intraoral scanner mounted on a Sirona® unit, in a University predoctoral clinic setting

These include the limited access to patient's oral cavity, existence of certain anatomic structures that may interfere (i.e., tongue, cheeks, lips), patient movement, gag reflex, highly reflective surfaces due to existing restorations and/or saliva, etc. The surge of photogrammetry in dentistry suggests in the most recent in vitro studies that this technology can overcome the potential scanning issues previously mentioned and was reported to present the best accuracy in terms of trueness and precision for complete-arch implant rehabilitation compared to the intraoral scanner and the conventional impression [86, 87].

4.8 Concluding Remarks

Although the accuracy of digital impressions is already very high, it will be further improved, as there is a lot of ongoing research both in the hardware and software areas. In the near future, digital impressions will be the dominant method of impression making for the fabrication of provisional and definitive dental and maxillofacial prostheses, occlusal and orthodontic appliances, as well as for surgical stents for implant placement. The evolution of the ultrasound digital impression will assist in simplifying impression making of subgingivally placed restorative margins, a procedure which is traumatic for the soft tissues and bothersome for both the patient and the dentist.

References

1. Rosenstiel S, Land M, Fujimoto J. Contemporary fixed prosthodontics. St. Louis: Mosby; 2016. p. 367–400.
2. Anusavice KJ, Shen C, Rawls HR. Phillips science of dental materials. St. Louis: Elsevier-Saunders. p. 151–181, 182–193, 194–230.
3. Ruel J, Schuessler PJ, Malament K, Mori D. Effect of retraction procedures on the periodontium in humans. J Prosthet Dent. 1980;44(5):508–15.
4. Bennani V, Aarts JM, Schumayer D. Correlation of pressure and displacement during gingival displacement: an in vitro study. J Prosthet Dent. 2016;115(3):296–300.
5. Duret F. Empreinte Optique. These Presentee a L Universite Claude Bernard, vol. 27. Lyon: Février; 1974.
6. Duret F. Vers Une prothese informatisee. Tonus. 1985:55–7.
7. Applications. Solid Modeling Today. 1986;1:6.
8. Duret F, Termoz C. Method of and apparatus for making a prosthesis, especially a dental prosthesis. US patent 4 663 720. May 1987.
9. News release. L' est republicain. Vienne: Hennson International; 1985.
10. Mörmann WH, Brandestini M, Lutz F, Barbakow F. Chairside computer-aided direct ceramic inlays. Quintessence Int. 1989;20:329–39.
11. Mörmann WH. Chairside computer-generated ceramic restorations: the CEREC third generation improvements. Pract Periodontics Aesthet Dent. 1992;4(7):9–16.
12. Chan KHS, Mai Y, Kim H, Tong KCT, Desmond NG, Hsiao JCM. Review: resin composite filling. Materials (Basel). 2010;3(2):1228–43.
13. Mörmann WH, Brandestini M. Method and apparatus for the fabrication of custom-shaped implants. U.S. Patent No. 4,575,805, March 11, 1986.
14. Brandestini M, Mörmann WH, Lutz F, Krejci I. Computer machined ceramic inlays: in vitro marginal adaptation [abstract]. J Dent Res. 1985;64:208.
15. Mörmann WH, Brandestini M. The fundamental inventive principles of CEREC CAD/CAM. In: Mörmann WH, editor. State of the art of CAD/CAM restorations: 20 years of CEREC. London: Quintessence; 2006. p. 1–8.
16. Mörmann W. The evolution of the CEREC system. J Am Dent Assoc. 2006;137:7S–13S.
17. Rekow D. Computer-aided design and manufacturing in dentistry: a review of the state of the art. J Prosthet Dent. 1987;58(4):512–6.
18. Mörmann W, Krejci I. Computer-designed inlays after 5 years in situ: clinical performance and scanning electron microscopic evaluation. Quintessence Int. 1992;23(2):109–15.
19. Patzelt SBM, Lamprinos C, Stampf S, Att W. The time efficiency of intraoral scanners: an in vitro comparative study. J Am Dent Assoc. 2014;145(6):542–51.
20. da Costa JB, Pelogia F, Hagedorn B, Ferracane JL. Evaluation of different methods of optical impression making on the marginal gap of onlays created with CEREC 3D. Oper Dent. 2010;35(3):324–9.
21. Joda T, Brägger U. Patient-centered outcomes comparing digital and conventional implant impression procedures: a randomized crossover trial. Clin Oral Implants Res. 2016;27(12):e185–9.
22. Zimmerman M, Mehl A, Mörmann WH, Reich S. Intraoral scanning systems: a current overview. Int J Comput Dent. 2015;18(2):101–29.
23. Rekow ED, Erdman AG, Speidel TM. Computer-assisted system to automate production of posterior dental restorations. In: Biostereometrics 85, vol. B602. Washington: SPIE; 1985. p. 204–10.
24. Abdel-Azia YI, Karara HM. Photogrammetric potentials of non-metric cameras. Civil engineering studies, photogrammetry series No. 36. Urbana, IL: University of Illinois; 1974.

25. Grimson WEL. Computing shape using a theory of human stereo vision. PhD thesis. Boston. Massachusetts Institute of Technology, 1980.
26. Stereolithography Interface specification, 3D Systems Inc. 1988.
27. Chua CK, Leong KF, Lim CS. Rapid prototyping data formats. In: Rapid prototyping: principles and applications. 2n ed. Singapore: World Scientific Publishing Co; 2003. p. 237–90.
28. Turk G. The PLY polygon file format. 1994. The Board of Trustees of the Leland Stanford Junior University.
29. Chuembou Pekam F, Marotti J, Wolfart S, Tinschert J, Radermacher K, Heger S. High-frequency ultrasound as an option for scanning of prepared teeth: an in vitro study. Ultrasound Med Biol. 2015;41(1):309–16.
30. Marotti J, Broeckmann J, Chuembou Pekam F, Praca L, Radermacher K, Wolfart S. Impression of subgingival dental preparation can be taken with ultrasound. Ultrasound Med Biol. 2019;45(2):558–67.
31. Bohner L, Habor D, Radermacher K, Wolfart S, Marotti J. Scanning of a dental implant with a high-frequency ultrasound scanner: a pilot study. Appl Sci. 2021;11:5494.
32. Logozzo S, Zanetti EM, Franceschini G, Kilpelä A, Mäkinen A. Recent advances in dental optics-part I: 3D intraoral scanners for restorative dentistry. Opt Lasers Eng. 2014;54:203–21.
33. Richert R, Goujat A, Venet L, Viguie G, Viennot S, Robinson P, Farges JC, Fages M, Ducret M. Intraoral scanner technologies: a review to make a successful impression. J Healthcare Engineering. 2017;ID 8427595:1–9.
34. Ireland AJ, McNamara C, Clover MJ, House K, Wenger N, Barbour ME, Alemzadeh K, Zhang L, Sandy JR. 3D surface imaging in dentistry—what we are looking at. Br Dent J. 2008;205(7):387–92.
35. Geng J. Structured-light 3D surface imaging: a tutorial. Adv Opt Photon. 2011;3:128–60.
36. Frigerio F. 3-dimensional surface imaging using active Wavefront sampling. PhD Thesis, Massachusetts Institute of Technology, 2006.
37. Frigerio F, Hart DP. Calibrationless aberration correction through Active Wavefront Sampling (AWS) and multi-camera imaging. Proceedings of the 13th International Symposium on Applications of laser techniques to Fluid Mechanics, Lisbon, Portugal. 2006.
38. Heber S. 3D image reconstruction using active Wavefront sampling. Diploma thesis, Technical University of Graz. 2010.
39. van der Meer WJ, Andriessen FS, Wismeijer D, Ren Y. Application of intra-oral dental scanners in the digital workflow of implantology. PLoS One. 2012;7(8):e43312. https://doi.org/10.1371/journal.pone.0043312.
40. Minsky M. Microscopy Apparatus. 1957 U.S. Patent no. 3013467 (awarded 1961).
41. Minsky M. Memoir on inventing the confocal scanning microscope. Scanning. 1988;10:128–38.
42. Zint M, Stock K, Claus D, Graser R, Hibst R. Development and verification of a snapshot dental intraoral three-dimensional scanner based on chromatic confocal imaging. J Med Eng. 2019;6(3):033502–1.
43. Elliott AD. Confocal microscopy: principles and modern practices. Curr Protoc Cytom. 2020;92(1):e68. https://doi.org/10.1002/cpcy.68.
44. Mulliken JB. Repair of bilateral cleft lip. In: Rodriguez E, editor. Plastic surgery. Volume 3: craniofacial, head and neck surgery and pediatric plastic surgery. St. Louis: Elsevier; 2018. p. 546–64.
45. Hartley R, Zisserman A. Multiple view geometry in computer vision. Cambridge: Cambridge University Press; 2003.
46. Bocklet C, Renne W, Mennito A, Bacro T, Latham J, Evans Z, Ludlow M, Kelly A, Nash J. Effect of scan substrates on accuracy of 7 intraoral digital impression systems using human maxilla model. Orthod Craniofac Res. 2019;22(Suppl. 1):168–74.
47. Wei D, Di P, Tian J, Zhao Y, Lin Y. Evaluation of intraoral digital impressions for obtaining gingival contour in the esthetic zone: accuracy outcomes. Clin Oral Investig. 2020;24:1401–10.
48. Revilla-León M, Jiang P, Sadeghpour M, Piedra-Cascón W, Zandinejad A, Özcan M, Krishnamurthy VR. Intraoral digital scans-part 1: influence of ambient scanning light conditions on the accuracy (trueness and precision) of different intraoral scanners. J Prosthet Dent. 2020;124:372–8.
49. Alzahrani SJ, El-Hammali H, Morgano S, Elkassaby H. Evaluation of the accuracy of 2 digital intraoral scanners: a 3D analysis study. J Prosthet Dent. 2021;126:787–92.
50. Imburgia M, Logozzo S, Hauschild U, Veronesi G, Mangano C, Mangano FG. Accuracy of four intraoral scanners in oral implantology: a comparative in vitro study. BMC Oral Health. 2017;17(1):92. https://doi.org/10.1186/s12903-017-0383-4.
51. Kim RJ, Park JM, Shim JS. Accuracy of 9 intraoral scanners for complete-arch image acquisition: a qualitative and quantitative evaluation. J Prosthet Dent. 2018;120(6):895–903.e1. https://doi.org/10.1016/j.prosdent.2018.01.035.
52. Diker B, Tak Ö. Comparing the accuracy of six intraoral scanners on prepared teeth and effect of scanning sequence. J Adv Prosthodont. 2020;12(5):299–306. https://doi.org/10.4047/jap.2020.12.5.299.
53. Diker B, Tak Ö. Accuracy of six intraoral scanners for scanning complete-arch and 4-unit fixed partial dentures: an in vitro study. J Prosthet Dent. 2021;S0022–3913(20):30797–6. https://doi.org/10.1016/j.prosdent.2020.12.007.
54. Mangano FG, Veronesi G, Hauschild U, Mijiritsky E, Mangano C. Trueness and precision of four intraoral scanners in oral implantology: a comparative in vitro study. PLoS One. 2016;11(9):e0163107. https://doi.org/10.1371/journal.pone.0163107.
55. Gardner FM. Margins of complete crowns-literature review. J Prosthet Dent. 1982;48:392–400.

56. Jacobs MS, Windeler AS. An investigation of dental luting cement solubility as a function of the marginal gap. J Prosthet Dent. 1991;65:436–42.
57. Walter JN, Gardner FM, Agar JR. A survey of crown and fixed partial denture failures: length of service and reasons for replacement. J Prosthet Dent. 1986;56:416–21.
58. Goldman M, Laosonthorn P, White RR. Microleakage-full crowns and the dental pulp. J Endod. 1992;18:473–5.
59. Sorensen SE, Larsen IB, Jorgensen KD. Gingival and alveolar bone reaction to marginal fit of subgingival crown margins. Scan J Dent Res. 1986;94:109–14.
60. Bosniac P, Rehmann P, Wöstmann B. Comparison of an indirect impression scanning system and two direct intraoral scanning systems in vivo. Clin Oral Investig. 2019;23:2421–7.
61. Güth JF, Keul C, Stimmelmayr M, Beuer F, Edelhoff D. Accuracy of digital models obtained by direct and indirect data capturing. Clin Oral Investig. 2013;17:1201–8.
62. Powers JM, Sakaguchi RL. Craig's restorative dental materials. 12th ed. St. Louis, Mosby: Elsevier; 2006. p. 323.
63. Lee WS, Kim WC, Kim YH, Kim WH, Kim JH. Evaluation of different approaches for using a laser scanner in digitization of dental impressions. J Adv Prosthodont. 2014;6:22–9.
64. International Organization for Standardization. Accuracy (trueness and precision) of measurement methods and results—Part 1: general principles and definitions (ISO 5725e1:1994). 1994.
65. Goracci C, Franchi L, Vich A, Ferrari M. Accuracy, reliability, and efficiency of intraoral scanners for full-arch impressions: a systematic review of the clinical evidence. Eur J Orthod. 2016;38(4):422–8.
66. Rubio RR, Shehata J, Kournoutas I, Chae R, Vigo V, Wang M, El-Sayed I, Abla AA. Construction of neuroanatomical volumetric models using 3-dimensional scanning techniques: technical note and applications. World Neurosurg. 2019;126:359–68. https://doi.org/10.1016/j.wneu.2019.03.099.
67. Ender A, Zimmermann M, Attin T, Mehl A. In vivo precision of conventional and digital methods for obtaining quadrant dental impressions. Clin Oral Investig. 2016;20(7):1495–504. https://doi.org/10.1007/s00784-015-1641-y.
68. Hajjar LG. Accuracy of photogrammetry, intraoral scanning, and conventional impression techniques for full-arch implant-supported prostheses: an in-vitro study. 2022. https://hdl.handle.net/2144/44996.
69. Flügge TV, Att W, Metzger MC, Nelson K. Precision of dental implant digitization using intraoral scanners. Int J Prosthodont. 2016;29(3):277–83. https://doi.org/10.11607/ijp.4417.
70. Rotar RN, Jivanescu A, Ille C, Podariu AC, Jumanca DE, Matichescu AM, Balean O, Rusu LC. Trueness and precision of two intraoral scanners: a comparative in vitro study. Scanning. 2019;2019:1289570. https://doi.org/10.1155/2019/1289570.
71. Ender A, Attin T, Mehl A. In vivo precision of conventional and digital methods of obtaining complete-arch dental impressions. J Prosthet Dent. 2016;115(3):313–20. https://doi.org/10.1016/j.prosdent.2015.09.011.
72. Andriessen FS, Rijkens DR, van der Meer WJ, Wismeijer DW. Applicability and accuracy of an intraoral scanner for scanning multiple implants in edentulous mandibles: a pilot study. J Prosthet Dent. 2014;11:186–94.
73. Giménez B, Özcan M, Martínez-Rus F, Pradíes G. Accuracy of a digital impression system based on parallel confocal laser technology for implants with consideration of operator experience and implant angulation and depth. Int J Oral Maxillofac Implants. 2014;29(4):853–62. https://doi.org/10.11607/jomi.3343.
74. Winkler J, Gkantidis N. Trueness and precision of intraoral scanners in the maxillary dental arch: an in vivo analysis. Sci Rep. 2020;10(1):1172. https://doi.org/10.1038/s41598-020-58075-7.
75. Lee SJ, Gallucci GO. Digital vs. conventional implant impressions: efficiency outcomes. Clin Oral Implants Res. 2013;24(1):111–5. https://doi.org/10.1111/j.1600-0501.2012.02430.x.
76. Wismeijer D, Joda T, Flügge T, Fokas G, Tahmaseb A, Bechelli D, Bohner L, Bornstein M, Burgoyne A, Caram S, Carmichael R, Chen CY, Coucke W, Derksen W, Donos N, El Kholy K, Evans C, Fehmer V, Fickl S, Fragola G, Gimenez Gonzales B, Gholami H, Hashim D, Hui Y, Kökat A, Vazouras K, Kühl S, Lanis A, Leesungbok R, van der Meer J, Liu Z, Sato T, De Souza A, Scarfe WC, Tosta M, van Zyl P, Vach K, Vaughn V, Vucetic M, Wang P, Wen B, Wu V. Group 5 ITI consensus report: digital technologies. Clin Oral Implants Res. 2018 Oct;29(Suppl 16):436–42. https://doi.org/10.1111/clr.13309.
77. Derksen W, Tahmaseb A, Wismeijer D. A randomized clinical trial comparing the clinical fit of CAD/CAM monolithic zirconia fixed dental prostheses (FDP) on ti-base abutments based on digital or conventional impression techniques. One year follow-up. Int J Prosthodont. 2021;34(6):733–43. https://doi.org/10.11607/ijp.7074.
78. Papaspyridakos P, Vazouras K, Chen YW, Kotina E, Natto Z, Kang K, Chochlidakis K. Digital vs conventional implant impressions: a systematic review and meta-analysis. J Prosthodont. 2020;29(8):660–78. https://doi.org/10.1111/jopr.13211.
79. Tan MY, Yee SHX, Wong KM, Tan YH, Tan KBC. Comparison of three-dimensional accuracy of digital and conventional implant impressions: effect of Interimplant distance in an edentulous arch. Int J Oral Maxillofac Implants. 2019;34(2):366–80. https://doi.org/10.11607/jomi.6855.
80. Giménez B, Özcan M, Martínez-Rus F, Pradíes G. Accuracy of a digital impression system based on active triangulation technology with blue light for implants: effect of clinically relevant parameters. Implant Dent. 2015;24(5):498–504. https://doi.org/10.1097/ID.0000000000000283.

81. Giménez B, Özcan M, Martínez-Rus F, Pradíes G. Accuracy of a digital impression system based on active wavefront sampling technology for implants considering operator experience, implant angulation, and depth. Clin Implant Dent Relat Res. 2015;17(Suppl 1):e54–64. https://doi.org/10.1111/cid.12124.
82. Giménez B, Pradíes G, Martínez-Rus F, Özcan M. Accuracy of two digital implant impression systems based on confocal microscopy with variations in customized software and clinical parameters. Int J Oral Maxillofac Implants. 2015;30(1):56–64. https://doi.org/10.11607/jomi.3689.
83. Gimenez-Gonzalez B, Hassan B, Özcan M, Pradíes G. An in vitro study of factors influencing the performance of digital intraoral impressions operating on active Wavefront sampling technology with multiple implants in the edentulous maxilla. J Prosthodont. 2017;26(8):650–5. https://doi.org/10.1111/jopr.12457.
84. Huang R, Liu Y, Huang B, Zhang C, Chen Z, Li Z. Improved scanning accuracy with newly designed scan bodies: an in vitro study comparing digital versus conventional impression techniques for complete-arch implant rehabilitation. Clin Oral Implants Res. 2020;31(7):625–33. https://doi.org/10.1111/clr.13598.
85. Tohme H, Lawand G, Chmielewska M, Makhzoume J. Comparison between stereophotogrammetric, digital, and conventional impression techniques in implant-supported fixed complete arch prostheses: an in vitro study. J Prosthet Dent. 2021;S0022–3913(21):00269. https://doi.org/10.1016/j.prosdent.2021.05.006.
86. Ma B, Yue X, Sun Y, Peng L, Geng W. Accuracy of photogrammetry, intraoral scanning, and conventional impression techniques for complete-arch implant rehabilitation: an in vitro comparative study. BMC Oral Health. 2021;21(1):636. https://doi.org/10.1186/s12903-021-02005-0. PMID: 34893053; PMCID: PMC8665494.
87. Sallorenzo A, Gómez-Polo M. Comparative study of the accuracy of an implant intraoral scanner and that of a conventional intraoral scanner for complete-arch fixed dental prostheses. J Prosthet Dent. 2021;S0022–3913(21):00083–4. https://doi.org/10.1016/j.prosdent.2021.01.032.

CAD/CAM Systems

5

Petros Mourouzis and Kosmas Tolidis

5.1 Introduction

Computer-aided design and computer-aided manufacturing (CAD/CAM) define the cooperation of a CAD with a CAM system in order for the first part to guide the second part of the system, to produce a digitized design [1, 2]. Concerning the dental CAD/CAM systems, the primary data are originated by the scanning of the patient mouth by an intraoral scanner (IOS). Following the scan, the dentist with the help of a dental design software can finalize the dental prosthesis restoration and use a milling unit to fabricate it from a variety of dental materials [3]. The milling unit can be a separate unit located in the dental office or it could be located in a dental technician lab [3].

In the previous years of dental prosthesis, the only method of reproducing the dental and oral tissues was the use of traditional methods like the use of impressions and fabrication of gypsum casts. This method has not been changed at all over the years, with the only exception being the improvement of impression materials [4].

On the contrary, the CAD/CAM systems eliminate the need for time-consuming or unpleasant silicone, alginate, or polyurethane impressions, making a dental prosthesis a matter of a single visit without the loss of quality [5, 6].

The conception and introduction of CAD/CAM in dentistry were accomplished by François Duret in the 1970s with the Sopha System. The first restoration that Dr. Duret fabricated with the Sopha System was milled in 1983 at the French Dental Associations' International congress in November 1985. The CAD/CAM technology was later refined in the 1980s by Dr. Werner Mörmann and Marco Brandestini with the development of the CEREC System. The word CEREC is an acronym for Ceramic Reconstruction or Chairside Economical Restoration of Esthetic Ceramics. The first chairside treatment was performed in 1985 at the University of Zurich Dental School.

5.2 Early CAD/CAM Systems

5.2.1 Sopha System

The Sopha system consisted of an intraoral camera which was documented as a "optical probe," an image processing system, the digital controller, and the micro-milling machine. The intraoral camera could digitize dental tissues to 3D struc-

P. Mourouzis (✉)
Division of Operative Dentistry, Faculty of Dentistry, Department of Tissues Pathology and Therapeutics, Aristotle University of Thessaloniki, Thessaloniki, Greece
e-mail: pmourouzis@dent.auth.gr

K. Tolidis
Department of Dental School, Aristotle University of Thessaloniki, Thessaloniki, Greece
e-mail: ktolidis@dent.auth.gr

A. Delantoni, K. Orhan (eds.), *Digital Dentistry*, https://doi.org/10.1007/978-3-031-52826-2_5

tures with a triangulation process with an accuracy of 20 µm. The image processing system was connected to the intraoral camera and recorded the scanned structures. The data were transmitted by a Charged Coupled Device (CCD) and applied to the software in order to produce the dental restoration. The software for the creation of dental restoration was called EUCLID MATRA and could design the internal surface of the restoration, considering the spacer and the retention with the dental tissues. With the software, the operator could design the external part of the restoration and modify the margins and the occlusal of the restoration. Finally, the micro-milling machine had several burs and mold supports while the machining of the material was executed by lathes with sliding steps or liner displacements. The final polishing of the restorations was done by the dentist, depending on the material used.

5.2.2 Celay System

The Celay system of Mikroma Technologie was a CAD/CAM system developed by Stefan Eidenbenz in 1988. This system which is rather a copy milling device consisted of two parts: the first part was for data acquisition using a mechanic touching probe, and the second part was a milling unit with 6 degrees of freedom. This CAD/CAM system could fabricate inlays including the occlusal surface. The main disadvantage of the system was that it required an already made restoration created from resin or wax which was sprayed with powder, inserted into a compartment of the system in which a pantographic arm linked to the reading tool was used to follow the profile of the resin/wax restoration, thus reproducing the same shape on the final ceramic or resin material.

5.2.3 Procera System

The Procera system was invented by Dr. Matts Andersson in 1987 from Nobel Pharma. This system was a duplicating and milling system that used a pantograph similar to the Celay system, while it also used a second milling process by electro-erosion. Two applications were available: the first used a copy milling approach to replicate a die, which was automatically traced with a probe, contact digitized, and afterwards with the help of 1–3 carbon-electrodes was copy milled and reproduced the tooth form. The second application was in the production of a high-strength ceramic coping. The material used was a Al_2O_3, which due to its high strength was difficult to be milled, so the CAD/CAM system first produced an image of the die, which later expanded three dimensionally by a computer program. The whole procedure lasted about an hour, and there was scientific literature with good evidence that supported the Procera system.

5.2.4 DSC-Titan

The DSC-Titan system was created in 1991 originally developed in Israel (Tavor and Co) and was presented and manufactured in Germany (Gim-Alldent, Varel Germany). It was combined by a manual contact digitizing station, a CAD station, and a CAM milling machine. It was designed to produce titanium copings using an industrial-type milling machine with carbide burs. The system was capable of machining titanium and ceramic materials. The system was presented in Cologne in April 1992 and was promoted that could mill bridge infrastructures using user-friendly two-dimensional software. Manipulation was slow, it could digitize a case in 20 min, and the accuracy was approximately 100 µm. The system was easier to use than the Procera system, while scientific data reported accuracy levels ranging between 100 and 140 µm from the margin.

5.2.5 Cerec System

It was invented in 1980 by Dr. Werner Moerman and Marco Brandestini. In the early versions, the system used opto-electronic techniques. The system was compact and was composed of a

256 × 256 Charge Coupled Device (CCD) camera (CEREC 1) or a 512 × 512 CCD camera (CEREC 2), an image processing station, and a 2.5-axis micro-milling machine driven by electrical motors. With this system the dentist could produce one surface and multi-surface inlays and veneers but without having the ability to produce the occlusal surface of the inlays. The dentist could scan intraorally using powder, or could scan the stone model of the patient. The accuracy of the CEREC system was detected to be 100 μm, and the time to fabricate a restoration (inlay) was 45 min. The materials that the CEREC system used were blocks of feldspathic porcelain made by Vita. The main disadvantage of the system was that the occlusal surface had to be produced by hand.

5.2.6 Bego-Rekow DentiCAD System

This system was manufactured by Dr. Diane Rekow in 1986 and in the beginning was designed exclusively for laboratories for producing crowns, inlays, and fixed partial dentures. This system consisted of a Bego electro-mechanical probe, a semiautomatic program, and a numerically controlled machine tool. Moreover, the system was semiautomatic; the milling part was turned by air pressure, while the tools were changed manually. The tracing probe resembled a periodontal probe, and the intraoral information of the tooth preparation was transferred to the CAD system to create the desired form. The system could mill resin, ceramic, or metal materials.

5.3 Conclusion

The first dental CAD/CAM system was presented in 1983, while the first crown was created in 1985. Many of the above systems did not survive through the years. However, those which survived improved in versatility, accuracy, and cost-effectiveness and were integrated into daily practice of several dental offices.

5.4 New CAD/CAM Systems

The need for automatization and elimination of human errors has driven the dental scientific community and manufacturers to discover new ways of dental restoration production [7]. CAD/CAM was an innovation of a few dental pioneer scientists who develop the first CAD/CAM systems. The computer limitations were an issue, the processor power was limited, the storage drive was poor, and yet the restorations design with the complex geometries was intensive [8]. Moreover, the material companies perceived that the CAD/CAM system would not involve their product line. However, the increase in computer power was the reason for the progress of the newer CAD/CAM systems. As stated by Gordon Moore in 1965, the power of computer processor will double every 2 years [9]. The "Moore's law" is responsible for the CAD/CAM benefits, making the systems faster, more accurate, and more cost effective. Since the first CAD/CAM systems were incorporated in the dental clinics, millions of restorations have been fabricated and produced, while CAD/CAM systems were part of many dental schools' curricula [8, 10]. Early CAD/CAM systems were limited to the variety of restorations; they could only fabricate inlays, onlays, or single crowns. Nowadays, there is no limit to the type of dental restoration that can be fabricated [11]. Single-unit crowns, inlays, onlays, veneers, implant abutments, and restorations to fixed and removable dental prostheses for partially or completely edentulous patients are routinely fabricated [6].

The newer CAD/CAM systems used several new methods to collect 3-dimensional data of the prepared tooth. The milling units have evolved and the conventional milling discs were replaced with a variety of diamond burs of different shapes, resulted in major improvements in milling technology [12]. The new CAD/CAM systems have enabled dentists and dental technicians to design, fabricate, and characterize a final restoration within minutes. Additionally, the integration of other new technologies like cone beam computed tomography combined with digital intraoral scanning or facial scanning has given additional tools and enhancements to the daily routine dentistry for other specialties besides prosthodontics like endodontics, implantology, and orthodontics [13].

The new CAD/CAM systems that have evolved from the early versions can scan, design, and mill. The outcome of the advancement of those systems is the fact that the CAD/CAM systems are installed in the dental practice, where the dentist can deliver dental restorations in one dental appointment [13, 14]. Moreover, dental laboratories, where dental technicians can enhance their dental restorations, can benefit from the time efficiency and the level of accuracy of CAD/CAM systems. Finally, there is an increase of milling centers where dentists or dental technicians can forward their dental impressions or restoration designs from the intraoral scanner or from the dental software, and the personnel of the milling center will mill and deliver the restoration.

5.4.1 Dental Chairside CAD/CAM Systems

The components of the new CAD/CAM systems are basically the same with the older systems. They consist of three major parts: (1) a unit that acquires the data from the prepared tooth structure, the adjacent tissues, and the opposite dental arch, (2) the software for designing the virtual dental restoration, (3) the milling device for manufacturing the restoration form a block of material [13]. The chairside CAD/CAM system is classified into systems in which the company provides a scanner and a milling unit, or systems in which the company has only an intraoral scanner without the restoration designing option.

5.4.2 Basic Technological Principles of New CAD/CAM Systems

The fundamental principle of all CAD/CAM systems is the transmission from the scanner of light that reflects from the dental or oral tissues and is received by the scanner's sensor. The software encodes the signal to 3D coordinates for each scanned point; a very large number of points will be produced, resulting in a cloud mesh from which the impression will be produced. There are four basic principles that different intraoral scanners use: (1) Triangulation, (2) Accordion fringe interferometry, (3) Parallel confocal imaging, (4) Video 3D in-motion [15].

5.4.2.1 Triangulation

The scanners that use triangulation as a basic principle emit the light which is reflected differently according to the distance of the scanned object. When it is received by the sensor it contacts a different zone which creates a 3D coordinate.

5.4.2.2 Accordion Fringe Interferometry

The emitted light in this category of intraoral scanners is projected onto the surface of the dental or oral tissues into parallel bands of different width. Those bands are distorted since the surface to be scanned is irregular and their distortions are recorded by an HD video camera while the software creates the 3D coordinates of the generated points.

5.4.2.3 Parallel Confocal Imaging

In this principle of scanning, the emitted light is projected and passes through a small aperture. Then it is reflected by a mirror which is placed toward the sensor of the scanner and passing through another small aperture. The result is that only the same focal distance points are registered by the sensor and the scanned object is assembled by only those.

5.4.2.4 Video 3D In-Motion

Finally, the video 3D in-motion use a white light source or laser and two high-definition cameras which are placed to a specified distance and have different perspectives. Those cameras record the intraoral tissues through the scanning procedure while the 3D image will be reassembled from the scanner software.

5.5 Dentsply Sirona

The new CAD/CAM system from Sirona has been introduced in 2019. It consists of a new scanner named Primescan with an updated version of the Cerec software (CEREC SW 5.0) and a new milling unit named Primemill. The main aspect of this CAD/CAM system is the accuracy, the ease of use, and the speed that the intraoral camera and the milling unit have acquired after years of research. Additionally, artificial intelligence has been integrated to the system software providing excellent restoration proposals and automation recognition of margin preparation. This CAD/CAM system is composed of an acquisition center which is a workstation equipped with a touchpad and a wide-format touchscreen. The design of the workstation has allowed for the optimization of sterilization protocols, because the user panel is flat without any physical raised cursor buttons or a trackball. Moreover, the sleeve of the intraoral scanner can be sterilized by high-level disinfection, and various hygiene protection sleeves have been incorporated for the dentist to choose from or to comply. Another feature of the intraoral scanner is that a smart scan has been introduced. Smart scan is an artificial intelligence feature which allows the automatic cutout of extraneous data in real time like cheek, finger, or tongue [16].

Dentsply Sirona has imported a new sensor in the Primescan intraoral scanner which can process more than 1.000.000 3D points per second. Also, the sensor has a dynamic depth scan technology which can enable the sharpness of the scanned tissues, even at a measuring depth up to 20 mm. The software can process the images very quickly because of the upgraded computer systems, processor, RAM memory, and graphical card of the acquisition center. The CAD/CAM system can scan full-arch edentulous arches in less than 25 s. There is a variety of dental restoration materials that can be scanned with ease like zirconia, gold, amalgam, or porcelain without any artifact or missing data. It can also be used for implant restorations with the use of a scanbody, or the scanner can be used extraorally in order to duplicate a denture. Some studies have reported that the CAD/CAM system has the required accuracy to be used for full-arch implantology cases, full and partial dentures, and efficient orthodontic scans [16].

As for the milling unit, the difference between the milling unit of this CAD/CAM system and other systems is that it can mill zirconia and lithium disilicate in less than 5 min, utilizing new machining algorithms using the Super-Fast Mode. There are new tool geometries integrated to the milling unit, along with new electronic and mechanical components resulting in fewer adjustments by the dentist after the placement of the restoration and better margin-edge stability. In addition to this super-fast milling, the dentist has the ability to mill zirconia, lithium disilicate, or any glass ceramic restorations in an extra fine mode which means that the milling unit will incorporate an extra-detailed anatomy to the morphology of the finished restoration. This extra fine approach can be used when "non-prep" restorations are to be fabricated and used by the dentist. The Primemill can mill in dry mode and in wet mode according to the material and preference of the dentist [17].

Until now, there have been few studies available about the efficiency and accuracy of the milling unit of this CAD/CAM system, finding that the Primemill can accomplish dental restorations with marginal gaps within the clinically acceptable range even in the super-fast mode.

Overall, this CAD/CAM system by Dentsply Sirona is until now a very promising system that has outstanding scanning accuracy and if combined with the Primemill milling unit can utilize dental restorations with exceptional margins and fit (Fig. 5.1).

5.5.1 Planmenca Emerald and Planmill

Planmenca introduced the Emerald scanner in 2017; Emerald is a complete chairside system combining the Emerald scanner with the PlanMill milling unit. The Emerald S scanner had been added to the armamentarium of Planmenca CAD/CAM systems along with the Emerald scanner.

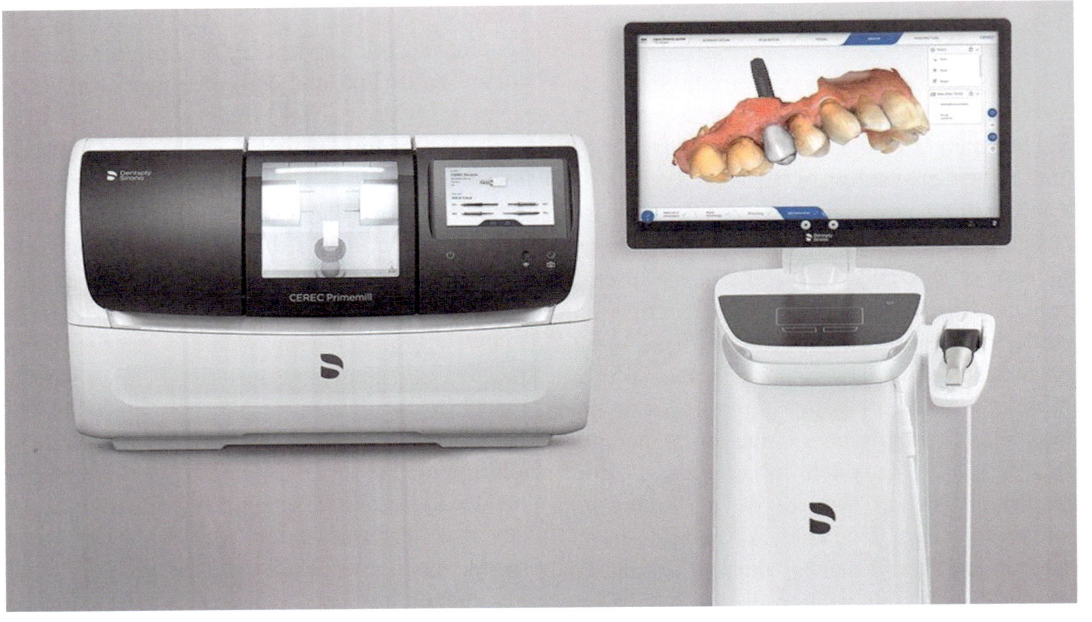

Fig. 5.1 The Dentsply Sirona chairside CAD/CAM systems

Both scanners are powder-free and provide true color images. Both scanners can scan dental tissues and capture an entire arch under a minute. The Emerald scanner has a slim design, is compact, and has good ergonomics which helps the dentist during the intraoral scanning. Both scanners have additional camera tips beside the basic one, in order to capture dental tissues in hard-to-reach areas. Moreover, there is a tip that operates as a tool to detect caries. However, the most differentiating innovation of this system is that it relies on an open architecture software which enables any integration of the scanner with the software and the milling unit according to the dentist preferences. The scanner can import and export STL (Standard Tessellation Language format) and PLY (Stanford Polygon Format) file formats; it also has a shade match capability and automatically can show the correct tooth shade when is necessary. There have been few studies about the trueness and accuracy of the Planmenca Emerald and Emerald S scanners showing that the above properties are affected by the updates of the current software [18]. In addition, there are two integrated versions of the scanners: the first version is the mounted scanner system on the Planmenca dental chair and the second version is the integration with a laptop through a USB.

As for the milling units PlanMill 40S and PlanMill 30S of Ivoclar Vivadent which are compatible with the 3Shape software, they can support a variety of materials such as ceramic, resin-ceramic, and zirconium. Both milling units can fabricate a variety of restorations like implant abutments, crowns, inlays, onlays, veneers, and up to 6-unit bridges. The average milling time for a molar crown is 9 min, while Planmenca Planmill 30S is considered as an entry level milling unit and the Planmenca 40S is considered a more advanced and powerful choice. Both have 4-axis motors, but they can only process in a wet environment. There are studies that have investigated the margins created by both milling units, finding that they had the same performance but different processing times, with Planmill 40S being the fastest. A difference in the milling units is the number of tools that can integrated to them. Planmill 40S has an automated 10-tool changer while Planmill 30S has 5-tool changer. Both milling machines have an integrated water tank, but they require an external compressed air supply.

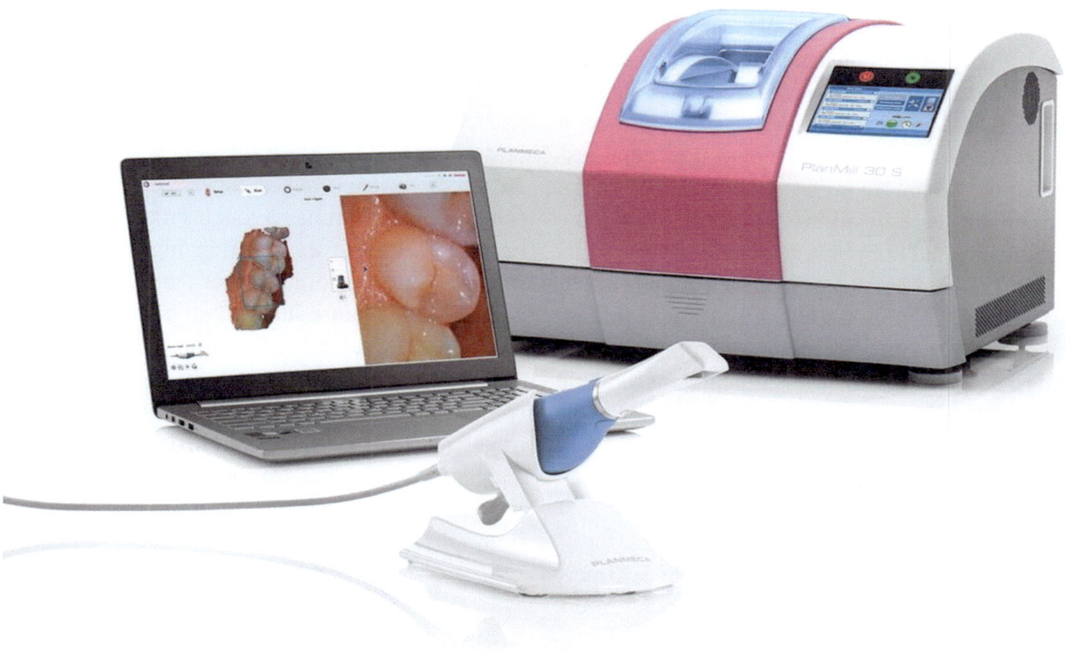

Fig. 5.2 The Planmenca chairside CAD/CAM system

Overall, this CAD/CAM system by Planmenca is a validated system that has good scanning accuracy, combining it with one of the PlanMill units, and the dentist can fabricate dental restorations with excellent margin and fit (Fig. 5.2).

5.5.2 Dental Wings

This CAD/CAM system was presented at a previous International Dental Show in Cologne; it consisted of an intraoral scanner and a laser milling machine. The company has evolved the intraoral scanner and presented the Virtuo Vio Scanner, laser milling. They deserted the milling concept and introduced a dental software which is compatible with the most popular open chairside milling machines. The manufacturers have incorporated a different scanning technology than the other manufacturers, named Multiscan Imaging, which is a further development of the triangulation principle. The scanner uses 4 miniature cameras in the handpiece and is able to record black points projected by one projector onto the tooth surfaces from multiple perspectives and multiple orientations simultaneously capturing difficult to see areas with minimal effort. The manufacturers have integrated a luminescent ring which in combination with the audible signals gives the dentist an indication when the scan data are being correctly captured. There are also integrated voice and gesture controls for the scanner, which in combination with the sterilization sleeves promotes infection control.

The STL output file is open for any open system milling machine, or any other third-party systems. The system supports a wide range of indications like crowns, inlays, onlays, and veneers along with short-span bridges and implant crowns. The software allows the automatic margin proposal, and the dentist can easily modify the margin and the insertion access for better fit. After the automated proposal of the dental restorations the software computes the shape and the anatomy (cusps, marginal ridges) by comparing the anatomy and occlusal pattern of the suggested proposal with the anatomy and occlusion of the adjacent teeth. With the software the dentist or dental technician can also design partial frameworks, full dentures, and bite splints. The intraoral scanner has a cart and laptop option; it is powderless and produces true color images. Since dental wings is nowadays a Straumann group brand, for the production of the dental restorations Dental Wings systems support the Straumann centralized milling centers and the Straumann CAD/CAM services.

There have been a few studies available about the accuracy of this CAD/CAM system, finding that dental restorations can be accomplished with marginal gaps within the clinically acceptable range [19, 20].

5.5.3 Fona Dental

Fona dental was founded in 2000 under BlueX name, in 2007 became a brand of Sirona Group, and in 2011 was merged into the brand FONA. The company has a CAD/CAM system with the name myCrown. The system is a complete chairside system which has many similarities with the Dentsply Sirona system. The scanner is a heated camera, and all tooth surfaces must be lightly powdered before scanning. The digital models are created using video sequences based on stereophotogrammetry. The system can design and create veneers, inlays, onlays, crowns, and bridges up to 3 teeth. All the scan and restoration data can be exported in open STL files. The acquisition system has a touchscreen that can be operated with gloves ensuring high-level disinfection. The restorations of the system are designed by NatureShape Design software and the user can send the restorations for milling to a 4-axis milling unit. The milling unit has a dual spindle technology and can mill in wet or dry mode, up to 40 mm blocks in length. The materials that can be milled are zirconia, glass ceramics polymers for permanent and temporary restorations (Fig. 5.3).

5.5.4 Carestream Dental

Carestream Dental has a CAD/CAM system which consists of an intraoral scanner (CS 3800) and a milling unit (CS 3000). The intraoral cam-

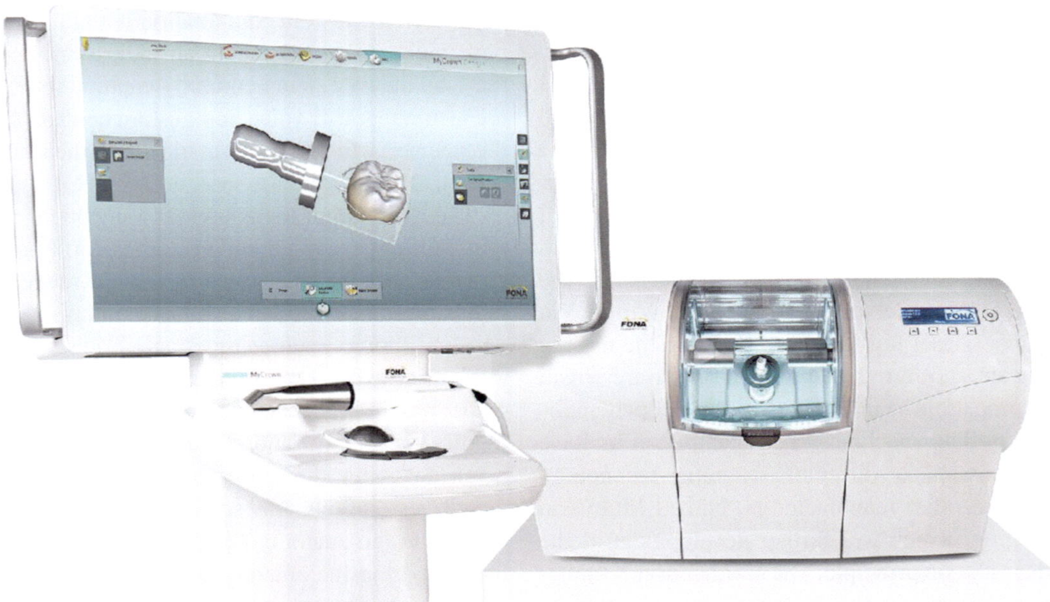

Fig. 5.3 The Fona MyCrown CAD/CAM system

era is a wireless scanner which uses triangulation technology which captures video. It is powder-free and has a true-color display of the scanned areas. The scanner can be integrated with a laptop or into the treatment unit. It is very light and compact since it weighs only 240 g and has a scanning time of 25 s for a single arch. The enlarged field of view (16 mm × 14 mm) from the previous versions of the intraoral scanner of Carestream and the broader (−2 to +16 mm) depth of field capture very fine details of intraoral dental tissues and can take care of subgingival margins. The intraoral scanner has a 1/2.9-inch CMOS sensor technology with LED technology which uses red, green, and red light. The scanner uses an anti-foggy technology by airflow so the scanner lenses will be clear when it is used intraorally.

This system also has a gesture motion control which is controlled by an embedded sensor integrated in the scanner that allows the dentist to control the digital model on the screen. This feature along with the autoclaved tips (up to 110 times) ensures proper sterilization. The company's software is named CS ScanFlow Premium and enables a laboratory-based workflow or a STL data export for the completion of the chairside workflow. Advanced scanning features include the denture mode for smooth edentulous scanning, high-definition 3D digital impressions, and recorded scans that can be used for referral purpose or training. Additionally, the CAD/CAM workflow is unified with CS connect which is a cloud service. The CAD/CAM system can export STL, PLY, OBJ, and Dentalproject files that can be used by any lab. The scanner can also serve as a communication tool because it can be used as a camera capturing images and videos. The CS3000 milling unit uses a 4-axis brushless motor with a spindle speed of 60.000 rpm; it can fabricate single-unit restorations that are made from zirconia, glass ceramic or resin-ceramic, PMMA, and composite materials. The milling unit has already an integrated water spray system and compressed air supply while the average milling time is 15 min with a milling accuracy of ±25 µm.

Studies that have investigated the accuracy of the Carestream 3600 found equal trueness and precision values compared with the conventional methods of impression [21, 22] (Fig. 5.4).

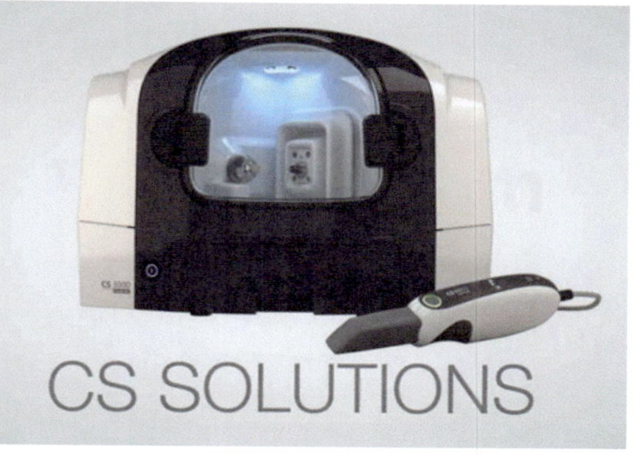

Fig. 5.4 The Carestream CAD/CAM system

5.5.5 Zfx Intrascan and Inhouse 5x

Zfx Birmingham has provided a CAD/CAM system which consists of a scanner (Intrascan) and a milling unit (Inhouse 5x). The scanner is a lightweight handpiece (600 g) and can connect via a USB port to a laptop. It is a powder-free scanner with an open system software which captures the oral tissues with video sequency by confocal microscopy by Moire effect recognition, integrated with smart pixel sensor for fast and precise scanning. After the scan, the STL export can be transferred using the Zfx Dental-Net online platform with the Zfx CAD design software. This CAD/CAM system is an open system, with a scan field of 10.4 × 9.6 × 18 mm and a typical scan speed of 18 scans/second. As for the Zfx inhouse 5x milling unit, this is a compact 5-axis milling unit which is controlled by the CAM software. The unit can mill in wet and dry mode and is equipped with a high frequency spindle (60.000–100.000 rpm). The milling unit can fabricate dental restorations from zirconia, glass ceramic, composite, PMMA, wax, and with the addition of an optional spindle, it can mill cobalt chrome and titanium materials. One originality of this chairside system is the automatic changer for blanks, blocks, and tools. The milling unit can hold up to 15 blocks and up to 28 cutting tools. It

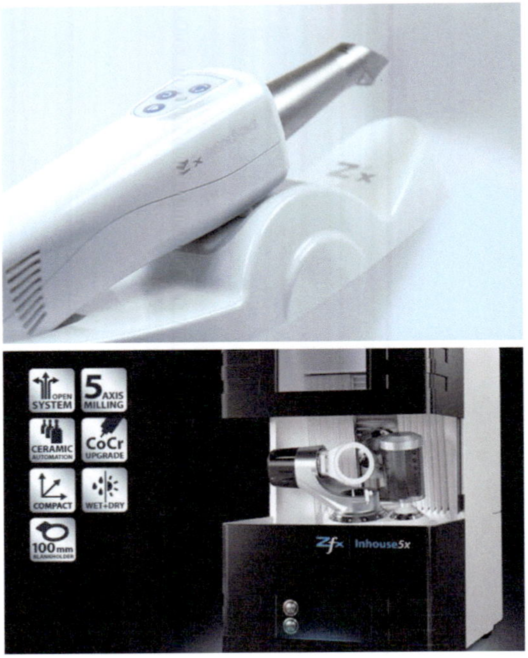

Fig. 5.5 The Zfx Intrascan and Inhouse 5x CAD/CAM system

can mill bridges of any span length and implant abutments, but the manufacturer recommends excluding the fabrication of metal frameworks and structures which have complex geometries. Drawbacks of the system are the weight of the milling unit with over 200 kg and the requirement of external water and compressed air.

Studies that have investigated the accuracy of the Zfx system have found acceptable values of accuracy compared with the accuracy of conventional impressions when there is a short-span scanning and interocclusal records [22, 23] (Fig. 5.5).

5.5.6 Trios 3Shape

The 3Shape Danish company has introduced Trios 4, a wireless intraoral scanner which captures video sequences by means of confocal microscopy. This high-accuracy, powder-free scanner with realistic scan colors is an open dental system and, at this time, supports 3 different cooperation partners, so that a chairside workflow can be implemented at the dental clinics. The partners are Straumann, Ivoclar Vivadent, and Lyra. The scanner has an automatic scan clean-up of unwanted scanned regions like cheeks, tongue, etc. and has integrated a built-in caries detection mode using fluorescent technology. This new generation of Trios scanner features an instant heat technology for the de-fogging of the scanner lenses and many software modules are integrated with the hardware. Modules as 3Shape Implant Studio, 3Shape Orthodontics, and Digital Patient Monitoring are unique tools for the dentist and for the patients in order to visualize the final outcome of the treatment or to plan implant cases. The scanner can be purchased as a stand-alone scanner connected to a laptop, as a cart version which includes a touchscreen, or it can be integrate into the dental unit. One particular feature of the scanner is the blocking function in which the previous scanned area can be protected and not altered during a later scanning. The company has recently introduced a communication platform in order for the management of the dentist cases and communication with dental lab, clear aligners companies, or dental restoration design services.

Overall, this intraoral scanner by 3Shape is one of the top scanners with outstanding accuracy. The company has not introduced a milling unit, and this is the reason for the cooperation of the company with other dental partners. One milling unit compatible with Trios 3Shape is from the manufacturer LYRA, which is Lyra Mill. Lyra is a French company which collaborates with 3Shape for a chairside workflow. This milling unit is a 4-axis milling unit which uses the 3Shape LAB Praxis CAD/CAM software. Lyra milling unit is equipped with a frequency spindle of 60.000 rpm. The overall precision is 15 μm as the company claims, and can mill several types of materials like glass ceramic, PMMA, and composite CAD/CAM blocks up to 40 mm in length. The dentist can use only the wet mode, and it has an integrated water and compressed air supply. The types of restorations are inlays, onlays, veneers, crowns, and bridges up to 3 units. The average time for the fabrication of dental restorations is 15–20 min for an inlay-

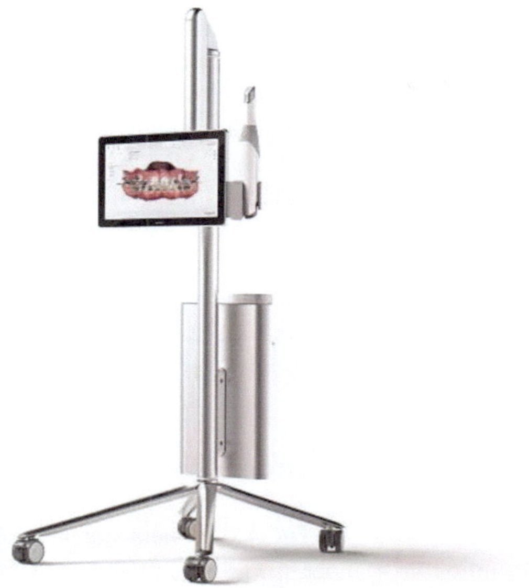

Fig. 5.6 The cart option for the Trios 3Shape intraoral scanner

onlay, 20–30 min for a crown and veneer restoration, and 35–50 min for a 3-unit bridge.

Studies that have investigated the accuracy of the Trios 3shape system have found that the scanner was more precise than other scanners [24], and more accurate in terms of trueness regardless of the scanning field [25] but showed less than expected repeatability on measuring different dental shades along with other scanners [26] (Fig. 5.6).

5.5.7 Amann Girrbach System

Amann Girrbach has introduced a CAD/CAM chairside system with an intraoral scanner and a milling unit named Ceramill map DRS and Ceramill motion DRS, respectively. The software that is used for the design of the restorations is Ceramill Mind DRS. While there are not many details about the technology the intraoral scanner uses for the acquisition of the intraoral tissues, the manufacturer claims that the scanning process is fast, with the full jaw scan taking about one minute. The dentist can scan dentulous partial and full jaws, and can take bite impression or implant positions with the help of scan bodies.

The Ceramill software can delete the excessive data like cheek, tongue, or fingers of the dentists that are acquired by mistake during the digital impression, while there is also a verifying sound of correct data acquiring during the impression. The impressions are displayed in true-color and there is a tooth shade option for the dentist convenience. The software has a virtual articulator which can perform the dynamic movements and be calculated during the initial proposal of the dental restoration in order to have less or no interfering contacts. Moreover, the software determines automatically the nesting of the restoration inside the block of the material and the placement of the sprue support which is important during the milling of the restoration.

The dentist can mill the design restorations with the aid of the milling unit or can send the design file or impression scan data to the AG Life portal to be manufactured in a laboratory or milling center.

The milling unit which is suitable for a dental office is the Ceramill motion DRS; it is a compact 4-axis unit, equipped with a 5-field RFID tool changer, a spindle speed of 100.000 rpm, and a 5 μm accuracy. The milling unit has a capability of fast milling and denture fabrication. Moreover, it recognizes the milling time of each cutting tool and notifies the dentist for replacement. There is also an integrated camera which documents the milling process via video, allowing technical support if needed.

5.5.8 Roland DG Shape

An open architecture clinical CAD/CAM solution for chairside solution is presented by Roland DG Shape, with the DWX-42 W system. It is an open system which allows the dentist to use the scanner of their choice to obtain intraoral impressions and then with the use of the Millbox CAM software to design the dental restorations. The milling unit can mill in the wet mode up to three different glass ceramic or composite blocks at once. It has an automatic pin rotation and a tool

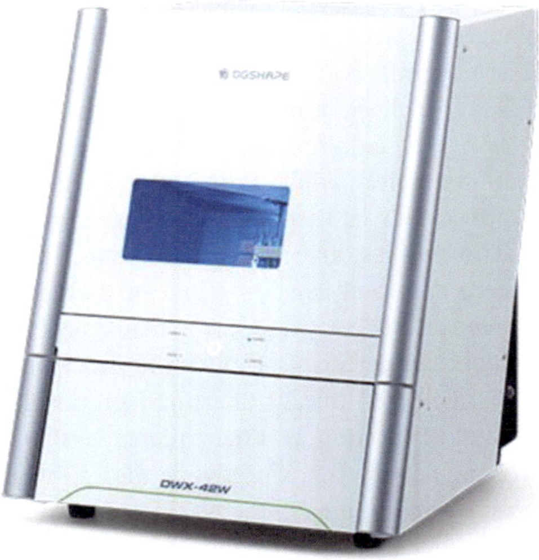

Fig. 5.7 The Roland CAM system

changer of 6 tools. The software can direct the milling unit to mill without interruption resulting in quick to produce restorations. The software can export and import STL files, can mill up to 3-unit bridges, and is designed for glass ceramic and resin-ceramic or resin CAD/CAM blocks up to 40 mm in length. It has an integrated water tank, but it requires an external compressed air supply (Fig. 5.7).

5.6 Laboratory CAD/CAM Systems

CAD/CAM systems that are used by dental technician, laboratories, and milling centers are considered that they have higher level of accuracy than chairside systems [27]. However, studies are inconsistent, with some demonstrating that intraoral impressions have higher accuracy, others finding extraoral laboratory scanning of impressions to be more accurate and other studies finding no statistically significant difference between intraoral and laboratory scanners [28, 29].

The components of the laboratory CAD/CAM systems are basically the same with the chairside systems; however they are different in size. They consist of three components: (1) a scanner that acquire the data from the analog impression, (2) the software for designing the virtual restoration, (3) the milling unit for manufacturing the restoration from a block of material, like in the chairside systems, or a disc of material which can be integrated in the laboratory milling unit [21]. Another difference of the laboratory CAD/CAM systems with the chairside systems is the ability to mill sintering metal and wax discs, which gives the opportunity for the dental technicians for further restorative applications like partial dentures, complete dentures, bars, surgical guides, impressions trays, and bite splints [30, 31].

5.6.1 Dentsply Sirona System

This laboratory CAD/CAM system consists of the inEos X5 scanner, the inLab software, and the MC X5 milling unit.

5.6.1.1 InEos X5 Scanner

The laboratory scanner of Dentsply Sirona has a demonstrated accuracy of 2.1 ± 2.8 μm for a bridge test specimen and an accuracy of 1.3 ± 0.4 μm for a standard inlay test specimen, according to DIN EN ISO 12836.2015. The scanner consists of a working area where the model or analog impressions trays are placed, integrated with a robot arm, and a 5-axis scanning technology which is used in order to digitize the impressions. Several articulators can be positioned within the scanner, while the scanner is suited for the capture of functional impressions and bite registration for the fabrication of full dentures.

The scanner can digitize impression of implants with the use of one-piece scan bodies and triple tray impressions. Different shapes and sizes of impression trays can be implemented in the scanner, while there is a multi-die scanning strategy in which up to four prepared dies are scanned automatically and implement in the digital model with no manual interaction. The scanner is very fast since it has the ability to digitize impressions in less than 60 s, while the scanning technique is a digital light stripe projection.

Studies about the InEos X5 scanner have demonstrated that the restorations that were made from a digital impression with this extraoral scanner had a lower gap value compared to intraoral scanners [32].

5.6.1.2 InLab CAD/CAM Software

The software of the laboratory CAD/CAM system is an independent software that can be used with or without the scanning and milling unit. The inLab software has modules that can be purchased independently, according to the dental technicians needs. There are three software modules, the basic module which covers the basic dental indications, as inlays, onlays, veneers, full crowns, full anatomical bridges, anatomically reduced bridge, copings and multilayer and models. Additional features of the inLab software include tooth databases, virtual articulator, a smile design feature, and gingival elements for producing restorations that require gingival components. A new feature that Dentsply Sirona has implemented to the new version of inLab is the Jaw Orientated Biogeneric Settings (J.O.B.S.). This feature can reconstruct the teeth true to nature by analyzing the position and morphology of the existing teeth and using this data to generate patient-specific anatomical proposals. The implantology module consists of tools and functions for the fabrication of single and multiple implants as well as surgical guide designs. Finally, the removable module can design splints, impressions trays, telescopes, and several designs of attachments. The software interface is an open system, exporting and importing several kinds of files like STL, 3ox (3Shape), and constructioninfo (exocad).

5.6.1.3 MC X5 Milling Unit

The MC X5 is a 5-axis milling unit for dry and wet milling of blocks and disc materials. It has a fully automated tool changer with the capacity of 6 tools per process. The milling unit can process standard discs and block materials. It is equipped with a multi-block holder which can handle up to 8 blocks of different materials and sizes. Dentsply Sirona has implemented a spindle touch technology which captures the workpiece position ensuring that the dental material can be gently prepared with optimal efficiency. For dry milling, the milling unit can be equipped with a suction and a cleaning system so the deposits of the materials can be removed efficiently.

Studies have found that the MC X5 milling unit produces the smallest marginal gap of lithium disilicate restorations than other combinations [33] (Fig. 5.8).

5.6.1.4 Shape System

3Shape first dental lab scanner and dental software was introduced in 2005; later in 2008 the company brought D700 lab scanner, and in 2009 it created an orthodontics software. The company does not have a laboratory milling unit, but as in the case of chairside system of 3shape, the software is compatible with many milling machines from other manufactures. The new lab scanner that was introduced recently is E4. This scanner is a very compact in size, but efficient in both accuracy and speed. The scanner uses 4 MP cameras and can be used for scanning impressions or dies, with a scan speed of 45 s for a full arch. The dental software that is used with the scanner can be divided into modules so the lab technician will purchase only the ones in need or preference. There are three modules for the lab technician, the "crown-bridge" module, the premium module, and the complete module which includes the full range of dental treatment workflows like dentures, partial dentures, implant surgical guides, orthodontic appliances, smile design, implant bars, etc.

5.6.2 Ivoclar Vivadent System

Ivoclar Vivadent has implemented a PrograMill CAM software for the calculation and nesting of dental restorations, ensuring an automated processing of the design. The software is fully compatible with 3Shape Dental System and Exocad software, allowing the design parameters, the preferred materials, the defined restoration type, the designed occlusal surfaces, and the processing strategy to be embedded to the exported file. The lab scanners that Ivoclar Vivadent has introduced are the PrograScan PS5 and PS3. Both lab scanners have two high-resolution cameras with 2 MP resolution and use white LED light source.

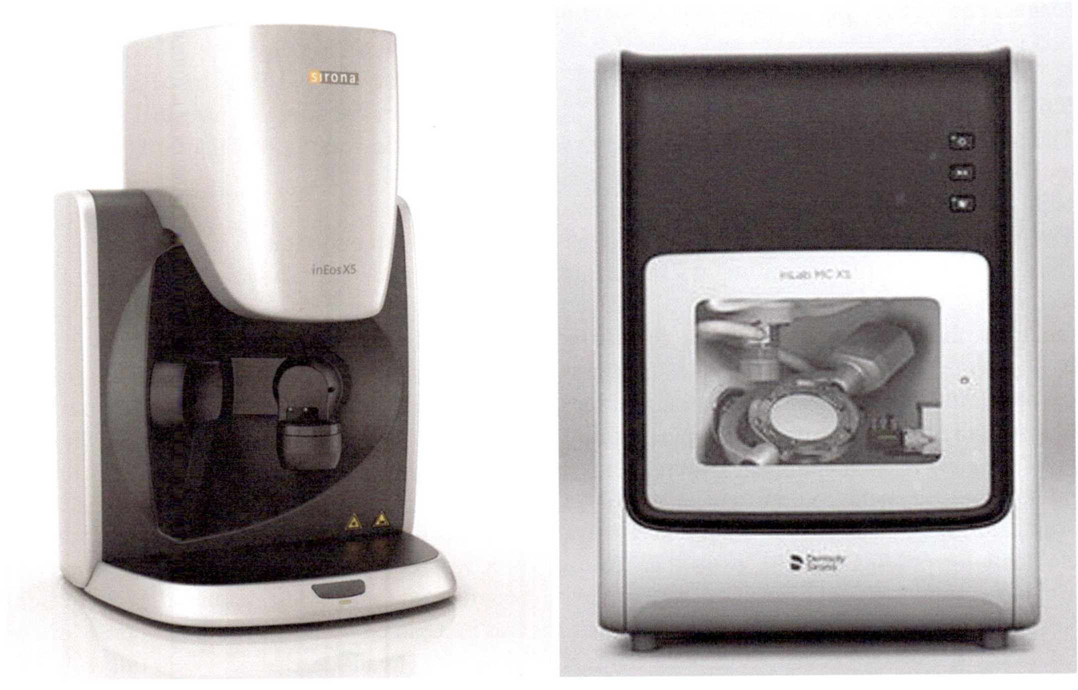

Fig. 5.8 The laboratory CAD/CAM system by Dentsply Sirona

The full scan arch for the PrograScan PS5 is 16 s while the PrograScan PS3 time is 20 s. The accuracy for both scanners according to the ISO 12836 is 5 μm. Both scanners have the ability to scan gypsum casts with the articulator. The difference among the scanners is the color of the digitized images, because PrograScan PS5 produces color images while the PrograScan PS3 produces black and white images. Additionally, the PrograScan PS5 has a fully automated process using a third scanning axis and can scan a full arch in 16 s while it can scan impression trays, and exporting in STL and PLY files. On the contrary, PrograScan PS3 can only export STL files and cannot scan impressions trays. The areas of applications are crowns, bridges, and bite guard splints for both scanners.

As for the milling units, Ivoclar Vivadent has introduced Programill PM7, Programill PM5, Programill PM3, and Programill Dry. The above milling units have a broad spectrum of applications and are intended to be used by dental laboratories with different needs. All the milling units use 5-axis milling technology; however, Programill PM7 is a more powerful unit and uses an in-built ionizer in order to neutralize the static charge of the material residuals and a self-cleaning function. Programill PM7 and PM5 have an automatic material changer of 8 discs, while Programill PM3 and Programill Dry do not support automatic material changer. All the milling units have an automatic tool changer except the Programill Dry. Programill PM7 can manage 20 cutting tools; Programill PM5 and Programill PM3 can control 13 cutting tools. The restorations that can be fabricated include the full range of dental restorative treatments, including veneers, inlays, onlays, complete dentures, primary telescopes, models, abutments, occlusal splints, impression trays, bridges, etc. The materials that the milling unit can use are in the form of discs and blocks, containing RFID labels so that they can be registered, managed, and identified automatically by the CAM software during the manufacturing phase. As for the Programill Dry, this is a compact CAD/CAM milling unit that can only fabricate zirconium oxide restorations and PMMA material in dry mode (Fig. 5.9).

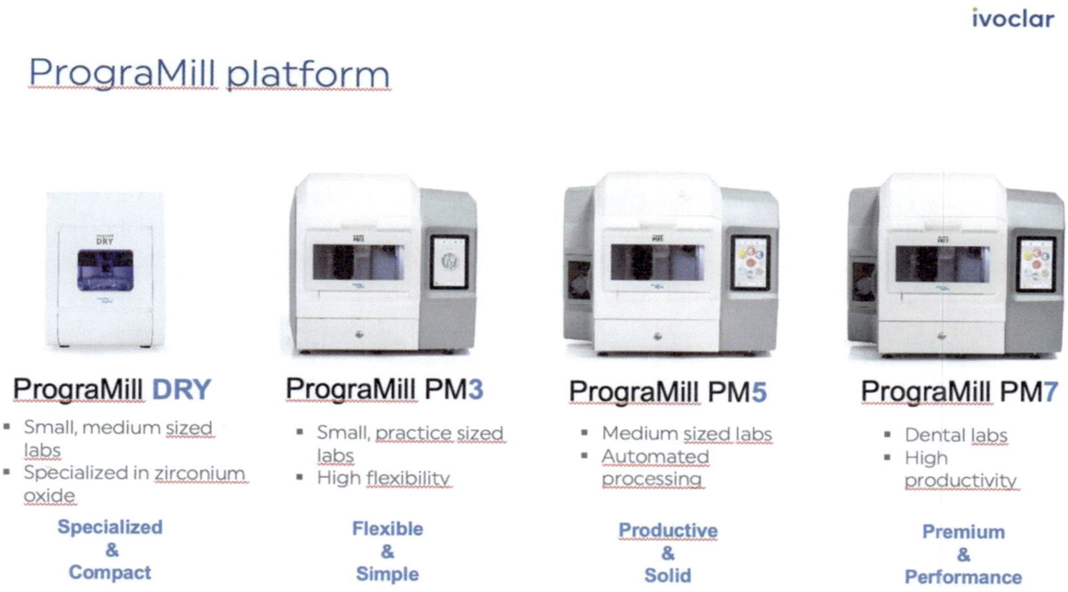
ivoclar
PrograMill platform
PrograMill DRY
Small, medium sized labs
Specialized in zirconium oxide
Specialized & Compact
PrograMill PM3
Small, practice sized labs
High flexibility
Flexible & Simple
PrograMill PM5
Medium sized labs
Automated processing
Productive & Solid
PrograMill PM7
Dental labs
High productivity
Premium & Performance

Fig. 5.9 The group of laboratory CAM systems by Ivoclar Vivadent

5.6.3 Amann Girrbach Laboratory System

Amann Girrbach has introduced in the dental market two laboratory scanners, Ceramill MAP 200+ and Ceramill MAP 600 and 5 milling units, Ceramill matik, Ceramil Motion 3 and Ceramill Motion 2, Ceramil mikro ic, and Ceramill mikro.

Ceramill MAP 200+ is characterized as an entry fully automatic 2-axis stripe light scanner. It has high-resolution 3D sensors and newly developed scanning strategies named "DNA Speed Scanning." The accuracy of the scanner as reported by the manufacturer is 6 μm and can perform a full-arch scan in 20 s. It uses blue light technology and has optical autofocus capability.

Ceramill MAP 600 is a 3-axis scanner with a 4 μm accuracy and an 18 s time for a full-arch scan. The scanner has a universal carrier plate for all common types of articulators. The scanner uses blue light technology, ensuring an outstanding depth of field.

Amann Girrbach has a variety of modules for the laboratory CAM construction. There is a software module for esthetic planning of anterior restorations, a bar module, a framework module for the fabrication of partial frameworks, a split module, etc.

As for the laboratory milling units, the Ceramill Matik is the leader among the milling units of Amann Girbach. This milling unit is a combination of three machines in one, since it combines a milling unit, a stock management system, and a machine cleaning device. It has a 10-axis control for activating the mechanics, and a spindle of 100.000 rpm frequency speed. It has a patented carving mode which saves processing time and a speed milling of acrylic, zirconium, and metal materials. There is an integrated tool manager of 26 tools, a camera for remote monitoring of the production process, while the cleaning system has a coolant and an extraction system. The Ceramill motion 3 is a 5-axis milling unit with an automated carving and detailing technology due to the C-Clamp and an automatic calibration system. There is also an integrated patent of the Carving mode which allows the glass ceramics, resin-ceramics, and resin materials to be processed with a saving time of 60%, by removing excess material in its entirety without the need to mill the block to its actual geometry. Thus, a milling time of 15 min is required to fabricate a crown, with the choice of high-precision milling strategy and the use of ultra-thin cutting burs to produce a very detailed restoration surface. There is also Ceramill motion 2 which is a 5-axis milling unit, the ceramil mikro and ceramil mikro ic. The later milling units are more compact 4-axis for wet milling or 5-axis for dry milling combining the features of the above milling machines. Studies about the extraoral scanners have showed higher trueness and precision regarding the Ceramill Map 600 than intraoral scanners [34].

5.6.4 Roland DG Shape

Like the chairside system Roland DG shape has developed a laboratory open architecture CAD/CAM solution. The company has manufactured two CAM systems, the DWX-52DCi and the DWX-52D. The DWX-52DCi has a 6-slot Automatic Disc Changer and a 15-station Automatic tool changer. It can mill a variety of materials like zirconia, PMMA, gypsum, PEEK, resin, resin-ceramic, and glass ceramic materials with the addition of CoCr sintered metal. It has a spindle speed of 6.000–30.000 rpm and is considered a 5-axis milling unit. It can hold up to eight pin-type blocks and optional carbide, diamond, and milling tools of 0.3, 0.6, and 1.0 mm. The automated regulator that is integrated to the milling unit eliminates the need for manual air control adjustments by changing air volume based on material data based on information obtained by the CAM software. The DWINDEX CAM software is a very unique tool than informs the dental technician about the milling machine productivity, since it offers data about the operation time per tool, per disk, and per unit. It can produce a log file for common errors and warnings, and export a file about the number of materials used and the deliverables of the restorations produced. One advantage that the DWX-52DCi has is that it uses a replaceable spindle that can be replaced by the user without the need for a technician. Finally, it can be loaded with a brush tool in order to sweep away the milling debris, while there are internal dust collection systems which automatically start to keep the dust away from lab surfaces and an ionizer reducing the static of the debris resulting in a clean air environment.

The DWX-52D has the same specifications with the DWX-52DCi milling unit but it has a more compact form. It has a Snap-In clamp system for disc changing and 6 material adapters with a secure and fast set up. It is a 5-axis milling machine and it can be used for the fabrication of temporary and provisional crowns, single and multiple bridge, veneers, inlays, onlays, abutments with a Tibase, frameworks, implant bars, bite splints, and surgical guides (Fig. 5.10).

5.6.5 Zfx Laboratory CAD/CAM Systems

Laboratory CAD/CAM systems from Zfx include the Evolution and Evolution plus scanning devices and the Zfx utramill 5-axis milling unit. The laboratory scanning unit is an open system which can digitize from a variety of articulated models and also can detect photometric surfaces like hand marked preparation margins. The scanning unit has 2 cameras with 1.296 × 964 pixels and a CCD camera sensor system and has a minimum scan time of 1.2 min for a model and 20 s for a die stump. The scanner accuracy is less than 9 μm according to the European laboratory validation test and has an "open scan technology" which includes a 128-line pairs which are projected with an LED light source. There is an enhanced Quick Scan option, and the algorithms of the image processing times of the scanner have been reduced to 30%. The scanner can also digitize up to 12 individual dies in under 10 min, and the dental technician can use realistic color reproduction. There is an integrated virtual articulator and the CAD software can be used to design abutments, bars, therapeutic splints, and also smile design cases and also there are a lot of modules which are supplied by the manufacturer which can installed in the basic software.

As for the milling units the Zfx provides the SAUER-Ultrasonic 20 linear machine, which has a considerable reduction of the process forces by incorporating a special actuator system, by means of which an ultrasonic frequency is transmitted

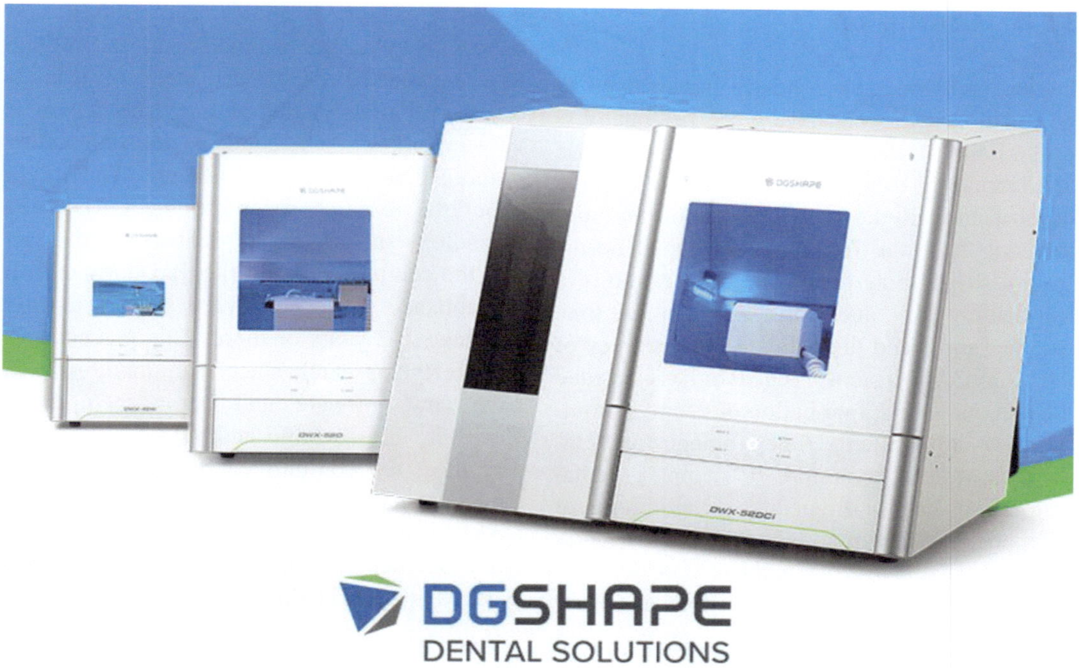

Fig. 5.10 The Roland DG shape CAD/CAM laboratory system

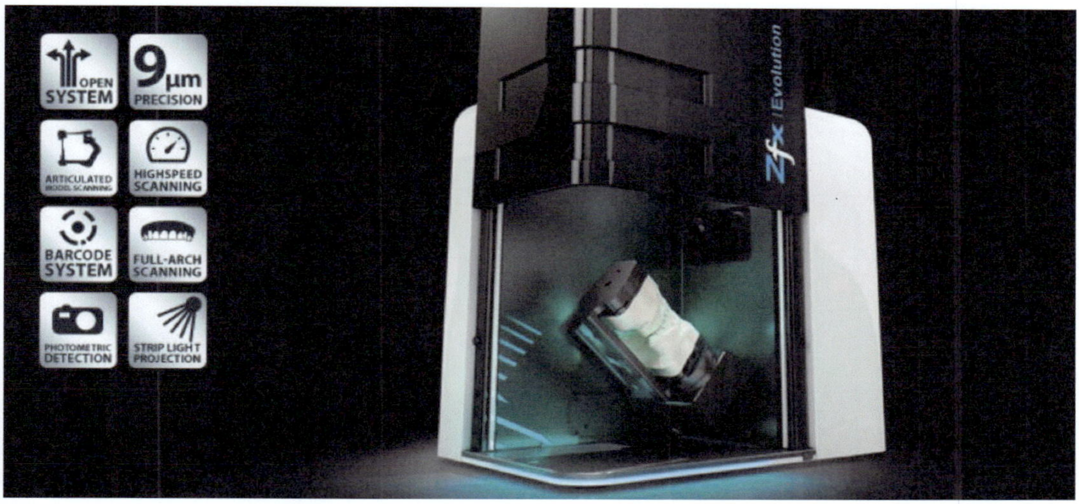

Fig. 5.11 The Zfx extraoral laboratory scanner

from the spindle to the tool. The result is a significant increase in the chop removal rate and a very smooth surface for the dental prosthesis. Zfx Ultramill has the same technology as the SAUER-Ultrasonic 20 but is more rigid and has low vibration characteristics due to the structure of the milling machine. Those milling units can increase the productivity of the laboratory due to the Zfx milling strategies compared to the conventional systems. The milling units can be used for the fabrication of inlays, onlays, and dental bridges from a variety of materials like PMMA, titanium, cobalt-chromium, glass ceramics, zirconium, wax, and composite (Fig. 5.11).

5.7 Conclusion

Digital technology in dentistry has evolved to powerful systems that have made personal and professional lives easier [11, 35]. The chairside and laboratory CAD/CAM systems are capable of fabricating all the dental restorations in order to rehabilitate the full range of dental needs, from a single inlay [36] to the fabrication of a full denture [37], and with less effort and time for the dentist and the patient. The accuracy of the CAD/CAM systems is equal or has exceeded the manual way of fabrication of dental restorations [38–40] while the time efficiency and predictable results of simple or complex dental restorations have shortened the rehabilitation of the patients. The materials that are currently being used exclusively with the CAD/CAM systems have been the materials of choice for many dental CAD/CAM clinics and laboratories, because they are more biocompatible [41] and have enhanced chemical and mechanical properties [42] with increased longevity which is very crucial when it concerns the demanding intraoral conditions [43]. The most difficult task about the research regarding the CAD/CAM technology in the field of dentistry is the fact that the completion of a scientific study until it is published to a peer-review journal usually will take 1–2 years or more. This process will outdate the research since manufacturers will have new software and hardware updates. However, the scientific and academic community have the commitment to prove the efficiency and reliability of digital dental CAD/CAM systems to the dental community. A summary of chairside and laboratory CAD/CAM systems is given in Table 5.1 and 5.2.

Table 5.1 Summary of chairside CAD/CAM systems

CAD/CAM system	Intraoral scanner	Milling unit	Real color scans	Powder-free	Shade analysis	Virtual articulation	Smile Design	STL export	Artificial Intelligence	Software Updates	Wirelesss
Dentsply Sirona	✓	✓	✓	✓	✓	✓	✓	✓	✓	✓	X
3Shape	✓	X	✓	✓	✓	✓	✓	✓	✓	✓	✓
Planmenca	✓	✓	✓	✓	✓	✓	X	✓	✓	✓	X
Dental Wings	✓	X	✓	✓	X	X	X	✓	X	✓	X
Fona Dental	✓	✓	X	X	X	✓	X	✓	X	✓	X
Carestream	✓	✓	X	✓	✓	X	X	✓	✓	✓	✓
Zfx	✓	✓	✓	✓	X	X	X	✓	✓	✓	X
Amann Girrbach	✓	✓	✓	✓	X	✓	X	✓	✓	✓	X

Table 5.2 Summary of laboratory CAD/CAM systems

CAD/CAM system	Extraoral scanner	Milling unit (5-axis)	Automated tool change	Tool capacity milling unit	Automated material change	Material Capacity milling unit	Open System files	Articulation scanning	Smile Design	Artificial Intelligence	Software Updates
Dentsply Sirona	✓	✓	✓	6	X	1 disc 8 blocks	✓	X	✓	✓	✓
3Shape	✓	X	✓	X	X	X	✓	X	✓	✓	✓
Ivoclar Vivadent	✓	✓	✓	13-20	✓	1-8 discs/ 48 blocks	✓	✓	✓	✓	✓
Roland	X	✓	✓	15	✓	6 discs 8 blocks	X	X	✓	X	✓
Zfx	✓	✓	✓	24	✓	2 discs/ 24 blocks	✓	✓	✓	✓	✓
Amann Girrbach	✓	✓	✓	6-27	✓	36 discs 4 blocks	✓	✓	✓	✓	✓

References

1. Zaruba M, Mehl A. Chairside systems: a current review. Int J Comput Dent. 2017;20:123–49.
2. Mormann WH. The evolution of the CEREC system. J Am Dent Assoc. 2006;137:7S–13S.
3. Miyazaki T, Hotta Y. CAD/CAM systems available for the fabrication of crown and bridge restorations. Aust Dent J. 2011;56(Suppl 1):97–106.
4. Chochlidakis KM, Papaspyridakos P, Geminiani A, et al. Digital versus conventional impressions for fixed prosthodontics: a systematic review and meta-analysis. J Prosthet Dent. 2016;116:184–90.
5. Blatz MB, Conejo J. The current state of chairside digital dentistry and materials. Dent Clin N Am. 2019;63:175–97.
6. Alghazzawi TF. Advancements in CAD/CAM technology: options for practical implementation. J Prosthodont Res. 2016;60:72–84.
7. Rekow ED. Digital dentistry: the new state of the art—is it disruptive or destructive? Dent Mater. 2020;36:9–24.
8. Li RW, Chow TW, Matinlinna JP. Ceramic dental biomaterials and CAD/CAM technology: state of the art. J Prosthodont Res. 2014;58:208–16.
9. Moore GE. Cramming more components onto integrated circuits. Electronics. 1965;38(6):82.
10. Patzelt SB, Lamprinos C, Stampf S, Att W. The time efficiency of intraoral scanners: an in vitro comparative study. J Am Dent Assoc. 2014;145:542–51.
11. van Noort R. The future of dental devices is digital. Dent Mater. 2012;28:3–12.
12. Bohner L, Gamba DD, Hanisch M, Marcio BS, Tortamano Neto P, Laganá DC, Sesma N. Accuracy of digital technologies for the scanning of facial, skeletal, and intraoral tissues: a systematic review. J Prosthet Dent. 2019;121:246–51.
13. Tapie L, Lebon N, Mawussi B, Fron-Chabouis H, Duret F, Attal JP. Understanding dental CAD/CAM for restorations—accuracy from a mechanical engineering viewpoint. Int J Comput Dent. 2015;18:343–67.
14. Park JH, Lee GH, Moon DN, Kim JC, Park M, Lee KM. A digital approach to the evaluation of mandibular position by using a virtual articulator. J Prosthet Dent. 2021;125:849–53.
15. Fung L, Brisebois P. Implementing digital dentistry into your esthetic dental practice. Dent Clin N Am. 2020;64:645–57.
16. Skramstad MJ. Welcome to Cerec Primescan AC. Int J Comput Dent. 2019;22:69–78.
17. Skramstad MJ. A new milling unit for an efficient workflow. Int J Comput Dent. 2020;23:83–91.
18. Vág J, Renne W, Revell G, Ludlow M, Mennito A, Teich ST, Gutmacher Z. The effect of software updates on the trueness and precision of intraoral scanners. Quintessence Int. 2021;52:636–44.
19. Sannino G, Gloria F, Schiavetti R, Ottria L, Barlattani A. Dental wings CAD/CAM system precision: an internal and marginal fit sperimental analisys. Oral Implantol (Rome). 2009;2:11–20.
20. Amornvit P, Rokaya D, Sanohkan S. Comparison of accuracy of current ten intraoral scanners. Biomed Res Int. 2021;13:2673040.
21. Zimmermann M, Ender A, Mehl A. Local accuracy of actual intraoral scanning systems for single-tooth preparations in vitro. J Am Dent Assoc. 2020;151:127–35.
22. Abduo J, Elseyoufi M. Accuracy of intraoral scanners: a systematic review of influencing factors. Eur J Prosthodont Restor Dent. 2018;26:101–21.

23. Fraile C, Ferreiroa A, Romeo M, Alonso R, Pradíes G. Clinical study comparing the accuracy of interocclusal records, digitally obtained by three different devices. Clin Oral Investig. 2022;26:1957–62.
24. Michelinakis G, Apostolakis D, Tsagarakis A, et al. A comparison of accuracy of 3 intraoral scanners: a single-blinded in vitro study. J Prosthet Dent. 2020;124:581–8.
25. Alzahrani SJ, El-Hammali H, Morgano SM, et al. Evaluation of the accuracy of 2 digital intraoral scanners: a 3D analysis study. J Prosthet Dent. 2021;126:787–92.
26. Ebeid K, Sabet A, Della BA. Accuracy and repeatability of different intraoral scanners on shade determination. J Esthet Restor Dent. 2021;33:844–8.
27. Dupagne L, Tapie L, Lebon N, et al. Comparison of the acquisition accuracy and digitizing noise of 9 intraoral and extraoral scanners: an objective method. J Prosthet Dent. 2021;S0022–3913(21):00076–7.
28. Sim JY, Jang Y, Kim WC, et al. Comparing the accuracy (trueness and precision) of models of fixed dental prostheses fabricated by digital and conventional workflows. J Prosthodont Res. 2019;63:25–30.
29. Papadiochou S, Pissiotis AL. Marginal adaptation and CAD-CAM technology: a systematic review of restorative material and fabrication techniques. J Prosthet Dent. 2018;119:545–51.
30. Baghani MT, Shayegh SS, Johnston WM, et al. In vitro evaluation of the accuracy and precision of intraoral and extraoral complete-arch scans. J Prosthet Dent. 2021;126:665–70.
31. Lo Russo L, Salamini A, Troiano G, et al. Digital dentures: a protocol based on intraoral scans. J Prosthet Dent. 2021;125:597–602.
32. Ekici Z, Kılıçarslan MA, Bilecenoğlu B, Ocak M. Micro-CT evaluation of the marginal and internal fit of crown and inlay restorations fabricated via different digital scanners belonging to the same CAD-CAM system. Int J Prosthodont. 2021;34:381–9.
33. Su S, Dudley J. The marginal gaps of lithium disilicate crowns constructed by different scanner and milling unit combinations. Aust Dent J. 2022;67:125–31.
34. Ellakany P, Aly NM, Al-Harbi F. A comparative study assessing the precision and trueness of digital and printed casts produced from several intraoral and extraoral scanners in full arch and short span (3-unit FPD) scanning: an in vitro study. J Prosthodont. 2022;31:521.
35. Miyazaki T, Hotta Y, Kunii J, et al. A review of dental CAD/CAM: current status and future perspectives from 20 years of experience. Dent Mater. 2009;28:44–56.
36. Kassis C, Khoury P, Mehanna CZ, Baba NZ, Bou Chebel F, Daou M, Hardan L. Effect of inlays, onlays and endocrown cavity design preparation on fracture resistance and fracture mode of endodontically treated teeth: an in vitro study. J Prosthodont. 2021;30:625–31.
37. Diker B, Tak Ö. Accuracy of six intraoral scanners for scanning complete-arch and 4-unit fixed partial dentures: an in vitro study. J Prosthet Dent. 2021;S0022–3913(20):30797–6.
38. Kernen F, Schlager S, Seidel Alvarez V, et al. Accuracy of intraoral scans: an in vivo study of different scanning devices. J Prosthet Dent. 2021;S0022–3913(21):00145–1.
39. Pattamavilai S, Ongthiemsak C. Accuracy of intraoral scanners in different complete arch scan patterns. J Prosthet Dent. 2022;S0022–3913(22):00046–4.
40. Nedelcu R, Olsson P, Nyström I, Rydén J, Thor A. Accuracy and precision of 3 intraoral scanners and accuracy of conventional impressions: a novel in vivo analysis method. J Dent. 2018;69:110–8.
41. Mourouzis P, Andreasidou E, Samanidou V, Tolidis K. Short-term and long-term release of monomers from newly developed resin-modified ceramics and composite resin CAD-CAM blocks. J Prosthet Dent. 2020;123:339–48.
42. Prpić V, Schauperl Z, Ćatić A, Dulčić N, Čimić S. Comparison of mechanical properties of 3D-printed, CAD/CAM, and conventional denture base materials. J Prosthodont. 2020;29(6):524–8.
43. Wierichs RJ, Kramer EJ, Reiss B, Schwendicke F, Krois J, Meyer-Lueckel H, Wolf TG. A prospective, multi-center, practice-based cohort study on all-ceramic crowns. Dent Mater. 2021;37(8):1273–82.

Part II

Novelties and Advances in Digital Dentistry

6 Digital Caries Detection Systems

İsmail Hakkı Baltacıoğlu, Gülbike Demirel, and Kaan Orhan

6.1 Introduction

Dentistry started to move away from aggressive surgery to minimally invasive procedures as well as placing more emphasis on prevention and early detection. Dentistry has evolved in terms of caries detection devices, and these devices have been introduced on the market to make it easier to catch caries early and reverse this condition before it costs patients their teeth. This chapter discusses some of the shortcomings of traditional caries detection technology and also explores the benefits that digital caries detection devices bring to the field of dentistry.

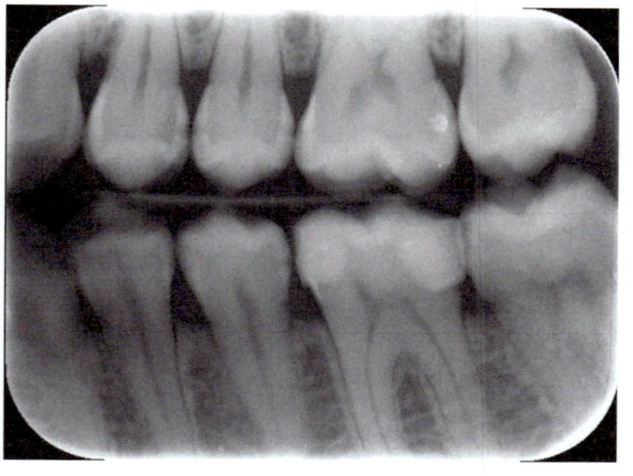

Fig. 6.1 Bitewing radiograph of aproximal caries lesions. (#24 distal RA 3, #25 mesial RA 2, distal RA 1,#35 distal RA 1 according to the ICDAS/ICCMS radiographic scoring system)

6.2 X-Rays

6.2.1 Digital Bitewing Radiographs

Intraoral radiography and especially bitewing radiographs are the most widely used method in the diagnosis of interface caries in the world. This method is also used as a standard for evaluating the effectiveness of newly developed methods. Conventional screen-film radiography has been surpassed by digital radiology since its introduction. While the exposure technique of digital bitewing radiographs resembles that of traditional radiographs (Fig. 6.1), the creation and evaluation of the radiographic images differ significantly from conventional ones [1, 2].

İ. H. Baltacıoğlu · G. Demirel (✉)
Faculty of Dentistry, Department of Restorative Dentistry, Ankara University, Ankara, Turkey
e-mail: baltacioglu@ankara.edu.tr; gdemirel@ankara.edu.tr

K. Orhan
Faculty of Dentistry Department of Oral and Maxillofacial Radiology, Ankara University, Ankara, Turkey

Ankara University Medical Design Application and Research Center (MEDITAM), Ankara, Turkey

Department of Oral Diagnostics, Faculty of Dentistry, Semmelweis University, Budapest, Hungary

A. Delantoni, K. Orhan (eds.), *Digital Dentistry*, https://doi.org/10.1007/978-3-031-52826-2_6

Digital systems have many advantages. First, these systems have very sensitive receivers to obtain the image, which provides less irradiation time and less radiation requirement. Since the image is created digitally, it does not need film developer solutions and time. Therefore, the image is formed very quickly, and the polluting and costly "development" process is eliminated. At the same time, the new system prevents errors during the development process, ensuring a correctly shot film does not result in an inadequate and low-quality image, which is due to the completely digital and standard process. While traditional films can be used only once, sensors and plates in digital systems can be used hundreds or even thousands of times. This again prevents environmental damage and film consumption [3, 4].

In the traditional system, the films that can be handled physically and evaluated with a negatoscope have been replaced by computer monitors, tablets, and phones in the digital system. In these environments, properties such as the size, color, and brightness of the image can be changed during evaluation, so that a more detailed examination can be made with images that are more comfortable to the eye [3, 5].

Today, in digital bitewing radiography, the image is acquired by two different receiver systems. The first of these is the "RadioVisioGraphy (RVG)" system, and the other is the "Photostimulable storage phosphor plate (PSP)" system. RVG technology started to be used earlier than PSP. These rigid systems had receivers with non-bendable cables and were slightly larger and thicker than conventional films. RVG systems collect X-rays passing through teeth and other tissues with Charge-Coupled Devices (CCD) or Complementary Metal Oxide Semiconductor technology (CMOS) solid-state sensors. Because of these sensors and the silicon wafer, they are placed on, RVG systems are thicker than conventional films. The beam detected by the sensors is sent to the computer with the help of a cable or wirelessly and an image is quickly formed on the screen. The situation differs in phosphorus plaques, these plates are thinner and wireless. The beams reaching this plate after exposure make the electrons excited in the phosphor lattice. Then this phosphor plate is scanned by a laser scanner and the resulting image is transferred to the computer environment. Although this two-step process takes more time than the RVG system, it is much faster than the traditional film system. The most important advantage of this system against RVG is that it is smaller and more flexible; it can be applied more easily in the oral environment and angulated more easily [1, 3, 6].

When compared to the first RVG systems and traditional film radiography in terms of caries diagnosis, although the traditional technique was found to be more successful, the latest RVGs and phosphor plates currently show similar diagnostic efficiency with conventional radiography. The storage file format for the raw image acquired through the digital technique is a distinct consideration. Although the image can be evaluated in its best form in the dedicated programs used with these systems, there may be a loss of detail in the converted file formats, especially when storing and sharing these images [6, 7]. Another emerging advantage of the digital bitewing technique is that these images can be used in caries detection programs using artificial intelligence. Although potential caries areas are marked on the digital radiograph with these techniques, the decision whether caries are present in these areas should be made by the human observer-operator [8, 9].

6.2.2 Dental Cone Beam Computed Tomography

Although the purpose of digital Dental Cone Beam Computed Tomography (CBCT) in dentistry is not to detect caries, caries can still be detected in some cases from already taken images. Since the subject of this section is not the working logic and exposition techniques of CBCT, the relationship between CBCT and caries diagnosis will be discussed.

First, if CBCT is to be used in caries diagnosis, it would be more appropriate to use it by its dedicated program and not by printed films (Fig. 6.2). It is not always possible to detect small lesions in these printed films because the slices used in the printed films were selected and organized by another operator and mostly these slices were chosen for planning surgical procedures such as implant planning or impacted tooth extraction [10, 11].

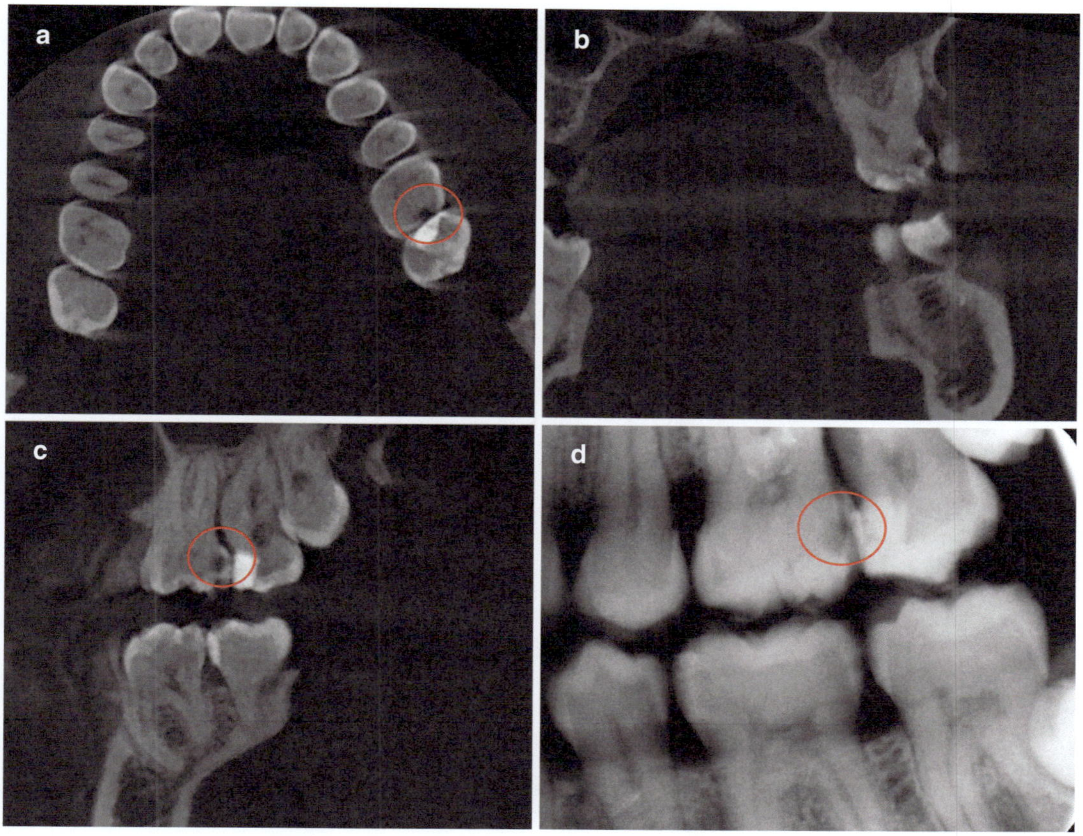

Fig. 6.2 (**a**) Axial CBCT image of caries lesions (#26 distal). (**b**) Inappropriate view for a segment to evaluate caries lesions. (**c**) Coronal CBCT image of same caries lesion. (**d**) Bitewing radiograph of same caries lesion

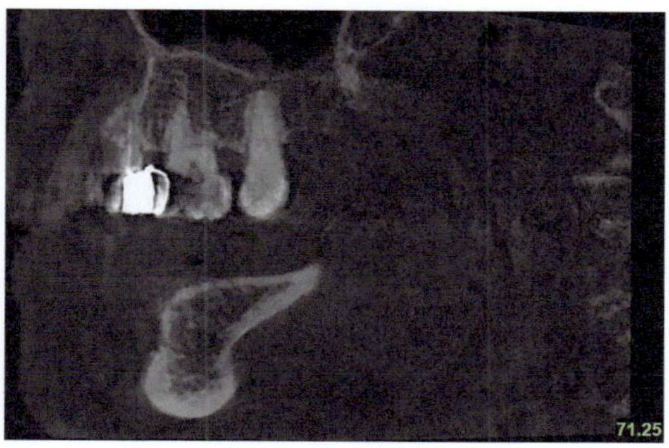

Fig. 6.3 Beam hardening artifact not allowing caries assessment

The biggest disadvantage of the digital CBCT technique as imaging is the artifacts that occur as a result of the scattering of the rays as they pass through dense materials. Especially in teeth with restoration, in areas with adjacent teeth with restoration, as a result of excessive scattering of rays from these dense materials, the density of the surrounding tissues may be reflected incorrectly on the image (Fig. 6.3). In studies in which the presence of secondary caries was evaluated with CBCT, this technique was found to be more unsuccessful than intraoral bitewing radiography [11, 12].

In the absence of restoration in both the related tooth and adjacent teeth, CBCT is a good digital caries detection method. In the presence of caries, a lesion can be located buccolingual in the axial section of the CBCT image. We can also define the depth and volume of the lesion from CBCT images, especially in areas without restoration. In summary, nowadays, although CBCT is not the primary method for caries diagnosis, it is an important tool that can give detailed data about caries in the presence of existing images [13–15].

6.3 Visible Light

6.3.1 Quantitative Light-Induced Fluorescence

Quantitative light-induced fluorescence (QLF) is the first optical technology used in clinical dentistry for the early detection of carious lesions [16]. QLF technology can simultaneously measure mineral content and bacterial activity on dental hard tissues. Like all light-based devices developed for the detection of carious lesions, QLF uses light of a certain wavelength [17]. By evaluating the loss of fluorescence of dental hard tissues by irradiation with blue light with a wavelength of 370 nm, a clear distinction can be made between initial carious lesions and sound tissues. Detection of initial caries lesions by QLF is due to the induction of fluorescence of visible blue light penetrating dental hard tissues and amplification by fluorophores at the enamel-dentin junction. Thus, the carious lesion appears as dark spots in the surrounding yellow to green sound enamel tissue [18]. The loss of fluorescence detected in dental hard tissues can be digitally visualized and the physical properties of carious lesions can be measured non-destructively from these images by converting them into numerical values thanks to the QLF's image analysis.

Besides the detection of carious lesions, an advantage of the latest generation of QLF devices is that they can detect dental plaque [19]. During the growth phase of dental plaque, secondary colonizer bacteria such as *fusobacterium, veillonella, haemophilus, campylobacter, neisseria, gemella, granulicatella, capnocytophaga, and Bacteroides* produce a metabolite called porphyrin [20]. QLF technology displays porphyrin-containing dental plaque as red fluorescence. Because of the positive correlation between mature dental plaque and carious lesions, this red fluorescence may be considered a red flag for clinicians. Besides the detection of primary carious lesions, QLF technology can also be used to evaluate the integrity of the restoration margins by assessing increases and decreases in red fluorescence around the margins. Despite all these positive features of QLF devices, various distractive factors need to be controlled to evaluate these devices quantitatively. Professional cleaning is essential before the examination to remove dental plaque and possible calculus. In the presence of periodontal diseases, the sensitivity of the fluorescent image may decrease due to gingival bleeding. It is necessary to provide standard conditions for obtaining comparative images, such as ambient light and camera angle standardization. QLF has been employed to detect a range of lesion types such as occlusal [21], proximal [22], smooth surfaces [23], root caries [24], and even caries adjacent restorations and sealants (CARS) [25]. For occlusal caries, sensitivity has been reported at 0.68 and specificity at 0.70 [16].

The QLF has additional benefits beyond very early caries detection and quantification. The device could be a useful tool for the clinician during caries removal [26]. Based on the fact that OLF uses bacterial metabolites for caries detection, the same mechanism can be used during caries excavation, instead of using caries-detecting dyes. This method might be very efficient, with less time needed to apply chemical agents, to test the cavity with an explorer. The major important feature is decreasing possible over-preparation during caries removal [27].

6.3.2 Digital Fiber-Optic Transillumination (DIFOTI)

Digital fiber-optic transillumination (DIFOTI) was formed as a result of digitizing the logic of fiber-optic transillumination (FOTI). Use of the digitalized system, images can be transferred to the computer environment and stored, and with sensitive sensors, the technique can be performed more comfortably without being affected by ambient light conditions [28, 29].

Like the FOTI system, in the DIFOTI system, a light is first sent to the tooth and then this light is reflected from the tooth. Unlike the FOTI system, light is collected by a sensor, not by the eye, and reflected on the monitor screen as a grayscale. These devices have two adjustable ends. One end sends the light from the labial or palatal sides of the teeth, and the sensor at the other end collects the light that can pass through the tooth. While the evaluation is made on the monitor, dark areas reflect the presence of caries, and light areas reflect non-carious tissues. This system is noninvasive as it does not use X-rays. In this way, it can be used repeatedly and for as long as desired [30, 31].

Operator knowledge and experience are important while acquiring and evaluating images in this system, so the use of the system is somewhat subjective and may differ for novice users. DIFOTI is very effective in detecting initial lesions. Experienced users can also detect lesions such as cracks and fractures. One of the disadvantages of this system is that the restorations on the teeth will affect the light transmission, so the lesions in the light route but behind the restoration area may not be visible on the monitor [30, 32, 33].

This system can be considered economical since it is not consumable once purchased, but this technology is outdated today and has been replaced by versatile FOTI devices and Near-Infrared Light Transillumination systems that work similarly to the DIFOTI technique.

6.3.3 Near-Infrared Light Transillumination (NILT)

Alternative methods have been sought in newly developed caries detection devices in order to prevent the harmful effects of X-rays. Near-Infrared Light Transillumination (NILT) sends light at a wavelength of approximately 780 nm to the dental tissue, allowing the diagnosis of caries based on the difference in the translucency of the dental tissues [34–36].

This technique was started to be used commercially in the Diagnocam device of the Kavo company. Although it is technically similar to the FOTI and DIFOTI systems, in the NILT system, light is sent from both the buccal and oral surfaces of the teeth, and images are collected by a CCD sensor from the occlusal surface. The resulting images can be viewed on the computer in grayscale mode and can be saved in both image and video formats. If desired, the whole mouth can be scanned in a few minutes. Both the occlusal and proximal regions can be evaluated with this imaging system. Because of the high wavelength, enamel, dentin, and the enamel-dentin junction can be distinguished. In this way, for caries lesions, their severity can be coded in systems such as ICDAS and different treatment methods can be decided by clinicians [37, 38].

Another advantage of this technique, which provides vision from the occlusal region, shows the exact buccolingual location of the caries lesion in the approximal region. Thus, in operative procedures, the access cavity will be prepared from the most preferred point to remove caries, and the loss of healthy tissue will be minimized.

When compared with digital bitewing radiography, the NILT system also showed similar values in sensitivity (Fig. 6.4). The validity of this system has been proven in many clinical studies

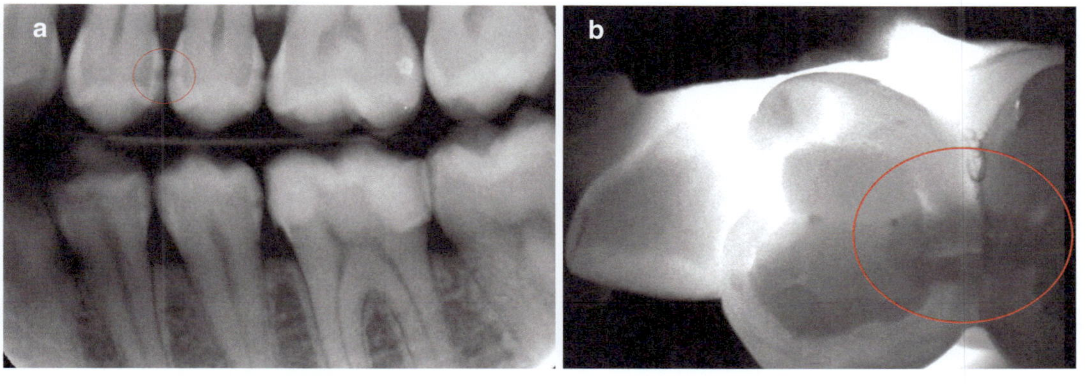

Fig. 6.4 (**a**) Bitewing radiograph of aproximal caries lesions. (#24 distal, #25 mesial). (**b**) NILT image capture of the same region

with patients. Like FOTI systems, the biggest disadvantage of the NILT system is that the tissue under restoration cannot be evaluated [35, 36, 39]. After the successful results of the Diagnocam product, companies that make intraoral scanners also started to provide caries detection in NILT mode by changing the tip of their cameras.

6.4 Laser Light

6.4.1 Laser Fluorescence

DIAGNOdent pen (KaVo, Germany) is a relatively new laser-based caries detection device [16]. Laser light with a wavelength of 655 nm is absorbed by the hard tissues of the teeth and is emitted as fluorescent [40]. Unlike the QLF system, the DIAGNOdent pen does not generate an image of the surface; instead, it displays a numerical value on the LED screen. In the presence of a caries lesion, fluorescence increases, and this increase is detected by the device as a digital number (Table 6.1). Although the reason for the increased fluorescence effect in the presence of caries lesions is not defined completely, it is thought that the bacterial metabolite porphyrin is responsible for this effect [41].

Since it is the basic requirement of all caries detection methods, the device should be used on a clean and dry tooth surface. In addition, the paste or powder used for prophylaxis must be completely removed to avoid a false fluorescence signal. Different tips should be used to detect occlusal (round-ended tip) and approximal (wedge-shaped tip) caries lesions. It should be kept in mind that since these tips are quite rigid, they may break due to pressure and bending. The device should be calibrated each time tips are changed and on a new patient. Diagnodent is a promising tool for clinical use; the correlation with the histological depth of lesions was at 0.85 and the sensitivity and specificity for dentin caries lesions were 0.75 and 0.96, respectively [42].

Similar to QLF, Diagnodent can be useful not only in caries lesion detection but also in determining the caries removal end-point [26]. According to a comparison with a histological examination in the confocal microscope, a DIAGNOdent reading of 15 was determined to best predict the presence of residual caries at the cavity [43]. Alleman and Magne [44] speculated that a Diagnodent reading of approximately 12 indicates virtually bacteria-free superficial dentin and a reading of 24 (acceptable range 12–36) indicates a bacteria-free region in intermediate to deep dentin (Fig. 6.5).

6.4.2 Laser-Induced Infrared Photothermal Radiometry (PTR) and Modulated Luminescence (LUM)

The Canary System (Quantum Dental Technologies, Ontario, Canada) projects the intensity-modulated low-energy laser light onto the tooth surface at a constant frequency (2 Hz);

Table 6.1 DIAGNOdent pen value thresholds for various tooth surfaces according to the manufacturer

Aspect	DIAGNOdent pen value threshold	Diagnosis
Fissure and smooth surface caries	0–12	Sound tissue
	13–24	Initial demineralization
	>25	Strong demineralization
Proximal caries	0–7	Sound tissue
	8–15	Initial demineralization
	>16	Strong demineralization

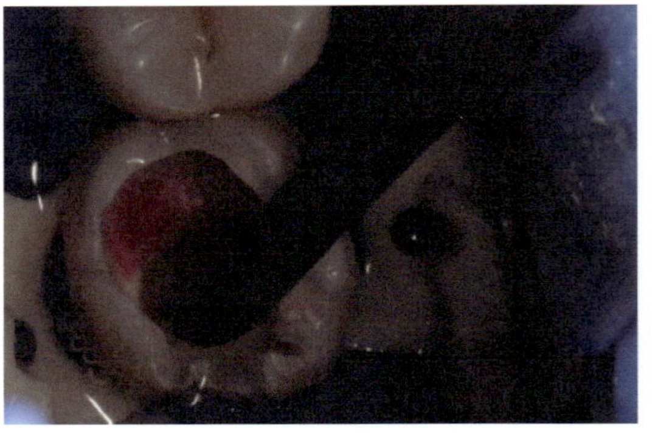

Fig. 6.5 Diagnodent used for caries removal end-point

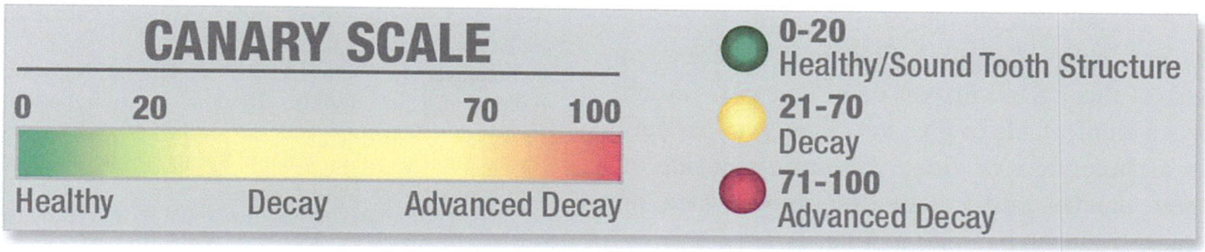

Fig. 6.6 Manufacturer provides a scale for interpretation of Canary Numbers

this laser light interacts with the crystal structure of the dental tissue and transforms into heat (< 1 °C) (PTR) and longer wavelength (LUM), producing infrared and optical emissions at the same frequency. The canary system collects the emitted luminescence and infrared radiation signals. Following the interpretation of luminescence and infrared radiation signals, the Canary system converts these signals into numerical values known as Canary Numbers (CN) [45] (Fig. 6.6). CN gives information from a hemispherical area beneath the laser beam that is 1.5 mm in diameter by 5 mm in depth. According to the manufacturer, a very heavy brown stain would affect the Canary Number but biofilm and plaque do not affect it. There is no need to prophy or polish the tooth surface if the food debris can be removed with a toothbrush or gauze square.

Jeon et al. [46] reported that the sensitivity of PTR–LUM was much higher than laser-induced luminescence, visual inspection, and radiographs in occlusal caries lesions. The Canary system can also be used for proximal caries detection.

6.5 Electrical Current

6.5.1 Electrical Impedance Spectroscopy (EIS)

The ancestor of the Electrical Impedance Spectroscopy devices, the Electronic Caries Monitor (ECM), uses a fixed frequency (23 Hz) alternating current to measure the current resistance of the teeth as close to zero frequency as possible [47]. Like all materials, the basic electrical properties of dental tissues include inductance, resistance, and capacitance. However, only resistance and capacitance are the main parameters in unrestored teeth. Unlike the ECM, the EIS measures the resistance of the dental hard tissues using a range of electrical frequencies. Thus, a more detailed analysis of the presence and extent of caries can be made. The working principle of EDS is the change of electrical conductivity in dental tissue due to the increase in porosity caused by caries. However, physical factors such as tooth temperature and hydration level (teeth should not be dried before examination), enamel thickness, surface area, and fluid ionic concentration can affect EIS results [16]. To date, EIS techniques have been used to assess the smear layer, detect early enamel caries lesions, and characterize the demineralization and remineralization of enamel [48].

Electrical current methods have higher sensitivity but lower specificity than clinical visual examination, visible light, and laser light-based caries detection technologies. Furthermore, this method is currently limited to occlusal and smooth surface caries detection [47, 49].

6.6 Other Methods

6.6.1 Digital Photographs and Videos

Digital photos have become the tools that we use in every aspect of our lives. Almost all people have smartphones that can take pictures. Mobile phones, digital extraoral cameras, intraoral cameras, and intraoral scanners have come to a very important place in patient evaluation and inform patients today.

Similar to visual examination, possible caries can be evaluated in photographs taken from the oral region. These photos can also be easily shared with colleagues or patients. Patients can also evaluate these images themselves. It is much more comfortable to give information to patients in a photograph or video showing the inside of their mouth, rather than describing caries or sound tissue on a radiology image.

Just like visual examination, caries evaluation from digital images will not give very accurate results without the tactile method or other methods such as radiography. The images show only the superficial part of the possible lesion and do not give information such as the depth and hardness of the tissue. On the other hand, it has been shown that demineralized regions can be detected in studies with photographs. Again, with photo editing software and artificial intelligence software, improvements have been made in the detection of caries from photographs. There are also studies showing that these methods give much more sensitive results besides just visual inspection [50, 51].

Popular and advanced intraoral scanners are among the exciting tools of today. Thanks to its artificial intelligence, potential caries areas can be easily examined by both the dentist and the patient with images that are free of saliva and tissues, showing all the arches of the patients, and can be rotated. Again, with the fluorescence modes of these scanners that show the plaque on the tissues, patients and dentists can obtain information not only about possible caries regions but also regions which can develop caries lesions [52, 53].

In the new era where prevention is more important than detecting, determining the spots where caries can start and more importantly being able to educate the patient should be the main goal of today's dentistry. These radiation-free and increasingly widespread devices will perhaps be the leader of preventive dentistry.

References

1. Wenzel A, Møystad A. Work flow with digital intraoral radiography: a systematic review. Acta Odontol Scand. 2010;68(2):106–14.
2. Neuhaus K, Ellwood R, Lussi A, Pitts N. Traditional lesion detection aids. Detection, assessment, diagnosis and monitoring of caries. Monogr Oral Sci. 2009;21:42–51.
3. Göstemeyer G, Schwendicke F. Digital bitewing radiographs. In: Ferreira Zandona A, Longbottom C, editors. Detection and assessment of dental caries: a clinical guide. Cham: Springer International Publishing; 2019. p. 119–26.
4. Mestriner SF, Vinha D, Mestriner JW. Comparison of different methods for the occlusal dentine caries diagnosis. J Appl Oral Sci. 2005;13:28–34.
5. Schlee M, Schad T, Koch JH, Cattin PC, Rathe F. Clinical performance of self-assembling peptide P11-4 in the treatment of initial proximal carious lesions: a practice-based case series. J Investig Clin Dent. 2018;9(1):e12286.
6. Wenzel A. A review of dentists' use of digital radiography and caries diagnosis with digital systems. Dentomaxillofac Radiol. 2006;35(5):307–14.
7. Wenzel A. Radiographic display of carious lesions and cavitation in approximal surfaces: advantages and drawbacks of conventional and advanced modalities. Acta Odontol Scand. 2014;72(4):251–64.
8. Yasa Y, Çelik Ö, Bayrakdar IS, Pekince A, Orhan K, Akarsu S, et al. An artificial intelligence proposal to automatic teeth detection and numbering in dental bite-wing radiographs. Acta Odontol Scand. 2021;79(4):275–81.
9. Başaran M, Çelik Ö, Bayrakdar IS, Bilgir E, Orhan K, Odabaş A, et al. Diagnostic charting of panoramic radiography using deep-learning artificial intelligence system. Oral Radiol. 2022;38(3):363–9.
10. Price JB. Caries detection with dental cone beam computed tomography. In: Ferreira Zandona A, Longbottom C, editors. Detection and assessment of dental caries: a clinical guide. Cham: Springer International Publishing; 2019. p. 127–38.
11. Baltacıoğlu İH, Eren H, Yavuz Y, Kamburoğlu K. Diagnostic accuracy of different display types in detection of recurrent caries under restorations by using CBCT. Dentomaxillofac Radiol. 2016;45(6):20160099.
12. Gaalaas L, Tyndall D, Mol A, Everett ET, Bangdiwala A. Ex vivo evaluation of new 2D and 3D dental radiographic technology for detecting caries. Dentomaxillofac Radiol. 2016;45(3):20150281.
13. Melo SLS, Belem MDF, Prieto LT, Tabchoury CPM, Haiter-Neto F. Comparison of cone beam computed tomography and digital intraoral radiography performance in the detection of artificially induced recurrent caries-like lesions. Oral Surg Oral Med Oral Pathol Oral Radiol. 2017;124(3):306–14.
14. Charuakkra A, Prapayasatok S, Janhom A, Pongsiriwet S, Verochana K, Mahasantipiya P. Diagnostic performance of cone-beam computed tomography on detection of mechanically-created artificial secondary caries. Imaging Sci Dent. 2011;41(4):143–50.
15. Aglarci OS, Bilgin MS, Erdem A, Ertas ET. Is it possible to diagnose caries under fixed partial dentures with

cone beam computed tomography? Oral Surg Oral Med Oral Pathol Oral Radiol. 2015;119(5):579–83.
16. Pretty IA. Caries detection and diagnosis: novel technologies. J Dent. 2006;34(10):727–39.
17. Ando M, Hall A, Eckert G, Schemehorn B, Analoui M, Stookey G. Relative ability of laser fluorescence techniques to quantitate early mineral loss in vitro. Caries Res. 1997;31(2):125–31.
18. De Jong EJ, Sundström F, Westerling H, Tranaeus S, Ten Bosch J, Angmar-Månsson B. A new method for in vivo quantification of changes in initial enamel caries with laser fluorescence. Caries Res. 1995;29(1):2–7.
19. Lee ES, de Josselin de Jong E, Kim BI. Detection of dental plaque and its potential pathogenicity using quantitative light-induced fluorescence. J Biophotonics. 2019;12(7):e201800414.
20. Lee E-S, Kang S-M, Ko H-Y, Kwon H-K, Kim B-I. Association between the cariogenicity of a dental microcosm biofilm and its red fluorescence detected by quantitative light-induced fluorescence-digital (QLF-D). J Dent. 2013;41(12):1264–70.
21. Alammari MR, Smith PW, de Josselin de Jong E, Higham SM. Quantitative light-induced fluorescence (QLF): a tool for early occlusal dental caries detection and supporting decision making in vivo. J Dent. 2013;41(2):127–32.
22. Ko H-Y, Kang S-M, Kim HE, Kwon H-K, Kim B-I. Validation of quantitative light-induced fluorescence-digital (QLF-D) for the detection of approximal caries in vitro. J Dent. 2015;43(5):568–75.
23. Zandoná AF, Zero DT. Diagnostic tools for early caries detection. J Am Dent Assoc. 2006;137(12):1675–84.
24. Kreher D, Park K-J, Schmalz G, Schulz-Kornas E, Haak R, Ziebolz D. Evaluation of quantitative light-induced fluorescence to assess lesion depth in cavitated and non-cavitated root caries lesions—an in vitro study. Photodiagn Photodyn Ther. 2022;37:102675.
25. Pretty IA, Smith PW, Edgar WM, Higham SM. Detection of in vitro demineralization adjacent to restorations using quantitative light induced fluorescence (QLF). Dent Mater. 2003;19(5):368–74.
26. de Almeida NA, Coutinho E, Vivan Cardoso M, Lambrechts P, Van Meerbeek B. Current concepts and techniques for caries excavation and adhesion to residual dentin. J Adhes Dent. 2011;13(1):7.
27. Lennon A, Attin T, Buchalla W. Quantity of remaining bacteria and cavity size after excavation with FACE, caries detector dye and conventional excavation in vitro. Oper Dent. 2007;32(3):236–41.
28. Macey R, Walsh T, Riley P, Hogan R, Glenny AM, Worthington HV, et al. Transillumination and optical coherence tomography for the detection and diagnosis of enamel caries. Cochrane Database Syst Rev. 2021;1:CD013855.
29. Strassler HE, Pitel ML. Using fiber-optic transillumination as a diagnostic aid in dental practice. Compend Contin Educ Dent. 2014;35(2):80–8.
30. Hogan R, Pretty IA, Ellwood RP. Fibre-optic Transillumination: FOTI. In: Ferreira Zandona A, Longbottom C, editors. Detection and assessment of dental caries: a clinical guide. Cham: Springer International Publishing; 2019. p. 139–50.
31. Pretty IA, Maupomé G. A closer look at diagnosis in clinical dental practice: part 5. Emerging technologies for caries detection and diagnosis. J Can Dent Assoc. 2004;70:540–1.
32. Ástvaldsdóttir Á, Åhlund K, Holbrook WP, de Verdier B, Tranæus S. Approximal caries detection by DIFOTI: *in vitro* comparison of diagnostic accuracy/efficacy with film and digital radiography. Int J Dent. 2012;2012:326401.
33. Bin-Shuwaish M, Yaman P, Dennison J, Neiva G. The correlation of DIFOTI to clinical and radiographic images in class II carious lesions. J Am Dent Assoc. 2008;139(10):1374–81.
34. Söchtig F, Hickel R, Kühnisch J. Caries detection and diagnostics with near-infrared light transillumination: clinical experiences. Quintessence Int. 2014;45(6):531.
35. Baltacioglu IH, Orhan K. Comparison of diagnostic methods for early interproximal caries detection with near-infrared light transillumination: an in vivo study. BMC Oral Health. 2017;17(1):130.
36. Near-Infrared KJ, Transillumination L. In: Ferreira Zandona A, Longbottom C, editors. Detection and assessment of dental caries: a clinical guide. Cham: Springer International Publishing; 2019. p. 151–8.
37. Abdelaziz M, Krejci I. DIAGNOcam—a near infrared digital imaging Transillumination (NIDIT) technology. Int J Esthet Dent. 2015;10(1):158–65.
38. Błażejewska A, Dacyna N, Niesiobędzki P, Trzaska M, Gozdowski D, Turska-Szybka A, et al. Comparison of the detection of proximal caries in children and youth using DIAGNOcam® and bitewing radiovisiography. Dent Med Probl. 2016;53(4):468–75.
39. Ortiz MIG, de Melo AC, De Paula BLF, Magno MB, Maia LC, Silva CM. Accuracy of near-infrared light transillumination (NILT) compared to bitewing radiograph for detection of interproximal caries in the permanent dentition: a systematic review and meta-analysis. J Dent. 2020;98:103351.
40. Neuhaus KW, Lussi A. DIAGNOdent. Detection and assessment of dental caries. Cham: Springer; 2019. p. 171–5.
41. Ástvaldsdóttir Á, Tranæus S, Karlsson L, Peter HW. DIAGNOdent measurements of cultures of selected oral bacteria and demineralized enamel. Acta Odontol Scand. 2010;68(3):148–53.
42. Shi X-Q, Tranæus S, Angmar-Månsson B. Validation of DIAGNOdent for quantification of smooth-surface caries: an in vitro study. Acta Odontol Scand. 2001;59(2):74–8.
43. Lennon A, Buchalla W, Switalski L, Stookey G. Residual caries detection using visible fluorescence. Caries Res. 2002;36(5):315–9.
44. Alleman DS, Magne P. A systematic approach to deep caries removal end points: the peripheral seal

concept in adhesive dentistry. Quintessence Int. 2012;43(3):197–208.
45. Amaechi BT. Photothermal radiometry and modulated luminescence: the canary system. Detection and assessment of dental caries. Cham: Springer; 2019. p. 177–86.
46. Jeon RJ, Han C, Mandelis A, Sanchez V, Abrams SH. Diagnosis of pit and fissure caries using frequency-domain infrared photothermal radiometry and modulated laser luminescence. Caries Res. 2004;38(6):497–513.
47. Longbottom C, Huysmans M-C. Electrical measurements for use in caries clinical trials. J Dent Res. 2004;83(1_suppl):76–9.
48. Liao Y-M, Feng Z-D, Chen Z-L. In situ tracing the process of human enamel demineralization by electrochemical impedance spectroscopy (EIS). J Dent. 2007;35(5):425–30.
49. Huysmans M-C, Longbottom C, Pitts N, Los P, Bruce P. Impedance spectroscopy of teeth with and without approximal caries lesions-an in vitro study. J Dent Res. 1996;75(11):1871–8.
50. Prapayasatok S, Janhom A, Verochana K, Pramojanee S. Digital camera resolution and proximal caries detection. Dentomaxillofac Radiol. 2006;35(4):253–7.
51. Duong DL, Kabir MH, Kuo RF. Automated caries detection with smartphone color photography using machine learning. Health Informatics J. 2021;27(2):14604582211007530.
52. Michou S, Lambach MS, Ntovas P, Benetti AR, Bakhshandeh A, Rahiotis C, et al. Automated caries detection in vivo using a 3D intraoral scanner. Sci Rep. 2021;11(1):1–9.
53. Róth I, Czigola A, Fehér D, Vitai V, Joós-Kovács GL, Hermann P, et al. Digital intraoral scanner devices: a validation study based on common evaluation criteria. BMC Oral Health. 2022;22(1):1–17.

7 Digital Shade Matching in Dentistry

Pantelis Kouros

7.1 Colorimetry in Dentistry

7.1.1 Importance of Proper Shade Matching

Shade matching is a constant everyday challenge for a clinical dentist. Failure to match a part of a tooth to a restorative material often leads to extension of restoration, so that it completely covers the aesthetic surface, meaning that instead of matching restoration to tooth, converting tooth appearance to the one of the restoration materials. This is not lacking biological cost, as unnecessary removal of healthy tissues is often needed to fit restoration material in limits of tooth's clinical crown, or to cover minimum material thickness requirements for mechanical strength. Additionally, appearance matching of a single crown in the aesthetic zone is considered one of the most difficult tasks, and this leads clinicians to a 2-4-6 crowning approach. This leads to further healthy tissue loss, which for a single tooth may reach up to 70% loss of crown volume, depending on the preparation design [1].

The past, present, and future of shade selection regarding materials, techniques, and practices in daily dental practice to maximize aesthetics.

P. Kouros (✉)
Operative Dentistry, Aristotle University of Thessaloniki, Thessaloniki, Greece
e-mail: kourosp@dent.auth.gr

A. Delantoni, K. Orhan (eds.), *Digital Dentistry*, https://doi.org/10.1007/978-3-031-52826-2_7

Crowning of teeth for aesthetic reasons only is opening a cycle which includes a high possibility of loss within years, as has been described from Elderton [2] and Simonsen [3] and recently has been verified by Burke [4]. Proper shade matching to satisfy patient's social needs at minimum could prove beneficial for the patient and cost-effective for both the patient and insurance companies, as it eradicates the need for bigger interventions and the possibility of unfavorable future events.

7.2 Current Practices

Most of dental clinicians today are using shade tabs to visually match hard tissues to materials. Shade tabs may be either universal and refer to a commonly accepted shade system (e.g., Vita Classical, or Vita 3D), or alternatively, specific corresponding to a shade series of materials produced by the same manufacturer. For cost reasons, most of such tabs are made of acrylic rather than a material similar in molecular structure to the final product (composite of ceramic). This is initiating issues related to metameristic properties and visual behavior of materials.

7.2.1 Metamerism

Metamerism is a physical property of materials to appear different in color when wavelengths of incident light change. It depends on molecular structure for translucent tissues or materials and on surface properties for completely opaque materials. Changing the wavelength of the incident light means that there are alterations to interaction on a surface or in the volume of a material or tissue, due to differences in the way that photons collide and refract to atoms or penetrate through, thus, altering the wavelength that returns towards observer's visual receptors. Consequently, an acrylic shade tab that appears the same shade to a composite or a ceramic in each illumination condition may differ when this condition changes even slightly. The same claim stands when comparing hard tissues to shade tables.

A way to overcome metameristic issues between tabs and final restorative product is constructing shade tabs from the same material (ceramic or composite). The problem is that this would be too costly and would still be valid only for materials and tabs manufactured by the same manufacturer. Such a system is offered for composites selection of Micerium S.p.A. (Via Marconi, 83, 16036 Avegno (Ge) Italy) related to HRi composites series.

A different approach to overcome metamerism would be construction of custom shade tabs, directly from the composite or the combination of that the dentist is aiming to use. Silicone matrices for the purpose are offered by Smile Line (PO Box 229, Z.I La Clef 5, 2610 St-Imier, Switzerland) or from GC (3-2-14 Hongo, Bunkyo-ku, Tokyo 113-0033, Japan) along with Essentia composites kit. Those are used to produce a tab by the same material to be used next for the final restoration and are even allowing construction of tabs consisted of dentin and enamel shades. The disadvantages of the method are the great waste of costly materials, the time-consuming procedure, and the visual estimation of matching.

7.2.2 Shade Tabs Consistency

Shade tabs are made of acrylic, a synthetic material which is cheaper than composites or ceramics, but it does not demonstrate optical stability over time. In fact, the repeatable use of disinfectants and UV-aging are altering the shade in a slow, constant rate, which is difficult to be noticed. There are data suggesting that changing of shade tabs every two years is necessary. Consistency issues may be also present at the production line; thus slight differences in shade are possible.

7.2.3 Observer Subjectivity

Visual shade matching is directly observer dependent. However, color perception may differ for individuals as it is the translation of the optical stimulus from the optical apparatus.

7.2.3.1 Cornea

Cornea covers the pupil, iris, and front chamber of the eye, and ideally it should be glass-transparent, not affecting wavelengths passing through. However, physiological conditions such as aging or a series of severe or less severe corneal disorders may change wavelengths, causing an individual to see "through a colored filter," similar to wearing colored glasses. This may alter shade perception or affect the ability of perceiving slight color differences.

Aging causes both structural and functional changes and affects the ability to refract light [5]. Usually, it is accompanied by "yellowing," which causes objects to appear more yellow to the observer. This in a representation would appear same as the picture … where on the right side are teeth of a young individual depicted as perceived by a DSLR camera, while on the left side a yellow filter has been digitally added to demonstrate the difference in perception of a young eye versus an aged one.

7.2.3.2 Retina

Vision in humans is considered to be trichromatic, meaning that all colors that we see is a result of proportional combination of red, blue, and green. This is because the human retina contains three types of cone cells, each type responsible for perceiving a color, namely L-cones for red, S-cones for blue, and M-cones for green. The perception of colors is a combination of neural response and response intensity of each type of cones.

Tetrachromacy is a condition where an individual possesses 4 types of cone sensitivity [6], enabling to see via 4 channels. In nature, it is common among certain species, but in humans it is a rare condition that has been described in relation to 2 opsin genes, OPN1MW and OPN1MW2, which are present in the X-chromosome; therefore, it is linked to people with a pair of X-chromosome (females). In humans, up to 50% of women and 8% of men are reported with increased color differentiation. A study suggests that 15% of women worldwide might be tetrachromats [7]; however, despite they differentiate colors better than trichromats, there is a possibility that most of them are not fully functional tetrachromats. There is however an established case of a fully functional tetrachromat woman [7].

Color vision may also be negatively influenced by a series of conditions related to congenital conditions, diseases, or medical treatments. Achromatopsia, or color blindness, is a congenital lack of functionality of one or more classes of rode cells. It can be partial, related to a specific color group, or total, when the individual is unable to see colors and usually is related also to decreased visual acuity and light sensitivity (photophobia). In its less severe versions, coping mechanisms allow adaptation and the individual is likely unaware of his condition. However, related to dental profession, a color blindness test is advisable, as vision is important to shade matching. Conditions that may lead to the development of color blindness are also glaucoma, Alzheimer's disease, injuries, or some medications, such as hydroxychloroquine which is used against malaria, lupus erythematosus, and rheumatoid arthritis.

7.2.3.3 Visual Cortex

Humans, like all other species, are a result of evolution over centuries. During this, men have adapted to hunting which gave them the ability to calculate distance and speed, while women were responsible for gathering and acquired the ability to distinguish slight color differences. Given that the visual cortex is rich in testosterone receptors, combined with a high level of androgens in males and polymorphic nature of genes related to cones cells, Abramov et al. support the neurological nature of differences in color perception. In their publications, they have tested sex-related vision differences, and according to that, men require slightly longer wavelengths to experience the same hue and are less adept at distinguishing among the shades at the center of the visible spectrum (yellows, greens, and blues), but are better in perceiving sizes from a far space [8, 9]. These conclusions indicate that women are expected to perform better in shade matching, especially in dentistry since they can distinguish smaller deviations in wavelengths in yellows, as has been previously said.

Lehmann et al.'s publication affirms these expectations, testing the reliability of shade matching using Vita shade tabs among sexes and concluding that females can significantly match better than males. Additionally, they found that better results were for both sexes in reddish-yellowish hue (Vita B-group). Most importantly, they demonstrated a success as low as 72.5% for visual shade matching, while for digital matching with the use of a spectrophotometer this success rose up to 98,9% [10].

Experience

It seems that a dentist's experience is an important factor in deciding on shade. A study has demonstrated greater success on experienced dentists, compared to dental students. This result was not to be expected considering aging alterations in cornea; however it seems that most important values in shade matching are translucency and luminosity rather than hue, and there could be a learning curve on distinguishing those color qualities related to experience [11].

7.3 Protocols for Visual Shade Matching

Recommendations of actions and setups for optimizing visual shade matching in dentistry are not always feasible for everyday clinical practice, especially for busy surgeries. They are as follows:

1. Remove any presence of make-up or lipstick from the patient. Lipstick, especially in dark colors, is increasing perception of contrast and may lead to the selection of a brighter shade than that of natural dentition.
2. Cleaning and polishing of teeth. Use of ultrasound devices and pumice paste on the teeth surface, surgical suction, and the need for the patient to open their mouth during procedures can lead to the dehydration of hard tissues. This will lead to misperception of color as teeth will appear more bright and less translucent. Consequently, it is advisable to perform those procedures one or two days before final shade decision.
3. Maintain an arm-length distance from the subject.
4. Position the dental chair so that the patient's eyes are level at dentist's eyes.
5. To perceive luminosity squinting of eyes will activate rods and responsible retina cells for vision in low-light conditions.
6. Calibrate eyes staring on a blue subject. To perceive color, a photo-switchable protein named rhodopsin that is contained in retina cones is activated, passes from trans to cis form, produces the signal received from optical nerve, and transfers to the visual cortex. Prolonged staring at a specific object consumes all cis rhodopsin molecules; thus nerve stimulus becomes weaker and distinction of different wavelengths difficult. Eye calibration aims to provide time to cis form return to trans and restore the ability to distinguish colors. Staring at a blue object aims to restore trans rhodopsin forms in L and M-cones (red and green) thus increasing sensibility to yellow. However, it fatigues S-cones (blue) and deviates the vision of neutral colors slightly towards yellow. Consequently, updated guidelines is to calibrate vision in a neutral gray surface.
7. Selection must be made within 5 s. Cone fatigue, as described above is the reason.
8. Color match at early morning. Color vision is psychotropic and is influenced not only by psychological condition, but also by fatigue.
9. Incident light should be between 5000 and 6000 °K. Better lighting conditions are Northern lights through big windows.

7.4 Button-Try Technique for Composite Shade Selection

Utilizing this technique is a way to overcome metameristic issues or issues related to inconsistencies of shade tabs color or inconsistencies among tabs and composites. It is only utilizable for direct restorations, and it has its merits and drawbacks as well.

Description: Small pieces of composites from the intended to be used range are polymerized directly on the tissues to be matched. Dentin shades should be placed near the cervical area of the tooth, while enamel shades should be evaluated below the incisal edge and not over it, because translucency is the most important quality to be matched (Picture 7.1). Decision for the best material can be made visually but is better to be estimated in an intraoral photography. Ideally, best information for shade is obtained in a cross-polarized image (Picture 7.2). Polarization is filtering glare from a picture and is being used by photographers to depict objects below surfaces with glare (e.g., water surface). Circular polarization is removing the majority of glare, but complete removal can be achieved with cross

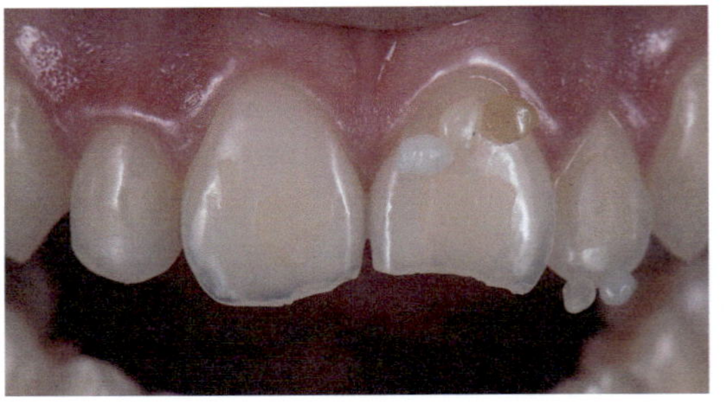

Picture 7.1 Buttons of composite polymerized on teeth surfaces for better shade selection. Dentin shades are positioned on the cervical area, while enamel shades hanging below incisal edge of teeth to be matched

polarization. To be achieved, linear polarizers (sheet filters) are positioned in front of light sources (flashes), complemented by a linear polarizer positioned in front of the lenses in an angulation of 90 degrees related to one of the flashes.

Some simple post-processing of digital image file with software available for all personal computers might help achieve the best shade selection. Reducing exposure and increasing chromaticity is best displaying dentin shade composites relation to dentin tissue (Picture 7.3). To better match enamel, color should be removed, and image should be converted to black/white. Removing of color aids to better understand translucency (Picture 7.4).

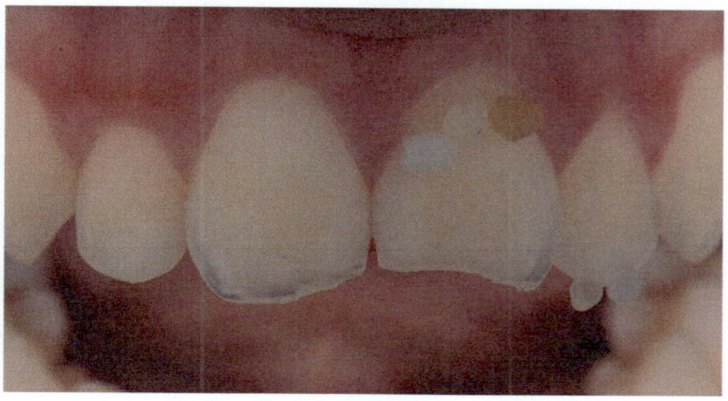

Picture 7.2 Same case and buttons, photographed with picture cross polarization

Button-try technique, despite overcoming metamerism, remains a qualitative way of deciding shade and relies on dentists' artistic capabilities and subjective vision specifications. Furthermore, both tissues and materials are relatively translucent; thus, color has thickness-dependent values. Buttons directly made on teeth surfaces cannot be equally thickly constructed, and this can lead to misinterpretation of their optical characteristics. Additionally, the time required to position and polymerize composite buttons and accompanied heat emitted by polymerization unit are enough to dehydrate hard tissues and rapidly change appearance, leading to a mistaken decision for a brighter and more opaque material. The best way to minimize the dehydration effect is to prepare buttons in a tool, then retract lips, position buttons with minimal air-drying, and block-polymerize all buttons not more than 3 s. Camera should be ready to capture a polarized picture, and all procedure should be completed within 1 min.

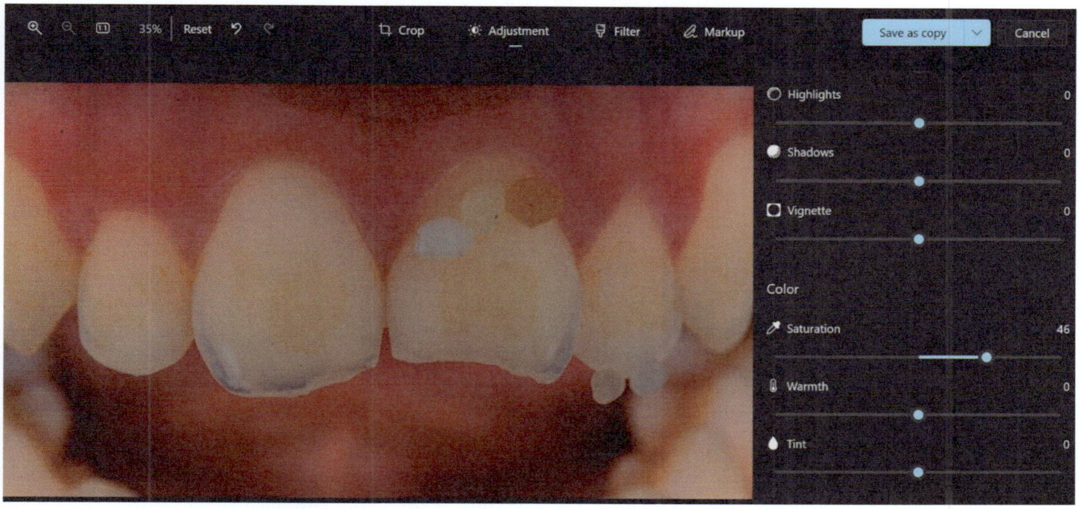

Picture 7.3 Oversaturated version provides more information on dentin shade selection

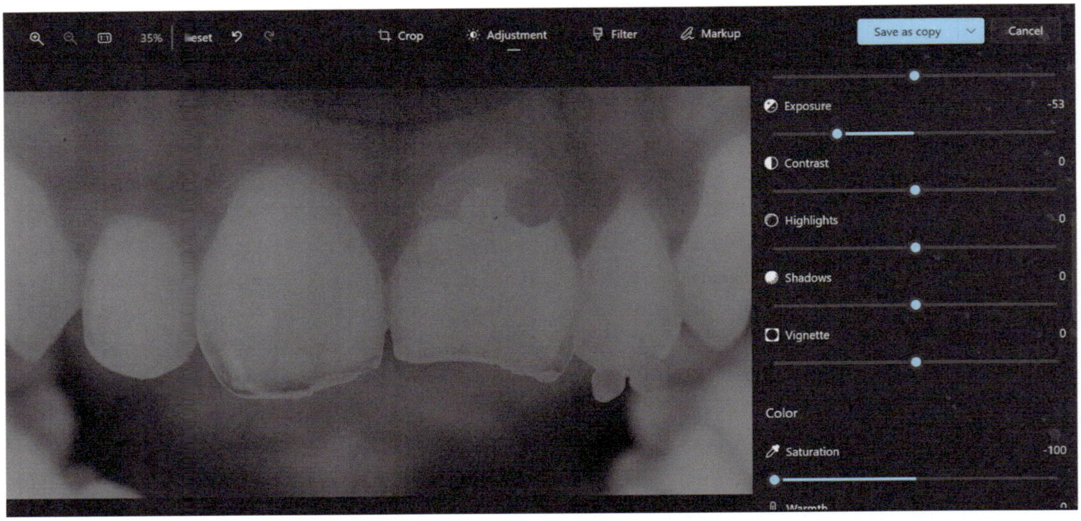

Picture 7.4 Complete removal of color aids to better select enamel shades, based on translucency only

7.5 Digital Shade Matching

7.5.1 Color Spaces

Despite that the majority of dental practicioners are relying on qualitative methods to match color, color is an objectively measurable quality. Foundations of Colorimetry has been set by Albert H. Munsell, a teacher of art at Massachusetts Normal Art School. Munsell published three books *A Color Notation* (1905), *Atlas of the Munsell Color System* (1915), and *A Grammar of Color: Arrangements of Strathmore Papers in a Variety of Printed Color Combinations According to The Munsell Color System* (1921). In his publications, he suggested a way to organize colors in a sphere positioning natural colors (grayscale) according to luminosity on a vertical axis (value axis, V), chromaticity (C) has been expressed in an analogic distance at the periphery of value axis, while hue (H) is expressed in different angles on the sphere's perimeter. In this way, color was able for the first time to be expressed with numerical values (HVC). The main disadvantage of Munsell's color space was uniformity, despite updates suggested by the Optical Society of America and later (1950) doubling the number of hues from 20 to 40.

In 1948, Hunter suggested Lab color space [12] based on the complementary color theory, as a uniform color scale. It is based on the theory of opponent color space as suggested by Ewald Hering [13], assuming that colors are perceived as pairs of opponent colors, light vs dark (L axis), red vs green (a axis), and blue vs against yellow (b axis). Colors positioned on L axis are all zero valued for a and b axes. Positive values for a and b correspond to red and yellow colors, while negative values to green and blue respectively. Hunter's system is compatible to be used with a tristimulus photoelectric colorimeter and utilizing the Euclidean distance formula, difference in color (ΔE) can be calculated. Today, most of the industry and applications are compliable with a 1976 modification suggested by the International Commission of Illumination (CIE). CIELab1976 values (L^*, a^*, b^*), differ to Hunter's values (L, a, b) to that the latter, are square roots in relation to CIEXYZ color space (a standard color space reference), while for CIELab1976 are cube roots. When comparing spaces in the yellow area that mostly concerns use in dentistry, Hunter's Lab color space is contracted, while CIELab color space is slightly overexpanded. Most of color-measuring systems and devices today are based on CIELab, 1976 modifications.

CIELab1976 color space remains today the most uniformly distributed and objective in terms of device-measuring system. However, the sensitivity of human eye to distinguish differences is higher for certain colors than others. The International Commission of Illumination introduced in 1994 CIE94 color space by adding application-specific weight coefficients in an extension to 1976 color space to address perceptual uniformities [14]. However, applications available were only graphic arts and textiles. Addition of five extra corrections in 2000 introduced CIEDE2000 color space which improved perceptual uniformity. Compensations added included a coefficient for neutral colors, lightness, chroma and hue, and a rotation term, to correct perception in blue [15]. Today, spectrophotometers, intraoral scanners, and photographic methods of shade recording entirely are based on the device-dependent CIELab1976 color space, despite there is evidence that to a human eye of a dentist, perceptual-oriented CIEDE2000 formulas perform better [16].

7.5.2 Colorimeters and Spectrophotometers

A colorimeter is a device equipped with a digital sensor capable of capturing tristimulus intensity, namely measuring chromaticity intensity for RGB color space (widely used in computer and television screens) individually for red, green, blue, and white (white represents luminosity). Digital sensors are supplied with Color Filters Array (CFA) or Color Filters Mosaic (CFM), which are responsible for color detection and wavelength specificity. A full-color image is formed adding the intensity of RGB wavelengths captured by CFA sheets. Differentiation on distribution and density of each element on CFA filters are manufacturer and model specific and configure RGB profile for each device. Colorimetric devices or cameras need to be satisfying Luther's condition, according to which spectral transmittance in connection with the spectral sensitivity of the sensors is in linear combination with the standard spectral value curves [17], which translates to that digital perception of color from a device should match average visual human color perception.

Colorimeters are less accurate compared to spectrophotometers; thus, their use was limited to monitor calibration. Recently digital photography, with the combination of a reference point of known color values depicted near an item to be assessed in color and picture processing software, gave rise to applications of digital cameras for colorimetric purposes. Methods used in dentistry for colorimetric applications of digital image capturing devices will be described in the following sections.

While a colorimeter is performing tristimulus measurements to measure color, a spectrophotometer utilizes wavelength-to-wavelength spectral analysis to indirectly calculate color values; consequently, spectrophotometers provide more accurate results. Both kinds of devices are illumination dependent; this means that wavelengths recorded are a result of reflection of transmission through the object of a particular wavelength, or a wavelength range. For colorimeters illuminant/observer pair is only one, while spectrophotometers can utilize more combinations. Spectrophotometers equipped with double or more illuminants are available to calculate different reflective curves for each transmitted wavelength and to determine metamerism. This is because for simplicity reasons, dental spectrophotometers are single-beam instruments. Unfortunately, double-beam spectrophotometers, although widely used in physics, chemistry, molecular biology, and other fields, are not yet available for clinical dentistry. Spectrophotometers are also capable of calculating reflectance, absorption, and translucency of an object. Similarly, some dental spectrophotometers only provided qualitative representation of areas of teeth, but there is not yet the option or the potential to a calculable translucency estimation.

7.5.3 Cameras and Digital Image Capturing Devices as Colorimetric Tools

A DSLR (Digital Single Lens Reflex) camera is equipped with a digital sensor. Digital sensor's surface is a diode-covered non-color-specific surface which can only transcript light to current. Diodes are only sensitive to light intensity independently on wavelength. Color is being reproduced thanks to CFA filters which have been previously described. Light is filtered to wavelengths and for each wavelength, the diode receives the correspondent intensity. Incorporation of intensities and wavelengths is expressing the final color in an additive (tristimulus) way. CFA's individual characteristics provide the sensors' RGB profile. This means that a different sensor produces different colors among the two pictures even if subject, frame, lens distance, exposure time, diaphragm opening, white balance, and lighting are kept the same. This issue is well known to photographers, especially when trying to reproduce real colors. The development of digital imaging allows for post-processing of an image file close to real colors. For doing so, an object of known optical dimensions must be depicted in the image file. Using an image processing software, such as Adobe Photoshop or Adobe Lightroom, is possible to alter digital image so that the depicted optical dimensions of the known object correspond to real ones. In compliance to this, all depicted objects are considered to be in real colors. Objects used for color reference most usually are gray cards. Gray cards are optically neutral surfaces which correspond to a* = 0, b* = 0, and a known L*. Most image processing software programs include a neutralization tool. In Adobe software, it appears as an eyedropper. Using this over a neutral surface (gray card), colors of the entire image are converted so that the area selected is neutralized. Then, the exposure tool is utilized to adjust luminosity of the same area to the actual L* value of the gray card according to it's known values. At this stage, the image is considered as calibrated and moving cursor over an area is considered to display real colors.

A disadvantage using this technique is that objects depicted in different distance related to light source than gray card, or objects depicted behind elements that may drop shadow on them, accept different amount of light and may appear more luminous or darker than actually are. This is why for dental applications, a gray card ideally is positioned directly below the incisal edge of tooth to be colorimetrically evaluated. Also, this is a colorimetric method of color measurement, which in relation to phasmatophotometric methods and instruments is illuminant-dependent, thus considered less accurate.

7.5.3.1 Smart Phones as Colorimetric Devices

A smartphone is a device which inside a small amount of space, combines photographic lenses, sensors, processors, and a display screen. In terms of photography, this constitutes a complete range of photography gear, compressed inside a single device. High marketing interest boosted orientation of manufacturers to invest towards cell phone development and favored rapid technology advancements. Current devices are in some respects equal or even better than expensive photographic equipment, yet volume limitations require software compensation.

Comparison of DSLR cameras and mobile phones as photographic devices:

Lenses: A DSLR camera has the ability of using different lenses according to its use. Lenses corresponding to human vision are considered to be those of focal length of 50 mm, while real macro (depiction of the real subject size) are considered to be a combination of a 100 mm lens and a full-frame sensor. Despite that objective documentation due to distortion factor and real size depiction should always require 1:1 shooting ratio; this in dentistry is most of the times not possible because of small frame size that would only include two central incisors. Thus, acceptance of existence of distortion factor is unavoidable. Smartphone lenses are not interchangeable and with fixed and short focal distance. Earlier models had

had a single lens for all kinds of photography, but current versions come with multiple lenses, each lens responsible for different shooting conditions. A sensor is coupled to each lens. Sensors are axiomatically smaller in size compared to a DSLR. Small lens and sensor sizes are responsible for poor performance in low light conditions. This does not affect smartphone use for dental photography, since in dental surgery conditions external light sources can provide adequate amount of light intensity. However, manufacturers have developed smart software which can enchase and—to a grade—correct prementioned issues. To describe cooperation of optics and software to compose a picture, the term used is computational photography. An example of such is multiple exposures automatically stitched in a single picture to overcome low lightning, known as HDR (High-Definition Range) technique. This is a known photography technique, which compensates areas of different exposure needs in a single frame. This in smartphones with a single lens is performed digitally. A single image file is used to patch areas selected from different exposure levels. Current smartphones are taking advantage of multiple lenses. Some phones produce a single file from continuing takes, by patching several pictures utilizing stable light sources depicted and blurring moving objects. The HDR mode is model and manufacturer dependent and differs for individual phone models. The main disadvantage of computational photography in smartphones is that it is an automated procedure that removes selection from operator; thus it is not advisable to be used in dentistry.

Documentation of a dental case requires a stable distortion factor. This is dependent on the distance of lens from the object. For DSLR's stable focal distance lenses such as ones used in dentistry, reproduction of distance is relatively easy. It only requires selection of manual focus and repetition in each picture of aspect ratio selected according to case. For smartphones this procedure is more difficult, mainly due to intervention of computational photography and focus and zoom utilities of each model. Most lenses in smartphones are of stable focal distance and zoom is performed digitally. A digital zoom is equal to post-acquiring image crop which means that it does not affect distortion factor, but only reduces image resolution, as it uses a smaller area on the sensor. Some more advanced phones have a limited capacity of optical zoom, using moving parts. Limited thickness of those devices does not allow a significant amount of optical zoom. Some models have integrated extruding lenses for optical zoom. Current smartphones switch automatically between standard, ultrawide, and telephoto cameras, depending on the users' manipulations, yet without user's control upon. This might create repeatability issues for documentation of a dental case, since distortion factor is not equal and depends on the lens utilized. A way to overcome those issues is to use the pro mode with full manual settings, maintaining identical adjustments, zoom indications, and exercising caution for frame reproduction in each picture throughout the procedure. Overall, DSLR cameras excel smartphones in terms of ease of use, but have significantly larger operation learning curve and cost.

The resolution of sensors that smartphones are equipped with is significantly higher compared to ones of conventional cameras with interchangeable lenses. This aims to compensate the significantly lower amount of light received from smaller lenses to smaller sensors. While a premium camera equipped with a full-frame sensor may bear resolutions of 20.2MP (Cannon 6D), there are smartphones that are reaching up to 108MP for the primary lens, assisted by 48MP on telephoto lens and 12MP on ultrawide lens (Samsung Galaxy S20 Ultra). For dental photography, given controlled lightning conditions, any smartphone with above 12MP primary lens sensor will be adequate.

Light Source

Options available for DSLR cameras in dentistry are mainly external flashes for macro-photography, which are positioned in front of the lens. Use of integrated flash in the camera is not indicated due to shadow produced by the lens. Macro flashes mostly used in dentistry are either positioned in a circle around lens (ring flashes) or provide a double light source, usually positioned on the right and left of the lens. Smartphones are also supplied with a light source, used in a stable (flashlight) rather than flashing mode. Integrated DSLR flashes provide a uni-directional beam, potentially leading to the depiction of more illuminated and shadowed areas, despite that for smartphones there is no lens shadow present. Great progress has been made in documentation with smartphones in dentistry, with the development of external illumination devices (Smile Lite MDP and similar). Those are continuous lights (usually produced by multiple LED lights) provided for use in live mode photography of with a smartphone which is mounted in a way that lenses are positioned in the specific hole on the device. They can produce results similar to a ring light when LEDs around the hole are activated, or similar to twin flashes, when side LEDs are on.

In terms of color documentation and measurement, areas that reflect light appear more luminous (higher L* values) than actually are. In photographic terms, areas that reflect light directly (similar to a mirror) are described as "burned areas" and appear as white areas with no color information. Cross-polarization technique is used to completely remove reflections and make all color dimensions of an object appear without reflection misinterpretation. Cross-polarizing filters are available in the market for each flash or can be made with the use of linear polarizer sheets positioned in front of flash and in front of the lens. To do so, lens polarizer sheet should be oriented in 90° linear polarization direction in relation to flash polarizer. For smartphones, polarizing filters usually accompany external illumination devices for mobile dental photography; therefore, it is an option available also to dentists using mobile documentation.

7.6 Image Post-Processing

Image files that are produced from image capturing devices do not correspond to real colors and bear characteristics of individual CFA filters. Also, images may appear less or more luminous compared to reality, dependent on the amount of light that reached the sensors which is reliant on the selected parameters while shooting. Calibrating images to what are considered as real colors requires simultaneous depiction of an object of known optical parameters and software post-processing. The object ideally should be equally illuminated and reflect light at the same amount as the area of interest does. Objects implied for this purpose are usually gray photographic cards. Gray cards are usually located on the central axis of CIELab1976 color space, which means they have $a^* = 0$ and $b^* = 0$ values. They may differ in terms of luminosity values, but L* should always be known. Any image processing software may be used, under the prerequisite that the software can process individually L* a* and b* parameters. The software used may be general photographic or specific to dental applications. The second variant is usually complete photographic protocols where specific gray cards accompany corresponding software and once the operator points at the gray neutral area, they automatically calibrate the image. Afterwards, software algorithms, are providing recipes for mixing of ceramic powders to better correspond to natural shades. Recipes are available for indirect restorations and those methods are marketed as communication with the lab tools. The most used non-dental-specific software are Adobe Photoshop and the lighter and more user-friendly Adobe Lightroom. An example of stages to calibrate an image in Lightroom follows in the pictures.

Unprocessed files (RAW files) consists of uncompressed (binary) data captured by the sensors and of all accompanying metadata such as date, exposure time, camera model, lens attached, etc. RAW files are not actually pictures but large files with lossless quality of raster images and info. RAW files can only be opened and processed and are significantly large, occupying lots of storage space in hard disks and memory cards. Most cameras, smartphones, and other capturing and reproduction devices and software are by default preset to shoot and read in the JPEG (Joint Photographic Experts Group) format. JPEGs are compressed image files that reduce original RAW data usually to 1:10 of storage volume. DSLR cameras can be set to shoot in the RAW format or even set to acquire dual files, both on RAW and JPEG. Both types of files can be processed in Lightroom for colorimetric reasons since they result in equal measurements. This is a result of the way that algorithm of JPEG format has been built. JPEG compression does not perform equally well when sharp contrasts are present in adjacent pixels. This is the case of diagrams, line drawings, etc. For depiction of human tissues (such as teeth) JPEG algorithm performs excellently. While JPEG is a lossy compression (meaning it is nonreversible), RAW files can be losslessly compressed, allowing reversible processing while keeping the original binary file intact. Therefore, they are preferred by professionals of photography. It does seem though that they do not offer any important advantage in colorimetric applications. Spectrophotometers that function with image processing read pixels color on a pre-calibrated image acquired by a calibrated system. Image files that are measured are low-quality JPEG images.

7.6.1 Accuracy

All imaging-based methods of defining color calculate color values over pixels. However, a single pixel may significantly differ from the average color of the included area. Therefore, the final displayed measurement does not correspond to a single pixel's color values, but average from values of pixels contained inside an area. The area size can usually be decided from an user when an image processing software has been used. The most frequent area size used for colorimetric purposes is a quadrant sized 5X5 = 25 pixels. Some phasmatophotometers are accompanied with software that offers the option to calculate average color out of complete tooth surface, or cervical, incisal, and middle third of a tooth, or even from small areas of 25 pixels.

It is inevitable that average CIELab values displayed when navigating over an image will deviate. Usually, when scouting over a relatively stable color area (such as gray card), this deviation ranges around 1–2% in terms of luminosity. This is because of small differences in reflectance and scattering of minor surface irregularities that may cause some pixels to appear brighter than others. The selection of a larger sample area is of benefit in such case of large color-uniform surfaces since it increases the sample size for extrapolating average values; however it will result in greater inaccuracies for non-uniform color areas. Thus, in such cases (teeth for instance), the smaller area option leads to more accurate measurements.

7.6.2 Image Processing

Any kind of picture processing software can be used to calibrate an image to what is considered true color and measure an object's color value. Adobe Photoshop is the most complete and complex available software. Also it requires more sources by computed processor; therefore, a simpler and "light" version is available and often is used for the purpoce. Steps followed in Adobe Lightroom are displayed in Pictures 7.5, 7.6, 7.7, 7.8, 7.9 and 7.10.

7.6.2.1 Translucency

All the abovementioned colorimetric methods perform well for completely opaque objects, where the actual value of Luminosity is not influenced by the amount of light absorbed or transmitted through its volume. However, this is not the case for teeth or human tissues in general. Teeth are semi-translucent, which means there is

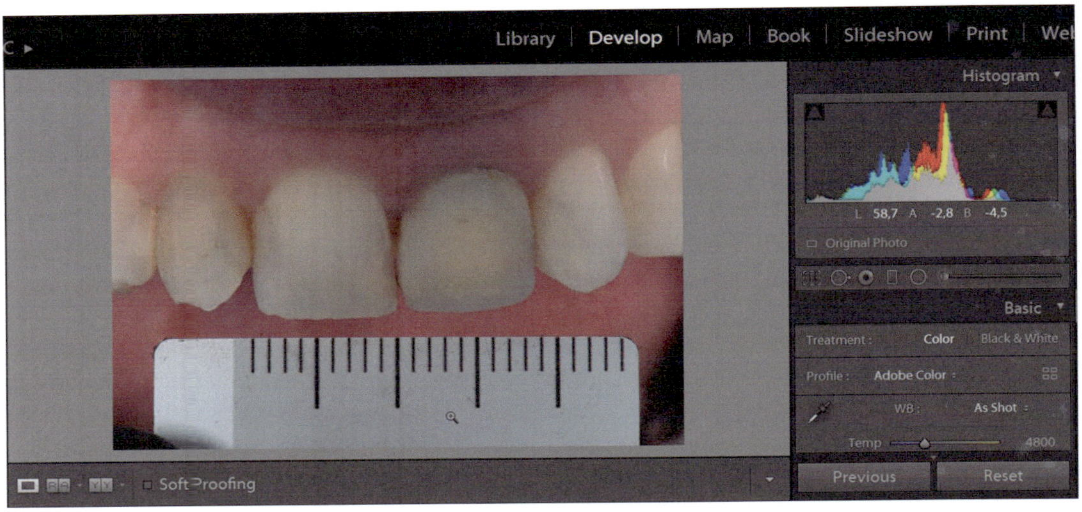

Picture 7.5 Importing a cross-polarized image in a picture processing software (in this case, Adobe Lightroom). Positioning the cursor above gray card is displaying L* = 58,7, a* = −2,8 and b* = −4,5. Known actual values of the object are L* = 75, a* = 0, and b* = 0. This actually means that the picture is underexposed and due to CFA filter characteristics, it appears more green and more blue than actual teeth colors

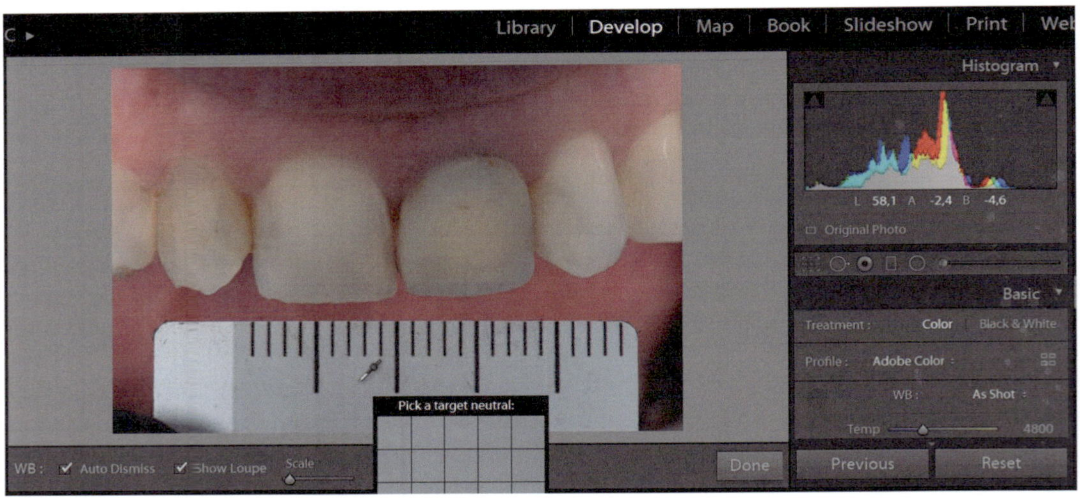

Picture 7.6 Eyedropper tool allows neutralization of colors. Clicking over a neutral area causes a* and b* values to be adjusted close to 0

a substantial percentage of light that is not scattered or refracted towards observer but absorbed from dentin mass and even illuminates soft tissues through its transmission into the root (optical fiber phenomenon).

In colorimetric of phasmatophotometric applications which are based on measurements in pixel values during reproduction of an image, the more translucent areas of an object appear less luminous. Even more, for dental applications, background is essential, since it influences teeth appearance during image acquiring. This means that when a black background (contrastor) is used, teeth appear different in color compared to the natural background (Pictures 7.11 and 7.12); translucent areas, mainly in incisal edge, appear

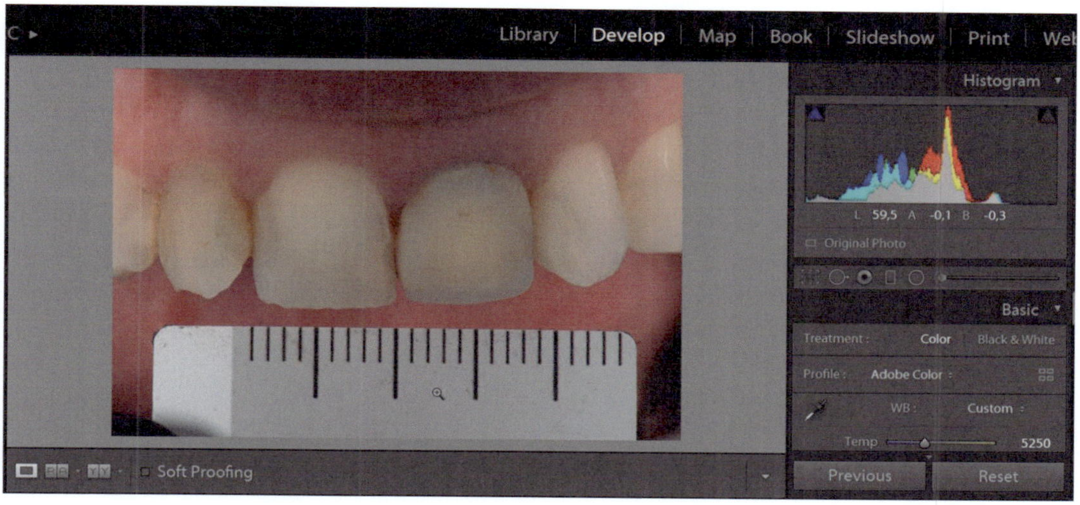

Picture 7.7 Neutralized image. Complete neutralization is not possible, since it is the average of area of 25 pixels that gets neutralized

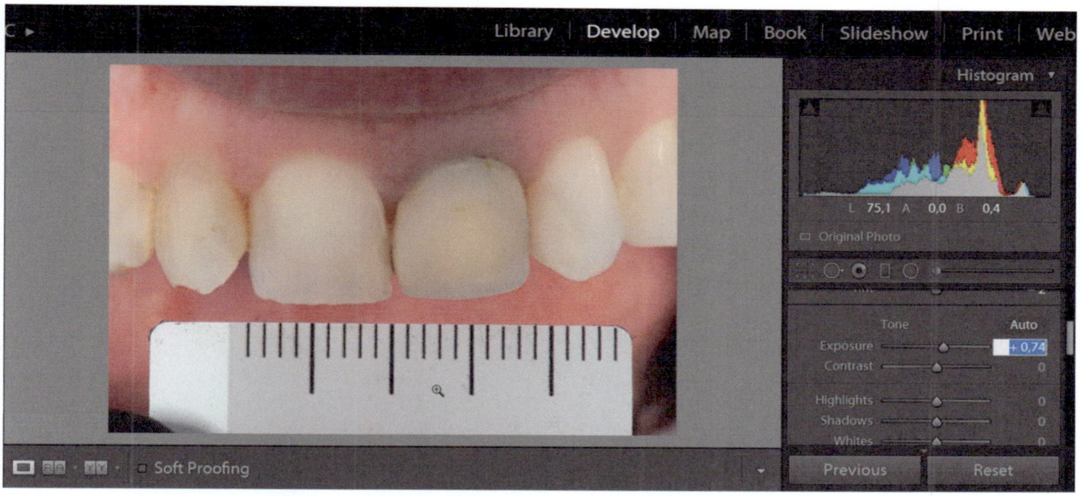

Picture 7.8 Adjustment of exposure occurs manually changing the value of exposure up to the point that a near to L* = 75 is displayed on histogram. Now the image is considered as neutralized and colors depicted as the real ones

dark, less luminous, while cervical areas are less influenced. This effect is linked to that for a semi-translucent object; optical values are directly dependent on its thickness. The thicker the object, the opaquer it becomes, while the more it becomes thin, the more it is influenced by the background it is placed.

The same principles are also applied in composite resins which are built with different grades of translucency by different manufacturers. Even more, composites despite in their microstructure are heterogenous masses (organic matrix and inorganic fillers in different sizes and shapes); they constitute a homogeneous mass regarding their optical behavior, and this makes them more translucent, since less scattering of light occurs when it interacts with the material.

Colorimetric applications are calculating pixel's average values. A tooth's incisal translucency is depicted as a black (or a substantially less

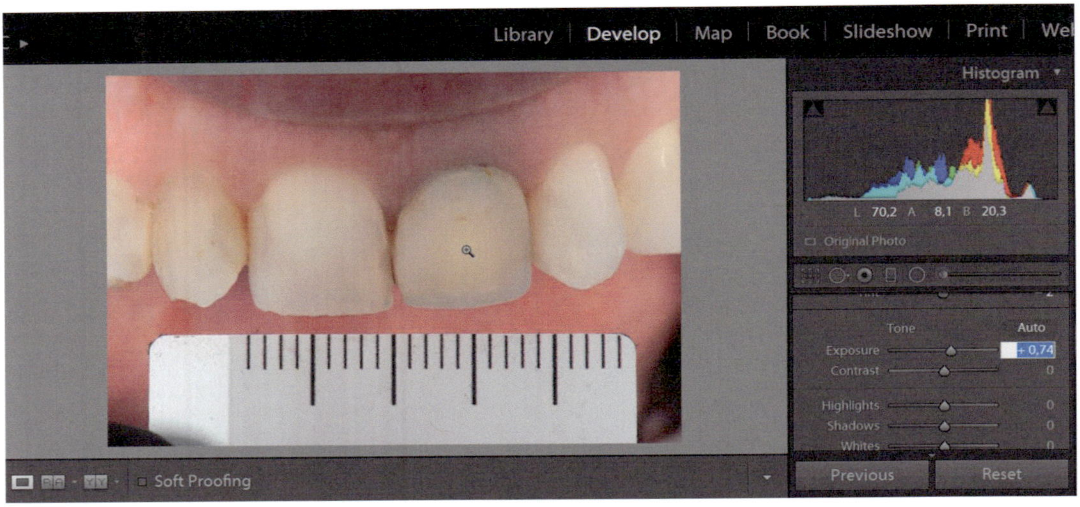

Picture 7.9 Positioning the cursor over restoration, values displayed on histogram are considered the actual restoration values

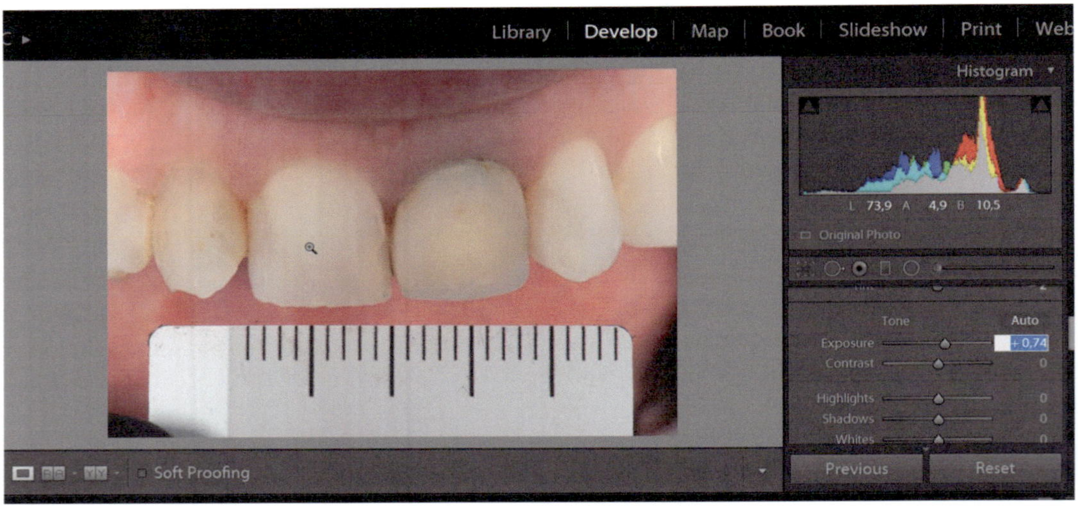

Picture 7.10 In the same way we can measure the adjacent natural tooth and calculate ΔE (in this case ΔE = 14,4)

luminous) area in dental photography. For a processor and running software, those are counting as low in L-value pixels, despite interpretation for a human brain indicating a "translucent" area. Subsequently, for colorimetry applications, completely opaque objects can be accurately represented in color values and replicated, using only 3 dimensions of CIELab1976 scale. But for a semi-translucent object, using only those 3 color dimensions would result in a 2-dimensional reproduction of a 3-dimensional object, like what a painter does with its models, or to what a photography does in relation to actual depictions. Accurate 3-dimensional reproduction of a semi-translucent object requires calculation of the fourth dimension of color, translucency.

Currently, only in Spectroshade Phasmatophotometer has been incorporated an algorithm that is approximately estimating translucency providing a rather qualitative representation. However, a quantitative estimation of translucency is possible, using the Euclidean distance

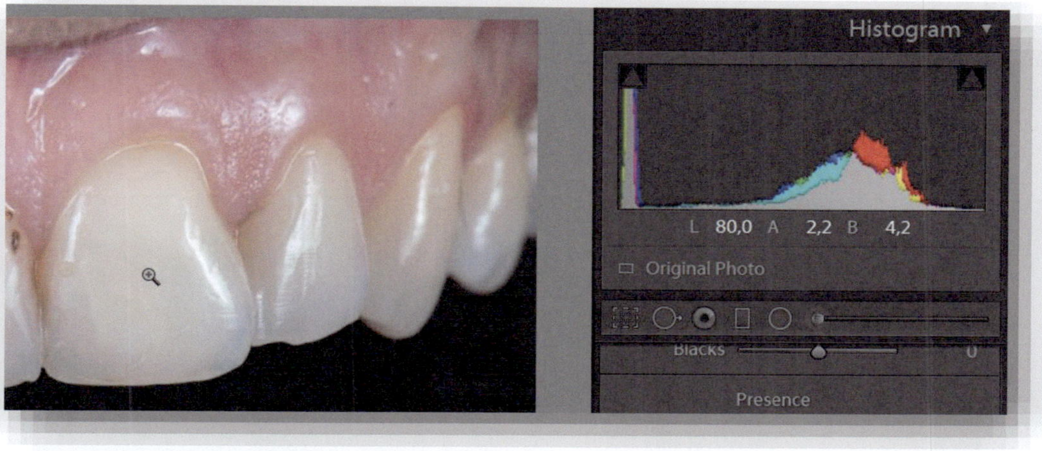

Picture 7.11 Tooth photographed against a contrastor (artificial black background is displayed significantly more luminous related to natural background)

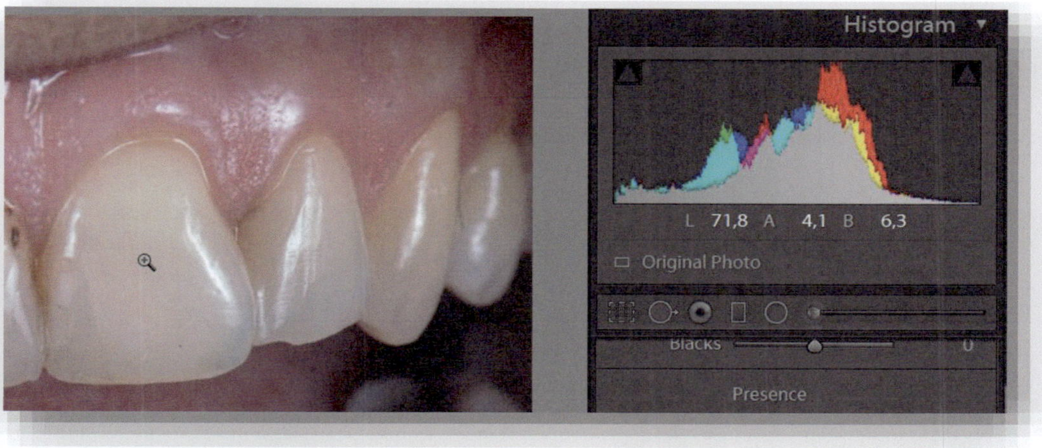

Picture 7.12 Same tooth, photographed under the same conditions and at the same time with previous picture. Its appearance is significantly affected by background and tooth now appears darker

formula for Lab values of the same object against black versus values against white background. Namely, translucency is defined as such, meaning the color differences of an object against white and black. A completely opaque material would not change its color values, meaning that TP will be counted as 0. Euclidean formula for translucency would be expressed as $TP = [(Lb - Lw)^2 + (ab - aw)^2 + (bb - bw)^2]^{1/2}$.

where Lb, ab, and bb represent values against black background, while Lw, aw, and bw against white.

For measuring translucency over a picture, a gray card that functions as a calibration tool should be able to provide the ability of modifying background in the same picture. Therefore, a gray card which is small in dimensions and contains a black and a white subsequent area that can be positioned directly behind the incisal edge can be utilized for translucency calculations. Such a card has been developed by the author (DSN card) (Picture 7.16), and together with a dedicated software presented next (Dental Shade Navigator—DSN) a translucency and color matching tool for use with direct restorations has been provided. Translucency measurement is presented in Pictures 7.13, 7.14 and 7.15.

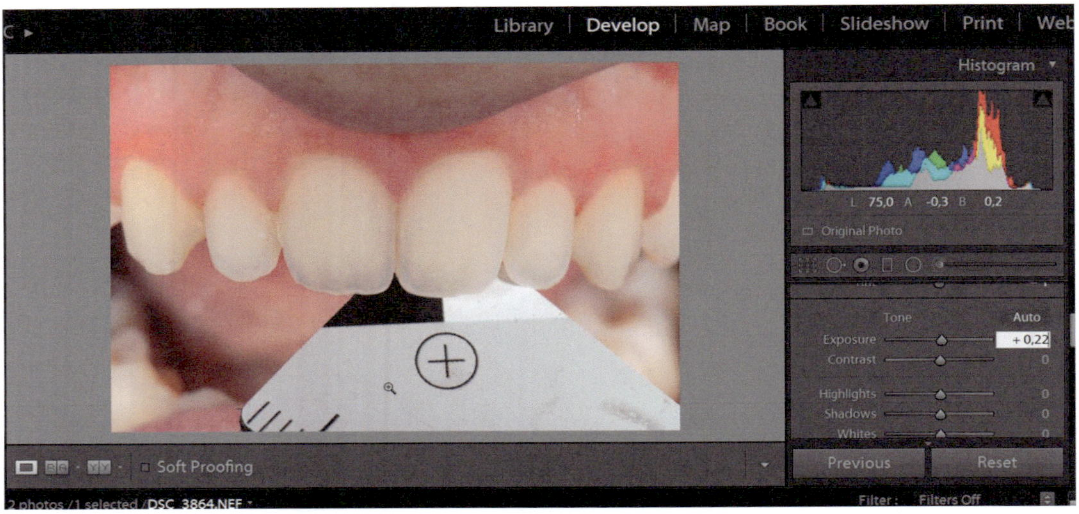

Picture 7.13 Translucency measurement, step one, image calibration

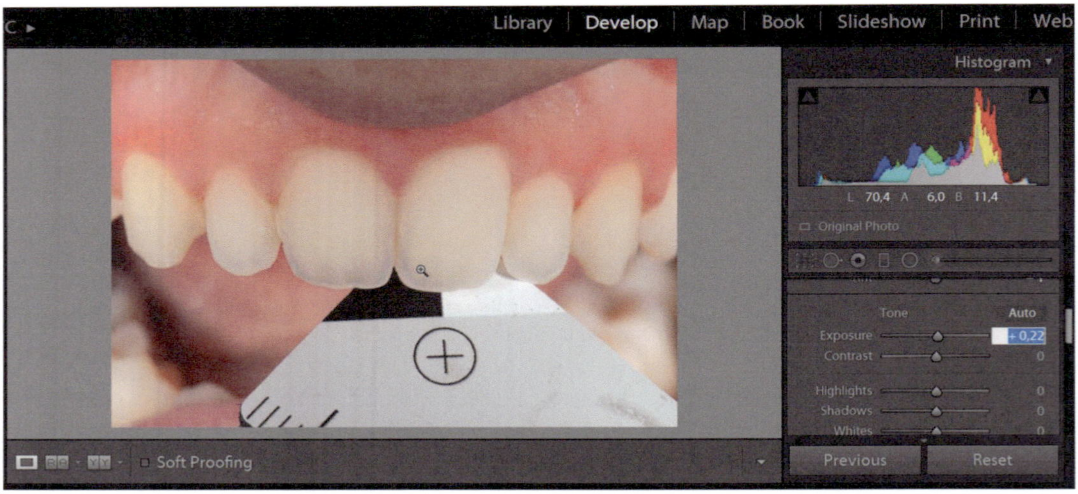

Picture 7.14 Translucency measurement, step two, measurement of values against black background

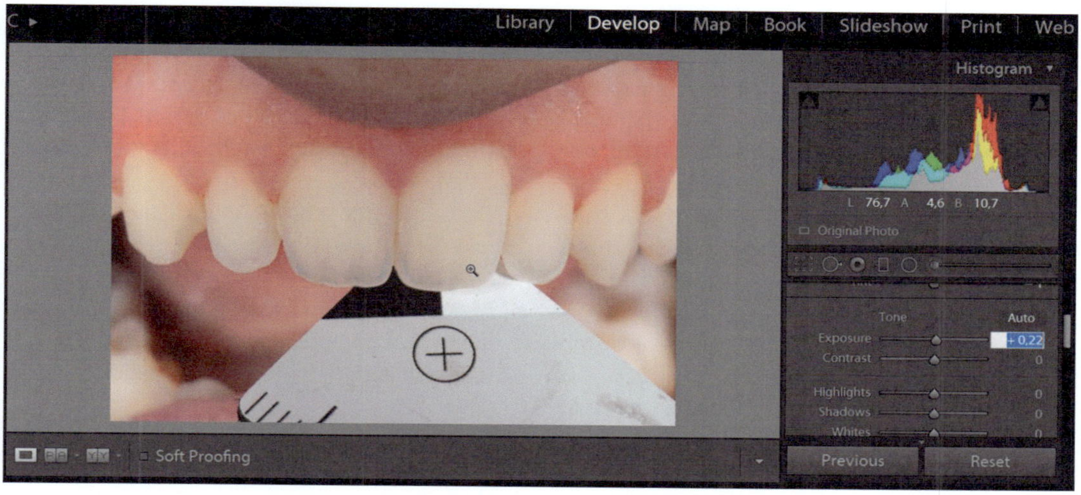

Picture 7.15 Translucency measurement, step two, measurement of values against white background. In this case, translucency has been calculated as TP = 6,49

7.7 Dedicated Dental Software for Color Matching

Based on the above presented sequence, available on the market are software applications which not only calibrate images acquired with the use of a gray card, but they also guide a dental technician to a powder-liquid mixing recipes that lead to the desired shade of indirect feldspathic ceramic restoration.

7.7.1 Direct Restorations

In contrast to pressed ceramic restorations which can be manufactured in various mixes and shades according to each case, patient's and dentist's will, shades of composites are predetermined by the manufacturer. In addition to that, there is no uniformity or an ISO standard that functions as reference point to a dentist. Each manufacturer follows his own decisions, mainly based on marketing purposes rather than actual human teeth representations, regarding shades range approach. This requires dentists to invest a significant amount of time and resources in familiarizing themselves with each new shade system to achieve satisfactory results, especially when applied to anterior restorations.

Furthermore, blending effect or chameleon effect as mostly is known, meaning the ability of two mases, in this case composite and teeth, that are distant in terms of color when separate, to appear more color-similar when they are adhered to each other, is popular among dental professionals. This property is directly linked to translucency of composite [18]. The more translucent this is, the more it absorbs color from adjunct tissues. This property is often marketed as an advantage and is popular among dentists. Popularity drives manufacturers towards marketing more transparent materials compared to real translucent properties of dental hard tissues. However, blending properties of a material which are beneficial when a cavity with a high number of tissue walls is restored (Class III cavities), may cause serious issues when the tissue deficiency is of full thickness (Class IV, or fractures). Blending of color with the dark background of the mouth will lead to a displeasing greyish result of the restoration, most of the times with unacceptable results. Namely, the most difficult to exactly match is the color of a restoration for class IV lesions.

7.7.1.1 An Additional Difficulty

According to what was explained so far, the ideal approach for direct restorations is the use of a composite with high blending properties for cases where restoration is surrounded by hard tissue walls. On the contrary, a material that carries its own optical properties, meaning a characterized and less transparent material, is preferrable when restoring a full-thickness lesion. Given those, a software providing a recipe after a colorimetric calculation of tissues to be restored should (Picture 7.16):

- Take into account all 4 dimensions of restorative materials (L, ab and TP).
- Prioritize most important optical property (translucency or luminosity) in a case-driven sense.
- Relate restoration thickness to optical properties of the result.
- Suggest for a single-shade or a layering approach, according to operator's preferences.

The main issue regarding shades of composites is that manufacturers do not follow similar approach or international standards (ISO). Consequenlty, composites labeled under the same Vita-corresponding shade, demonstrating different optical properties. Differences on composites appearance are not only on three color dimensions of CIELab 1976 space but are even more substantial regarding translucency (Pictures 7.17, 7.18, and 7.19).

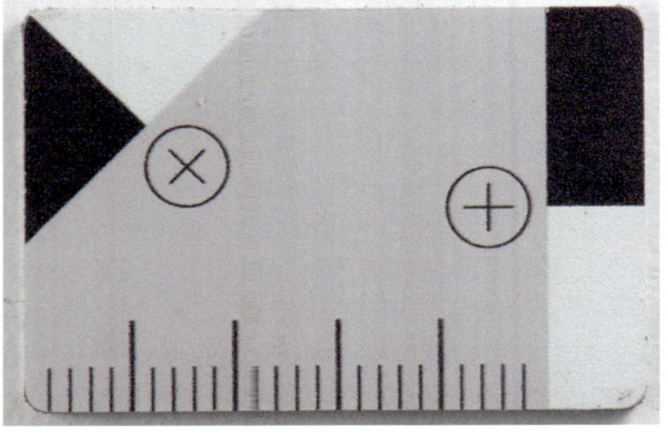

Picture 7.16 A gray card developed for translucency calculation. Contains adjacent black and white areas and a gray calibration area

Optimal shade-related material selection, should be taking under consideration thickness-related color dimensions of each individual composite and relate it to actual lesion dimensions clinical measurements on healthy tissue to be matched.

Based on the above, a dedicated software should then

- Make suggestions based on actual, thickness-dependent composite optical properties rather than a material's vita-reference label.

Following this scheme, an application operating in smartphones has been developed and currently is in beta testing stage. The application is operating based on a data base of measurements made for each individual shade of included composite brands for 0.5, 1, 1.5, and 2 mm thickness. Results underwent statistical correction and values on the linear regression and least square lines have been used and entered in data base. The software runs on smartphones and functions as follows (Pictures 7.20, 7.21, 7.22 and 7.23).

- Operator at first use creates a profile, providing information regarding what calibration method (gray card) is used. All cards are possible to be implied, yet only the correspondent DSN card with the white and black adjacent areas can be utilized to measure translucency.
- Followingly, the operator is selecting out of the included in the database composites, which ones are available in his armamentarium. This is so that the software will only suggest the best option amongst the materials available to user.
- In the case, the operator can select between class III, class IV, or veneer case. On the case selection tab, the operator can choose between class III, class IV or veneer case. This decision is related to the number of surrounding tissue walls and results in prioritizing either Translucency, or Luminosity for shade matching. Luminosity will be prioritized for class III lesions, while Translucency will be matched first for class IV or veneers.

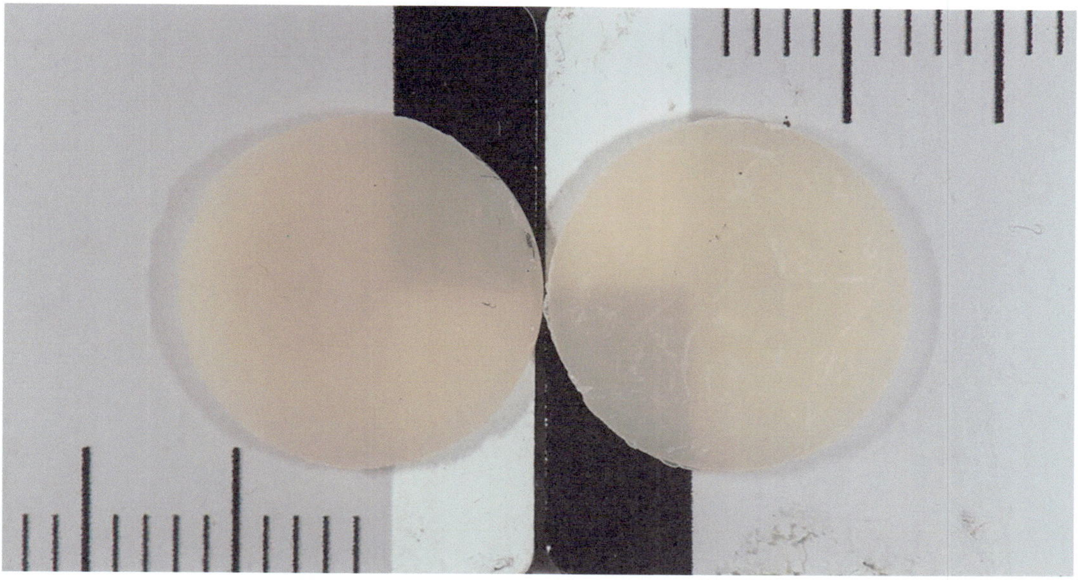

Picture 7.17 Calibrated, cross-polarized image. Equal thickness samples (1 mm), both labeled as A3 but from different manufacturers. All color dimensions are varying significantly

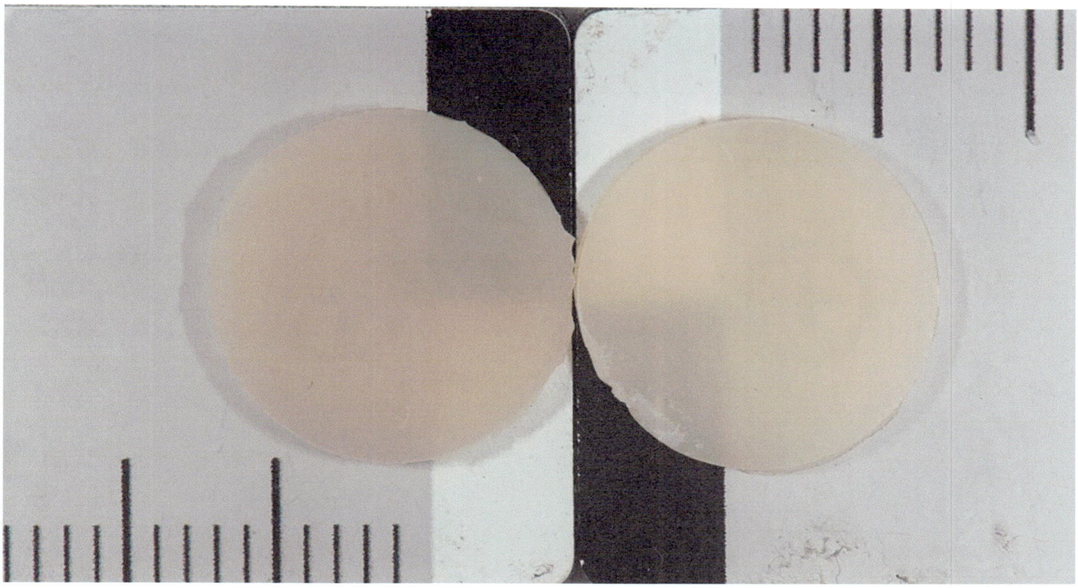

Picture 7.18 Calibrated, cross-polarized image. Equal thickness samples (1 mm), both labeled as A2 but from different manufacturers. All color dimensions are varying significantly

- Following, the operator can make a choice between a single layer of layering approach.
- Next, estimation of lesion thickness is asked. Clinically, this can be measured with a periodontal probe or a thickness caliper.
- Software asks for a picture to be made. A picture may be acquired in spot or transferred from a DSLR camera. A cross polarized image is suggested for best results. Cross polarized images for smartphones can be acquired with

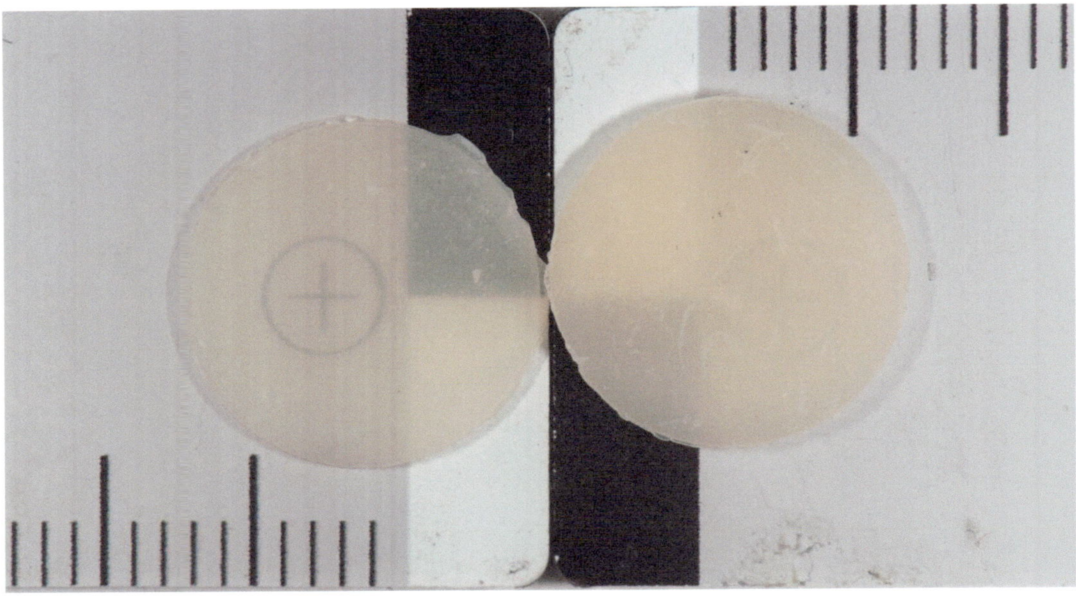

Picture 7.19 Calibrated, cross-polarized image. Influence of thickness to a material's optical properties. Same materials on different thicknesses (Left 0.5 mm, Right 1 mm)

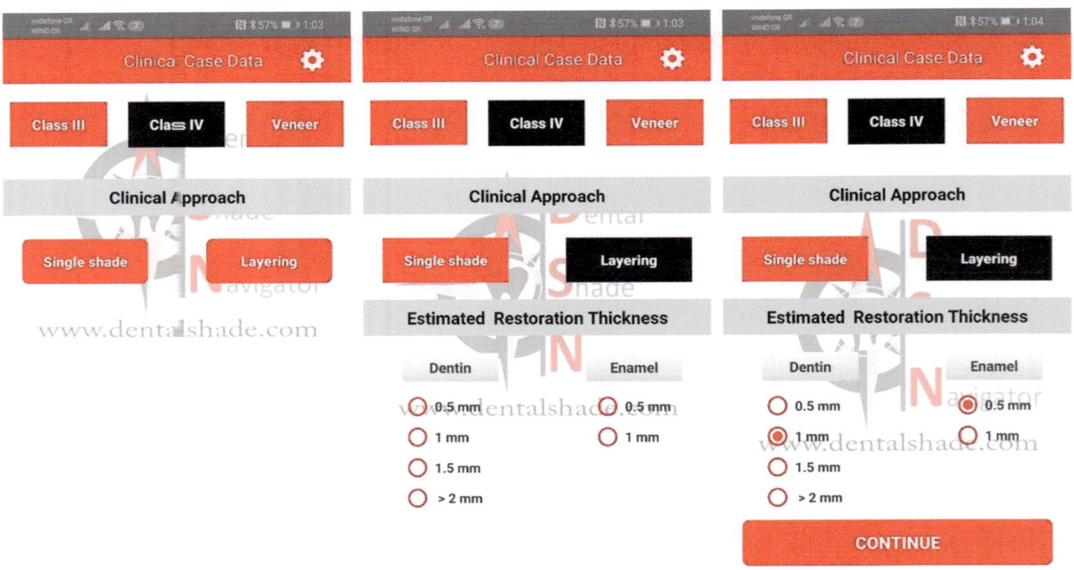

Picture 7.20 Application loading with clinical case data. Example was a class IV case which has been treated with layering approach contributing 1 mm to dentin shade and 0.5 mm to enamel shade

the use of lightning devices dedicated for this purpose, such as MDP (Smile Line).

- Then, software asks to point at the neutral spot, this means gray card area. Calibration of image to real colors occurs automatically.
- Then, information regarding the exact tissue spot to be matched will be asked. Better choice will be a spot with a natural background and at the same cervico-incisal height compared to the lesion, so that tissue thickness is similar.

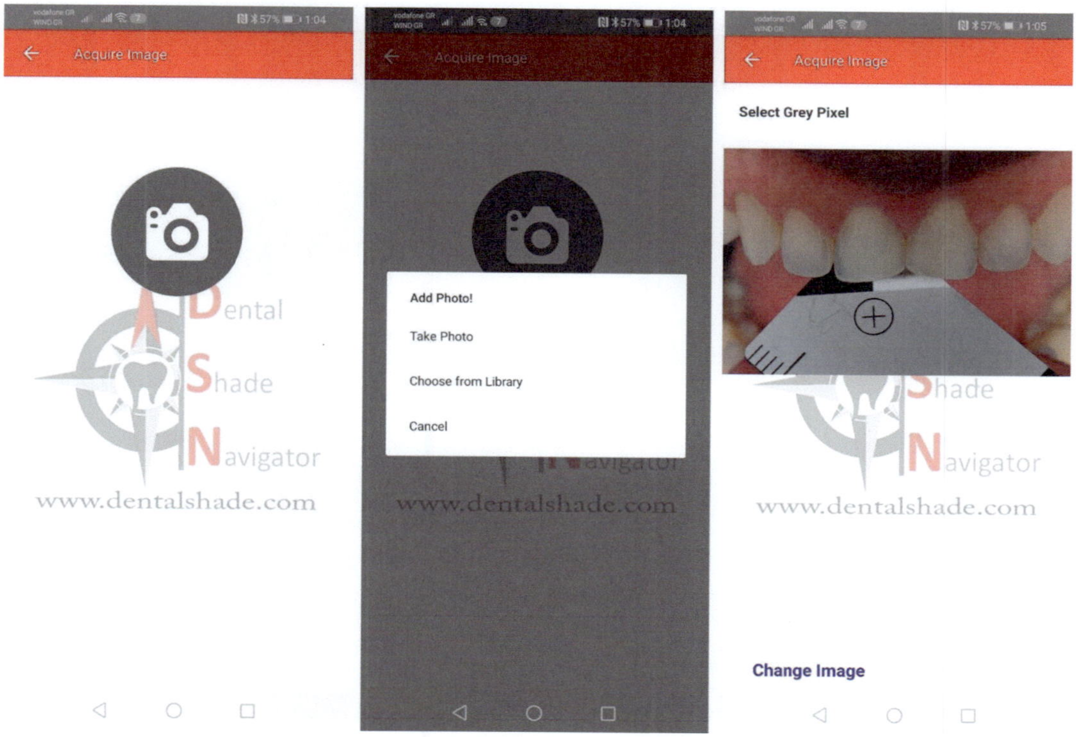

Picture 7.21 Loading of image to software. Calibration

- When a DSN card is used, and positioned behind incisal edge, software will consequently ask to point a tooth area against the white and black background. This is to calculate translucency and to better match to it.
- When all needed information is provided, the user is requesting the best shade suggestion. Prioritizing as described, software will provide best shade selection out of the available composites and the ΔE between material and tissues.

Blending effect is not considered, but according to definition, this will function in favor of the operator, minimizing the initial ΔE.

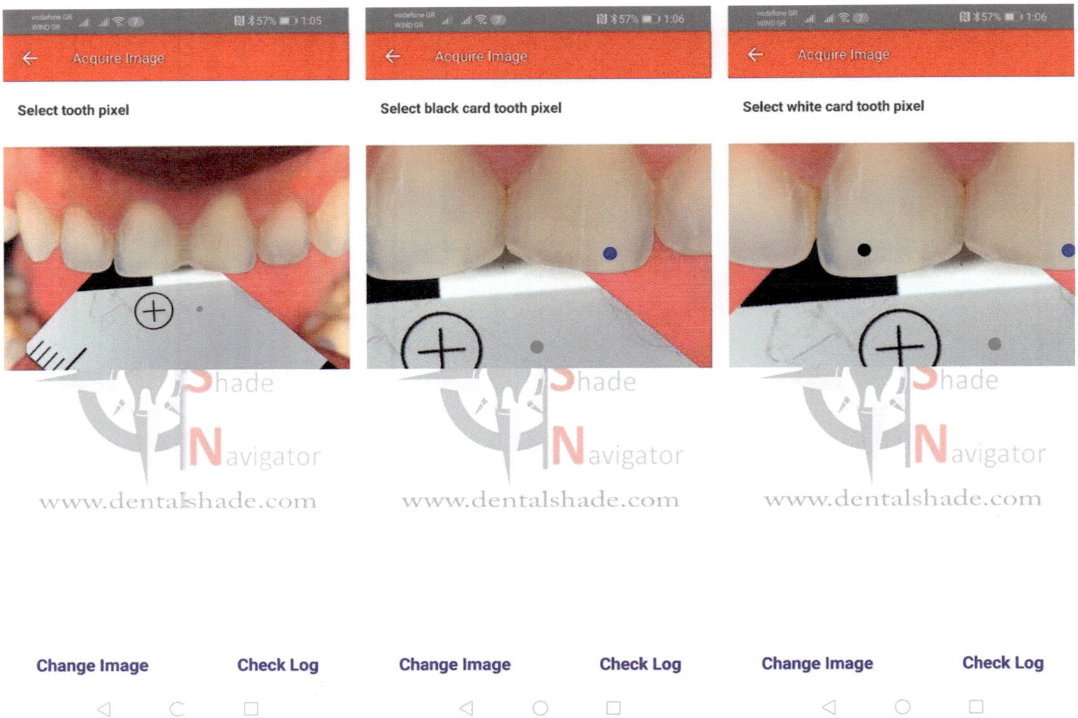

Picture 7.22 Positions of measurements for color dimensions and translucency

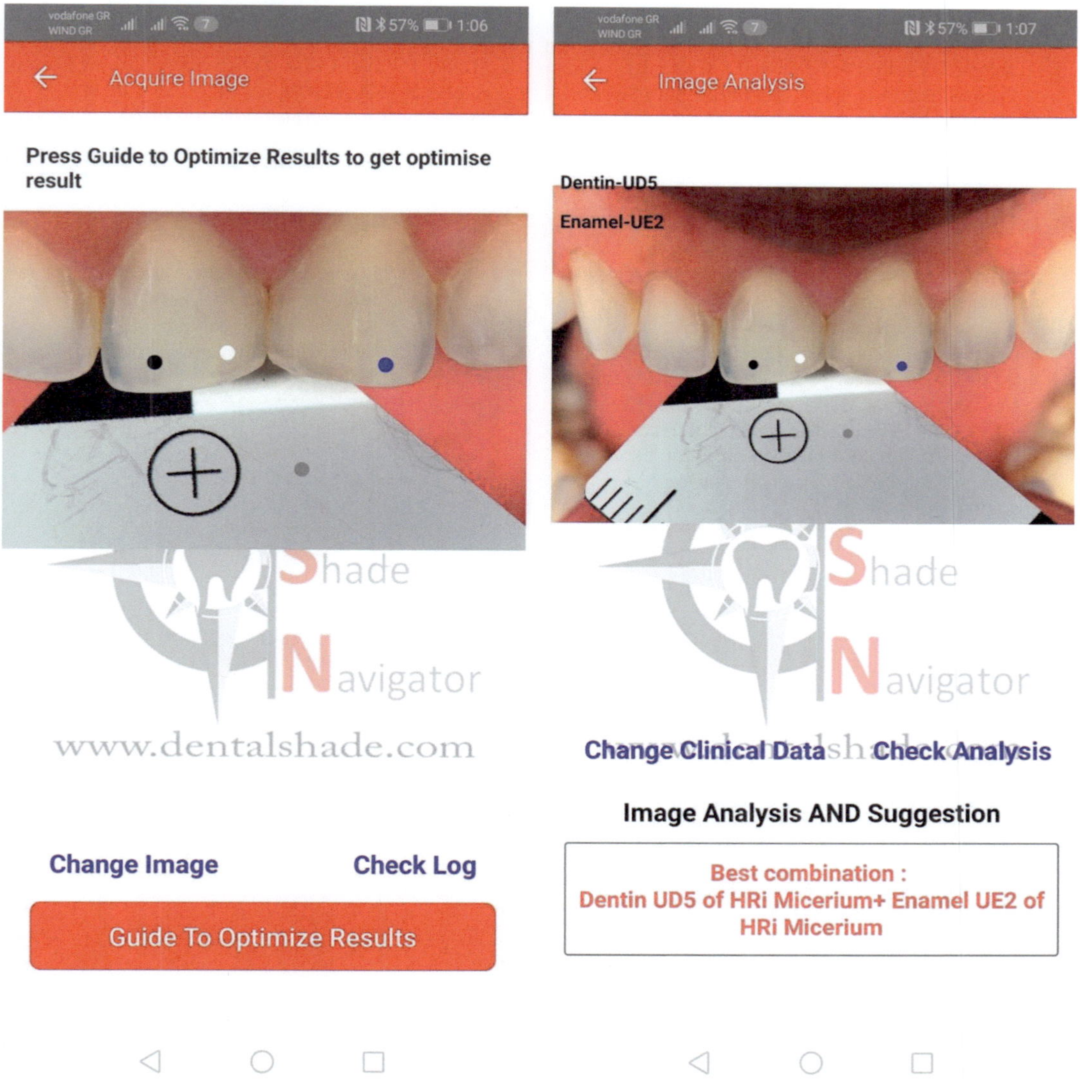

Picture 7.23 Results suggesting the closest option out of the preselected composite kit (Micerium ENA composites)

References

1. Al-Fouzan AF, Tashkandi EA. Volumetric measurements of removed tooth structure associated with various preparation designs. Int J Prosthodont. 2013;26:545–8.
2. Elderton RJ. Restorations without conventional cavity preparations. Int Dent J. 1988;38(2):112–8.
3. Simonsen RJ. New materials on the horizon. J Am Dent Assoc. 1991;122(7):24–31.
4. Burke F, Lucarotti P. The ultimate guide to restoration longevity in England and Wales. Part 5: crowns: time to next intervention and to extraction of the restored tooth. Br Dent J. 2018;225:33–48.
5. Greiner JV, Kenyon KR. Chapter 52. In: Albert DM, Jakobiec FA, editors. Principles and practice of ophthalmology—basic sciences. Philadelphia: WB Saunders; 1994.
6. Jameson KA, Highnote SM, Wasserman LM. "richer color experience in observers with multiple photopigment opsin genes" (PDF). Psychon Bull Rev. 2001;8(2):244–61.

7. Jordon G. A study of women heterozygous for colour deficiencies. Vision Res. 1993;33(11):1495–508.
8. Abramov I, Gordon J, Feldman O, Chavarga A. Sex & vision I: spatio-temporal resolution. Biol Sex Diff. 2012;3:20.
9. Abramov I, Gordon J, Feldman O, Chavarga A. Sex and vision II: color appearance of monochromatic lights. Biol Sex Diff. 2012;3:20.
10. Lehmann K, Devigus A, Wentaschek S, Igiel C, Scheller H, Paravina R. Comparison of visual shade matching and electronic color measurement device. Int J Esthet Dent. 2017;12(3):396–404.
11. Della Bona A, Barrett AA, Rosa V, Pinzetta C. Visual and instrumental agreement in dental shade selection: three distinct observer populations and shade matching protocols. Dent Mater. 2009;25(2):276–81.
12. Hunter RS. Photoelectric color-difference meter. JOSA. 1948;38(7):661. (Proceedings of the Winter Meeting of the Optical Society of America).
13. Hering E. 1868. Die Lehre vom binokularem Sehen. Leipzig.
14. “Delta E: The Color Difference”. Colorwiki.com. Accessed 16 Apr 2009.
15. The "Blue Turns Purple" Problem, Bruce Lindbloom.
16. Gómez-Polo C, Montero J, Gómez-Polo M, Martin CA. Comparison of the CIELab and CIEDE 2000 color difference formulas on gingival color space. J Prosthodont. 2020;29(5):401–8.
17. Xie Hao and Fairchild Mark. The Luther condition for all: evaluating colorimetric camera design for personalized color imaging. 2022.
18. Paravina RD, Westland S, Kimura M, Powers JM, Imai FH. Color interaction of dental materials: blending effect of layered composites. Dent Mater. 2006;22(10):903–8.

Digital Orthodontic Systems

8

Olga-Elpis Kolokitha and Ioannis A. Tsolakis

The use of digital technology is one of the most recent advancements in the field of Dentistry. Three-dimensional technologies have been widely used in different areas of dentistry including orthodontics. The implementation of these systems has gradually changed the way clinicians perform their diagnosis, treatment plans, case monitoring, and outcome assessment.

In 1974, the advent of computerized scheduling marked the beginning of digital technology's entry into dentistry and orthodontic practices. The orthodontic field has followed a significant transition from an analog status to the almost entirely digital one. Most practices have gone paperless, and digital photography and radiography have taken the place of their analog equivalents as industry standards. The evolution of digital technology resulted in a three-dimensional representation of anatomical structures. These technologies replicate anatomical structures to present tridimensional anatomy with accuracy. Study casts and two-dimensional radiography are being quickly replaced by digital intraoral images and three-dimensional radiography. Digital technology has now impacted every element of orthodontic therapy, not only the gathering and maintenance of records. With the use of numerous imaging and CAD/CAM techniques, including 3D printed models, indirect bonding trays, custom-made brackets, and robotically bent wires, it is now commonplace to undertake virtual treatment planning and translate the plans into treatment execution [1–4].

The most popular 3D techniques in orthodontics are CBCT (cone beam computerized tomography), the digitization of 3D facial, intraoral and model scans, and 3D printing devices with CAD/CAM (computer-aided design and manufacturing) technology.

8.1 Cone Beam Computed Tomography

Cone beam computer tomography (CBCT) was created by Robles RA in 1982 for angiography purposes. CBCT was first used in dentistry in Europe in 1998 and was licensed for use in the United States in 2001. An early appraisal of the anticipated future impact of this technology upon dentistry, specifically in orthodontics, was first discussed and reported in the proceedings of a symposium on "Craniofacial Imaging in the Twenty-First Century" held in 2002 in Pacific

O.-E. Kolokitha (✉)
Faculty of Health Sciences, Department of Orthodontics, School of Dentistry, Aristotle University of Thessaloniki, Thessaloniki, Greece
e-mail: okolok@dent.auth.gr

I. A. Tsolakis
Faculty of Health Sciences, Department of Orthodontics, School of Dentistry, Aristotle University of Thessaloniki, Thessaloniki, Greece

Department of Orthodontics, School of Dental Medicine, Case Western Reserve University, Cleveland, OH, USA

A. Delantoni, K. Orhan (eds.), *Digital Dentistry*, https://doi.org/10.1007/978-3-031-52826-2_8

Grove, CA. Since that time, CBCT technology has advanced quickly, partly due to the demands of each specialty for precise, repeatable, and secure three-dimensional (3D) images. In orthodontics, 3D imaging can aid in the deciphering of the complexities of dental and skeletal malocclusions, as well as improving diagnosis and treatment planning in specific case types [5, 6].

The CBCT machine is composed of a cone-shaped X-ray bundle, with the X-ray source and detector (Image Intensifier or Flat Panel Detector) rotating around a point (or field) of interest to the patient (Fig. 8.1). In a manner similar to computed tomography (CT), CBCT rotates around the patient's head while taking several images, creating a three-dimensional (3D) volume. However, CBCT uses a volumetric approach that only requires one rotation, resulting in far lower radiation exposure. In a single scanner sweep during CBCT (Cone Beam Computed Tomography) imaging, the radiation source and 2D sensor rotate synchronously around the patient's head by 180° or 360° depending on the CBCT apparatus being utilized. Recent advancements in CBCT imaging techniques have made it possible to expose patients to less radiation than with conventional two-dimensional radiography. Computer software is used by CBCT to create a three-dimensional volume from a collection of 160–600+ two-dimensional images received by the detector. This process is called primary reconstruction. The term CBCT reflects this emphasis. For example, as it refers to volume rather than two-dimensional space, the term voxel is used rather than the pixel. The image files follow the DICOM (Digital Imaging and Communications in Medicine) standard, which is the industry-standard three-dimensional image format for the medical industry. A three-dimensional CBCT image will therefore have the file extension "dcm," as opposed to a digital image, which would have an extension like "tif," "jpeg," etc.

The three-dimensional volume that the doctor wants to assess is called the region of interest (ROI). The ROI is, for instance, the area around the mandibular incisors when requesting a periapical radiograph of those teeth. The resolution of that image is improved the smaller the ROI. The size of the field of view (FOV), which determines the size of the produced image, and the resolution are frequently connected (Fig. 8.2). For instance, if a large FOV that encompasses the entire head is used and the clinician wants to see a cyst in the mandibular incisor area, the image quality will not be as excellent as a FOV that was focused solely on that incisor location. All radiographic pictures can be acquired in under a minute thanks to CBCT technology. Dental practitioners can access images with high diagnostic value such as periapical radiographs, panoramic radiographs, cephalograms, occlusal radiographs, and TMJ images, as well as views

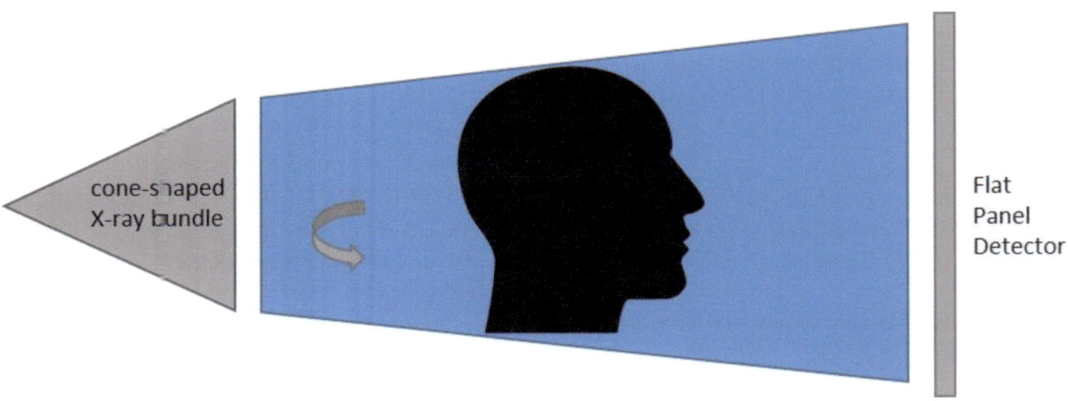

Fig. 8.1 CBCT machine rotates around a field of interest to the patient, and it is composed of a cone-shaped X-ray bundle, with the X-ray source and Flat Panel Detector

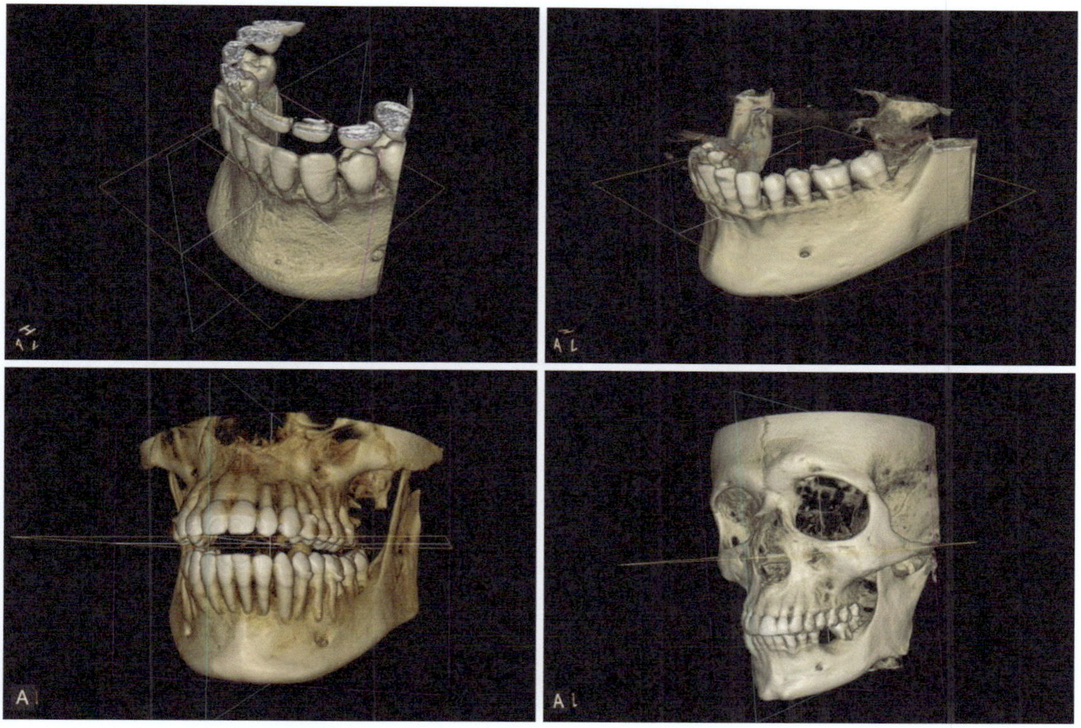

Fig. 8.2 Different fields of view (FOV) in CBCT captions

that are not possible with conventional radiography equipment, like axial and cross-sectional views [7–9].

There are various applications of CBCT in clinical orthodontic practice. The cephalometric analysis is a tool of orthodontics as it helps assess the etiology of malocclusion; to determine whether the malocclusion is due to skeletal or dental relationship or both. It is used primarily in orthodontic diagnosis and treatment planning but can also be used during treatment to assess progress and for research purposes. Incorrect positioning of the head, structure overlay, geometrical distortions, and craniofacial asymmetries can all hinder two-dimensional assessment accuracy [10]. Three-dimensional cephalometry, which is done using a CBCT exam, allows for a more detailed evaluation of the craniofacial structure. With this method, the clinician can more easily detect and quantify craniofacial asymmetries, longitudinal growth, and subtle occlusal changes. Additionally, the current literature does not state if 3D cephalograms can be used on every orthodontic patient [11–14]. More recently, new criteria for the use of CBCT specifically directed at dentists and orthodontists disclosed from the European Academy of Dental and Maxillofacial Radiology [15]. CBCT has been shown to be extremely important in the treatment of patients with impacted teeth (Fig. 8.3). The information provided by the CBCT grants a more accurate location of the impacted tooth location and the adjacent structures [16–20]. This contrasts with the two-dimensional imaging method where several images of the impacted tooth from different perspectives are required, making the lower resolution imaging method unreliable. The extent of the pathology connected to the ectopic tooth can be more precisely assessed thanks to the CBCT. Clinical studies employing three-dimensional imaging have revealed that root resorption of teeth next to impacted teeth occurs more frequently than previously believed. The specific location of ectopic cuspids can be determined using CBCT imaging, which can also be

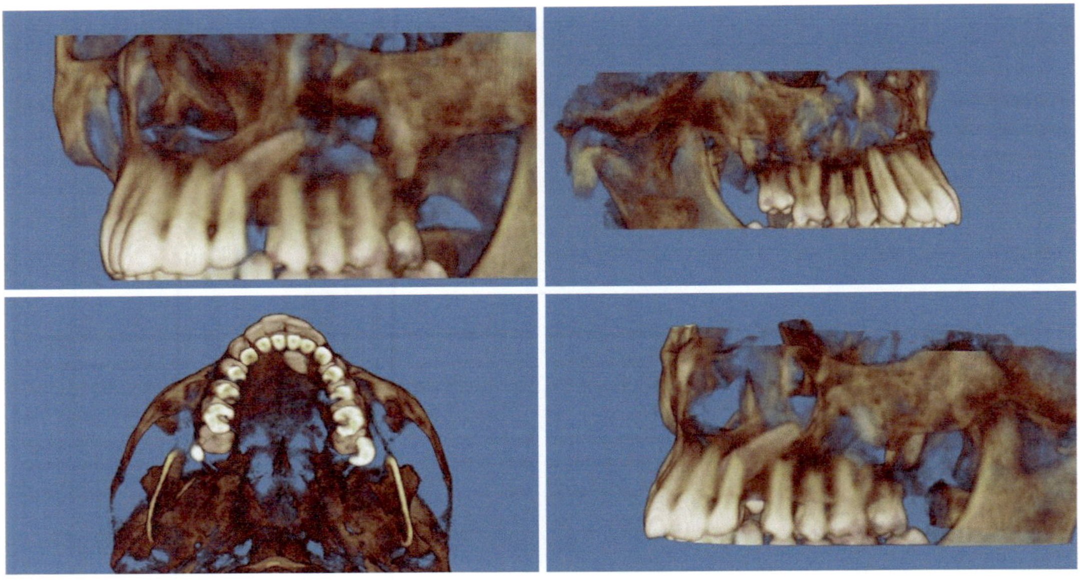

Fig. 8.3 Impacted cuspid

utilized to develop treatment plans that need less invasive surgical intervention. Smaller incisions, more conservative flap design, and overall lower surgical morbidity are all benefits of computer- and image-guided surgical exposure. Another use of CBCT in the Orthodontic field is the accurate placement of mini-implants. CBCT is used to assess the bone density, the alveolar bone height as well as the exact position of the adjacent teeth roots compared to the area of mini-implant placement. The evaluation and effectiveness of CBCT imaging of the temporomandibular joint have been studied in the past [21]. The results of these studies show that CBCT offers superior imaging compared to helical CT and conventional radiography. When it came to detecting anomalies in the mandibular condyle, the CBCT outperformed the helical CT in terms of sensitivity and accuracy. Three-dimensional measurements of the airway can be accurately obtained with the use of a CBCT [22]. The examination of the airway is significantly improved by CBCT technology, which enables three-dimensional and volumetric measurements. CBCT has proven to be as accurate as other gold standard methods to measure the upper airway volume and constricted area (Fig. 8.4) [22]. Some orthodontic patients appear with airway constriction. CBCT examination has been proven a useful tool for these patients, allowing for a comparison of airway constriction before and after undergoing different types of treatment plan. The comprehension of more complicated disorders including obstructive sleep apnea (OSA) and enlarged adenoids would benefit from three-dimensional airway analysis. The nasal cavity can also suffer changes in situations of maxillary expansion, as nasal base width increase, which can be assessed by measuring different variables to accurately assess the treatment success [23, 24]. Also, with CBCT imaging, it is possible to assess the ossification stage of the spheno-occipital synchondrosis. The improper fusion or growth of this synchondrosis influences the antero-posterior dimension of the cranium and can lead to the development of malocclusion [25]. Another use of CBCT is to scan dental plaster models and digitize them. Lastly, all radiographic data required for an orthodontic diagnosis can be captured in less than a minute thanks to CBCT technology. A more detailed assessment of the outcome can be made possible

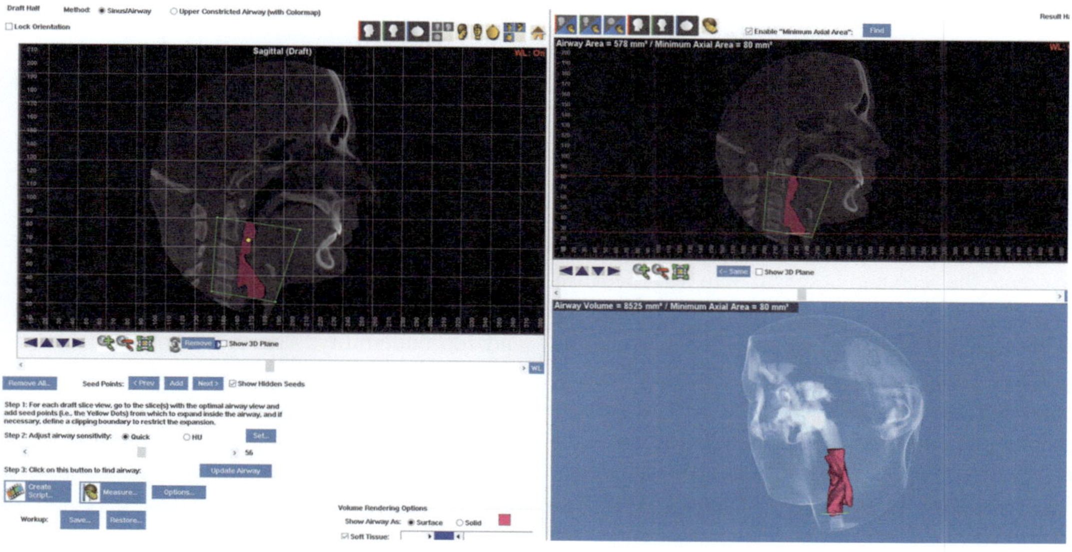

Fig. 8.4 Airway volume analysis and minimum cross-section area

by a three-dimensional vision of the patient, which enables a more accurate assessment of both dental and skeletal asymmetries.

8.2 Scanners

Scanners in orthodontics have played an important role in digital diagnosis, treatment planning, and research. All scanners use optical scanning methods. They are all composed of at least one camera, and they are used to scan the face, the dental arches, and the dental casts.

8.2.1 Facial Scanners

Facial scanners use optical scanning methods to digitally record and display a precise three-dimensional representation of a subject's face and head. The information can then be used for numerous analyses, such as patient care planning, diagnostics, and communication. Combining image files from a facial scanner, intraoral scanner, and CBCT to create a virtual patient can speed up diagnostic processes, enable accurate patient analysis, and serve as an effective communication tool for relaying information to the lab technician and simulating treatment outcomes for the patient. Face scanners use photogrammetry, stereophotogrammetry, structured light scanning, and laser scanning as their four scanning techniques. There are two approaches within these mechanisms: passive and active. The patient's face is scanned using two or more photos in the passive approaches (photogrammetry and stereophotogrammetry). In the active technique, laser beam and structured light are utilized to triangulate 3D sensors to collect light patterns actively. Despite the scanning technique, photogrammetry, stereophotogrammetry, laser beam scanning, and structured light scanners have multiple advantages because they are noninvasive and are characterized by high accuracy and reproducibility [26–28].

To create a 3D image, photogrammetry, a technology that was initially used in topographic mapping, gathers data from many shots. In a manner like stereophotogrammetry, an object is photographed from two separate planes to produce a 3D model. It enables the measurement of volume, surface area, and distance.

Stereophotogrammetry, which is particularly helpful in maxillofacial prosthetics, is unable to reliably detect hair or reflective or bright skin surfaces. Stereophotogrammetry needs a certain area to set up two or more cameras from various angles surrounding the subject, as shown in Fig. 8.5, as well as a computer. This method requires specialized software that has been tuned to create the scan and is sensitive to light because it involves numerous photos. Since insufficient or excessive ambient light might affect the photographs taken, adequate lighting is required. A computer system then joins the several photographs to create a 3D facial model after the scan is finished. A structured light scanner may gather light patterns and produce a 3D shape of a subject's face using trigonometric triangulation. As shown in figure, this system needs a projector to cast a pattern of light onto the object and a calibrated camera to record the projection. Blue light or white light make up most conventional light scanners. However, blue light scanners are replacing white light scanners because they offer a more accurate scan because they produce a shorter wavelength and are less likely to reflect. White light scanners, which emit a shorter wavelength and are less likely to reflect light accurately, are, nevertheless, being phased out. A 3D mesh based on the displacement of the light pattern is used to record the light coming from different angles. Structured light technology has several benefits, including quickness, accuracy, and reproducibility. The scan, however, can be distorted by additional ambient light when using this scanning technique because it is sensitive to lighting conditions. Like light scanning, laser scanning works by photographing the laser's reflection off the object being scanned. A camera can determine a laser beam's geometry and calculate the laser's distance and three-dimensional shape. The laser scanner needs numerous, consecutive scans with the patient positioned in various directions for a thorough 3D facial scan, as shown in Fig. 8.5. Although laser scanning is

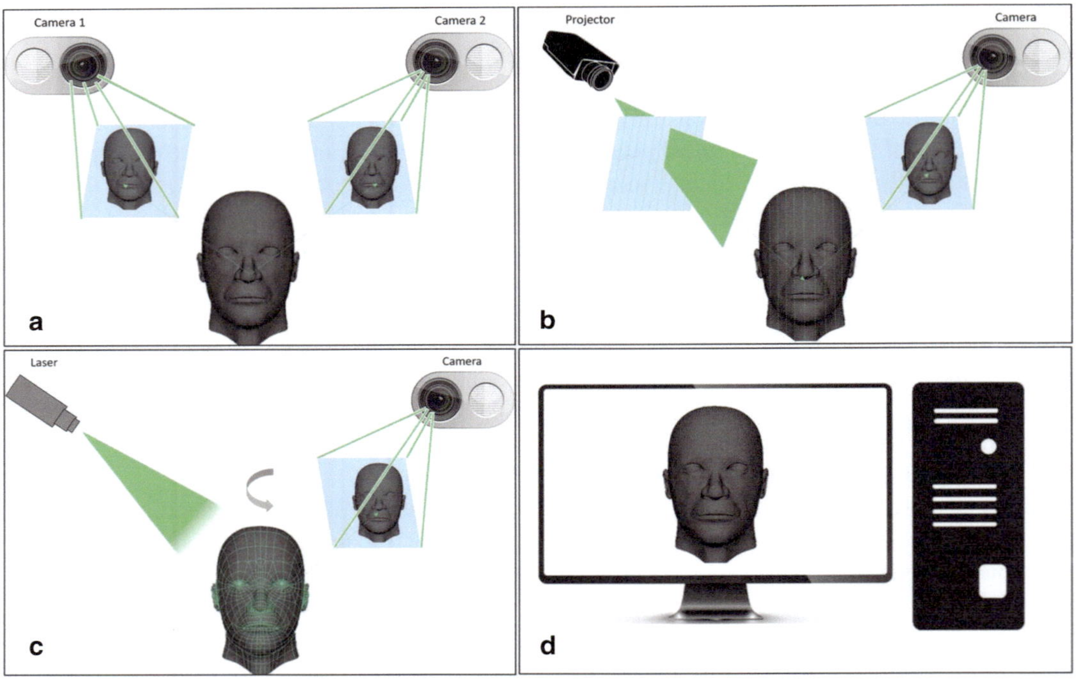

Fig. 8.5 Types of facial scanners. (**a**) Photogrammetry and stereophotogrammetry, (**b**) structured light scanning, (**c**) laser scanning, (**d**) digitized patient's face

quite accurate, additional light sources may reduce accuracy. When opposed to scanning with structured light, laser scanning is slower [29–32].

8.2.2 Intraoral Scanners

The first intraoral scanner came into production in 1985 and was developed by Dentsply Sirona (Charlotte, NC, USA). Its purpose was to take digital impressions for fixed prosthetic restorations. The introduction of 3D models into orthodontics came in 1999 from Orthocad (Czestochowa, Poland) with the first version of their software, which allowed the study of digital versions of orthodontic casts after proper scanning. Since then, scanners have improved significantly, providing high-quality mapping of both hard and soft tissues, being able to replace traditional plaster models. Significant benefits from intraoral scanners include more comfort, lower risk of allergic reactions, the streamlining of clinical procedures, easy storage, and the ability to record and share data between peers [33, 34].

The time it takes to scan the dental arches is variable and dependent on operator technique and experience. Thanks to their ability to do full arch scanning, indirect bonding, and digitally create fixed orthodontic equipment, their usage in the field of orthodontics has expanded in recent years. Additionally, they facilitate orthodontic diagnosis and treatment planning by providing quick and simple electronic data transfer, immediate access, and less storage space needs. Intraoral scanners use optical scanning to duplicate and recreate the patient's mandibular and maxillary dental arch architecture. A digital image that can be shared and duplicated is displayed on the screen after a patient's oral cavity has been scanned to show information about the patient's natural anatomical structures (Fig. 8.6). Intraoral scanners can be effectively employed in orthodontic practice for effective treatment planning, custom appliance fabrication like functional appliances or clear aligners, and orthognathic surgery simulation. Intraoral scanning's fundamental idea, alike all scanning methods, is based on optical phenomena such as optical triangulation, coherence tomography, accordion fringe interferometry, and three-dimensional motion video recording [35–37].

This optical triangulation method can be used to determine an object's distance from a few millimeters to a few microns. Where direct touch is undesirable and contraindicated, wet surfaces, soft and sensitive objects can be carefully scanned utilizing the built-in sensors. A laser-based light source, a powerful lens, and a very sensitive sensor plate make up a triangulation imaging system. A point spot image is created on the sensor plate once the region of interest to be scanned is exposed to radiation. Thereafter, it is possible to precisely establish the baseline angle and image length.

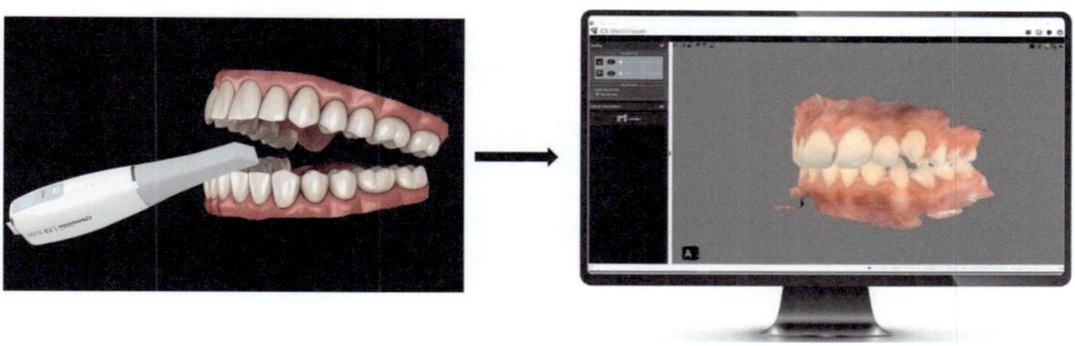

Fig. 8.6 Scanning of dental arch system

The optical coherence tomography (OCT) technology is just as effective as the ultrasonography technique; however, the former transmits and projects images using light, while the latter does so using sound waves. To create realistic and realistic images of microstructure with precise scale measurements of the item, backscattered radiations and reflected waves are used. One hundred times more detailed than an ultrasonographic image, this technology provides 1–15 mm resolution. Due to its long wavelength, it has the benefit of penetrating live tissues up to a depth of 3 mm.

Accordion fringe interferometry (AFI) projects three separate fringe patterns using two different light sources. This fringe design splits and reframes to take up a new pattern when it contacts the intended surface. The distinctive curve of the scanned object is what gave rise to the new form. The deformation in the original pattern of the object that underwent AFI is known as fringe curvature. Specific points and aspects of fringe curvature can be captured using a high-definition camera with a video feature.

The most predominant intraoral scanner technology nowadays is three-dimensional motion video recording. The intraoral scanner that uses this technology is composed of a 3-min video camera incorporated into the lens that uses trinocular imaging as its foundation. It employs a trinocular imaging HD video camera to record the recorded structure's intricate detail. With the use of complementary metal-oxide semiconductor (CMOS) based sensors located next to the cameras, light is converted to electric energy in the form of electric signals. To create an image with a realistic emotion, 3D data is collected. An additional benefit is scanning without a previous coating of abrasive powder and having a greater dynamic luminosity range. Exact models are used to determine the linear distance between two data points. With this technology, the clinician can create a three-dimensional image of the dental arches, either independently or in occlusion, by directly scanning the oral cavity. They can then be used as templates to create basic and sophisticated orthodontic appliances and retainers [38].

A systematic review done by Gabrielle Rossini et al. [39] concluded that digital models are as reliable as traditional plaster models, with high accuracy, reliability, and reproducibility. Landmark identification, rather than the measuring device or the software, appeared to be the greatest limitation. A recent systematic review done by Jedliński et al. [40] aimed to investigate the accuracy and efficacy of intraoral scanners for orthodontic purpose assumed that there are plenty of data available on accuracy and efficacy of different scanners. Scanners of the same generation from different manufacturers have almost identical accuracy. This is the reason why future similar research will not introduce much to the orthodontics. The challenge for the coming years is to find new applications of digital impressions in the orthodontic practice.

8.2.3 Model Scanners

The model scanners use the same types of technology as the intraoral scanners. These dental 3D scanners capture images not from a patient but rather at a dental lab by scanning a conventionally made plaster impression. The scanner gathers a point cloud, or the coordinates of an object in space, with the aid of directional structured light, and creates a 3D model from it. This is carried out automatically by the machine without human involvement. A digital image is produced on the monitor screen once the information is analyzed by specialized software. In the model scanners, the camera can picture the entire model. This scanning technique has excellent accuracy. The circumstances are particularly favorable in this instance due to the good lighting, complete access to every aspect of the object, and its stillness. As a result, the photographs have exceptional quality. Without any omission, every detail is communicated. Plaster casts, on the other hand, do not reveal the true color of the teeth. As a result, the doctor will choose the prosthesis or restoration's desired color and tint. However, most lab 3D scanners feature tools that let you adjust the image's color. Depending on the work

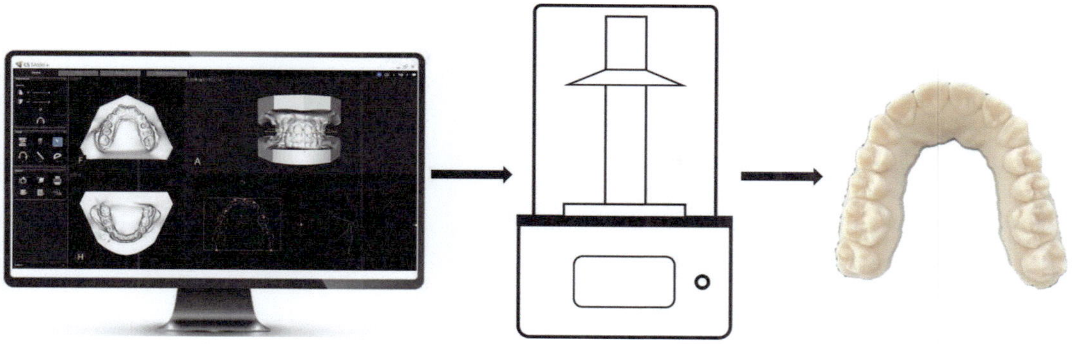

Fig. 8.7 Orthodontic software, dental cast processing, and 3D printing

at hand, there are other possibilities for "refining" a 3D model [41, 42].

8.2.4 Computer Software

Every scanning system is completed with the usage of special software. All scanners are connected to the computer, and the images are processed through computer software. In addition, the scanning images after they get processed can be used for multiple other software for diagnostic measurements or appliance fabrication. Those files can be exported in "STL," "OBJ," and "PLY" formats in order to be imported to other software or to be 3D printed (Fig. 8.7). The STL file is the most used file type that makes use of approximate mesh. Triangles, also known as facets, are the building blocks of STL files and are used to cover the surface of 2D shapes. The use of STL over other file formats has several benefits. First, collaboration is made simpler because it is widely accepted and used. Additionally, STL files are straightforward and compact, which speeds up processing. However, STL files have a significant drawback. Tessellation simply covers the surface; hence the files only describe surface geometry without color or texture representation. Resolution is another problem with STL files. More triangles are needed to maintain high resolution or to encode larger-sized objects, which increases the file size. Processing files takes longer the bigger they are. The following two file formats, OBJ and PLY, were developed to cover the downsides of STL files. Both are capable of storing attributes like color and texture. Both OBJ and PLY are well-known and frequently used for their capacity to contain color and texture together with other data, although not being as popular as STL files. Both files are seen as having greater relevance in the future than STL files and benefit from more advanced 3D printers [43].

8.3 Three-Dimensional Printing

One of the most cutting-edge technologies in the manufacturing field is three-dimensional printing. Producing dental casts was one of the very first applications for three-dimensional printers in orthodontics. Charles Hull presented the first three-dimensional (3D) printer in 1986. Hull discovered stereolithography (SLA) and created the first 3D printing technology in the same year. Scott Crump introduced fused deposition modeling (FDM) 4 years later. Due to SLA printing's precision and stiffness, it has gained significant traction in the dentistry industry. Nowadays, the SLA, Direct Light Processing (DLP), Liquid Crystal Display (LCD), Fused Filament Fabrication (FFF), and PolyJet Photopolymer (PPP) three-dimensional printers are used in orthodontics (Fig. 8.8) [43].

SLA 3D printers are composed of a UV laser that is used to build the printing model. The first step in the procedure is to place the building platform at a layer-height distance within the liquid

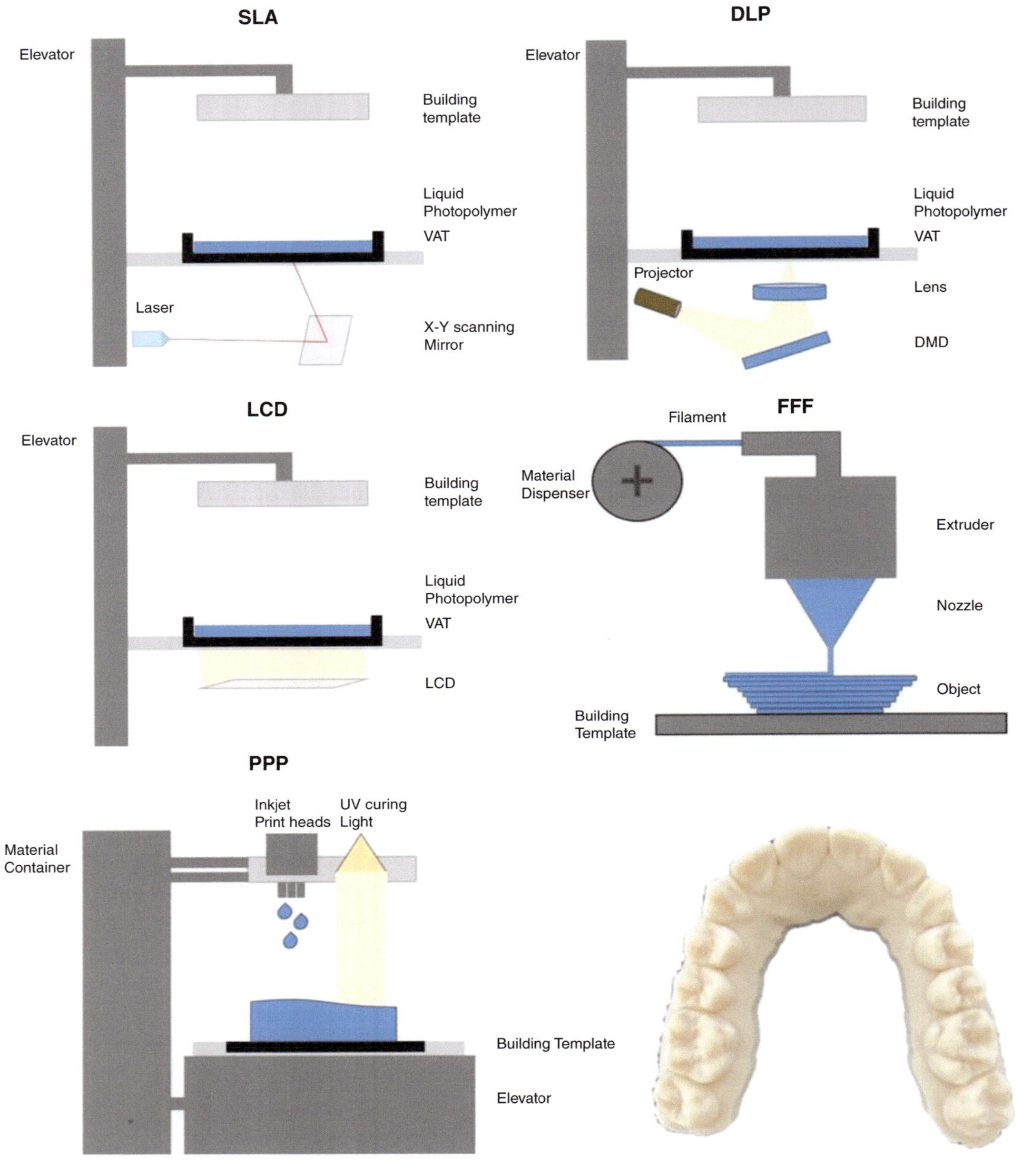

Fig. 8.8 Types of 3D printing technologies

photopolymer tank. The photopolymer resin is selectively cured by the UV laser to create the subsequent layer. The resin solidifies after curing. A system of mirrors is being used to direct the laser beam along a predefined route. Galvos are the name for the mirrors. The printed product is not entirely dried when the printing procedure is finished. The item needs to be exposed to UV light again for this reason. The object requires an ultrasonic bath with isopropyl alcohol to remove any remaining resin before the post-processing UV light cure [43].

DLP is a form of vat polymerization, just like SLA. Technologies for vat polymerization use a liquid photopolymer resin that is cured by light. Based on a digital light projector, DLP technology is a 3D additive manufacturing technique. A layer's image can be flashed at once using the DLP projector. As a result, a layer's many locations can all cure simultaneously. Due to this feature, the DLP printing technique is significantly faster than Laser-SLA. The DLP printer's LED screen, which is made up of a digital micromirror device (DMD), serves as its light source. Millions of tiny micromirrors are used in this apparatus to focus light onto the resin tank's bottom in the shape of a layered pattern. Like with SLA, the model needs to be washed and post-cured after printing [43].

LCD is a 3D printing technology that is based on vat polymerization technology. The light source in LCD printers is a liquid crystal display. In LCD 3D printers, the build area is illuminated in parallel by light passing through the LCD screens. A lens or other equipment is not used to magnify the light, either. Therefore when using an LCD 3D printer, pixel distortion is not a concern. The primary distinction between LCD printers and SLA printers is speed. Although LCD printers are as quick as DLP printers, they are more economical due to the low cost of the manufacturing components used to construct them. This is the primary cause of the increasing popularity of those printers [43, 44].

FFF is a method of additive manufacturing. To make an object, a thermoplastic material is pushed through an extruder (heated nozzle) during this procedure. The constructing platform is moved into a layer distance after the first layer has been installed to create the second layer. Layers are added one at a time until the printed product is completely constructed. Polylactic acid (PLA) and acrylonitrile butadiene styrene are the two thermoplastic substances that have been utilized most frequently in FFF printing technique (ABS). The first is renowned for its exquisite detailing, while the second is renowned for its toughness [43].

PPP is a 3D printing method that functions similarly to an ordinary inkjet printer. It creates parts by UV-solidifying tens of thousands of photopolymer droplets that are jetted onto a build platform. Photopolymer resin is applied for this kind of technology. The resin is placed into the container and heated before printing begins. The carriage moves across the X-axis and over the build platform to begin printing as soon as the resin reaches the proper viscosity. The resin is jetted into the build platform by the print heads in this process. UV light cures the resin once it has been jetted. The build platform lowers the height of the build platform when each layer is finished, and this process continues until the object is printed [43].

The various 3D printing technologies can have an impact on the accuracy of three-dimensional printed models. The PPP printing technology is the most accurate of them, and it is followed by the DLP, SLA, LCD, and FFF printing technologies in that order, according to the present literature. The design of the base appears to have an impact on the accuracy of 3D dental models as well. It has been established that the standard dental model base and a horseshoe model with a posterior connection are realistic, although the horseshoe design is susceptible to distortion. The printing materials used also have an impact on the precision of the 3D-printed dental models. The layer height or the model's placement on the building template has no effect on how accurate dental models are produced with any 3D printing technology. Whether the preferred shape is solid or hollow, the accuracy of the dental model's print is the same. It is important to mention that none of these variables have an impact on the clinical orthodontic result. Since none of the aforementioned criteria have a clinically significant impact on the clinical outcome, doctors can choose a printer based on how expensive and time-consuming it is to create dental models for orthodontic applications [43, 44].

8.4 Artificial Intelligence

All the aforementioned machines can be combined with artificial intelligence software in order to produce a faster and ideally more accurate diagnosis, treatment planning, and fabrication of various devices. Artificial intelligence (AI) is the capacity of a technology to imitate human intelligence or to arrive at conclusions that, according to established standards, are moral and effective. Due to improvements in analytics methods, computing power, and data accessibility, AI may now touch many aspects of modern culture. On a worldwide basis, we are already experiencing its repercussions. For social media, web searches, and consumer electronics like cameras, telephones, tablets, and even cars, it filters data. A significant area of artificial intelligence is machine learning. Machine learning makes predictions about new data and circumstances using the statistical patterns of previously learned data. Training data are necessary for machine learning to function. Machine learning cannot work without training data. With this approach, the computer model can develop over time by learning from experience rather than through conventional explicit programming. A model needs a lot of data to learn aspects about the data using abstractions from various processing levels. The benefit of deep learning is that little engineering effort is needed to prepare the data for analysis. Recognition of visual objects and item identification have seen the most use of deep learning techniques. Recent technological developments have made machine learning more crucial for the identification and categorization of certain diseases seen in medical imaging.

Artificial Intelligence is being used in orthodontics for cephalometric analysis, teeth segmentation, superimposition of dental arches, and airway analysis. There are various types of research done in terms of cephalometric measurements and the use of artificial intelligence. According to the present literature, automatic landmark detection and automatic cephalometric measurements using different cephalometric software are accurate [45]. Another usage of artificial intelligence software is the automatic tooth segmentation in digital dental models. Deep learning-based automatic tooth segmentation of a digital model demonstrates a great success rate, accuracy, and efficiency in tooth segmentation. Therefore, it may be used for orthodontic diagnosis and appliance fabrication [46]. A great application of artificial intelligence in orthodontics is the superimposition of dental casts in order to assess tooth movement during or after orthodontic treatment. According to the present literature, in comparison to other software types, semiautomatic best-fit registration software regularly shows outstanding agreement in superimpositions. Compared to other methods, automatic best-fit registration software consistently showed superior agreement for mandibular superimpositions. The quantification algorithm used in superimposition investigations can be credited with the accuracy of digital model superimpositions for tooth movements [47]. Lastly, artificial intelligence can be used to automatically segment and analyze the airway. Due to a successful AI technique, the pharyngeal airway may now be automatically segregated from CBCT images. Automatic segmentation can be employed in clinical settings, according to the existing literature. This is due to the fact that it seems to be quick and simple to use while also measuring the airway with great accuracy [48].

References

1. Francisco I, Ribeiro MP, Marques F, Travassos R, Nunes C, Pereira F, Caramelo F, Paula AB, Vale F. Application of three-dimensional digital technology in orthodontics: the state of the art. Biomimetics. 2022;7:23. https://doi.org/10.3390/biomimetics7010023.
2. Karatas OH, Toy E. Three-dimensional imaging techniques: a literature review. Eur J Dent. 2014;8:132–40.
3. Impellizzeri A, Horodynski M, De Stefano A, Palaia G, Polimeni A, Romeo U, Guercio-Monaco E, Galluccio G. CBCT and intra-oral scanner: the advantages of 3D technologies in orthodontic treatment. Int J Environ Res Public Healthy. 2020;17:9428.
4. Sannino G, Germano F, Arcuri L, Bigelli E, Arcuri C, Barlattani A. CEREC CAD/CAM chairside system. Oral Implant. 2015;7:57–70.
5. Mozzo P, Procacci C, Tacconi A, Martini PT, Andreis IA. A new volumetric CT machine for dental imaging based on the cone-beam technique: preliminary results. Eur Radiol. 1998;8:1558–64.
6. Hatcher DC. Operational principles for cone-beam computed tomography. J Am Dent Assoc. 2010;141(Suppl. 3):3S–6S.
7. Kapila S, Farman AG. Craniofacial imaging in the 21st century. Proceedings of the 2002 COAST Conference, Asilomar Conference Center, Pacific Grove, California. Orthod Craniofac Res. 2003;6:7–8.

8. Kapila S, Conley RS, Harrell WE Jr. The current status of cone beam computed tomography imaging in orthodontics. Dentomaxillofac Radiol. 2011;40:24–34. https://doi.org/10.1259/dmfr/12615645.
9. Kapila S. Contemporary concepts on cone-beam computed tomography in orthodontics. In: Kapila S, editor. Cone beam computed tomography in orthodontics: indications, insights and innovations. Hoboken, NJ: Wiley-Blackwell; 2014. p. 5–42.
10. Ludlow JB, Walker C. Assessment of phantom dosimetry and image quality of i-CAT FLX cone-beam computed tomography. Am J Orthod Dentofacial Orthop. 2013;144:802–17.
11. Juerchott A, Freudlsperger C, Weber D, Jende JME, Saleem MA, Zingler S, Lux CJ, Bendszus M, Heiland S, Hilgenfeld T. In vivo comparison of MRI- and CBCT-based 3D cephalometric analysis: beginning of a non-ionizing diagnostic era in craniomaxillofacial imaging? Eur Radiol. 2020;30:1488–97.
12. Pinheiro M, Ma X, Fagan MJ, McIntyre GT, Lin P, Sivamurthy G, Mossey PA. A 3D cephalometric protocol for the accurate quantification of the craniofacial symmetry and facial growth. J Biol Eng. 2019;13:42.
13. Pittayapat P, Limchaichana-Bolstad N, Willems G, Jacobs R. Three-dimensional cephalometric analysis in orthodontics: a systematic review. Orthod Craniofacial Res. 2013;17:69–91.
14. Swennen GR, Schutyser F. Three-dimensional cephalometry: spiral multi-slice vs cone-beam computed tomography. Am J Orthod Dentofacial Orthop. 2006;130(3):410–6.
15. European Commission. Radiation Protection No 172: cone beam CT for dental and maxillofacial radiology. Evidence based guidelines. 2012. http://www.sedentexct.eu/files/radiation_protection_172.pdf. Accessed 10 Nov 2021.
16. Walker L, Enciso R, Mah J. Three dimensional localization of maxillary canines with cone-beam computed tomography. Am J Orthod Dentofacial Orthop. 2005;128:418–23.
17. Mah J, Enciso R, Jorgensen M. Management of impacted cuspids using 3-D volumetric imaging. J Calif Dent Assoc. 2003;31:835–41.
18. Becker A, Chaushu S, Casap-Caspi N. Cone-beam computed tomography and the orthosurgical management of impacted teeth. J Am Dent Assoc. 2010;141:14S–8S.
19. Tsolakis AI, Kalavritinos M, Bitsanis E, Sanoudos M, Benetou V, Alexiou K, Tsiklakis K. Reliability of different radiographic methods for the localization of displaced maxillary canines. Am J Orthod Dentofacial Orthop. 2018;153(2):308–14.
20. Kalavritinos M, Benetou V, Bitsanis E, Sanoudos M, Alexiou K, Tsiklakis K, Tsolakis AI. Incidence of incisor root resorption associated with the position of the impacted maxillary canines: a cone-beam computed tomographic study. Am J Orthod Dentofacial Orthop. 2020;157(1):73–9.
21. Tsiklakis K, Syriopoulos K, Stamatakis HC. Radiographic examination of the temporomandibular joint using cone beam computed tomography. Dentomaxillofac Radiol. 2004;33:196–201.
22. Tsolakis IA, Venkat D, Hans MG, Alonso A, Palomo JM. When static meets dynamic: comparing cone-beam computed tomography and acoustic reflection for upper airway analysis. Am J Orthod Dentofacial Orthop. 2016;150(4):643–50.
23. Schendel SA, Broujerdi JA, Jacobson RL. Three-dimensional upper-airway changes with maxillomandibular advancement for obstructive sleep apnea treatment. Am J Orthod Dentofac Orthop. 2014;146:385–93.
24. Görgülü S, Gokce SM, Olmez H, Sagdic D, Ors F. Nasal cavity volume changes after rapid maxillary expansion in adolescents evaluated with 3-dimensional simulation and modeling programs. Am J Orthod Dentofac Orthop. 2011;140:633–40.
25. Vale F, Francisco I, Lucas A, Roseiro A, Caramelo F, Sobral A. Timing of spheno-occipital synchondrosis ossification in children and adolescents with cleft lip and palate: a retrospective case-control study. Int J Environ Res Public Heal. 2020;17:8889.
26. Piedra-Cascón W, Meyer MJ, Methani MM, Revilla-León M. Accuracy (trueness and precision) of a dualstructured light facial scanner and interexaminer reliability. J Prosthet Dent. 2020;124:567–74.
27. Hong C, Choi K, Kachroo Y, Kwon T, Nguyen A, McComb R, Moon W. Evaluation of the 3dMDface system as a tool for soft tissue analysis. Orthod Craniofac Res. 2017;20(Suppl. S1):119–24.
28. Heike CL, Upson K, Stuhaug E, Weinberg SM. 3D digital stereophotogrammetry: a practical guide to facial image acquisition. Head Face Med. 2010;6:18.
29. Tzou C-HJ, Artner NM, Pona I, Hold A, Placheta E, Kropatsch WG, Frey M. Comparison of three dimensional surface-imaging systems. J Plast Reconstr Aesthetic Surg JPRAS. 2014;67:489–97.
30. Gibelli D, Pucciarelli V, Poppa P, Cummaudo M, Dolci C, Cattaneo C, Sforza C. Three-dimensional facial anatomy evaluation: reliability of laser scanner consecutive scans procedure in comparison with stereophotogrammetry. J Craniomaxillofac Surg. 2018;46:1807–13.
31. Amornvit P, Sanohkan S. The accuracy of digital face scans obtained from 3D scanners: an in vitro study. Int J Environ Res Public Health. 2019;16:5061.
32. Pundir M, Sandhu JK, Kumar A. Quality-of-service prediction techniques for wireless sensor networks. J Phys Conf Ser. 2021;1950(1):012082.
33. Sehrawat S, Kumar A, Grover S, Dogra N, Nindra J, Rathee S, Dahiya M, Kumar A. Study of 3D scanning technologies and scanners in orthodontics. Mater Today Proc. 2022;56(Part 1):186–93.
34. Martin CB, Chalmers EV, McIntyre GT, Cochrane H, Mossey PA. Orthodontic scanners: what's available? J Orthod. 2015;42:136–43.

35. Nulty AB. A comparison of full arch trueness and precision of nine intra-oral digital scanners and four lab digital scanners. Dent J. 2021;9:75.
36. Mangano A, Beretta M, Luongo G, Mangano C, Mangano F. Conventional vs digital impressions: acceptability, treatment comfort and stress among young orthodontic patients. Open Dent J. 2018;12:118–24.
37. Aragón MLC, Pontes LF, Bichara LM, Flores-Mir C, Normando D. Validity and reliability of intraoral scanners compared to conventional gypsum models measurements: a systematic review. Eur J Orthod. 2016;38:429–34.
38. Christopoulou I, Kaklamanos EG, Makrygiannakis MA, Bitsanis I, Perlea P, Tsolakis AI. Intraoral scanners in orthodontics: a critical review. Int J Environ Res Public Health. 2022;19:1407.
39. Rossini G, Parrini S, Castroflorio T, Deregibus A, Debernardi CL. Diagnostic accuracy and measurement sensitivity of digital models for orthodontic purposes: a systematic review. Am J Orthod Dentofac Orthop. 2016;149:161–70.
40. Jedliński M, Mazur M, Grocholewicz K, Janiszewska-Olszowska J. 3D scanners in orthodontics—current knowledge and future perspectives—a systematic review. Int J Environ Res Public Health. 2021;18:1121.
41. Rheude B, Sadowsky PL, Ferriera A, Jacobson A. An evaluation of the use of digital study models in orthodontic diagnosis and treatment planning. Angle Orthod. 2005;75:300–4.
42. Möhlhenrich SC, Brandt M, Kniha K, Bock A, Prescher A, Hölzle F, Modabber A, Danesh G. Suitability of virtual plaster models superimposed with the lateral cephalogram for guided paramedian orthodontic mini-implant placement with regard to the bone support. J Orofac Orthop Fortschr Der Kieferorthopädie. 2020;81:340–9.
43. Tsolakis IA, Gizani S, Panayi N, Antonopoulos G, Tsolakis AI. Three-dimensional printing technology in orthodontics for dental models: a systematic review. Children (Basel). 2022;9(8):1106.
44. Tsolakis IA, Papaioannou W, Papadopoulou E, Dalampira M, Tsolakis AI. Comparison in terms of accuracy between DLP and LCD printing technology for dental model printing. Dent J (Basel). 2022;10(10):181.
45. Tsolakis IA, Tsolakis AI, Elshebiny T, Matthaios S, Palomo JM. Comparing a fully automated cephalometric tracing method to a manual tracing method for orthodontic diagnosis. J Clin Med. 2022;11(22):6854.
46. Im J, Kim JY, Yu HS, Lee KJ, Choi SH, Kim JH, Ahn HK, Cha JY. Accuracy and efficiency of automatic tooth segmentation in digital dental models using deep learning. Sci Rep. 2022;12(1):9429.
47. Adel SM, Vaid NR, El-Harouni N, Kassem H, Zaher AR. TIP, TORQUE & ROTATIONS: how accurately do digital superimposition software packages quantify tooth movement? Prog Orthod. 2022;23(1):8.
48. Tsolakis IA, Kolokitha O-E, Papadopoulou E, Tsolakis AI, Kilipiris EG, Palomo JM. Artificial intelligence as an aid in CBCT airway analysis: a systematic review. Life. 2022;12(11):1894.

Digital Prosthodontics

9

Luis DelCastillo, Hiroshi Hirayama, Lea Hajjar, and Konstantinos Michalakis

Recent digital revolutions affect our everyday life. Dentistry, especially in the field of Prosthodontics, is no exception from this digital explosion on our everyday practice. This bursting development of digital technologies has changed many aspects of the way we practice in Prosthodontics today. Most of the conventional materials and techniques have been or are being replaced by new digitally compatible materials and techniques; nevertheless, all the fundamentals of Prosthodontics still remain the same or have had minimal changes. This digital transformation ranges from the patient's data accruing, analyzing, and creating treatment options, to fabricating definitive restorations. An overview of digital developments in the field of Prosthodontics will be provided in this chapter.

L. DelCastillo · H. Hirayama
Department of Restorative Sciences and Biomaterials, Advanced Education Program in Prosthodontics, Boston University Henry M. Goldman School of Dental Medicine, Boston, MA, USA

L. Hajjar
Department of Prosthodontics, Tufts University School of Dental Medicine, Boston, MA, USA

K. Michalakis (✉)
Department of Restorative Sciences and Biomaterials, Boston University Henry M. Goldman School of Dental Medicine, Boston, MA, USA

Boston University Center for Multiscale and Translational Mechanobiology, Boston, MA, USA
e-mail: kmich@bu.edu

9.1 Digital Evolution in Prosthodontics Examination and Planning

According to a *Fortune Business Insight* report, the dental CAD/CAM field's global market growth was USD $2.36 billion in 2021 and is projected to increase from USD $2.72 billion in 2022 to USD $4.94 billion by 2029. The Compound Annual Growth Rate (CAGR) is expected 8.9% during the forecast period of 2022–2029 [1].

9.1.1 Intraoral Scanners (IOS)–Extraoral Scanners (EOS): CAD/CAM

Currently, digitalization in dentistry is a part of the dentist's everyday life, which ranges from practice and patient management software to total digital execution of an entire dental treatment process, such as full-arch implant restorations by using Computer-Aided Design and Computer-Aided Manufacturing (CAD/CAM). The evolution of digitalization in dentistry was further

A. Delantoni, K. Orhan (eds.), *Digital Dentistry*, https://doi.org/10.1007/978-3-031-52826-2_9

accelerated around 2010, especially in the field of Prosthodontics. Clinical chairside CAD/CAM (CEREC, E4D: current Planscan etc.) systems became much more accessible and popular [1]. Digitalization of intraoral structures can be done either directly by Intraoral Scanners (IOS) or indirectly by scanning the model/impression by Extraoral Laboratory Scanners (EOS), which utilize laser scanning or visible light source scanning technology (blue or white light). Both the IOS and EOS scanning methods have advantages and disadvantages. It is important however to mention that both have had significant improvements in speed and accuracy (precision and trueness) in the past 10 years. The IOS and the EOS are explained in detail in Chap. 4. The IOS systems became popular when they were sold independently from the chairside CAD/CAM systems. At the same time many commercial dental laboratories started engaging in CAD/CAM technology since the EOS and the dental laboratory software have made considerable advancements and became more accessible and user friendly. Additionally, existing and new dental materials were also made available for this emerging technology, as milling machines became more widely available and more accurate. Moreover, the advancement of 3D printing technologies paved the way for the development of 3D printing materials over the past 5 years in the dental industry.

Initially, the CAD/CAM software was mainly developed for the clinical chairside system such as CEREC for same-day type of restorations such as inlays and onlays. However, due to the increased number of CAD/CAM technologies used in dental laboratories and the versatility of the laboratory CAD software, the use of an open IOS system integrated with a laboratory CAD software, such as 3Shape (3Shape Dental system: 3Shape, Copenhagen, Denmark) and Exocad (exocad Dental CAD: exocad GmbH owned by Align Technology, San Jose, CA) with an additional open type milling machine and/or 3D printer, became extremely popular in the dental market.

The current trend of the dental CAD software could integrate with different digital file formats such as DICOM (Digital Imaging and Communications in Medicine developed by the National Electrical Manufacturers Association), STL (Standard Triangle Language/Standard Tessellation Language developed by 3D system in 1988), OBJ (a geometry definition file format developed by Wavefront Technologies), as well as other different file formats for creating a "Virtual patient" for digital treatment planning. Therefore, today the gap between the laboratory CAD software and the clinical chairside CAD software is becoming smaller.

9.1.2 Digital Radiography

Since the first dental radiograph was employed in 1896, conventional radiograph technique was used for nearly 100 years until the first digital radiographs were introduced by Trophy in 1987. In the late 1990s to early 2000s, digital panoramic radiography and cone beam computed tomography (CBCT) became also available in dentistry. Currently integration of CBCT data in DICOM file with dental arch scanning data in STL or DICOM file, as well as diagnostic planned restoration data in STL or DICOM file made it possible to do digital treatment planning for patients requiring implant placement. Pre-restorative orthodontics treatment planning has also benefitted from this technology.

9.1.3 Digital Photography

Conventional film-based clinical and laboratory photographs were used until mid-1990s, when digital technology in photographs became available, utilizing different formats, such as JPEG (Joint Photographic Experts Group), RAW (unprocessed and un-compressed data files), TIFF (Tag Image File Format), etc. [2].

Digital cameras became available to document and magnify the view of hard and soft oral tissues, which in turn became a very powerful treatment communication tool between the patient and the dentist, as well as between the dentist and the dental laboratory technologist. These provided a great service to dentists, when they were combined with 90–105 mm macro lenses and ring or side flashes. Extraoral 2D digital photographs taken with an SLA camera or even with smartphones have begun to be used for digital smile analysis of patients. In this way the dentists started creating and sharing with their patients esthetically ideal treatment plans, as well as designing maxillofacial prostheses [3].

9.1.4 3D Surface Imaging

Three-dimensional surface imaging methods, which are executed without exposing the patient to any radiation, are also an important advancement in dentistry. Currently, the available 3D imaging technologies include 3D Laser Scanning, the Structured Light Technique (3D White light scanning), and Stereophotogrammetry (3dMD) [4]. Technically, 3D laser scanning and the Structured Light Technique utilize the same technology as surface scanning of a dental model by a laboratory scan. A recent research study by Ye et al. has shown that both the structural light technique and the stereophotogrammetry techniques are accurate and reproductive [5]. Handheld type of 3D scanning equipment is commonly used for face surface scanning methods, which may present both advantages and limitations [5]. Advantages of the photogrammetry method can be the high cost and accessibility, since a camera (either SLA camera or smartphone) and a photogrammetry software are required [5]. It should be mentioned however that a single camera technique requires taking multiple pictures from different angles and then reconstructing them into a single 3D image. This procedure is time-consuming and may result in inaccuracies in the final 3D image, if the subject is not still.

The use of commercially available Stereophotogrammetry systems became widely popular with craniofacial clinics and research centers. These systems have two or more cameras that capture more than one image simultaneously, at a capture speed of approximately 1.5 ms, and are then processed through their proprietary software at an image rendering speed of 7 s to create a 3D image or even a 3D video (4D imaging) with videocameras (video Stereophotogrammetry) (e.g., 3dMD system) [6, 7] (Fig. 9.1). Currently,

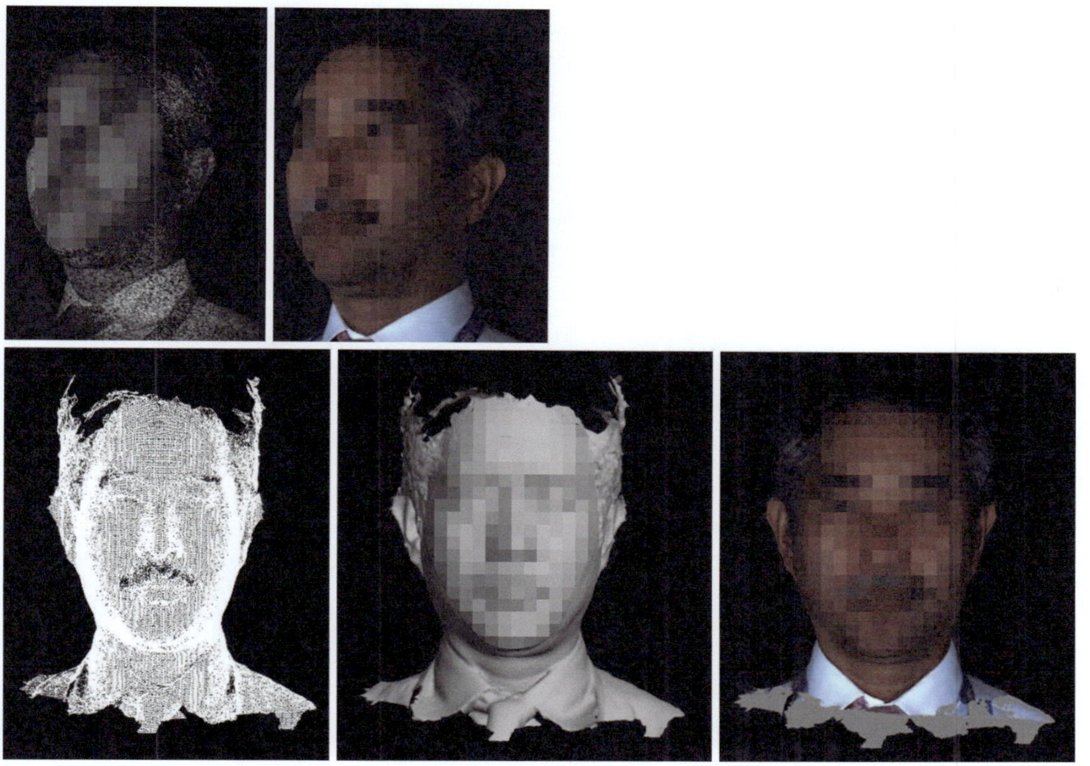

Fig. 9.1 Head and neck image taken with 3dMDface® system

some CBCT units have also integrated face image scanning functions that can superimpose hard and soft tissue images simultaneously (e.g., Galileos FaceScanner®: Dentsply Sirona, Planmeca ProFace®: Planmeca). One of the limitations of the Stereophotogrammetry systems however is that they may not register some objects accurately, particularly clear objects like the eyes, or reflective materials like teeth in the 3D image.

The accuracy of 3D image may vary, depending on the CBCT unit employed (Planmeca ProFace® Galileos FaceScanner®) (Fig. 9.2).

Besides the 3D scanning equipment available in the market, some companies have also introduced software that made possible 3D scanning with the use of a smartphone. A very popular one was that of Bellus3D (Bellus 3D Inc.), which was user friendly and allowed a 3D reconstruction at a very affordable cost. Sadly enough the company terminated their service in 2022 [8]. Today, there are several options for the restorative dentists who want to integrate a virtual 3D face reconstruction in their treatment planning. A recent study has reported that the esthetic treatment plan can be achieved without 3D face imaging devices, by using a virtual 3D face reconstruction from 2D conventional digital photographs. This process is based on a web-based online code repository, three-dimensional dense face alignment (3DDFA), and STL files via IOS/EOS before and after a digital wax-up [9]. It is worth mentioning that the majority of dental CAM software accept or have the ability to combine 3D facial image data with other 3D data such as DICOM file (CBCT) and STL/OBJ/PLY file (IOS/DLS/3D face scan) [10, 11]. However, there are still limitations in this area, restricting the use of 3D or 4D facial scan data in everyday clinical practice.

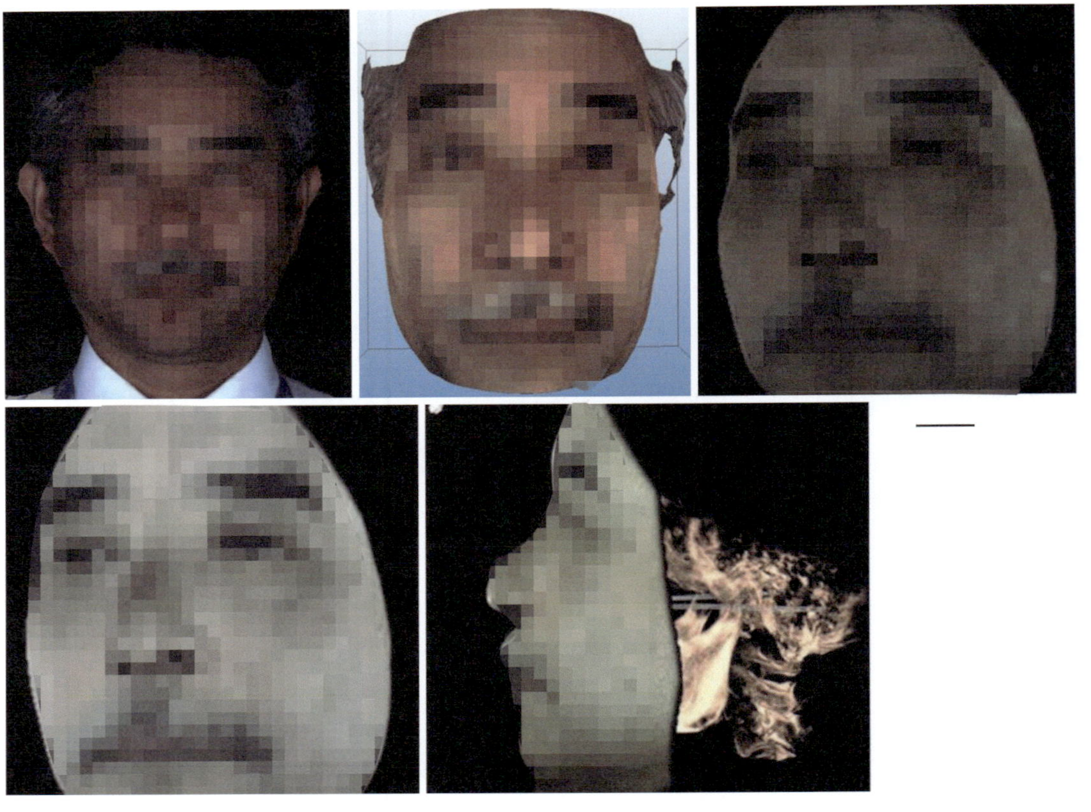

Fig. 9.2 Face image made with 3dMDface® system image, Planmeca ProFace® image, Sirona Dentsply Galileo FaceScanner® image (CBCT face images were not accurate and limited field)

9.1.5 Jaw Tracking

The evolution of digitized jaw tracking unit started with a *Mandibular Kinesiograph* (K7x jaw Tracking, Myotronics; Bio JT-3D™, Bioresearch Associates Inc.), which measures jaw movement using a magnet at the mandibular central incisor cervical area. Instead, the *Computerized Axiograph* measures jaw movement at the condyle level. However, presently, the magnetic jaw tracker systems have limitations in terms of transferring the jaw tracking information to CAD CAM systems. Currently, only a few systems can transfer jaw tracking information to CAD CAM systems. These can be grouped into three categories: (1) the *Computerized Axiograph* (CADIAX 2 and CADIAX 4, Gamma Dental), (2) the *Ultrasonic Axiograph* (JMA+ by Zebris GmbH; JMT+ by CICAT GmbH & Co. KG; Axioquick by SAM® Präzisionstechnik GmbH both of which are manufactured by Zebris GmbH) and the *Optical Axiograph* (ARCUSdigma™ 3 by KAVO Dental which is manufactured by Zebris GmbH and JMA Optic by Zebris GmbH), and (3) the *Stereophotogrammetry system* (MODJAW, MODJAW), which uses an STL file for static data. The latter can be used in the CAD software and the motion data is in XML (Extensible Markup Language) file format, which can be transferred to the Exocad software [12] (Fig. 9.3).

Currently all available systems can transfer information to CAD software like Exocad and three Shape. However, typically, all three categories of systems transfer only some parts of the jaw tracking information to CAD software, such as the Bennet angle and immediate mandibular lateral translation. Real integration of use of all vital Jaw tracking data, which includes functional jaw movements for diagnosis, treatment planning, and fabrication of definitive restorations, is not readily available but it would be necessary in the future. Digital file combination is available today, but not with full integration capabilities (Fig. 9.4).

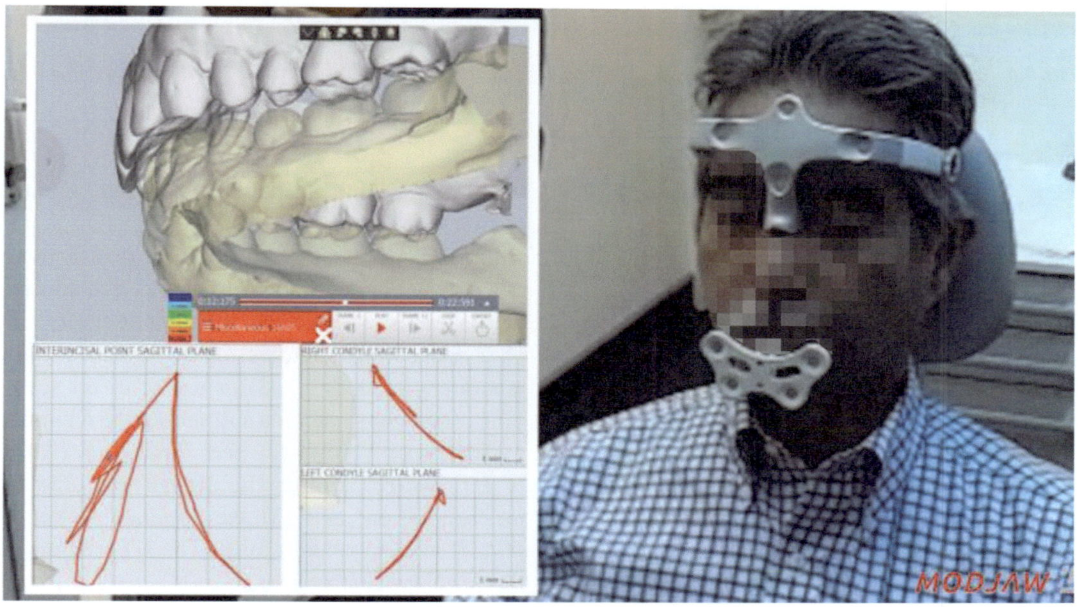

Fig. 9.3 MODJAW system and recording

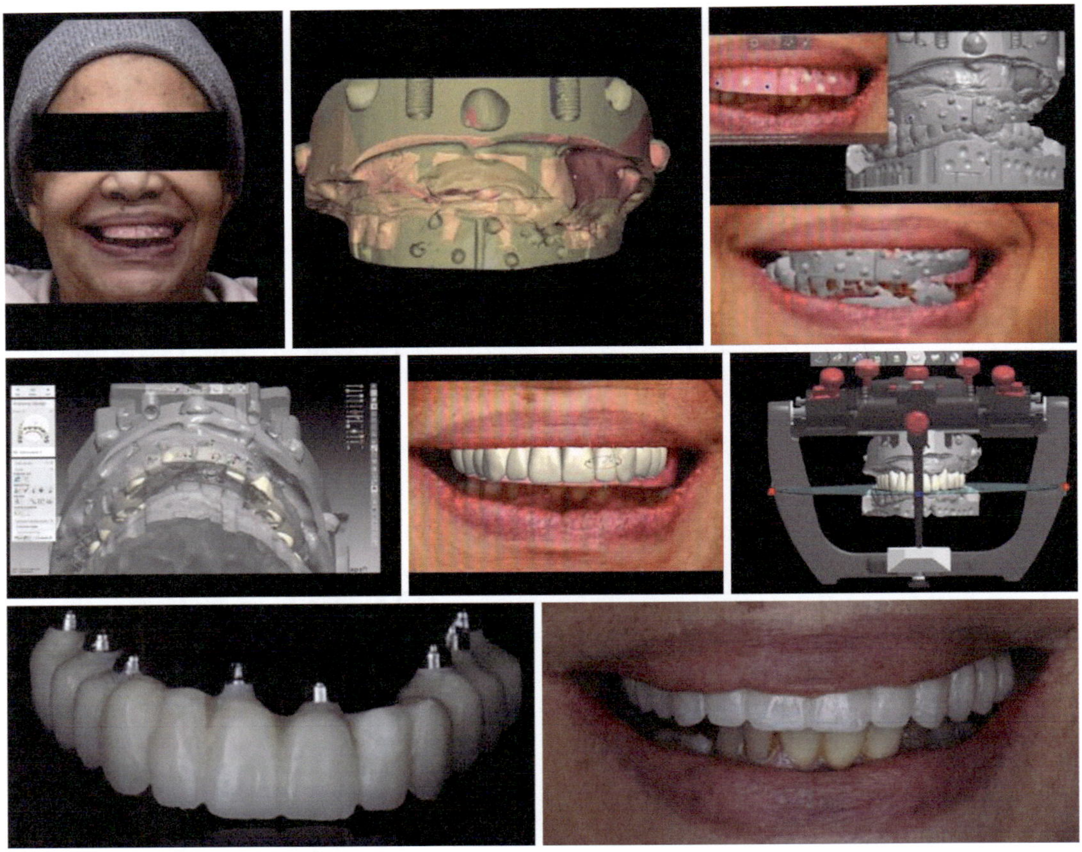

Fig. 9.4 Digital workflow using facial analysis and 2D and 3D data with virtual articulator for the fabrication of a full-arch implant-supported prostheses milled provisional. (Courtesy of Dr. Lea Hajjar)

9.2 Digital Fixed Prosthodontics

The evolution in digital dentistry in the field of fixed prosthodontics initiated with the development of a commercially available chairside Computer-Assisted Design/Computer-Assisted Manufacturing (CAD/CAM) system. Originally the CAD/CAM used in fixed prosthodontics was limited to the use of the chairside CAD/CAM systems for definitive fixed restorations, such as inlays, onlays, and full-coverage restorations. Today, digital technology products are delivered to dentists on a regular basis, even to those who have not incorporated the digital flow in their practices. This became a reality since the development of CAD/CAM zirconia restorations, which replaced a big number of metal ceramic restorations.

CAD/CAM technology in fixed prosthodontics can be divided into three phases that consist of: (1) the *Acquisition Phase*, which includes use of a conventional impression combined with a laboratory scanner (EOS) or use of direct scanning of patient's hard and soft tissues via an intraoral scanner (IOS), (2) the *Designing Phase (CAD)*, which involves the digital designing of the restoration, and (3) the *Production Phase (CAM)*, which includes milling or 3D printing of the definitive restorations.

The current bursting development of digital dentistry has positively impacted the field of fixed prosthodontics, from the initial phase of data collection with digital radiographs and images, treatment planning, digital diagnostic wax-up and implant surgery planning, fabrication of mock template and provisional restorations, to the fabrication of the definitive fixed restorations. This technology has impacted favorably the fit and accuracy of the definitive restorations. It has also helped to reduce the costs and time associated with the conventional fixed prosthodontics procedures.

Today fixed prosthodontic procedures can be completed with a purely digital flow or a combination of analog and digital steps. Usually the transition point is after obtaining a conventional definitive impression with an elastomer, which is then scanned before proceeding with the digital design and the fabrication of the definitive restorations.

9.2.1 Tooth Preparation for CAD/ CAM

During tooth preparation the practitioner needs to know the type of material that will be used for the definitive restoration. The basic concepts of tooth preparation should be followed with digital dentistry procedures. These in general include parallel axial walls, rounded internal line angles, and adequate space for the restorative material to guarantee the esthetic result and strength. However, the fact that different restorative materials can be utilized during the CAM process makes imperative the need to know the exact mechanical properties and requirements of each material. To that end, zirconia may require less tooth reduction, vertical preparation with thinner margins, but more axial wall parallelism than lithium disilicate [13]. It should be mentioned however that the literature suggests that in general a more favorable margin design for these restorations is a rounded shoulder or a chamfer [14]. Moreover, it has been shown that the preparation quality has a direct effect on the marginal fit of chairside CAD/CAM crowns [15].

9.2.1.1 Intraoral Scanners (IOS)

The definition, explanation, and description of intraoral scanners are covered in Chap. 4. However, as a brief introduction, there are different technologies available today to obtain a digital impression of the teeth and the surrounding soft tissues. These technologies are continuously being updated and refined. As a result, intraoral acquisition units have become smaller, making it easier to capture previously challenging areas. Obviously, this was beneficial for both the practitioner and the patient. Another important fact is that the intraoral scanners available today no longer need the antireflective powder used before and can easily capture colors, as well as assist with tooth shade selection.

Apart from eliminating the uncomfortable aspects of traditional dental impressions, one of the major advantages of intraoral scanning is that any area that during the initial scan may have not been adequately captured can be locally rescanned. Modern intraoral scanners function by using different image capturing technologies, and the oral structures are recorded as individual images or video. These images are compiled by the software, which recognizes certain specific points of interest and stitches the images.

9.2.1.2 Treatment Planning, Fabrication of Provisional and Definitive Restorations

The digital planning process for fixed prosthodontics should not deviate much from the conventional planning process, in the sense that a careful diagnosis needs to be established prior to any dental procedure. Traditional procedures which involve a careful clinical and medical evaluation of the patient, full mouth set of X-rays, preliminary impressions and properly mounted casts in a semi-adjustable articulator, and an occlusal analysis are still necessary. Diagnostic waxing can be performed either traditionally or digitally in order to visualize the final result before any irreversible intraoral modification is done.

In the digital realm, the oral cavity can be scanned and a digital model created and mounted on a digital articulator. Like the traditional method, this too can provide the necessary information for planning the prosthodontic treatment needed. As mentioned above, a digital wax-up can be created in conjunction with the intraoral and face scans, and this can help the clinician to make better clinical decisions, but can also serve as a tool for patient education, motivation, and case acceptance. The process is then completed by the so-called guided dentistry, which implies that digital guides, appliances, and restorations can be printed or milled to transfer the digital plan to the patient's mouth [16].

The software involved in this process can be classified as *pre-case Acceptance Software* (planning) and *post-case Acceptance Software* (execution). The pre-software needs to be able to incorporate all the necessary dental and facial information and integrate successfully all available data, in order to achieve a satisfactory result. Modern dentistry is interdisciplinary, and the impact of a procedure in one specialty over the others must not be underestimated. Therefore, the software should be used for diagnosis, treatment plan, design, and simulation of different solutions. Ideally the software should be capable of performing all interdisciplinary simulations, so one can judge the best combination of procedures for each patient.

The main goals of a *pre-case acceptance software* include: (a) data acquisition; (b) improvement of key medical/dental conditions and diagnosis; (c) case simulation, comparison of options, and promotion of team brainstorming for possible treatment options; (d) improvement of the decision-making and risk assessment processes; (e) presentation-explanation of treatment options, with patient participation in the decision-making process by using the pre-software as a 3D visual communication tool [17].

After treatment plan acceptance, data are exported from the pre-software and imported to the post-software. The post-software is the specialized software for each specialty area—i.e., orthodontics, orthognathic surgery, implant surgery, restorative—and its main goal is to assist in planning and executing specific disciplinary procedures. The main goals of a *post-case acceptance software* include: (a) import of files from the pre-software, including ideal design and simulation suggestions; (b) precise merging of files from pre-software to perform sub-specialty disciplinary operations; (c) design of devices needed for specific treatment procedures; (d) connection to manufacturing systems, such as milling and 3D printing machines [17].

9.2.2 CAD/CAM Materials

With the advent of digital dentistry, the increase in patients' esthetic demands and the desire for "metal free" restorations, ceramic alternatives to metal substructures have been developed. It is well documented that ceramic restorations present excellent esthetic properties, chemical stability, and biocompatibility [18, 19]. However, until quite recently ceramic dental restorations were limited to the anterior region, because of their brittle character [20]. The development of dental ceramic systems with very good mechanical properties has been followed by their use in the posterior regions. Zirconia ceramics, which present excellent biocompatibility and high fracture strength, are now used for fixed partial dentures in both anterior and posterior regions. Obviously, use of a fracture-resistant core material is necessary to withstand clinical functional and parafunctional forces [21].

Yttria-stabilized tetragonal zirconia (3Y-TZP) was initially brought into the dental field approximately 20 years ago, because of its outstanding strength and tooth-like color [22]. As this material presented high opacity, it was intended to be used for frameworks of full-coverage restorations and fixed partial dentures, which were then veneered with translucent porcelains, similarly to the traditional metal ceramic restorations. These zirconia ceramics were veneered with feldspathic ceramics and produced an acceptable esthetic result. A drawback of this technique was that the layered feldspathic porcelain was prone to fracture due to the residual thermal stresses induced during the production process [23]. Therefore, manufacturers created layered zirconia, in an effort to produce a material with the strength of monolithic zirconia combined with the esthetic outcome of feldspathic ceramics.

In order to improve the translucency of zirconia, different manufacturing techniques have been employed. This is usually achieved by altering its cubic content, which can be controlled by the sintering temperature and the yttria content. It should be noticed that, as the yttria content and the sintering temperature are increased, the final product becomes more translucent. Nevertheless, this comes to the expense of strength and toughness of the material. Currently there are three grades of monolithic zirconia available in the market, namely 3Y-TZP, 4Y-PSZ, and 5Y-PSZ (mol% yttria partially stabilized zirconia). There is a trade-off between the translucency and the strength of these three grades, and therefore they have different clinical indications [22, 23].

Zirconia is currently available in the format of discs, where the restorations are machined via a milling system and then sintered to produce the definitive restoration. Initially, the available monolithic discs were monochromatic, and therefore their esthetic result was unsatisfactory. Recently, multilayered zirconia systems have been developed, in an effort to upgrade the esthetic properties of zirconia dental restorations. The multilayered zirconia design mimics the shade gradient observed between the cervical and the occlusal (incisal) areas of natural teeth. Different grades of translucency are produced to cover a big spectrum of various indirect dental restorative applications. The first multilayered zirconia system introduced to the dental market was the Katana (Kuraray Noritake, Japan), which includes three zirconia grades: Ultra Translucent Multi Layered zirconia (UTML), Super Translucent Multi Layered zirconia (STML), and Multi Layered zirconia (ML). According to the manufacturer, these three materials can cover all monolithic restorative applications. Since its first introduction to the dental market, this multilayered monolithic zirconia system has received immense attention both from clinicians and researchers. Other products, such as the Cercon (Dentsply Sirona), have also been marketed with very successful results (Fig. 9.5).

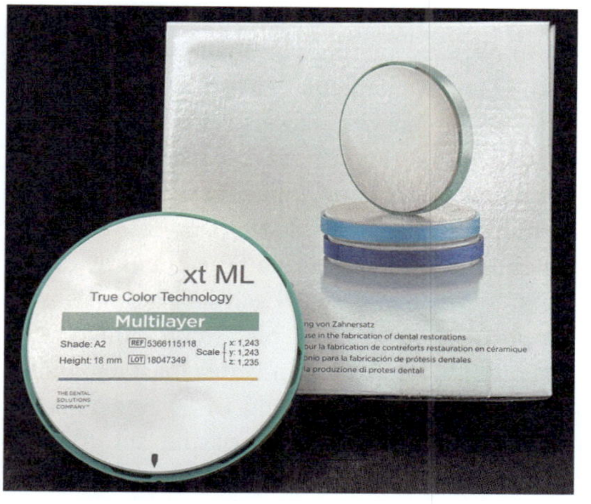

Fig. 9.5 Example of layered zirconia disc (Cercon®; Dentsply Sirona™)

Wear is also a significant factor when using zirconia restorations, particularly when the opposing teeth are natural. The amount of tooth wear caused to a natural tooth by a restorative material placed on the opposing arch should be a deciding factor in treatment planning. An ideal restorative material would produce tooth wear with the same rate with that of a natural tooth. Gundugollu et al. studied the wear of natural teeth when these had antagonists either monolithic or layered zirconia (multilayered). Varied surface treatments (unpolished-unglazed, polished-unglazed, and polished-glazed) were also studied in this research. The authors concluded that monolithic zirconia caused significantly less tooth wear when compared to layered zirconia. It was also found that polished-unglazed monolithic zirconia resulted in less tooth wear compared to polished-glazed monolithic zirconia [24].

One of the most common and challenging clinical conditions encountered in daily dental practice is the restoration of a discolored tooth. When managing this type of situation, the success of the procedure is highly dependent on the skills and experience of the treating dentist, as well as those of the dental technologist. This is due to the fact that the masking of a discolored substrate can sometimes be an unpredictable process. One advantage that zirconia has over other types of ceramic restorations is its inherent opacity and the ability to mask dark substrates. A recent study examined the masking ability of monolithic and layered zirconia full-coverage restorations on 11 discolored substrates by evaluating the middle, cervical and incisal thirds with a spectrophotometer. This study found that monolithic zirconia had a better masking ability compared to bi-layered and tri-layered zirconia restorations, independently of the substrate or tooth area. On the other hand, on moderately or severely discolored substrates at 1 mm thickness, monolithic zirconia showed insufficient masking ability [25].

9.2.3 3D Printing

3D printing is emerging in Dentistry as a promising technique for the fabrication of dental restorations and other dental appliances. A big advantage of 3D printing is that restorative material is not wasted during the fabrication process. Therefore, it is more economical than subtractive manufacturing techniques in terms of hardware investment and overall production costs [21]. With the advancement of digital technologies in dentistry, new 3D printing methods become commercially available very frequently [21, 26]. This fact makes the classification of current 3D printing methods especially challenging. A simplistic approach to define more common 3D printing technologies may categorize printing systems according to their fabrication process [27]. Under this classification, one may differentiate 3D printing methods under four broad categories: (1) extrusion printing; (2) inkjet printing; (3) laser melting/sintering; (4) lithography printing. In brief, in extrusion printing, a material is dispensed from a nozzle with computer-controlled movement in a three-axis stage [16, 28]. In inkjet printing, micrometer-sized droplets of an ink (typically a photopolymer) are dispensed, also using three-axis stages. Laser melting and sintering [29], on the other hand, typically do not dispense a material from a nozzle; rather, a laser light is used that creates an elevated temperature that can either sinter or weld specific regions in a powder bed. This technology is used in prosthodontics for the fabrication of FPD and RPD frameworks, as well as for metal copings. The material is added layer by layer, as a platform moves vertically, thus generating a 3D structure [30]. Lastly, light or lithography printing, which often also employs lasers as the light source, uses photopolymers that are kept in a *Z*-axis controlled vat. As the vat or sample holder moves vertically, a 3D structure results from direct exposition of the polymer to a light [31].

The impact that this technology has in the field of prosthodontics is broad, from the fabrication of dental models and provisional restorations to surgical guides, RPD frameworks, and metal copings. The impact of 3D printing has been immense, not only for the ease of use but also for the level of accuracy achieved and the minimal waste of material compared to the traditional process of fabrication. Another important advantage is the reduction in manufacturing time.

9.3 Digital Removable Prosthodontics

9.3.1 Digital Removable Complete Dentures (DRCDs)

The digitalization of the Removable Prosthodontics field has had remarkable improvements in both RCD and RPD areas. The first commercially available Digital Removable Complete denture (DRCD) system was from AvaDent™ (Global Dental Science LLC, Scottsdale, AZ), which uses a patented proprietary thermoplastic tray and occlusal registration system before proceeding to the milling of the denture. Dentca™ (Dentca Inc., Los Angeles, CA) is another manufacturer specializing in DRCD that works on their proprietary tray and gothic arch tracing system.

Until Dentsply Sirona and Ivoclar Vivadent (Ivoclar) came in the DRCD market in 2017, there was not much progress in the commercial use of digital dentures, except for the patented monolithic DRCD with denture base and teeth in one piece. This was initially developed by AvaDent™. Ivoclar followed with the Ivotion Denture system, which offered a monolithic DRCD in 2021. Although initially DRCDs were limited to subtractive manufacturing (milling) methods only, later on FDA approved the use of additive manufacturing (3D print) materials. Additive manufacturing (3D print) started with DENTCA in 2017. Dentsply Sirona released their 3D printed denture materials in 2019. Their method and materials were initially associated with Carbon 3D (Redwood City, CA) and 3 Shape software.

Currently, DRCDs became much more accessible to all dentists, and their construction can start from any of the steps of denture fabrication. This is mentioned in detail in one of the authors' publications [32]. Additional DRCD workflows have been proposed in the literature [33]. These are currently incorporated in some CAD software (3 Shape denture workflow), as well as in fully digitized DRCD workflows.

Today some companies offer a full line of DCDR fabrication methods, focusing especially on 3D printed DCDRs techniques. It should be pointed out that the properties of modern 3D printed materials have improved and are similar to those of conventional denture materials (Fig. 9.6).

Regarding the workflows of the subtractive and additive techniques, it can be understood that these differ significantly:

Subtractive DCDR fabrication workflows use rotary instruments mounted on a milling machine to carve pre-polymerized polymethylmethacrylate (PMMA) discs to monolithic Digital Removable Complete Dentures (DCRDs). The teeth used for these DCRDs can be either manufactured or milled and they are bonded to the DCDR base.

In the additive DCDR fabrication workflow, the denture base is fabricated by light polymerization of resins, specially fabricated for that purpose. The teeth can be manufactured, milled, or 3D printed and are bonded to the denture base. Pink colored composite resins can afterwards be applied to the facial/buccal aspects of the DCDR to mimic natural gingival tissues, with excellent esthetic results (Fig. 9.7).

Although the traditional fabrication of a removable complete denture had one workflow, with small variations, the digital fabrication offers many different paths:

9.3.1.1 Conventional Removable Complete Denture (RCD) Clinical Workflow

1. Preliminary impression
2. Secondary (final) impression with custom trays
3. Registration of maxillomandibular relation with wax rim trial base
4. Denture teeth try-in: Conventional RCD fabrication
5. Delivery

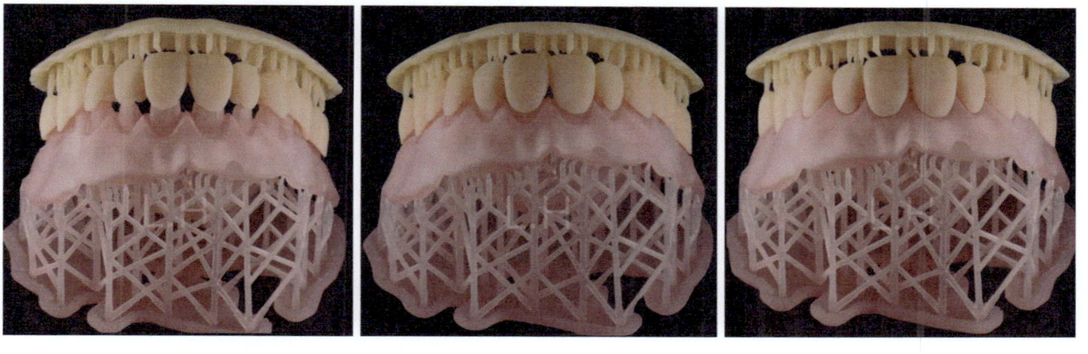

Fig. 9.6 3D printed denture digitally designed on InLab (Dentsply Sirona) and 3D printed using FormLabs2® printer. (Courtesy of Dr. Lea Hajjar)

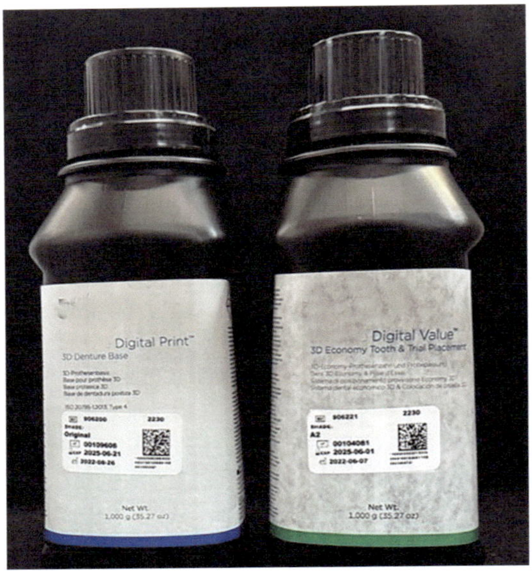

Fig. 9.7 Materials used for subtractive and additive methods of DCDR fabrication (Lucitone Digital Print™; Dentsply Sirona™)

9.3.1.2 DRCD Workflow 1: Digital Production of the Definitive DRCD

1. Preliminary impression
2. Secondary (final) impression with custom trays
3. Registration of maxillomandibular relation with wax rim trial base
4. Conventional wax denture try-in: DRCD fabrication (milled or 3D printed)
5. Delivery

It should be mentioned that DRCD workflow 1 is good when the dentist feels comfortable with the conventional workflow. However, this workflow does not provide a big advantage for clinical time reduction or smaller number of patient visits.

9.3.1.3 DRCD Workflow 2: Custom Tray Impression and Wax Rim Base Intra-occlusal Record (IOR) Technique

1. Preliminary impression
2. Secondary (final) impression with custom trays
3. Registration of maxillomandibular relation with wax rim trial base
4. 3D printed Denture try-in: DRCD fabrication (milled or 3D printed)
5. Delivery

Like the previous workflow, DRCD workflow 2 is good when the dentist feels comfortable with the conventional workflow. Nevertheless, this workflow too does not provide a big advantage for clinical time reduction or smaller number of patient visits.

9.3.1.4 DRCD Workflow 3: Wax Rim Impression Technique

1. Preliminary impression or IOS preliminary scan: Digitally/Conventionally fabricated Wax rim trial base
2. Wax rim impression technique (final impression followed by registration of maxillomandibular relation)
   (a) Scan maxillary wax rim and trial base: occlusal, polished and tissue surfaces along with final impression
   (b) Scan mandibular wax rim and trial base: occlusal, polished and tissue surfaces along with final impression
3. Maxillary and Mandibular wax rims and trial bases with a maxillomandibular relation registration
4. 3D printed denture try-in: DRCD fabrication (milled or 3D printed)
5. Delivery

DRCD workflow 3 is recommended when the patient does not have any previous dentures or the existing dentures are not of good quality in regard to peripheral extension, teeth position, or amount of occlusal wear (Fig. 9.8).

9.3.1.5 DRCD Workflow 4: Replication Denture Technique

1. Existing RCD Scan IOS or EOS for producing duplicate RCD (3D printed/milled): DRCD fabrication
2. Replication technique with copied RCDs (final impression, verification of maxillomandibular relation followed by new registration of maxillomandibular relation)

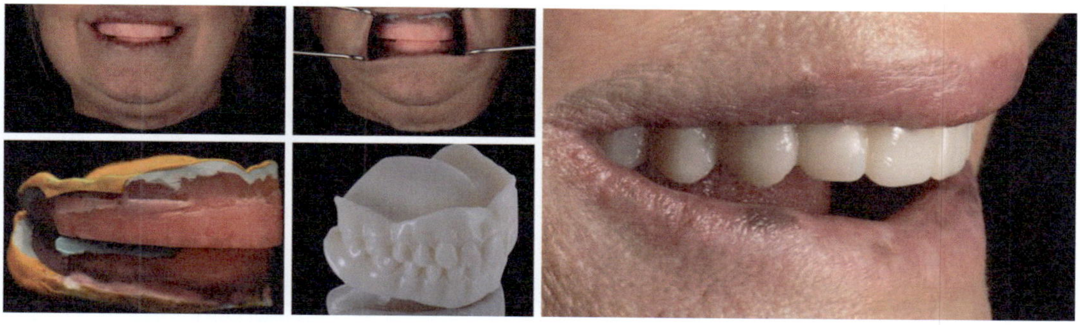

Fig. 9.8 DRCD workflow 3 with wax rim impression and Biofunctional try-in (Avadent™). (Courtesy of Dr. Lea Hajjar)

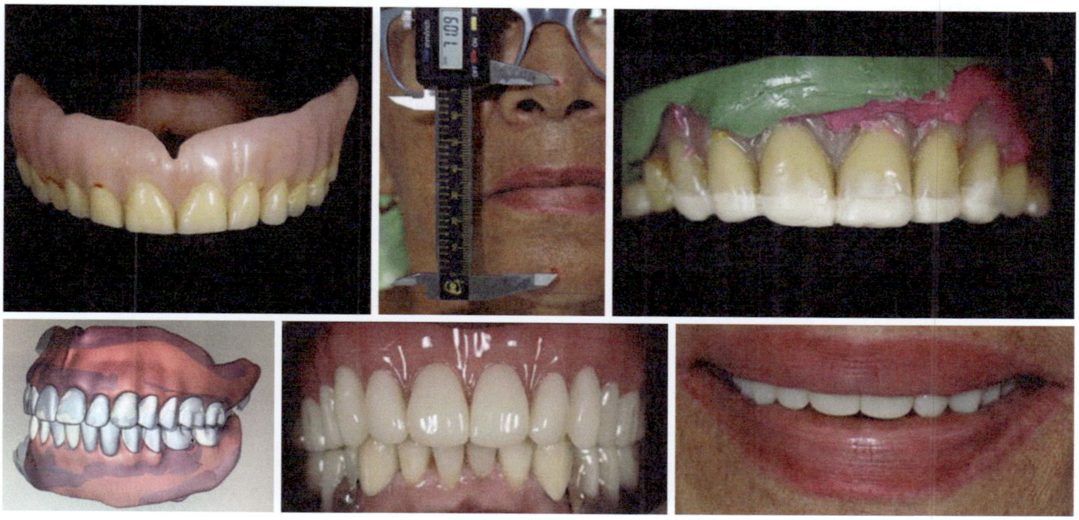

Fig. 9.9 DRCD workflow 4 using patient's existing dentures. Desired modifications were made before the final impression. Definitive dentures from Avadent™. (Courtesy of Dr. Esteban Molina)

   (a) Scan maxillary denture: occlusal, polish and tissue surfaces with final impression
   (b) Scan mandibular denture: occlusal, polish and tissue surfaces with final impression
   (c) Maxillary and mandibular dentures with a maxillomandibular registration
3. Optional 3D printed denture try-in: DRCD fabrication (milled or 3D printed)
4. Delivery

DRCD workflow 4 is recommended when the patient presents with removable complete dentures of reasonably good condition, but with the need of some modification before the final impression (Fig. 9.9).

9.3.1.6 DRCD Workflow 5: Reference Denture Technique

1. Reference denture technique (final impression and registration of maxillomandibular relation with existing RCD: Scan with IOS or EOS)
   (a) Scan maxillary denture occlusal, polished and tissue surfaces along with final impression
   (b) Scan mandibular denture occlusal, polished and tissue surfaces along with final impression
   (c) Maxillary and mandibular dentures with an occlusal registration

2. Optional 3D printed denture try-in: DRCD fabrication (milled or 3D printed)
3. Delivery

DRCD workflow 5 is recommended when the patient presents with existing dentures of a reasonably good condition with the exception of fitting and retention. A possible limitation of this technique is that frequently the dentist cannot modify the existing dentures without patient's consent. As a result, the digital modification of denture teeth setup is challenging.

9.3.1.7 DRCD Workflow 6: Fully Digitized DRCD Technique

1. IOS final impression (design final denture border) scans and a PVS putty, maxillomandibular registration with proper lip support, and plane of occlusion references. IOS scan design trial dentures based on anatomical references and averages and 3D printed try-in dentures
2. 3D printed denture try-in (border molding and wash impression, followed by maxillomandibular registration):
   (a) Scan Maxillary trial denture occlusal, polished and tissue surfaces along with final impression
   (b) Scan Mandibular trial denture occlusal, polished and tissue surfaces along with final impression
   (c) Maxilla and Mandibular trial dentures with a maxillomandibular registration
3. DRCD fabrication (milled or 3D printed)
4. Delivery

DRCD workflow 6 can be chosen when the patient presents with no existing dentures and has ideal oral conditions for denture fabrication: presence of reasonably well-developed alveolar ridges, presence of adequate inter-occlusal space, and good neuromuscular coordination. The IOS scan should cover the peripheral tissues, including all necessary anatomical landmarks for designing optimal denture extension for support, retention, and stability [33].

In case of immediate denture fabrication with pre-existing dentition, a chairside digital design of immediate complete dentures can be done on the STL file obtained. The design can then be sent to AVADENT™ or Dentca™ for the fabrication of the immediate dentures, following either milled or 3D print routes (Figs. 9.10 and 9.11).

9.3.2 Digital Removable Partial Dentures (DRPD)

The use of a general CAD software for designing removable partial dentures (RPDs) was first reported by Williams et al. in 2004 [34]. The authors developed a digital survey method, designed a simple RPD framework, and then produced a plastic pattern for casting, by employing 3D printing. Later Han and coworkers described the use of a specifically developed RPD design CAD software (the Tang Long CAD system). With this method the metal framework was fabricated by the Selected Laser Melting (SLM) 3D printer (Fig. 9.12) [35].

The RPD CAD software development was slow until the end of 2010. SensAble Technologies Dental division created a unique RPD design software using force-feedback haptic device technology and touch-enabled 3D design software around 2011. Exocad® America acquired SensAble® Dental division in 2014, while Geomagic acquired SensAble's haptic device assets in 2012 [36]. Currently, 3Shape, Exocad, Dental Wings, and Dentsply Sirona share the majority of RPD CAD software in the market [37].

RPD framework fabrication can be either subtractive (milling) or additive (3D printing). There are different types of materials for each fabrication method. Metals such as titanium, cobalt-chromium, and polymers such as polyetherketone (PEEK) are available for the milling method. The materials for 3D printing include Co-Cr alloys and resins for casting with metal alloys or pressing for PEEK [38, 39].

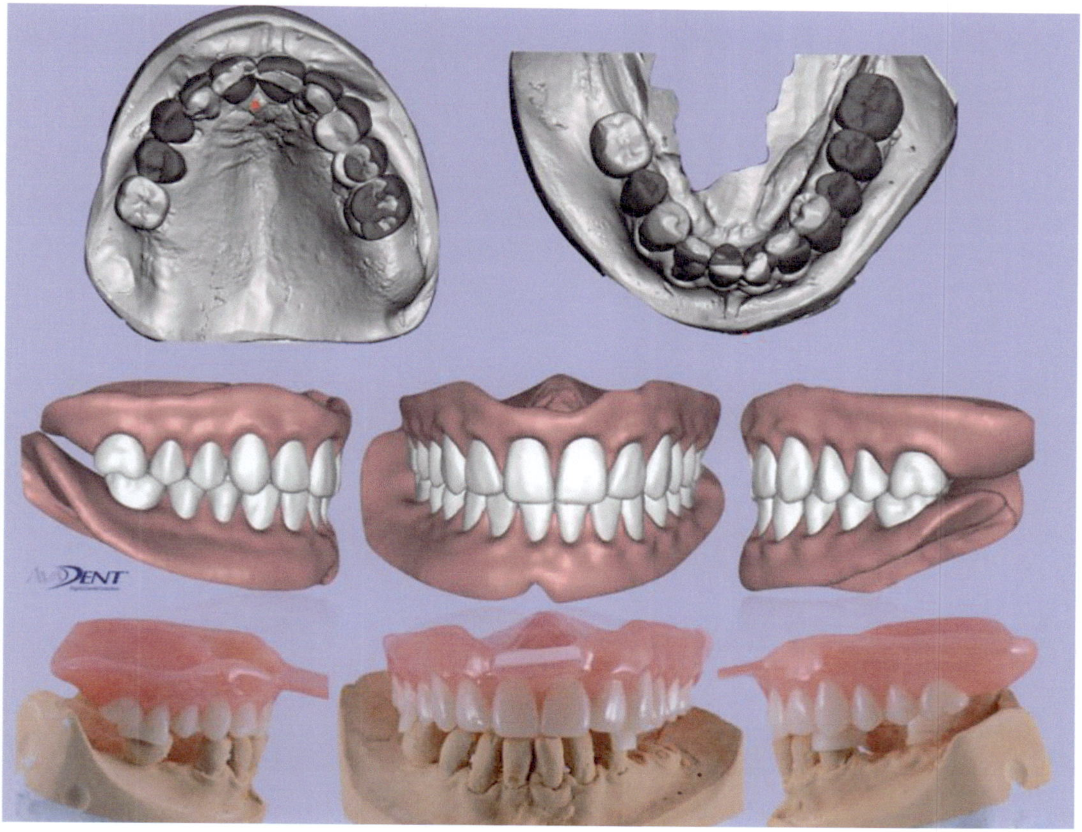

Fig. 9.10 Fabrication of maxillary immediate denture against patient's current mandibular natural dentition for correct positioning of the maxillary denture by clip utilization. Definitive maxillary denture milled by Avadent™. (Courtesy of Dr. Hajjar)

Workflow of RPD design and fabrication Although currently the digital workflow for RPD fabrication is limited to digital design and digital production of metal frameworks, a total digital workflow will soon become a reality.

9.3.3 The RPD Workflows: Conventional and Digital

9.3.3.1 Conventional RPD Design and Fabrication

1. Diagnostic cast: Preliminary survey and preliminary RPD design
2. Mouth preparation: Post preparation survey cast for verification purposes
3. Final impression
4. RPD design on definitive (master) cast (duplicated definitive cast)
5. Blocking of undercuts and model duplication for a refractory die material
6. RPD framework wax-up on the model as designed
7. Investing, casting, divesting, finishing and polishing
8. Framework try-in, denture teeth setup and wax-up of polished surfaces
9. Wax-up try-in and processing
10. Delivery

9.3.3.2 Digital RPD Design and Fabrication

1. IOS: Preliminary digital survey and preliminary RPD design

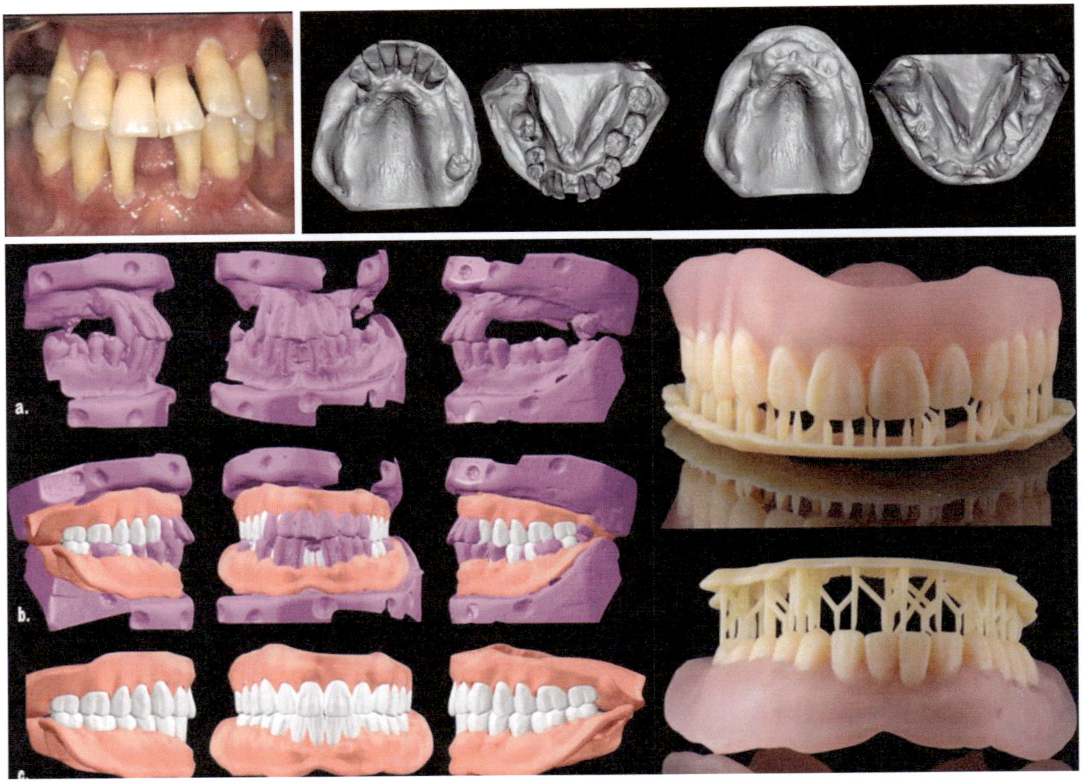

Fig. 9.11 Chairside digital design of immediate complete dentures: patient's initial clinical picture (top left). Models were scanned and teeth were digitally removed (top right). Chairside digital setup of immediate dentures using Dentca™ (bottom left): (a) scanned models in occlusion, (b) superimposed models with teeth setup, (c) definitive immediate denture setup. Denture base and teeth 3D printed using FormLabs 3D printer (bottom right). (Courtesy of Dr. Yousef Behbehani)

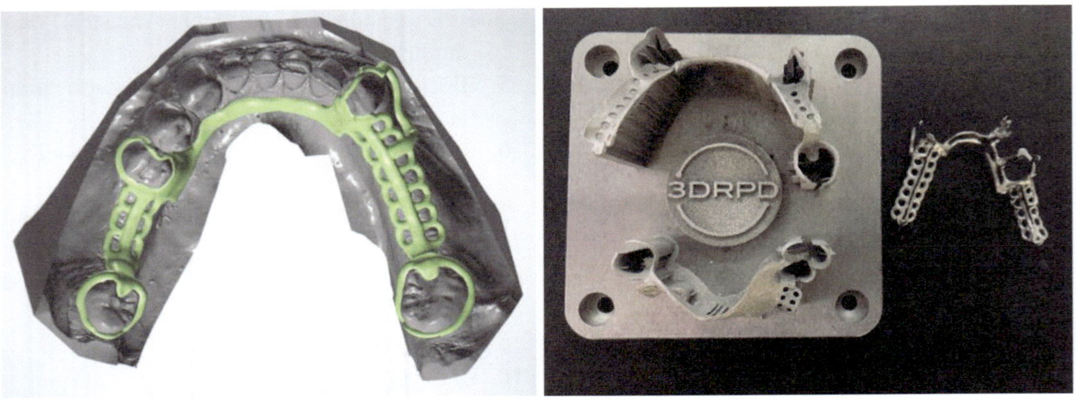

Fig. 9.12 Digitally designed and fabricated Removable Partial Denture framework

2. Mouth preparation; IOS for verification of mouth preparation
3. Final impression, cast fabrication, and EOS
4. Digital RPD design
5. 3D Print/Milling: CAM metal framework production
6. Framework try-in, denture teeth setup and wax up of polished surfaces on definitive (master) cast
7. Wax-up try-in and processing
8. Delivery

9.3.3.3 Total Digital RPD Design and Fabrication

1. IOS: Preliminary digital survey and preliminary RPD design
2. Mouth preparation; IOS for verification of mouth preparation
3. IOS; final digital scan
4. Digital RPD design including digital denture teeth setup and flange extension
5. 3D print/milling: CAM metal framework, 3D printed denture teeth and flange
6. Assembled RPD try-in/delivery

9.3.4 Summary of DRCD and DRPD

DRCD's complete digital workflow can now be incorporated in everyday clinical practice. This is due to the development of 3D printed denture teeth and base materials that have equal or better mechanical properties compared to conventional denture materials. Additionally, it has been clinically proven that the DRCD provides better fitting dentures, with less remakes compared to the conventional RCDs [40, 41]. As already mentioned, a complete digital workflow of DRCD is not yet feasible, and therefore a hybrid approach is still followed. 3D printed denture materials may soon change the landscape in DRCD fabrication. Although polymer RPD frameworks, like PEEK, are commercially available, there are still a number of challenging issues that must be resolved prior to being used on a daily basis. If the 3D printable RPD polymer framework materials could fulfill the required mechanical properties of the conventional metal RPD frameworks, it could be possible to print an one-piece RPD, by using a 3D printer capable of printing multiple materials with different colors.

9.4 Digital Technology in Implant Prosthodontics

9.4.1 Planning Software

During a prosthodontic dental treatment, the aim has always been to try to obtain the highest level of accuracy during both planning and execution, by trying to eliminate any guesswork and possible failure. Until quite recently, dentists and oral surgeons planned for implant placement with information obtained from bone-mapping and 2D radiographic images. Implants were placed free hand, with favorable or unfavorable results, depending on the practitioner's experience. With the advent of digital technology in the dental industry, most of this guesswork has been eliminated. The digital workflow in implant dentistry is constantly and rapidly evolving, reducing the number of analog steps that were previously taken and producing more accurate results [42, 43]. Regardless of the simplicity of the various stages of treatment, a digital workflow requires a steeper learning curve, as well as an understanding of the possible shortcomings, due to inherent hardware and software errors. These limitations may result in deviations in final implant position [44, 45].

The key in digital treatment always begins with proper planning. The available software used in implantology for virtual planning requires certain steps fundamental to achieve clinical success. These include segmentation, deletion of artifacts, superimposition of images (DICOM/STL), and virtual implant placement (Fig. 9.13). The accuracy of the surgical guides has been demonstrated to be strongly linked to both the printing device and printing method [46]. Therefore, it is evident that at the stages of guide planning and manufacturing, there are many points in which the sum of errors may lead to undesirable results [44, 47]. In general, guided

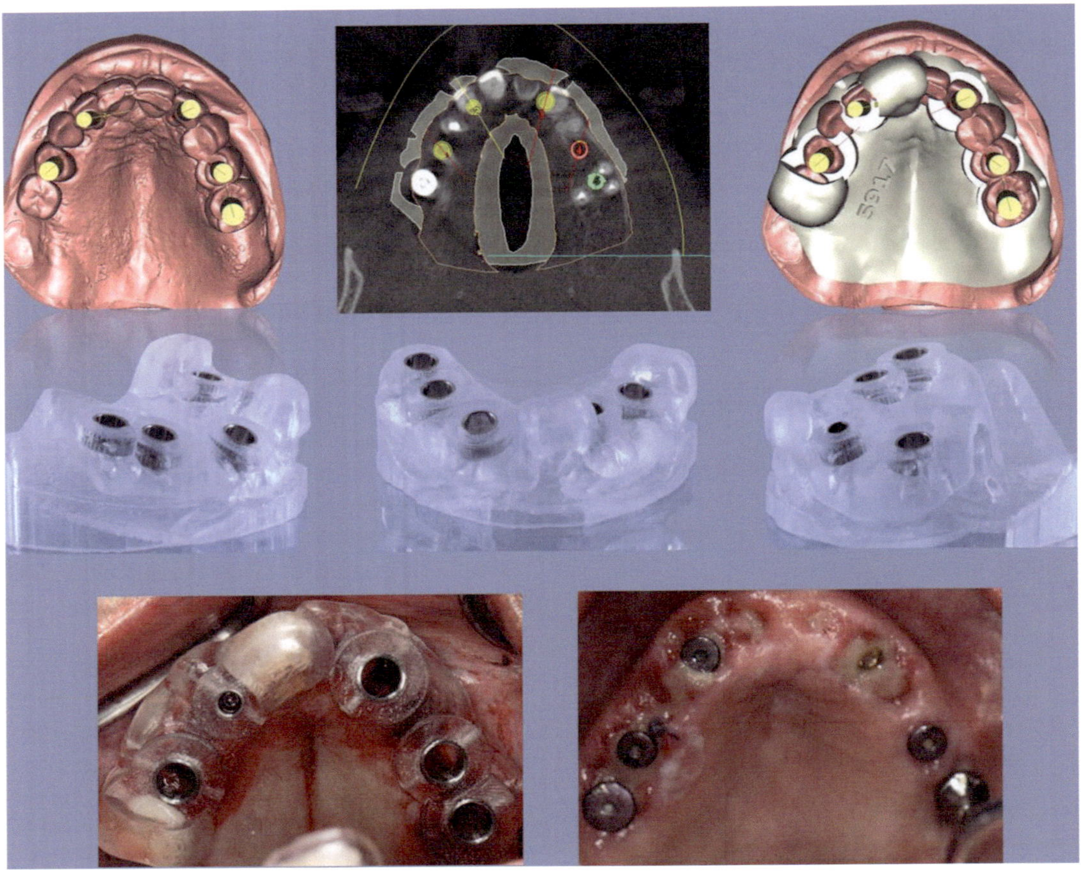

Fig. 9.13 Precise selection of implant positions based on the digital wax-up and patient's CBCT scan DICOM file. Simplant Implant planning software was employed for accurate implant placement. (Courtesy of Dr. Lea Hajjar)

implant surgery results in a faster procedure compared to conventional freehand surgery. Moreover, it usually provides better results in the postoperative period. Although guided surgery is generally indicated in cases of flapless implant placement, it can also be used in open flap surgeries, as well [48]. It should be mentioned however that extreme caution should be exercised in certain areas, where there is considerable risk of biologic and/or esthetic failure due to bone defects and possible postoperative gingival recession. When facing these situations, guided implant surgery is the preferred approach, ensuring precise implant placement [49]. The precision of the guided surgery has already been documented in the literature. However, some deviations should be anticipated and taken into consideration when developing a virtual plan [44, 50, 51].

Digital full-arch impressions acquired with intraoral scanners can have slight deviations in accuracy, especially when the midline is crossed [15]. There are some researchers, however, who have found similar accuracy levels among several scanners when full-arch scans were obtained [52]. A recent literature review article has concluded that, currently, the use of intraoral scanners should not be our first choice, when long-span restorations on teeth or implants are planned [53]. Researchers indicate that further investigation is necessary on digital impressions for dental implants [54].

The limitation of intraoral scanners when it comes to cross-arch digital impressions is that the technology relies on stitching images together. As the acquisition unit travels across the arch, some of these stitched images become unreliable, leading to inaccuracies in the full-arch scan. This has a negative impact in prosthodontics procedures, as accuracy is crucial when scanning for implant-supported complete fixed prostheses. Therefore, a verification jig should always be used to assess the accuracy of the designed restoration, before proceeding to prosthesis fabrication. It is always imperative to be aware of the limitations of the technology, in order to achieve the most satisfactory results.

The latest literature has shown that photogrammetry technology for full-arch implant restorations provides higher accuracy in terms of trueness and precision, compared to IOS and conventional impressions. This is explained in detail in Chap. 4.

Currently there are many different planning software options available to dentists. When these are used properly, they can achieve very satisfactory and predictable results. With the way technology has developed lately, it is not surprising that the level of accuracy has improved dramatically. This is especially true in the field of implant surgery planning, where guesswork and a large number of errors have been eliminated. In the field of prosthodontics or restorative dentistry, this aspect becomes crucial because the prosthodontist or restorative dentist, who is ultimately responsible for providing the definitive restoration, should carefully plan the final implant position. Thus, every minor detail needs to be evaluated in order for the highest level of accuracy that this technology can provide to be obtained.

9.4.1.1 Navigated Surgery

The goal for any prosthodontist or restorative dentist, when it comes to implant dentistry, is the ideal placement of the implant, in order to provide a functional and esthetic restoration free from any biological or technical complications for a long-term period. In that context, any tool or aid available to achieve such result is always desirable. Dentists and oral surgeons have several options when it comes to implant planning and placement. Dental implant treatment planning and placement has greatly benefited from in office-based imaging, as well as from complex simulation and planning software. The combination of software and imaging allowed for the development of static implant guides to achieve predictable accuracy in implant placement.

Dynamic navigation (DN) has improved the process by providing surgeons a real-time navigation tool to improve the accuracy of implant placement. Currently, DN is used by many medical specialties, including ophthalmology, otolaryngology, orthopedics, vascular surgery, neurosurgery, and surgical oncology. These specialties routinely use DN to perform simple and complex procedures with increased accuracy and precision [55, 56]. In the field of dentistry, primarily oral and maxillofacial surgeons have historically used DN, in hospital facilities. The medical DN systems used were designed primarily for craniofacial-based procedures, such as orthognathic surgeries, trauma, pathology, reconstructive procedures, as well as for locating foreign bodies within the head and neck areas [57, 58]. In the United States, Robodent was the first DN system and was introduced in the early 2000s to assist in the placement of dental implants. Since then, additional systems have been approved for this indication. The current DN workflow requires (1) obtaining a three-dimensional (3D) scan with rigidly fixed or predictably reproducible and accurate fiducial marking systems; (2) virtual implant planning; (3) calibration and registration of fiducial markers, implant drill, and drill lengths with attached tracking arrays; and (4) implant osteotomy and placement according to the 3D image on the navigation screen.

9.4.1.2 The Technology

The DN systems available in the United States are a type of Computer-Assisted Surgery (CAS) that uses optical tracking as a guide. Currently two types of optical motion tracking systems exist: (1) *active* and (2) *passive*. The *active* tracking systems emit an infrared light, which is then tracked by stereo cameras, while the *passive* tracking systems use reflective spheres to reflect an infrared light, which is emitted from a light source, back to a camera. The patient and drill must be positioned over the line of sight of the tracking camera [59]. Presently, the most commonly utilized DN technology is the *passive* type. A light is projected from a light emitting diode source above the patient. The light is then projected down to the patient and the surgical field. This projected light is then reflected off tracking arrays (passive patterned arrays) attached to the patient and the surgical instrument that is being tracked. A pair of stereo cameras located above the patient then captures the reflected light. The system calculates the position of the patient and the instruments relative to the pre-surgical plan. This is performed in real time. A virtual image is then shown on a monitor for the surgeon and staff. This virtual reality device gives the surgeon the ability to work dynamically on the patient and execute the planned implant surgery. At any time, the surgeon has the liberty to change the plan, based on the clinical situation [60].

It is important to always confirm the accuracy of the tracking system, by performing frequent system checks. Anatomical landmarks on the patient are touched with the instruments. The dentist then visually confirms that the radiographic landmarks on the screen are exactly correlating. The operator looks at the screen, as the drill is positioned over the surgical site. The navigation system screen allows viewing of a virtual drill with demonstration of the depth in tenths of a millimeter, angular deviation of the drill bit axis from the planned implant axis to the tenths of a degree, and the implant timing (Figs. 9.14 and 9.15).

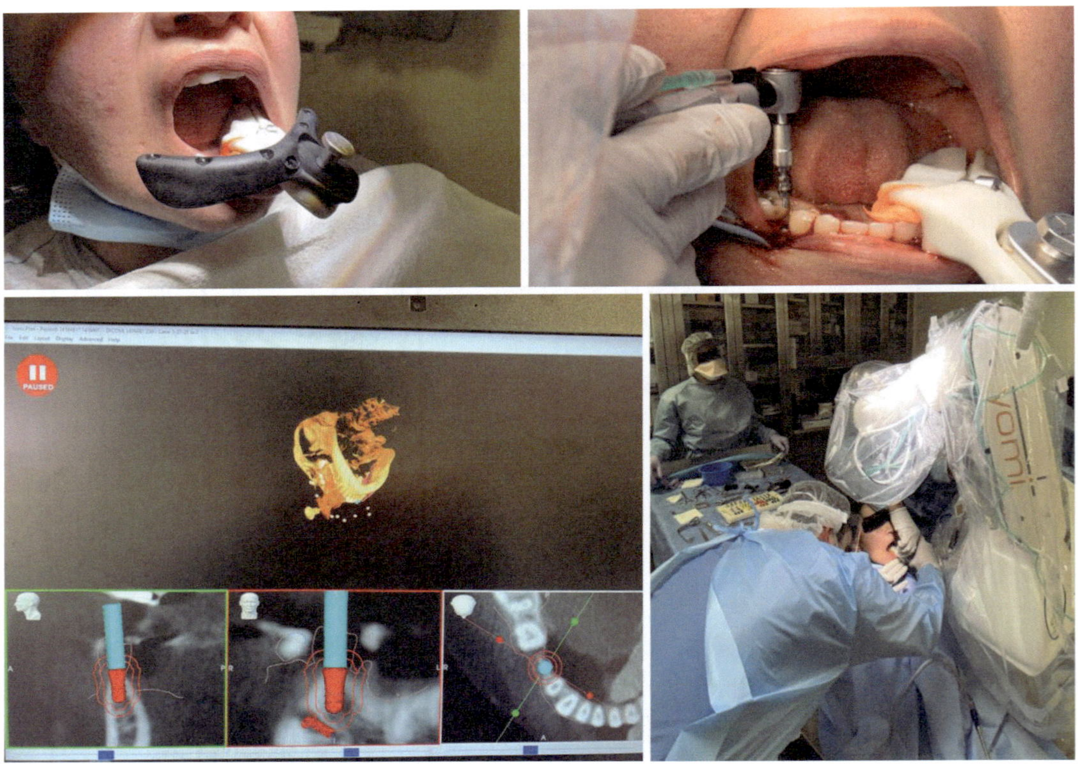

Fig. 9.14 Guided surgery for single implant placement with Yomi® Robotic System at Boston University Henry M. Goldman School of Dental Medicine. (Photos courtesy of Dr. Esteban Molina)

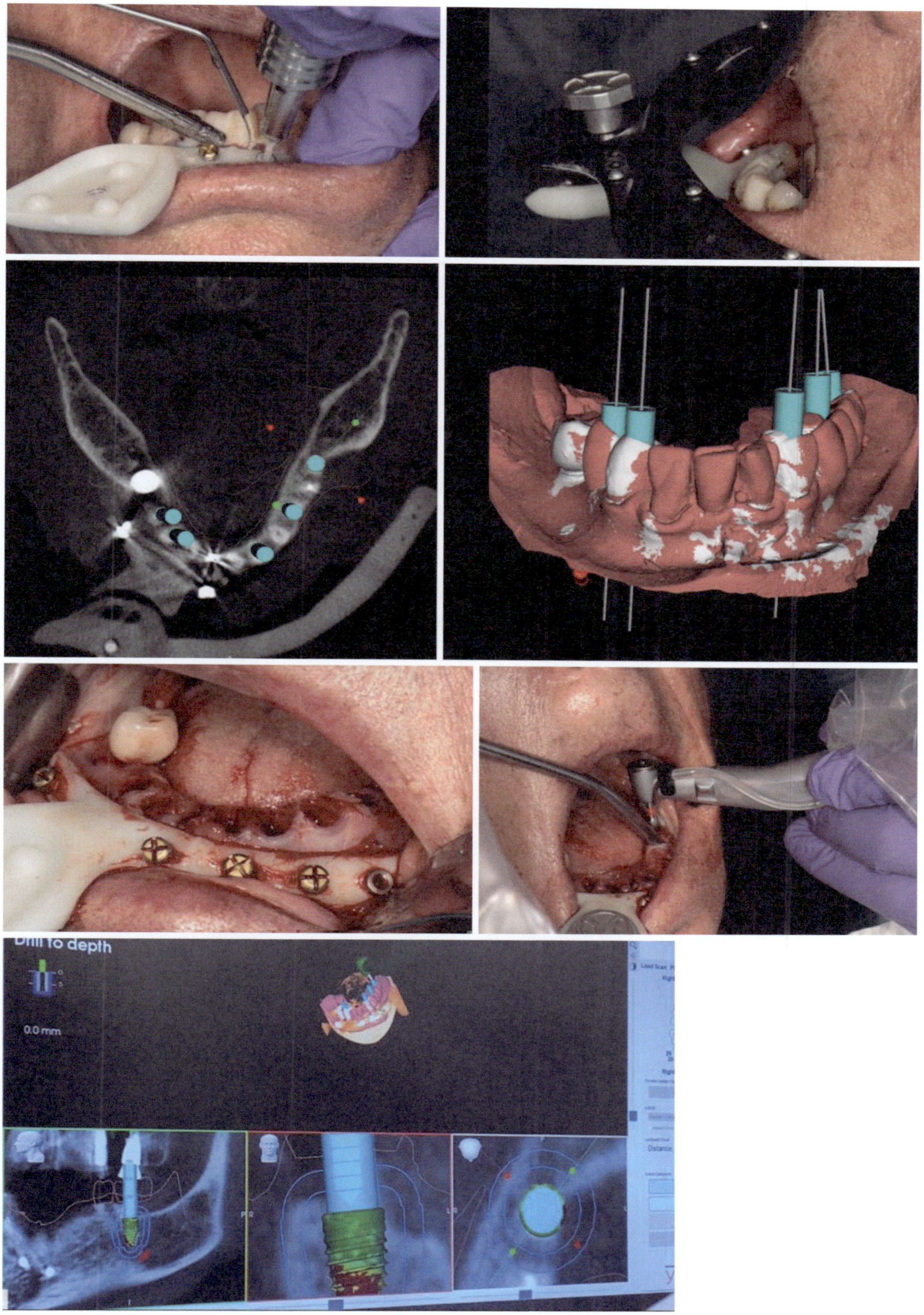

Fig. 9.15 Guided surgery for full-arch immediate implant placement with Yomi® Robotic System. (Photos courtesy of Dr. Lea Hajjar)

9.4.1.3 Dynamic Navigation Advantages

Implant surgeons are able to evaluate and scan the patient, plan for the final implant position, and perform the surgery in the same day without the delay or cost associated with the fabrication of a static surgical guide stent. This technology also allows the implant surgeon to change the implant size, system, and location parameters during the operation, when clinical situations dictate a change. DN allows oral surgeons to confidently acknowledge the implant is placed in the right position, without having to raise a flap, thus minimizing trauma to the patient. The major benefit of DN is that it allows the surgeon to verify accuracy at all times of the surgery, as opposed to the static technique, where, if the splint is not appropriately positioned and fixated, there can be significant errors in implant placement.

9.4.1.4 Dynamic Navigation Disadvantages

The implementation of DN requires a significant investment for the dental implant surgeon. In addition to a CBCT and an IOS, there is the capital cost of the DN system. There is also a per-case cost of fiducial clips, markers, and plates. Those surgeons with limited experience with technology and virtual image processing may find difficult the transition to a different modality of practice. There is also a big learning curve associated with the application of innovative technology. Another disadvantage is that during the operation patients have tracking arms attached to their mouth. As the DN systems' hardware and software develop further, these disadvantages will probably diminish.

The increased utilization of 3D technologies for both diagnostic and therapeutic modalities has allowed the dentist to see the limitations of free-hand implant placement and overcome this obstacle. The accuracy and precise execution of implant placement have increased and, consequently the restorative outcome has been more successful, as it is "prosthetically driven."

9.4.2 Robotic Surgery

Robotic surgery represents one of the valuable tools developed in the recent years to assist the dentists in accurate implant placement and long-lasting successful implant restorations. It should be mentioned that the amount of information found in the literature on robotic surgery is rather low. The first recognized digitally operated and programmable robot was an industrial one, called "Unimate" (Unimation, Inc., USA), which was used in the automotive industry in 1961 [61]. The Programmable Universal Machine for Assembly 200 (PUMA 200, Westinghouse Electric, Pittsburg, PA, USA) was the first robot to be used in medicine over 25 years later, in 1988. Its purpose was to align a needle during neurosurgical biopsies [59]. Since then, experiments with robot technology in many fields of dentistry have been described, including implantology, restorative dentistry, and education [62, 63]. Some robotic solutions have become commercially available in recent years and are marketed for use in the general dentist practice, such as the implantology robot "Yomi" (Neocis, Miami, Florida, USA) (Fig. 9.16).

Robotics in dentistry is a field that might be considered that it is in its infancy. There is not a large number of articles currently available in the literature on this topic. Most of the articles are research-oriented and not evidence-based. However, undoubtedly robotics will provide useful solutions in the future, and therefore clinical trials are needed to support its clinical use.

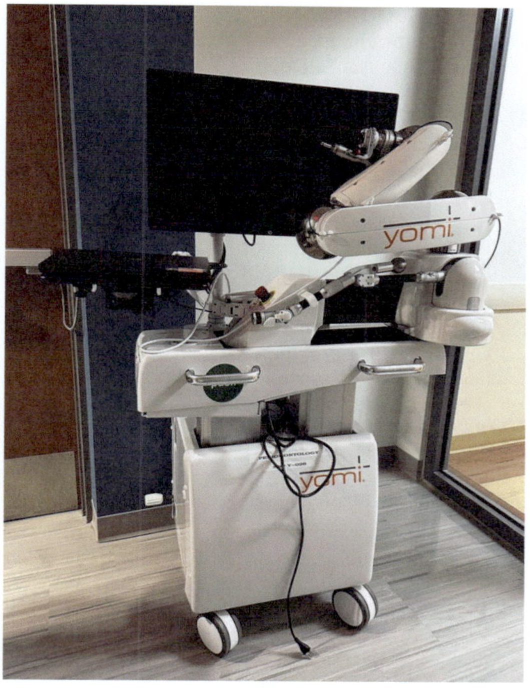

Fig. 9.16 Yomi® Robotic System used at Boston University Henry M. Goldman School of Dental Medicine

References

1. https://www.fortunebusinessinsights.com/dental-cad-cam-market-105080. Report ID: FBI 105080.
2. Tania Dworjan. Timeline of digital photography technology. 2022. https://photography.lovetoknow.com/Timeline_of_Digital_Photography_Technology.
3. Salazar-Gamarra R, et al. Monoscopic photogrammetry to obtain 3D models by a mobile device: a method for making facial prostheses. J Otolaryngol Head Neck Surg. 2016;45:33. https://doi.org/10.1186/s40463-016-0145-3.
4. Karatas OH, Toy E. Three-dimensional imaging techniques: a literature review. Eur J Dent. 2014;8(1):132–40.
5. Ye H, Lv L, Liu Y, Liu Y, Zhou Y. Evaluation of the accuracy, reliability, and reproducibility of two different 3D face-scanning systems. Int J Prosthodont. 2016;29(3):213–8.
6. Heike CL, et al. 3D digital stereophotogrammetry: a practical guide to facial image acquisition. Head Face Med. 2010;6:18.
7. Hallac RR, Feng J, Kane AA, Seaward JR. Dynamic facial asymmetry in patients with repaired cleft lip using 4D imaging (video stereophotogrammetry). J Craniomaxillofac Surg. 2017;45:8–12.
8. https://www.bellus3d.com/.
9. Liu Y, Chen D, Zhang R, Cui X, Zhou Y. The application of 3D dense face alignment in esthetic rehabilitation. J Prosthodont. 2022;31(2):171–4.
10. Joda T, Brägger U, Gallucci G. Systematic literature review of digital three-dimensional superimposition techniques to create virtual dental patients. Int J Oral Maxillofac Implants. 2015;30:330–7.
11. https://www.photomodeler.com/photogrammetry-vs-3d-scanning/.
12. Dental Tribune. MODJAW: a next-generation digital dentistry solution. 2021. https://www.dental-tribune.com/news/modjaw-a-next-generation-digital-dentistry-solution/.
13. Paniz G, Kang K-H, Kim Y, Kumagai N, Hirayama H. Influence of coping design on the cervical color of ceramic crowns. J Prosthet Dent. 2013;110(6):494–500. ISSN 0022-391.
14. Renne W, McGill ST, Forshee KVS, DeFee MR, Anthony S. Mennito, predicting marginal fit of CAD/CAM crowns based on the presence or absence of common preparation errors. J Prosthet Dent. 2012;108(5):310–5. ISSN 0022-3913.
15. Ender A, Zimmermann M, Mehl A. Accuracy of complete- and partial-arch impressions of actual intraoral scanning systems in vitro. Int J Comput Dent. 2019;22(1):11–9. PMID: 30848250.
16. Panwar A, Tan LP. Current status of bioinks for micro-extrusion-based 3D bioprinting. Molecules. 2016;21:685. https://doi.org/10.3390/molecules21060685.
17. Coachman C, Blatz MB, Bohner L, Sesma N. Dental software classification and dento-facial interdisciplinary planning platform. J Esthet Restor Dent. 2021;33(1):99–106. https://doi.org/10.1111/jerd.12713. Epub 2021 Jan 20. PMID: 33470496.
18. Christensen GJ. Choosing an all-ceramic restorative material: porcelain fused-to metal or zirconia based? J Am Dent Assoc. 2007;138:662–5.
19. Koçak EF, Uçar Y, Kurtoğlu C, Johnston WM. Color and translucency of zirconia infrastructures and porcelain-layered systems. J Prosthet Dent. 2019;121(3):510–6. https://doi.org/10.1016/j.prosdent.2018.08.001. Epub 2018 Nov 23. PMID: 30477923.
20. Seghi RR, Sorensen JA. Relative flexural strength of six new ceramic materials. Int J Prosthodont. 1995;8:239–46.
21. Johnston WM, O'Brien WJ, Tien T-Y. The determination of optical absorption and scattering in translucent porcelain. Color Res Appl. 1986;11:125–30.
22. Zhang Y. Making yttria-stabilized tetragonal zirconia translucent. Dent Mater. 2014;30:1195–203.
23. Zhang Y, Lawn BR. Novel zirconia materials in dentistry. J Dent Res. 2018;97:140–7.
24. Gundugollu Y, Yalavarthy RS, Krishna MH, Kalluri S, Pydi SK, Tedlapu SK. Comparison of the effect of monolithic and layered zirconia on natural

teeth wear: an in vitro study. J Indian Prosthodont Soc. 2018;18(4):336–42. https://doi.org/10.4103/jips.jips_105_18. PMID: 30449962; PMCID: PMC6180733.
25. Gasparik C, Manziuc MM, Burde AV, Ruiz-López J, Buduru S, Dudea D. Masking ability of monolithic and layered zirconia crowns on discolored substrates. Materials (Basel). 2022;15(6):2233. https://doi.org/10.3390/ma15062233. PMID: 35329684; PMCID: PMC8949301.
26. Stansbury JW, Idacavage MJ. 3D printing with polymers: challenges among expanding options and opportunities. Dent Mater. 2016;32:54–64. https://doi.org/10.1016/j.dental.2015.09.018. [PubMed: 26494268].
27. Obregon F, Vaquette C, Ivanovski S, Hutmacher DW, Bertassoni LE. Three-dimensional bioprinting for regenerative dentistry and craniofacial tissue engineering. J Dent Res. 2015;94:143S–52S. https://doi.org/10.1177/0022034515588885. [PubMed: 26124216].
28. Chang CC, Boland ED, Williams SK, Hoying JB. Direct-write bioprinting three-dimensional biohybrid systems for future regenerative therapies. J Biomed Mater Res B Appl Biomater. 2011;98:160–70. https://doi.org/10.1002/jbm.b.31831. [PubMed: 21504055].
29. Ayyildiz S. The place of direct metal laser sintering (DMLS) in dentistry and the importance of annealing. Mater Sci Eng C Mater Biol Appl. 2015;52:343. https://doi.org/10.1016/j.msec.2015.03.016. [PubMed: 25953576].
30. Tahayeri A, Morgan M, Fugolin AP, Bompolaki D, Athirasala A, Pfeifer CS, Ferracane JL, Bertassoni LE. 3D printed versus conventionally cured provisional crown and bridge dental materials. Dent Mater. 2018;34(2):192–200. https://doi.org/10.1016/j.dental.2017.10.003. Epub 2017 Oct 27. PMID: 29110921; PMCID: PMC5801146.
31. van Noort R. The future of dental devices is digital. Dent Mater. 2012;28:3–12. https://doi.org/10.1016/j.dental.2011.10.014. [PubMed: 22119539].
32. Hirayama H. Chapter 6: Digital removable complete denture (DRCD). In: Tamimi F, Hirayama H, editors. Digital restorative dentistry: a guide to materials, equipment, and clinical procedures. Berlin: Springer Nature Switzerland AG; 2019.
33. Goodacre BJ, Goodacre CJ. Using intraoral scanning to fabricate complete dentures: first experiences. Int J Prosthodont. 2018;31(2):166–70.
34. Williams RJ, Bibb R, Rafik T. A technique for fabricating patterns for removable partial denture frameworks using digitized casts and electronic surveying. J Prosthet Dent. 2004;91:85–8.
35. Han J, Wang Y, Lü P. A preliminary report of designing removable partial denture frameworks using a specifically developed software package. Int J Prosthodont. 2010;23:370–5.
36. Exocad®, America Acquires SensAble® Dental, Soon To Offer Partial Denture Design Software By Kelly Fessel Carr Posted Dec 02, 2014 in Industry News LMT. https://lmtmag.com/articles/exocad-r-america-acquires-sensable-r-dental-soon-to-offer-partial-denture-design-software.
37. Takaichi A, Fueki K, Murakami N, Ueno T, Inamochi Y, Wada J, Arai Y, Wakabayashi N. A systematic review of digital removable partial dentures. Part II: CAD/CAM framework, artificial teeth, and denture base. J Prosthodont Res. 2022;66(1):53–67.
38. Papathanasiou I, Kamposiora P, Papavasiliou G, Ferrari M. The use of PEEK in digital prosthodontics: a narrative review. BMC Oral Health. 2020;20:217.
39. Ali Z, Baker S, Sereno N, et al. A pilot randomized controlled crossover trial comparing early OHRQoL outcomes of cobalt-chromium versus PEEK removable partial denture frameworks. Int J Prosthodont. 2020;33(4):386–92.
40. Wang C, Shi Y, Xie P, Wu J. Accuracy of digital complete dentures: a systematic review of in vitro studies. J Prosthet Dent. 2021;125:249–56.
41. Goodacre B, Goodacre C, Baba N, Kattadiyil M. Comparison of denture base adaptation between CAD-CAM and conventional fabrication techniques. J Prosthet Dent. 2016;116:249–56.
42. Fasbinder DJ. Digital dentistry: innovation for restorative treatment. Compend Contin Educ Dent. 2010;31(Spec No 4):2–11.
43. Monaco C, Scheda L, Ciocca L, Zucchelli G. The prototype concept in a full digital implant workflow. J Am Dent Assoc. 2018;149(10):918–23.
44. Tatakis DN, Chien HH, Parashis AO. Guided implant surgery risks and their prevention. Periodontol 2000. 2019;81(1):194–208.
45. Kihara H, Hatakeyama W, Komine F, et al. Accuracy and practicality of intraoral scanner in dentistry: a literature review. J Prosthodont Res. 2020;64(2):109–13.
46. Sommacal B, Savic M, Filippi A, Kühl S, Thieringer FM. Evaluation of two 3D printers for guided implant surgery. Int J Oral Maxillofac Implants. 2018;33(4):743–6.
47. Vercruyssen M, Jacobs R, Van Assche N, van Steenberghe D. The use of CT scan based planning for oral rehabilitation by means of implants and its transfer to the surgical field: a critical review on accuracy. J Oral Rehabil. 2008;35(6):454–74.
48. Van Assche N, van Steenberghe D, Quirynen M, Jacobs R. Accuracy assessment of computer-assisted flapless implant placement in partial edentulism. J Clin Periodontol. 2010;37(4):398–403.
49. Wöhrle PS. Predictably replacing maxillary incisors with implants using 3-D planning and guided implant surgery. Compend Contin Educ Dent. 2014;35(10):758–62.
50. Younes F, Cosyn J, De Bruyckere T, Cleymaet R, Bouckaert E, Eghbali A. A randomized controlled study on the accuracy of free-handed, pilot-drill guided and fully guided implant surgery in partially edentulous patients. J Clin Periodontol. 2018;45(6):721–32.
51. Tahmaseb A, Wu V, Wismeijer D, Coucke W, Evans C. The accuracy of static computer-aided implant

surgery: a systematic review and meta-analysis. Clin Oral Implants Res. 2018;29(S16):416–35.
52. Patzelt SB, Emmanouilidi A, Stampf S, et al. Accuracy of full-arch scans using intraoral scanners. Clin Oral Investig. 2014;18(6):1687–94.
53. Mangano F, Gandolfi A, Luongo G, et al. Intraoral scanners in dentistry: a review of the current literature. BMC Oral Health. 2017;17(1):149.
54. Rutkūnas V, Gečiauskaitė A, Jegelevičius D, et al. Accuracy of digital implant impressions with intraoral scanners. A systematic review. Eur J Oral Implantol. 2017;10(Suppl 1):101–20.
55. Mezger U, Jendrewski C, Bartels M. Navigation in surgery. Langenbecks Arch Surg. 2013;398:501–14.
56. Clarke JV, Deakin AH, Nicol AC, et al. Measuring the positional accuracy of computer assisted surgical tracking systems. Comput Aided Surg. 2010;15(1–3):13–8.
57. Gerbino G, Zavattero E, Berrone M, et al. Management of needle breakage using intraoperative navigation following inferior alveolar nerve block. J Oral Maxillofac Surg. 2013;71:1819.
58. Bobek SL. Applications of navigation for orthognathic surgery. Oral Maxillofac Surg Clin North Am. 2014;26:587.
59. Strong EB, Rafii A, Holhweg-Majert B, et al. Comparison of 3 optical navigation systems for computer aided maxillofacial surgery. Arch Otolaryngol Head Neck Surg. 2008;134(10):1080–4.
60. Block MS, Emery RW. Static or dynamic navigation for implant placement—choosing the method of guidance. J Oral Maxillofac Surg. 2016;74:269.
61. Block MS, Emery RW, Cullum DR, et al. Implant placement is more accurate using dynamic navigation. J Oral Maxillofac Surg. 2017;75:1377.
62. Chauhan S, Coelho R, Kalan S, Satava R, Patel V. Robotic urologic surgery. In: Evolution of robotic surgery: past, present, and future. Berlin: Springer; 2011. p. 3–10.
63. Abe S, Noguchi N, Matsuka Y, Shinohara C, Kimura T, Oka K, et al. Educational effects using a robot patient simulation system for development of clinical attitude. Eur J Dent Educ. 2018;22(3):e327–36.

Digital Systems in Surgical Implant Placement

10

Antigoni Delantoni, Theodoros Lillis, and Georgios Giannelis

10.1 Introduction

The evolution in CBCT and the development of 3D imaging software have led to an evolution in digital planning and implant treatment.

The low radiation dose the patient is exposed to, the relatively low cost of the technique, and the selection of an appropriate field of view are the major advantages modern CBCT units offer.

Generally in the literature there are two techniques described when it comes to guided implant placement, the static and the dynamic protocol.

The static refers to the use of a stable in position surgical guide, which represents the virtual implant placement position, as it was selected during the presurgical guide by the surgeon and as is developed from the CBCT data [1].

The surgical guide is made from resin through 3D printers and prefabricated resin blocks with the use of CAD/CAM systems. This protocol does not allow the surgeon to change anything during the surgical procedures [2–4].

The dynamic protocol which is also referred to as stereolithic method uses a surgical guide that reproduces the exact position of the implant, directly from electronic tomographic data on a screen. The surgeon observes during the screen in real time and can manipulate and handle all the drills to establish an ideal location for the implant placement [5, 6].

Between the two protocols the static is the one more widely used and readily available.

10.2 The Rationale for Digital Systems Use in Implant Dentistry

The last 40 years dental implantology has shown significant evolution both on the type of implant and surgical technique selected, as well as positioning precision and accuracy. The primary objective, which was originally the successful achievement of a bone anchorage for restoration of complete edentulism in order to restore masticatory function, has been gradually extended to the development of prosthetic components and techniques that could rehabilitate partial edentulism or single missing teeth. Concomitantly, the initial challenge of successful osseointegration has been extended to the achievement of restorations with long-term complete functional and aesthetic stability.

A. Delantoni (✉)
Department of Dentoalveolar Surgery, Implant Surgery and Radiology, Faculty of Dentistry, Aristotle University of Thessaloniki, Thessaloniki, Greece
e-mail: andelant@dent.auth.gr

T. Lillis
Department of Dentoalveolar Surgery, Implant Surgery and Radiology, Aristotle University of Thessaloniki, Thessaloniki, Greece

G. Giannelis
Division of Periodontology, University of British Columbia, Vancouver, BC, Canada

A. Delantoni, K. Orhan (eds.), *Digital Dentistry*, https://doi.org/10.1007/978-3-031-52826-2_10

The surgical placement of dental implants in proper position has been recognized as an important parameter in the long-term success of implant-supported restorations [7, 8]. To adequately plan the placement of a dental implant and determine its ideal position, the height and width of the alveolar ridge and the neighboring anatomical structures (mandibular nerve, nasal floor, maxillary sinus, adjacent teeth, etc.) should be considered at first [9]. However, if the position and inclination of the implant would be determined solely according to the anatomy of the alveolar ridge, hard and soft tissue long-term stability would not be guaranteed, due to bone resorption after extraction [10]. Thus, the exact position of the implant should be determined in additional consideration to the ideal position and dimensions of the final prosthetic restoration (prosthetically driven implant placement) [11]. The aforementioned requirements indicate that a strict and precise diagnostic path should be followed preoperatively, in order to determine an individual treatment plan and ideal positioning of the dental implants. Moreover, the transfer of these information in the surgical field and the final placement of the dental implant in this ideal position can be a tricky procedure, especially when the placement is performed by freehand.

The diagnostic methods in dental implantology have also evolved over the years. Originally, the preoperative evaluation of edentulous alveolar ridge and neighboring anatomical structures was conducted in simple radiographs such as panoramic radiographs, while prosthetic planning was conducted in stone casts mounted on an articulator and diagnostic wax-up [12, 13]. The information gathered was integrated and transferred in a surgical template which was fabricated with several traditional techniques described in the literature [14–16]. This surgical template could be used as a guide during the drilling process in order to achieve ideal implant positioning. However, these traditional methods may have many manufacturing errors and they cannot always assure the precise final position of the implant.

The development of digital systems in surgical implant placement was emerged by the advancements in digital radiographic imaging, digital 3D scanning, and 3D printing technology. The development of computed tomography (CT) and special software that allows the mandible and maxilla to be imaged in three planes—axial, panoramic, and cross-sectional—can be considered as the first step in the late 1980s [17]. Following, the development of cone beam computed tomography (CBCT) in the late 1990s was further contributed to the advancement of digital imaging in dental implantology and more precisely in implant placement [18]. A special feature added in the software of radiographic digital image processing was the ability to place a digital image of a dental implant into the jawbone by overlapping [19]. In the same period, introduction of 3D scanning technology enabled the creation of digital 3D images of the oral structures that can be processed by special software.

Today, two computer-guided implant placement protocols can be described: the "static" and the "dynamic." The "static" protocol refers to the use of a surgical template that is fabricated according to the digital planning made in appropriate software which combines the CBCT radiographic data and the intraoral 3D scanning data. This surgical template fits firmly in the patient's mouth and it has properly oriented holes that guide the implant drills in the exact selected ideal position of the implant [20]. The "static" protocol represents the most widely used one in the everyday practice today. On the other hand, the "dynamic" protocol, which is also referred as "stereolithographic method," uses a surgical navigation system which displays the position of the implant on the tomographic image in a screen in real time [19]. The surgeon watches on the screen and guides the drills and the implant appropriately.

10.3 Static Computer-Guided Implant Placement

10.3.1 Preparation of the Surgical Template

The preparation of the surgical template for static computer-guided implant placement includes the following steps [21–23].

First step: A CBCT scanning is required in order to acquire the 3D digital radiographic imaging data of the patient's jawbone anatomy (DICOM format file) (Fig. 10.1a). Moreover, 3D digital data of the patient's intraoral anatomy should be obtained with the use of an intraoral scanner or by scanning the patient's diagnostic stone casts with use of an extraoral scanner (STL format file) (Fig. 10.1b).

Second step: Import of DICOM and STL files in appropriate planning software, in which the 3D data are registered and overlapped (Fig. 10.2). For the registration process, distinct anatomical landmarks of hard and soft tissues from the two 3D images respectively, such as dental cusps or palatine rugae, are matched.

Third step: Digital planning of the surgical template in the planning software (Fig. 10.3). For this purpose, a digital wax-up of the ideal final restoration precedes. Following, selection of the proper sized implant from the software's library and its placement in the ideal position considering both anatomical and prosthetic requirements is performed digitally. Then, digital planning of the surgical template is performed (support, extend, positioning of the holes for the sleeve guides, reinforcing bars, etc.) by taking into account the preselected ideal position of the implant (Fig. 10.4).

Fourth step: Fabrication of the surgical template. The final digital 3D model of the surgical template is used for the fabrication of a surgical template from acrylic resin either in 3D printer or in CAD/CAM device. This acrylic surgical template has properly oriented holes where metallic sleeve guides are used for the implant drills mounting (Fig. 10.5).

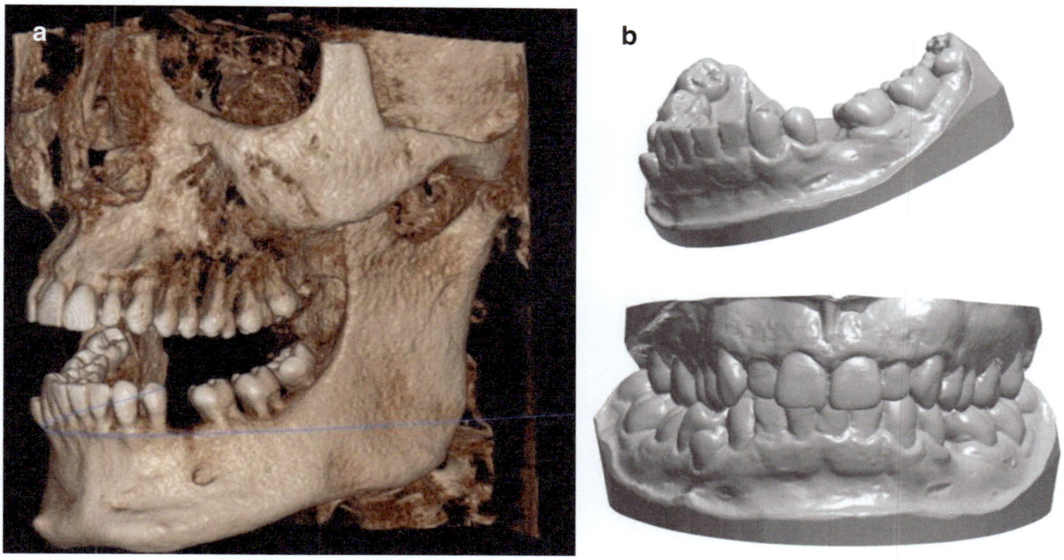

Fig. 10.1 3D digital radiographic image from CBCT (DICOM file) (**a**) and 3D digital image from extraoral scanning of the diagnostic stone casts (STL file) (**b**)

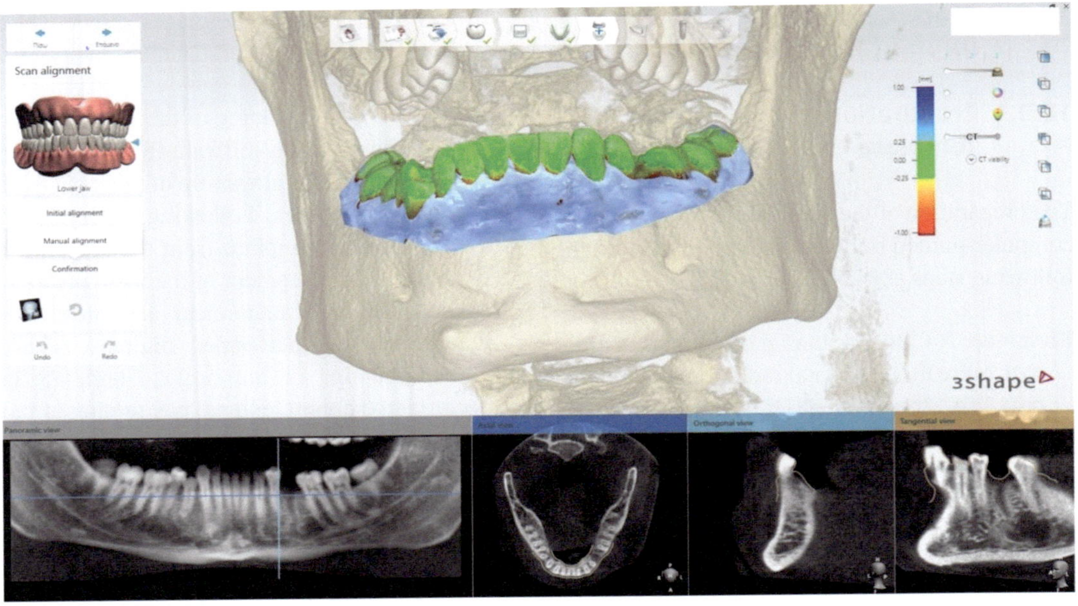

Fig. 10.2 Process of registration of DICOM and STL file in appropriate software

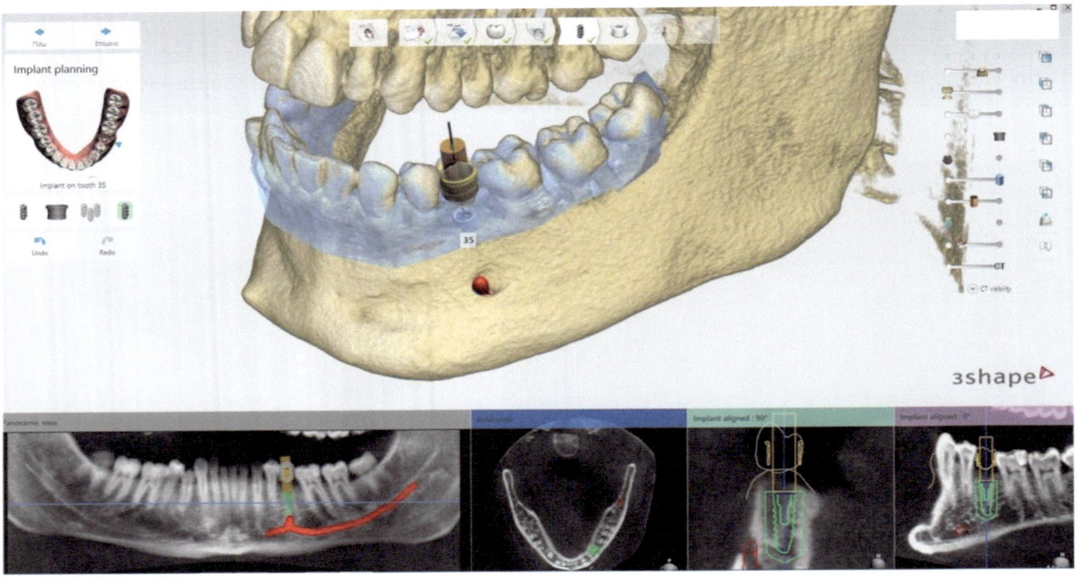

Fig. 10.3 Digital planning of the surgical template in the appropriate software

10.3.2 Types of Computer-Guided Surgical Templates

Firm sitting of the surgical template into the patient's mouth has a crucial role in the success of static computer-guided implant placement protocol. Computer-guided surgical templates may be designed digitally so that to be supported on several anatomical structures onto the mandible or the maxilla. Considering the

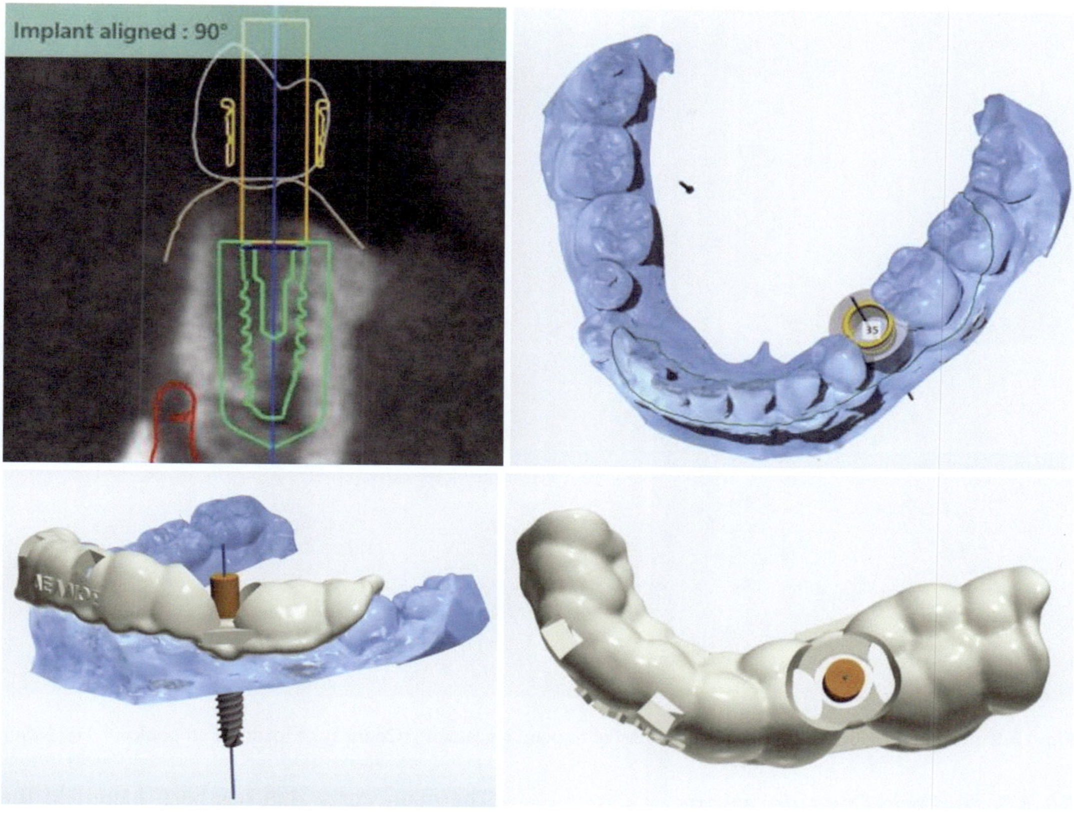

Fig. 10.4 Stages of digital planning of the surgical template. (Courtesy of Ioannis Fotopoulos, DDS, MSc)

type of support, the surgical templates may be [17] either:

- **Tooth-supported**. These templates fit on remaining teeth and they are used for placement of implants in single tooth or partially edentulous cases.
- **Mucosa-supported**. These templates fit on the mucosa of the mandible or the maxilla similarly to the removable prostheses. They are used in cases of complete edentulism and they need stabilization by special pins anchored in jawbone.
- **Bone-supported**. These templates fit immediately onto the bone of the alveolar ridge after flap raising. They are also used in cases of complete edentulism, where extended surface of the jawbone is exposed during surgery.
- **Specially supported**. This type refers to templates which fit on implants which have been inserted before surgery or to templates that are stabilized by pins anchored in the jawbone during the surgery.

The surgical templates can be used during the surgery for fully or partially guided implant placement. In **fully guided implant placement**, the template is used during the whole sequence of the drills and implant placement, providing full guidance in terms of drilling depth/width and inclination. In **partially guided implant placement**, the template is used to provide guidance only during the pilot drilling, while the rest of the procedure is completed freehanded. This protocol gives the advantage of changing the depth or inclination of the implant if any differences from the initial digital planning are perceived [24, 25].

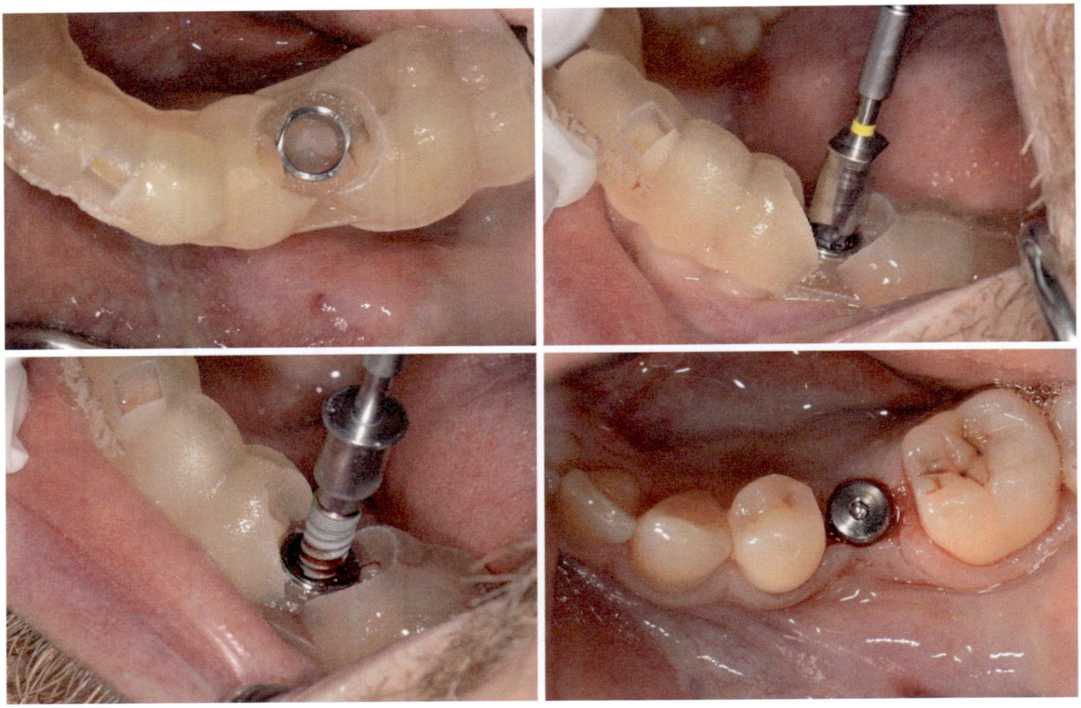

Fig. 10.5 Acrylic surgical template during surgery of implant placement. (Courtesy of Ioannis Fotopoulos, DDS, MSc)

10.3.3 Method Considerations

10.3.3.1 Accuracy

The accuracy of computer-guided dental implant placement refers to the level of matching between the digitally planed position of the implant and its final position into the alveolar ridge after completion of the surgical procedure. Deviation between digital and final position is a critical aspect of computer-guided implant placement in clinical practice. Several in vitro and in vivo studies have evaluated this deviation and found an acceptable discrepancy between the two positions in clinical practice [17]. On average, a discrepancy of 1.2 mm in entry point of the implants, 1.4 mm at the apex of implants, and a deviation of 3.5° in the central axis of the implants have been reported [20–22]. However, an important issue is the maximum deviation that can occur in clinical practice. In some cases, these outliers may exceed in unacceptable range and serious complications may occur.

The main factor that has been identified for the occurrence of the outliers is the fitting and stability of the surgical template during surgery [23–26]. In dentate cases, it has been proposed that the template should have unilateral support on the dental arch and fit on at least five teeth [20]. In edentulous cases where the template is bone- or mucosa-supported, special pins inserted during the implant surgery provide better stabilization [20].

10.3.3.2 Advantages

- More accuracy in the final position of the implant compared with free-hand placement or using traditional surgical templates fabricated on stone casts.
- Flapless implant placement may be performed safely providing less postoperative morbidity.
- Immediate loading of the implants may be less time-consuming, as provisional restoration may be prefabricated digitally.

10.3.3.3 Disadvantages

- Higher cost than traditional methods, including equipment.
- Incorrect fitting of the surgical template can lead to complications, especially in fully guided placement.
- Misfit or fracture of the template during surgery may create problems on their use.

10.4 Dynamic Computer-Guided Implant Placement

The evolutions in computed tomography and implant planning software allowed the development of static surgical guides that can predictably transfer the preoperative plans to the surgical site and provide accurate three-dimensional positioning of dental implants [16, 18, 27]. Dynamic navigation can further improve this process by providing surgeons "real-time" screen-based guidance and by allowing the surgeon to visualize any deviation from the original plan and adjust it intraoperatively [28, 29].

Although dynamic navigation has been routinely used by other medical specialties (i.e., ophthalmology, neurosurgery, or orthopedics) for decades, the first dynamic navigation system was introduced in implant dentistry in 2000 [16].

10.4.1 Dynamic Navigation Equipment

The dynamic navigation systems use optical tracking technologies to track a surgical tool (i.e., a surgical handpiece) relative to the patient, and to display on a monitor the real-time location of the surgical tool within the patient's preoperative CBCT [30].

The intraoperative tracking is based on an infrared light source and stereoscopic optical cameras attached to the overhead light (Fig. 10.6a). An LED light source above the patient projects light on the surgical field. Special tracking arrays (reflective spheres), attached both to the patient and to the handpiece being used, reflect off the light (Fig. 10.6b). The stereo cameras can optically identify the tracking arrays by capturing the reflected light. The position of the patient's head is tracked by a dynamic reference frame (patient tracker) with tracking arrays printed on it (Fig. 10.6c). The patient tracker is attached to a thermoplastic stent that is worn by the patient during surgery (Fig. 10.6d). The dynamic navigation technology that was described above is the passive one and is the most commonly used. In the active optical motion tracking systems, active system arrays emit infrared light themselves that is then tracked to the stereo camera [28–34].

This way the dynamic navigation software can track the position of both the patient and the handpiece relative to the predefined implant plan on the computed tomography data and have a dynamic virtual image projected onto the monitor screen. The handpiece and the patient should be within the line of sight of the overhead tracking stereo cameras [29, 30].

10.4.2 Scanning and Planning

A thermoplastic device (stent) with radiopaque markers (fiducials) and an attachment section for the patient tracker on the buccal side is fabricated. The stent will be attached to the teeth of the arch that is planned to receive the dental implants, and it should not interfere with the surgery area. The stent needs to be stable and firmly adapted on the patient's jaw during CBCT, because this specific radiographic location needs to be reproduced during the surgery. In edentulous jaws, mini screws are used as fiducials. These screws are placed and spread out throughout the arch prior to the CT scan and they will have the patient tracker arm anchored to them during the implant surgery. The field of view of the CBCT needs to cover the surgical site and the fiducials. The Dicom file is then imported into the dynamic navigation software for prosthetically directed digital planning of the case and proper selection of implant dimensions and implant alignment [28, 31, 32].

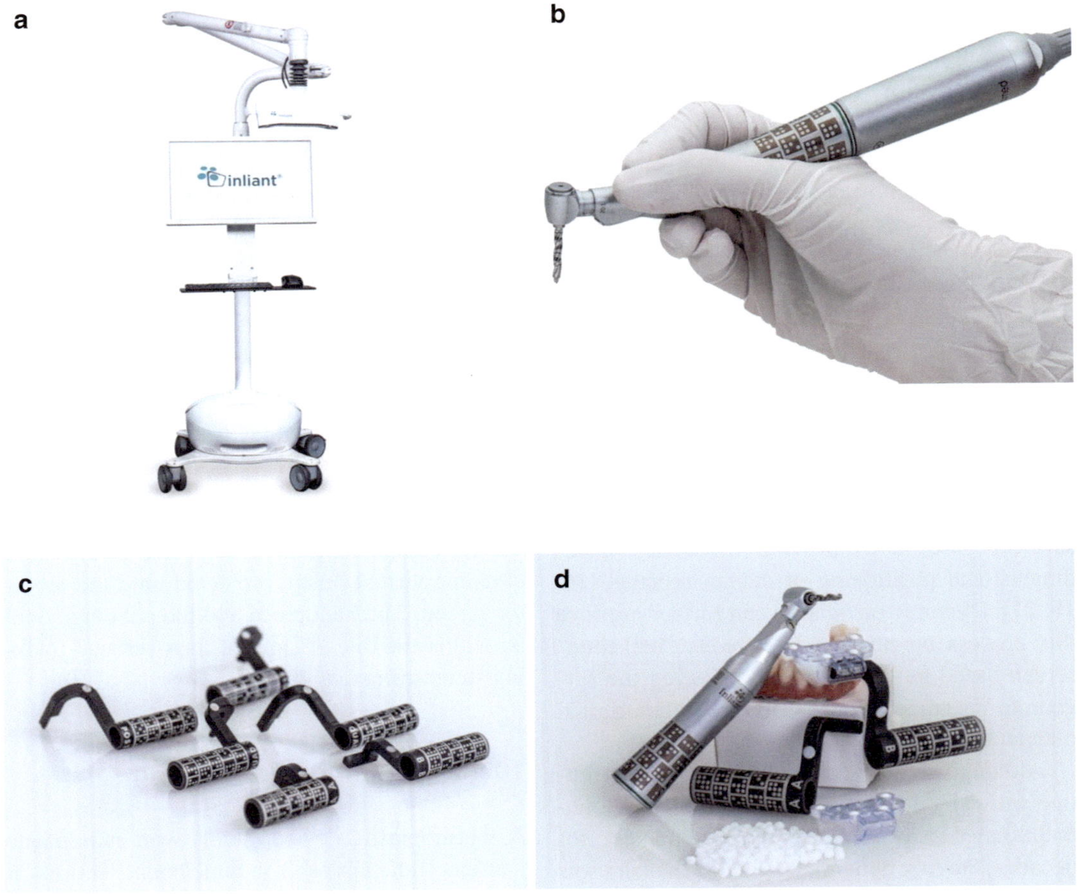

Fig. 10.6 Stereoscopic tracking camera (**a**). Surgical handpiece with tracking arrays that enable the stereo cameras to track the handpiece (**b**). Set of patient trackers (**c**). The patient tracker is attached to a thermoplastic stent with radiographic markers that is worn by the patient during surgery (**d**). (Courtesy of Inliant, Navigate Surgical Technologies, Vancouver, BC, Canada)

10.4.3 Registration and Navigation

At the beginning of the surgery, the stent with the patient tracker attached to it is mounted on the dentition. The markers of the stent act as the anchor point between the CBCT scan and the patient's anatomy and are used to register the patient. The registration process is the linking between the physical space coordinates of the patient (operative field volume at the time of surgery) and the patient's image coordinates (CBCT). A precise registration is the key point of a successful dynamic navigated implant surgery [28, 31, 32, 35, 36].

The dynamic navigation software identifies the tracking arrays both on the handpiece and the patient tracker and proceeds with a short calibration. The calibration accuracy is checked by placing the drill on anatomical landmarks in the patient's mouth and visually confirming their proper dynamic projection on the monitor (accuracy check) [27, 30, 32] (Fig. 10.7a).

The surgery is performed by focusing on the monitor (Fig. 10.7b). The dynamic navigation

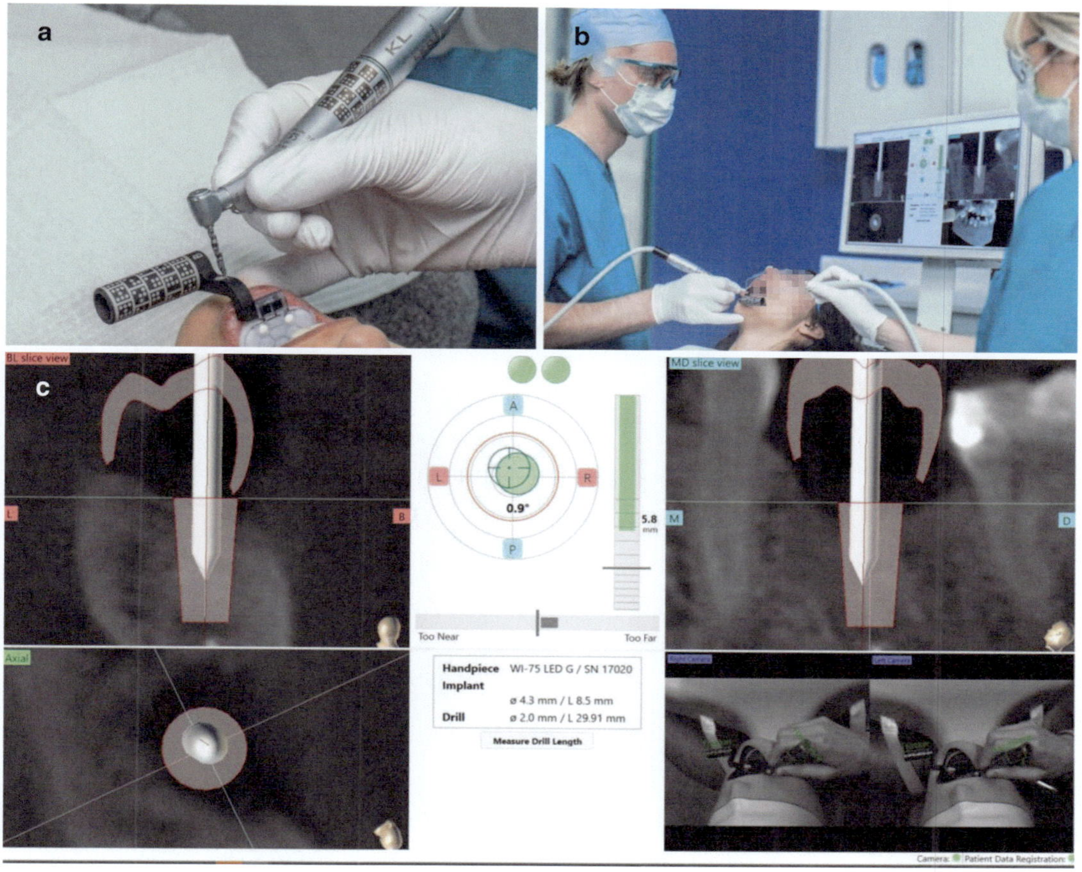

Fig. 10.7 Handpiece calibration process (**a**). The surgery is performed by focusing on the monitor (**b**). The dynamic navigation software shows a virtual drill on the monitor. Every time the position of the drill corresponds with the preplanned implant location, a cross-hair display is shown on the screen (**c**). (Courtesy of Inliant, Navigate Surgical Technologies, Vancouver, BC, Canada)

software shows a virtual drill on the monitor. Every time the position of the drill corresponds with the preplanned implant location, a cross-hair display is shown on the screen (Fig. 10.7c, d). Different color markers provide real-time visual feedback indicating if the osteotomy preparation coincides with the pre-planned or if real-time adjustments to the orientation of the drill need to be made. Dynamic guided surgery allows for intrasurgical changes in implant size, type, or location as there is no restrictive static guide involved [27, 30–32]. The previously described workflow is shown through a clinical case in Figs. 10.8 and 10.9.

10.4.4 Method Considerations

10.4.4.1 Accuracy

Several studies have evaluated the accuracy of dynamic navigated implant surgery. The accuracy can be assessed in vivo by comparing the virtually planned and final positions of implants as shown on preoperative and postoperative CBCT scans [33, 37].

In 100 consecutive implants placed by 3 surgeons, Block and coworkers evaluated the accuracy of dynamic guided implant placement and they reported a mean (SD) 0.87 (0.42) and 1.09 (0.69) mm lateral deviation at platform level and

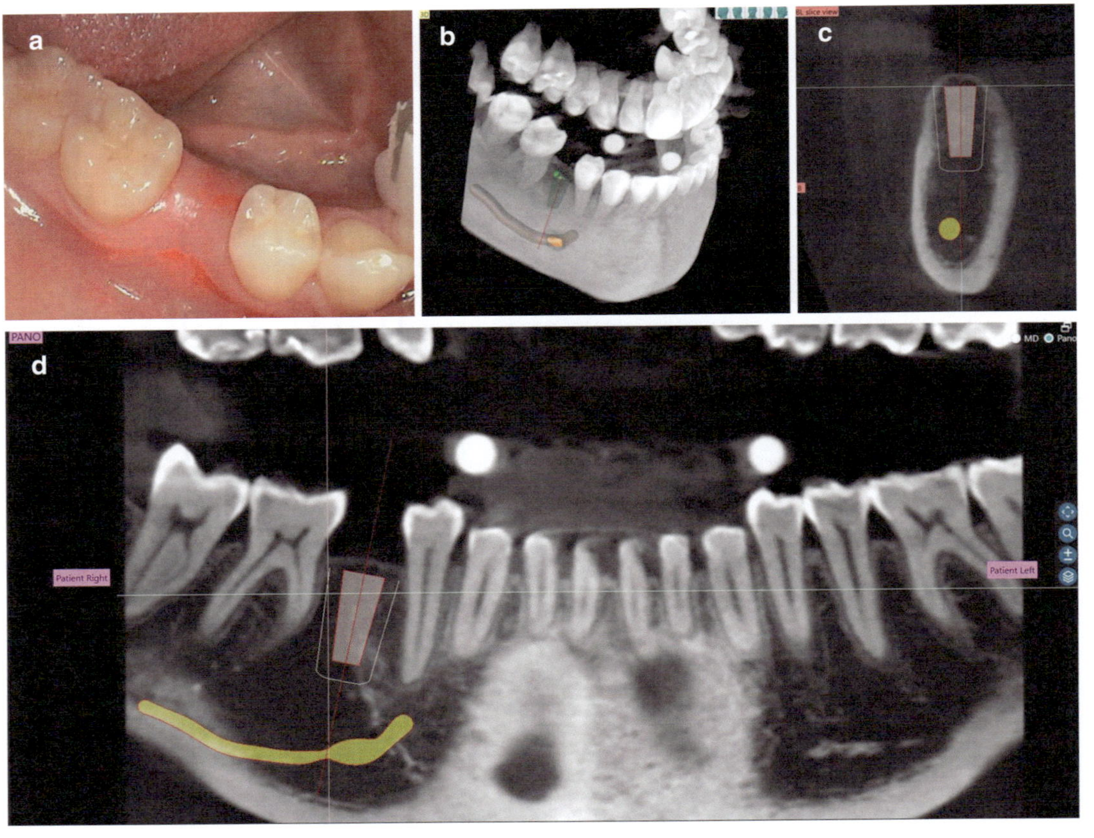

Fig. 10.8 Congenitally missing mandibular right second premolar (**a**). The case was planned with the Inliant Planning Software (Inliant, Navigate Surgical Technologies, Vancouver, BC, Canada). Cross-sectional CBCT image superimposed with a virtual (red) implant. The round radiographic markers (fiducials) are visible (**b–d**). (The pictures are courtesy of Dr. Jim Yeganegi, Private Practice, Vancouver, BC, Canada)

tip level, respectively, and a 3.62 (273) degree angular deviation. In 20 conventional implant insertion cases, a significant increase of discrepancies was reported with a mean 1.15 (0.59) and 2.21 (0.99) mm lateral deviation at platform level and tip level, respectively, and a 7.69 (4.92) degree angular deviation. The results also indicate that the three surgeons showed similar accuracy after the achievement of their learning curve. It seems that surgeons became proficient after the placement of 20 implants with the system [28].

Similar results were reported by Stefanelli and coworkers. In 231 consecutive implants placed in healed ridges under dynamic guidance, the mean (SD) discrepancies were 0.71 (0.40) mm at the platform lever and 1.00 (0.49) mm at the apex. The mean angular deviation was 2.26° (1.62°) from actual vs. planned implant positions. This study also concluded that the experience level of the surgeon with dynamic navigation can improve accuracy outcomes. All the outcome parameters were significantly improved in the last 50 implants (coronal deviation 0.59 mm, apical deviation 0.85 mm, and angular deviation 1.98°) compared with the first 50 implants (0.94 mm, 1.19 mm, and 3.48°, respectively) [30].

A study that compared the accuracy of implant placement between 30 implants placed with a dynamic guided approach and 30 implants placed with a static approach in single tooth spaces showed that both techniques provided similar implant placement errors. At implant platform

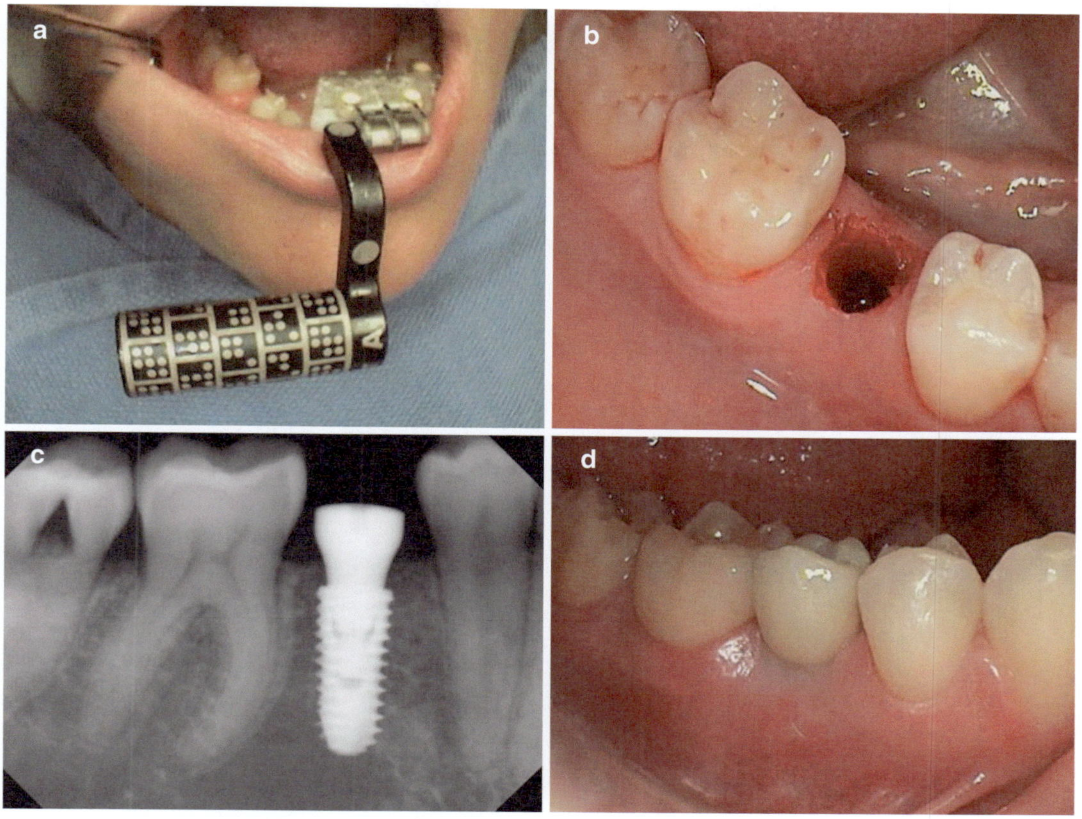

Fig. 10.9 An implant was placed in the mandibular right second premolar site with a flapless approach. A dynamic computer-guided navigation system was used (Inliant, Navigate Surgical Technologies, Vancouver, BC, Canada). In picture (**a**), the fiducial and the patient tracker (with tracking arrays printed on it) are visible. Flapless implant placement (**b**). Periapical radiograph confirming the correct implant placement (**c**). Final restoration 4 months post-surgery (**d**). (The pictures are courtesy of Dr. Jim Yeganegi, Private Practice, Vancouver, BC, Canada)

level the mean deviation was 0.97 (0.44) mm in the static group versus 1.05 (0.44) mm in the dynamic group. Similarly, at the apex the mean deviation was 1.28 (0.46) mm in the static group and 1.29 (0.50) mm in the dynamic group. The angular deviation in static and dynamic groups was 2.84 ± 1.71° and 3.06 ± 1.37°, respectively [38].

No significant differences in accuracy of implant placement were shown in another study by Guzman and coworkers. More specifically, the mean deviation at the coronal entry point and at the apical endpoint in the static group was 0.78 (0.43) mm and 1.20 (0.48) mm, while that in the dynamic group was 0.85 (0.48) mm and 1.18 (0.60) mm, respectively [39].

10.4.4.2 Accuracy of Guided Surgery vs. Conventional Surgery

In this chapter the authors aim to present various parameters that determine the surgical result. One of them by many authors in many studies reported as the most important is the degree of accuracy obtained when placing dental implants by guided surgery compared to conventional surgery.

In a systematic review by Elena Araujo-Corchado and Beatriz Pardal-Peláez [40] 12 measurements were analyzed. After analyzing all measurements and variables from other studies the authors concluded that in most studies the results were worse with conventional surgery than with guided surgery, and thus could be said that, in general terms, significant differences were found in all the measurements of all the included studies [41–46], except in three (apical vertical deviation and coronal and apical bucco-lingual deviation), in the studies by Smitkarn et al. and Chen et al. [41, 42]. However, although the differences were not significant, the results of these three measurements were also worse in conventional surgery than in guided surgery.

10.4.4.3 Accuracy of Different Guided Surgery Techniques

From the various studies available, it can be concluded that the most accurate surgeries were fully guided (FG) and half-guided (HG), as the implants placed with these two surgical techniques deviated the least from the planned position, in raw values (1479, [44–46]).

Some studies that included pilot drill-guided surgery (PD) performed worse than the other guided surgery techniques [43, 44, 46], since in them, the implants placed deviated the most from the planned position, in raw values.

Dynamic guided surgery (DG) was only performed in one study, that of Aydemir and Arisan [46], showing better results than conventional surgery when the deviations between implant axes and the distance between crowns and apexes of planned and laterally placed implants were measured.

10.4.4.4 Advantages

Both static and dynamic computer-guided implant surgeries are clearly superior to conventional implant placement. Computer-guided surgery offers predictable and accurate prosthetically driven implant placement by reducing surgical times.

However, dynamic guided surgery can provide some advantages over the static technique:

- Patient evaluation, CBCT, planning and implant surgery can be potentially performed in a single appointment.
- There is no delay or additional cost for the fabrication of a static surgical guide.
- Deviations from the original plan can be easily identified during the surgery.
- Intraoperative adjustments (implant size, system, location) can be easily facilitated.
- Better visibility of the surgical field and better perception of the bone density.
- Increased irrigation/cooling of the alveolar bone.
- Implant placement is feasible even if interdental or interocclusal space is limited.
- There is no need for specific implant-manufacturer equipment (guided kits).
- Elimination of failures due to guide fractures or poorly fitting guides [30, 32, 33, 37].

10.4.4.5 Disadvantages

One of the disadvantages of dynamic guided surgery is the significant initial investment (dynamic navigation equipment, stereo cameras, software, CBCT). Another disadvantage is that the bulky equipment (stents, fiducials, patient trackers) can sometimes make the surgery challenging. Furthermore, edentulous cases require an additional invasive procedure for fiducial screw placement [30, 32].

Navigation surgery has a learning curve associated with it. Since most clinicians are unfamiliar with the philosophy of the technique, training on models, mentoring with over-the-shoulder observation and hands-on mentoring during the first few cases are recommended [28, 30, 32, 47].

10.5 Indications for Guided Surgery

Computer-guided surgery may be more indicated in cases where the implant is planned to be placed in the vicinity of a critical anatomy (proximity of the inferior dental nerve, maxillary sinus, etc.) [24]. The most suitable technique in these cases is fully guided surgery, due to its great precision and fewer complications. However, in cases where fully guided surgery is not possible, the pilot drill-guided surgery technique could be indicated, as it would provide better results than conventional surgery [21].

10.6 Limitations of Guided Surgery

The issue of limitations of the techniques is as in many cases debatable. Though there are not many studies on the topic this major problem was addressed in one study by Smitkarn et al. [22, 44], and it was concluded that, although the accuracy obtained with guided surgery is higher than with conventional surgery, it has limitations, including higher costs and the need for favorable anatomical conditions. Two other trials [43, 46] also addressed this last limitation, and found that the stability of the guide position during implant placement is important particularly in fully edentulous patients. On the other hand, with regard to dynamic surgery, only addressed in one study [46], it was noted that surgeon familiarization with the procedure was necessary, as the entry point is visualized on the monitor instead of directly observing the patient's jaw. As the surgeon in this study was unfamiliar with the procedure, there were frequent starts and stops during the surgery. Furthermore, in this same study [46], it was concluded that in static guided surgery there are limitations in detecting deviations in implant position. This is due to the closed and restrictive structure of the static guides, which does not occur in dynamic surgery because it allows complete visibility of the surgical area and the final position of the implant.

10.7 Complications of Guided Surgery

Conventional surgery may involve more complications than guided surgery [21]. A reflection of this is that, in the large systematic review study [17], all the implants placed (both with guided surgery and conventional) were intended to be restored with a screw-retained restoration; however, 19.2% (5/26) of the implants that were placed conventional had to be restored with a cemented restoration, because deviations were observed and the screw holes were placed towards the buccal plane and the aesthetics were compromised. In relation to the guided surgery techniques, [43], only 4.2% (1/24) of the implants placed with pilot drill had to receive a screw-retained restoration.

None of the implants placed with fully guided surgery had to be screw-retained, as they could all be restored with a cemented restoration.

Another study [41] also showed a greater buccal deviation in implants placed conventionally, and therefore also stated that complications were lower in guided surgery than in conventional surgery. It is important to note that, apart from complications with regard to the type of restoration, no biological complications of invasion of neighboring structures such as perforation of the floor of the maxillary sinus, the inferior dental nerve, or the mental nerve were described for any of the techniques in any of the included studies [41–46, 48]. This leaves to a large number of debatable and unanswered questions that hopefully will be solved in the near future.

10.8 Conclusions

When it comes to evaluating the degree of precision with guided surgery compared to conventional surgery, overall most studies agree that the degree of precision obtained when placing dental implants in partially edentulous patients with guided surgery techniques is greater than with conventional surgery. The results however between the different studies show differences that are of statistical significance in many cases. Most authors agree that when it comes to static guided surgical techniques (fully guided, half guided and pilot drill-guided), fully guided and half-guided surgery are the most accurate, while pilot drill-guided surgery is the least accurate [18–24]. When one is debating on the use of dynamic guided surgery, it is not safe to conclude that it offers better results than static guided surgery. This is mainly since there is only one of the included studies that dealt with this issue and compared it only with conventional surgery. One could argue that the large variability in studies of all the measurements and the data supplied is insufficient and does not yet provide all the needed information. There are no standard measurements to be assessed that make it difficult to provide unified and homogeneous data in terms of the measurements evaluated.

The advantages of guided surgery include

- greater precision,
- reduced trauma to the patient,
- reduced duration of the surgical procedure;

The disadvantages include

- lower primary stability of the implants,
- higher cost.

The disadvantages of guided implant surgery are not frequently discussed and were addressed in two studies [43, 44]. While one study by Smitkarn et al. [43] addressed primary stability in static implant placement, it was noted that primary stability was lower in implants placed using fully guided surgery than those using conventional surgery, This was attributed to limited tactile perception of implant stability due to the splint used. In relation to costs which is the second study addressing disadvantages, Younes et al. [44] found that performing guided surgery increased the cost of treatment due to the need for a surgical guide, specific instruments and tools, as well as specific planning software.

Guided surgery is currently indicated and selected in situations of critical anatomy, such as proximity to the inferior dental nerve or maxillary sinus, as it offers greater precision and a lower probability of complications. The main limitations of this type of surgery are the higher cost compared to conventional surgery, the need for a good mouth opening, the visibility and adjustment of the surgical guides, and the need for prior familiarization with the procedure.

References

1. Benic GI, Bernasconi M, Jung RE, Hämmerle CH. Clinical and radiographic intra-subject comparison of implants placed with or without guided bone regeneration: 15-year results. J Clin Periodontol. 2017;44(3):315–25.
2. Thoma DS, Benić GI, Zwahlen M, Hämmerle CH, Jung RE. A systematic review assessing soft tissue augmentation techniques. Clin Oral Implants Res. 2009;20(Suppl 4):146–65.
3. Tahmaseb A, Wismeijer D, Coucke W, Derksen W. Computer technology applications in surgical implant dentistry: a systematic review. Int J Oral Maxillofac Implants. 2014;29(Suppl):25–42.
4. Bornstein MM, Al-Nawas B, Kuchler U, Tahmaseb A. Consensus statements and recommended clinical procedures regarding contemporary surgical and radiographic techniques in implant dentistry. Int J Oral Maxillofac Implants. 2014;29 Suppl:78–82.
5. Maeder MT, Weber L, Ammann P, Buser M, Ehl NF, Gerhard M, Brenner R, Haager PK, Maisano F, Rickli H. Relationship between B-type natriuretic peptide and invasive haemodynamics in patients with severe aortic valve stenosis. ESC Heart Fail. 2020;7(2):577–87.
6. Canullo L, Tallarico M, Radovanovic S, Delibasic B, Covani U, Rakic M. Distinguishing predictive profiles for patient-based risk assessment and diagnostics of plaque induced, surgically and prosthetically triggered peri-implantitis. Clin Oral Implants Res. 2016;27:1243–50.
7. Hammerle CHF, Tarnow D. The etiology of hard- and soft-tissue deficiencies at dental implants: a narrative review. J Clin Periodontol. 2018;45(20):S267–77.
8. Kageyama I, Maeda S, Takezawa K. Importance of anatomy in dental implant surgery. J Oral Biosci. 2021;63(2):142–52.
9. Winkler S. Implant site development and alveolar bone resorption patterns. J Oral Implantol. 2002;28(5):226–9.
10. Garber DA, Belser UC. Restoration-driven implant placement with restoration-generated site development. Compend Contin Educ Dent. 1995;16(8):796, 798–802, 804.
11. Wyatt CC, Pharoah MJ. Imaging techniques and image interpretation for dental implant treatment. Int J Prosthodont. 1998;11:442.
12. Lazzara RJ. Criteria for implant selection: surgical and prosthetic considerations. Pract Periodontics Aesthet Dent. 1994;6(9):55–62; quiz 64.
13. Wat PY, Chow TW, Luk HW, Comfort MB. Precision surgical template for implant placement: a new systematic approach. Clin Implant Dent Relat Res. 2002;4(2):88–92.
14. Adrian ED, Ivanhoe JR, Krantz WA. Trajectory surgical guide stent for implant placement. J Prosthet Dent. 1992;67:687–91.
15. Espinosa Marino J, Alvarez Arenal A, PardoCeballos A, Fernandez Vazquez JP, Ibaseta Diaz G. Fabrication of an implant radiologic-surgical stent for the partially edentulous patient. Quintessence Int. 1995;26(2):111–4.
16. D'haese J, Ackhurst J, Wismeijer D, De Bruyn H, Tahmaseb A. Current state of the art of computer-guided implant surgery. Periodontol 2000. 2017;73(1):121–33.

17. Gaêta-Araujo H, Alzoubi T, Vasconcelos KF, Orhan K, Pauwels R, Casselman JW, Jacobs R. Cone beam computed tomography in dentomaxillofacial radiology: a two-decade overview. Dentomaxillofac Radiol. 2020;49:20200145.
18. Jung RE, Schneider D, Ganeles J, Wismeijer D, Zahlen M, Hammerle C, Tahmaseb A. Computer technology applications in surgical implant dentistry: a systematic review. Int J Oral Maxillofac Implants. 2009;24:92–109.
19. Hämmerle C, Stone P, Jung R, Kapos T, Brodala N. Consensus statements and recommended clinical procedures regarding computer-assisted implant dentistry. Int J Oral Maxillofac Implants. 2009;24:126–30.
20. Tahmaseb A, De Clerck R, Wismeijer D. Computer-guided implant placement: 3D planning software, fixed intraoral reference points, and CAD/CAM technology. A case report. Int J Oral Maxillofac Implants. 2009;24:542–6.
21. Ozan O, Turkyilmaz I, Ersoy A, McGlumphy E, Rosenstiel S. Clinical accuracy of 3 different types of computed tomography-derived stereolithographic surgical guides in implant placement. J Oral Maxillofac Surg. 2009;67:394–401.
22. Gallucci G, Benic G, Eckert S, Papaspyridakos P, Schimmel M, Schrott A, Weber H. Consensus statements and clinical recommendations for implant loading protocols. Int J Oral Maxillofac Implants. 2014;29:287–90.
23. Lou F, Rao P, Zhang M, Luo S, Lu S, Xiao J. Accuracy evaluation of partially guided and fully guided templates applied to implant surgery of anterior teeth: a randomized controlled trial. Clin Implant Dent Relat Res. 2021;23(1):117–30.
24. Kraft B, Frizzera F, de Freitas RM, de Oliveira GJLP, Marcantonio JE. Impact of fully or partially guided surgery on the position of single implants immediately placed in maxillary incisor sockets: a randomized controlled clinical trial. Clin Implant Dent Relat Res. 2020;22(5):631–7.
25. Tahmaseb A, Wu V, Wismeijer D, Coucke W, Evans C. The accuracy of static computer-aided implant surgery: a systematic review and meta-analysis. Clin Oral Implants Res. 2018;29(Suppl 16):416–43.
26. Tallarico M, Xhanari E, Kim YJ, Cocchi F, Martinolli M, Alushi A, Baldoni EE, Meloni SM. Accuracy of computer-assisted template-based implant placement using conventional impression and scan model or intraoral digital impression: a randomised controlled trial with 1 year of follow-up. Int J Oral Implantol (Berl). 2019;12(2):197–206.
27. Vercruyssen M, Fortin T, Widmann G, Jacobs R, Quirynen M. Different techniques of static/dynamic guided implant surgery: modalities and indications. Periodontol 2000. 2014;66(1):214–27.
28. Block MS, Emery RW, Lank K, Ryan J. Implant placement accuracy using dynamic navigation. Int J Oral Maxillofac Implants. 2017;32(1):92–9.
29. Jayaratne YS, Zwahlen RA, Lo J, Tam SC, Cheung LK. Computer aided maxillofacial surgery: an update. Surg Innov. 2010;17(3):217–25.
30. Stefanelli LV, DeGroot BS, Lipton DI, Mandelaris GA. Accuracy of a dynamic dental implant navigation system in a private practice. Int J Oral Maxillofac Implants. 2019;34(1):205–13.
31. Strong EB, Rafii A, Holhweg-Majert B, Fuller SC, Metzger MC. Comparison of 3 optical navigation systems for computer aided maxillofacial surgery. Arch Otolaryngol Head Neck Surg. 2008;134(10):1080–4.
32. Panchal N, Mahmood L, Retana A, Emery R. Dynamic navigation for dental implant surgery. Oral Maxillofac Surg Clin North Am. 2019;31(4):539–47.
33. Pellegrino G, Ferri A, Del Fabbro M, Prati C, Gandolfi MG, Marchetti C. Dynamic navigation in implant dentistry: a systematic review and meta-analysis. Int J Oral Maxillofac Implants. 2021;36(5):e121–40.
34. Block MS, Emery RW. Static or dynamic navigation for implant placement-choosing the method of guidance. J Oral Maxillofac Surg. 2016;74(2):269–77.
35. Eggers G, Mühling J, Marmulla R. Image-to-patient registration techniques in head surgery. Int J Oral Maxillofac Surg. 2006;35(12):1081–95.
36. Ma F, Sun F, Wei T, Ma Y. Comparison of the accuracy of two different dynamic navigation system registration methods for dental implant placement: a retrospective study. Clin Implant Dent Relat Res. 2022;24(3):352–60.
37. Wei SM, Zhu Y, Wei JX, Zhang CN, Shi JY, Lai HC. Accuracy of dynamic navigation in implant surgery: a systematic review and meta-analysis. Clin Oral Implants Res. 2021;32(4):383–93. https://doi.org/10.1111/clr.13719.
38. Kaewsiri D, Panmekiate S, Subbalekha K, Mattheos N, Pimkhaokham A. The accuracy of static vs. dynamic computer-assisted implant surgery in single tooth space: a randomized controlled trial. Clin Oral Implants Res. 2019;30960:505–14.
39. Guzmán AM, Deglow ER, Zubizarreta-Macho A, Agustín-Panadero R, Montero SH. Accuracy of computer-aided dynamic navigation compared to computer-aided static navigation for dental implant placement: an in vitro study. J Clin Med. 2019;8(12):2123.
40. Putra RH, Yoda N, Astuti ER, Sasaki K. The accuracy of implant placement with computer-guided surgery in partially edentulous patients and possible influencing factors: a systematic review and meta-analysis. J Prosthodont Res. 2022;66(1):29–39.
41. Chen Z, Li J, Sinjab K, Mendonca G, Yu H, Wang H-L. Accuracy of flapless immediate implant placement in anterior maxilla using computer-assisted versus conventional surgery: a cadaver study. Clin Oral Implant Res. 2018;29:1186–94.
42. Younes F, Eghbali A, De Bruyckere T, Cleymaet R, Cosyn J. A randomized controlled trial on the efficiency of freehanded, pilot-drill guided and fully guided implant surgery in partially edentulous patients. Clin Oral Implants Res. 2019;30:131–8.
43. Younes F, Cosyn J, De Bruyckere T, Cleymaet R, Bouckaert E, Eghbali A. A randomized controlled study on the accuracy of free-handed, pilot-drill guided and fully guided implant surgery in partially

edentulous patients. J Clin Periodontol. 2018;45:721–32. Prosthesis 2022;4:553.
44. Smitkarn P, Subbalekha K, Mattheos N, Pimkhaokham A. The accuracy of single-tooth implants placed using fully digital guided surgery and conventional implant surgery. J Clin Periodontol. 2019;46:949–57.
45. Varga E, Antal M, Major L, Kiscsatári R, Braunitzer G, Piffkó J. Guidance means accuracy: a randomized clinical trial on conventional versus guided dental implantation. Clin Oral Implants Res. 2020;31:417–30.
46. Aydemir CA, Arısan V. Accuracy of dental implant placement via dynamic navigation or the conventional method: a split-mouth randomized controlled clinical trial. Clin Oral Implants Res. 2020;31:255–63.
47. Koch AD, Ekkelenkamp VE, Haringsma J, et al. Simulated colonoscopy training leads to improved performance during patient-based assessment. Gastrointest Endosc. 2015;81(3):630–6.
48. Araujo-Corchado E, Pardal-Peláez B. Computer-guided surgery for dental implant placement: a systematic review. Prosthesis. 2022;4:540–53.

Digital Craniofacial and Orthognathic Surgery

11

Kaan Orhan and Merve Berika Kadıoğlu

11.1 Introduction

Dentofacial deformities do not only affect functions, it can also influence quality of life, self-image, and social behavior due to aesthetic concerns regardless of age. This may lead to the perception that the individual is less attractive, less successful, and less socially acceptable according to social norms [1]. *For this reason, the combined application of orthodontic treatment and orthognathic surgery in adults with dentofacial deformities is considered a very powerful tool for both correcting functional abnormalities and improving facial aesthetics* [2].

Although intraoperative surgical technique is of great importance in the success of orthognathic surgical treatment, the accuracy of the skeletal and dental diagnosis of the deformity and the correct preoperative prediction of predicted jaw movements are also extremely important in the successful outcome of orthognathic surgical treatment [3, 4]. For this reason, making the correct diagnosis, creating a correct treatment plan, and transferring this plan to the operating room are of vital importance for the successful treatment of maxillofacial disorders that require orthognathic surgery. Therefore, for the successful treatment of maxillofacial disorders requiring orthognathic surgery, it is vital to make the correct diagnosis, create the correct treatment plan, and transfer this plan to the operating room accurately [5, 6].

After years of clinical validation and feedback, traditional orthognathic surgery planning has become the standard procedure before orthognathic surgery [7]. Traditional surgery planning (TSP) consists of many critical stages such as clinical examination, obtaining two-dimensional (2D) radiographs and dental models, face-bow transfer, placing models in the articulator, cephalometric surgery planning and predictions, performing model surgery, producing splints, and adapting them to the patient's mouth [4, 8].

In traditional orthognathic surgical planning, the direction and amount of movement of hard tissues and changes in soft tissues are determined by 2D cephalometric planning. In order to simulate these 2D predictions in three dimensions, model surgery must be performed and then final and/or intermediate splints for surgery must be produced [9, 10]. In order to start the model surgery, firstly, impressions of the maxillary and mandibular dental arches are taken and plaster models are obtained. These plaster models are

K. Orhan
Faculty of Dentistry, Ankara University, Ankara, Turkey

Ankara University Medical Design Application and Research Center (MEDITAM), Ankara, Turkey

Department of Oral Diagnostics, Faculty of Dentistry, Semmelweis University, Budapest, Hungary
e-mail: knorhan@dentistry.ankara.edu.tr

M. B. Kadıoğlu (✉)
Faculty of Dentistry, Department of Orthodontics, Ankara University, Ankara, Turkey

A. Delantoni, K. Orhan (eds.), *Digital Dentistry*, https://doi.org/10.1007/978-3-031-52826-2_11

subsequently mounted with a face-bow transfer onto an anatomic articulator to relate the maxilla to the cranial base. The face-bow transfer must accurately capture the orientation of the maxilla to assess the occlusal plane angle, occlusal cant, and horizontal arch rotation as well as the vertical movements desired with surgery [11].

Predictive movements in a three-dimensional (3D) model align the relationship of the maxilla and mandible as it relates to the Frankfort horizontal plane and then subsequently relate the maxillomandibular unit in the traditional yaw, pitch, and roll alignment in the *X*, *Y*, and *Z* coordinates [4]. The traditional model surgery has some drawbacks such as being time-consuming, labor-intensive, and having too much error potential due to head positioning errors [12]. Furthermore, it has inherent limitations due to the reduction of the assessment of the three-dimensional craniofacial complex to two dimensions. In traditional orthognathic surgical planning 2D cephalometric analysis is limited, facial asymmetry cannot be evaluated, superpositions of anatomical structures may cause misdiagnosis [13–15]. Moreover, due to the different planning steps for cephalometric tracing, face-bow transfer, model surgery, and surgical splint fabrication, there is a great risk for errors to transfer and accumulate in each of the subsequent steps.

It has been reported that dental models transferred to the articulator with face-bow registration are positioned 8° more vertically than the Frankfurt Horizontal Plane, and in addition, the face-bow transfer is made incorrectly up to 7–8° [16, 17]. Gateno et al. [18] identified up to 15% of systematic errors that could lead to incorrect projection of the maxilla [18]. For this reason, the control of the 3D position of the maxilla (anteroposterior, mediolateral, vertical, and rotation) relative to the basal skull is insufficient and this indirectly affects the mandible even more [19, 20]. In addition, it contains potential errors such as incorrect positioning of the plaster models on the articulator, incorrect placement of the reference lines of the models, and incorrect millimetric measurements of the surgical movements of the segments. And due to these errors, malpositions up to 5 mm have been reported [10]. Obviously, all these potential errors can be transmitted and even amplified between the multistep procedures during the acquisition of final and intermediate splints for surgical intervention [4].

For this reason, there are obvious limitations in traditional surgical planning (TSP), such as the complexity of the preoperative preparation that can lead to errors, the lack of three-dimensional control (especially in the transverse plane), and the inability to evaluate temporomandibular joint position changes [6, 21–23].

In orthognathic surgery, there has been a paradigm shift toward working virtually in 3D over the last decade because of the inherent limitations of visualizing, planning, and predicting three-dimensional (3D) structures in TSP [24]. With the development and easy accessibility of cone-beam computed tomography (CBCT), the use of virtual surgical planning (VSP) methods for 3D planning and analysis by using computer-aided design and computer-aided manufacturing (CAD-CAM) technology has become increasingly common [8, 23, 25–29].

These advances in the use of 3D software have provided clinicians with valuable tools to assist in diagnosis, treatment planning, and postoperative evaluation [27, 29, 30]. 3D simulation, 3D-printed surgical splints, 3D-printed metal plates, and sawing guides were introduced and adopted in clinical practice, providing practical advantages to orthognathic surgeons [31].

VSP consists of 3D analyzing the patient's skeletal deformity with CBCT which provides superior quality to 2D radiographs, aligning the maxilla and the mandible in the appropriate relationship by performing virtual surgery, and then fabricating a surgical splint using a 3D printing machine [4, 8]. It overcomes the main limitations of the conventional technique, which lies in its 2D nature and multiple steps requiring combinations of data gathered from different sources, including physical examination, anthropometric analysis and 2D cephalograms, face-bow registration, and mock surgery using a semiadjustable articulator [4, 27, 29].

Virtual surgical planning allows for more thorough analysis and surgical planning, especially in patients with complex facial deformities

[32]. VSP greatly improves the clinician's ability to diagnose and treat the facial form and position problems that prevent the patient from accomplishing the important functions such as eating, breathing, and communicating. It also enhances facial-skeletal orientation, maxillary and mandibular positioning, correction of asymmetries, and occlusal plane management [33]. VSP also provides an advantage because it allows the jaw movements to be measured in three planes of space and the simulation of multiple and different surgical operations on the same model in a comfortable way. Hence, it helps surgeons to simulate different surgical approaches to determine optimal outcome and communicate with patients [34]. Computer technology has certainly enhanced the ability of the clinician to deliver a more precise treatment outcome, reduce risk, and achieve better outcomes [2].

Just as small mistakes made in traditional surgical planning have big consequences, the same is true for the virtual surgical planning procedure. For this reason, in this part of the book, the points to be considered in the virtual surgery planning clinical and digital workflow will be explained in detail on the cases.

11.2 Image Acquisition for 3D Virtual Surgery Planning

Accurate 3D virtual treatment planning for orthodontics and orthognathic surgery primarily requires obtaining appropriate and accurate images to create an accurate model/database that can represent a realistic digital simulation. For this purpose, there are several different data collection methods such as surface scans, volumetric scans, and four-dimensional (4D) video scans/movements. The common goal in all this is to create a perfect replica of the patient for the preparation of a comprehensive diagnosis, treatment planning, treatment simulation, design and presentation for orthognathic surgical treatment [2].

For this reason, extreme care should be taken about how various data collection methods may affect the results of treatment simulation.

11.2.1 Image Acquisition of the Maxillofacial Region (Cone-Beam Computed Tomography)

For the proper planning of orthognathic surgery, cone-beam computed tomography (CBCT) images obtained in the patient's natural head posture and the resting position of the soft tissues are indispensable. All orthognathic surgical planning software requires Digital Imaging and Communications in Medicine (DICOM) data from either multislice computed tomography (MSCT) or CBCT devices. Once data are imported and displayed, surgical planning software enables virtual surgical simulations of the volumetric or surface-shaded renderings, including the facial soft tissue mask, underlying bony structures and dentition [26, 28].

CBCT is a volumetric image acquisition technique that offers excellent accessibility due to its low cost and use in small spaces compared to multislice computed tomography [35]. The benefits of CBCT in orthodontics include increased image accuracy by eliminating problems such as image magnification, anatomical structure superimposition, and image distortion commonly encountered in 2D radiographs such as traditional cephalometry [36].

One of the most important considerations when obtaining a CBCT image is the use of a cone-beam computed tomography (CBCT) device, which has a large scanning potential to capture the entire face consisting of hard, soft tissues and teeth with the lowest possible radiation dose [37]. For this reason, CBCT devices with a wide field of view (FOV) including all necessary anatomical structures should be preferred to plan orthognathic surgery [15, 35]. The field of view for the exposure should include the soft tissue chin and nose cephalo-caudally and the left and right temporomandibular joints (TMJs) laterally, with a border extension of 10 mm to avoid beam distortion affecting significant structures [24]. The FOV (field of view) range of many CBCT devices is vertically too short to capture all types of maxillofacial deformities and does not allow scanning of the patient from the upper thyroid border to 2 cm above the superior orbital rim (Fig. 11.1).

The FOV depth is also important and there should be an adequate free margin to accommodate both the Porion and the tip of the nose. The image volume of CBCT is dependent on the shape of the X-ray beam and the size of the flat panel detector. Since the relatively small detector size of the CBCT device will limit the scanned volume it is preferable to use devices with large detectors [35]. Although CBCT is advantageous in terms of cost and radiation dose, it should be considered that compared with MSCT imaging CBCT imaging has some limitations as higher noise level, lower contrast and poor image quality. Because most tissue segmentation algorithms are based on thresholding, some anatomical structures (e.g., sella turcica, condyles, orbital walls) are difficult to visualize anatomically in the 3D viewer (Fig. 11.1).

Another important issue is the image acquisition time. Patient movement is more likely when the patient is upright rather than supine (i.e., swallowing, breathing, head movement). The time interval to take the CBCT scans can vary among machines from 5 to 70 s, and a longer interval allows more potential for patient movement. A long scan time or the process of obtaining two separate images and combining them may cause patients to move during image acquisition [2]. This may result in the deterioration of the natural head posture and various motion artifacts, resulting in poor quality and useless data. This brings with it additional radiation dose, additional cost, and additional loss of time. For this reason, it should be ensured that the image is obtained as soon as possible by well-informing the patients beforehand by experienced technician (Fig. 11.2).

Another important issue in obtaining CBCT is scatter-related artifacts. As it is known, many of the orthognathic surgical treatments require preoperative orthodontic treatment, which requires decompensation of the teeth. Although clear aligner treatment has become widespread nowadays, orthodontic treatments are routinely carried out using metal bands, brackets, and wires. All these metallic structures cause serious scatters, especially in CBCT images, negatively affecting the image quality. For this reason, arch wires used in orthodontic treatment must be removed during CBCT scanning to reduce scatter-related artifacts. In addition, the increasingly widespread surgery-first applications and the application of preoperative orthodontic treatment with clear aligners provide a great advantage in this regard by preventing the formation of artifacts due to brackets (Fig. 11.3).

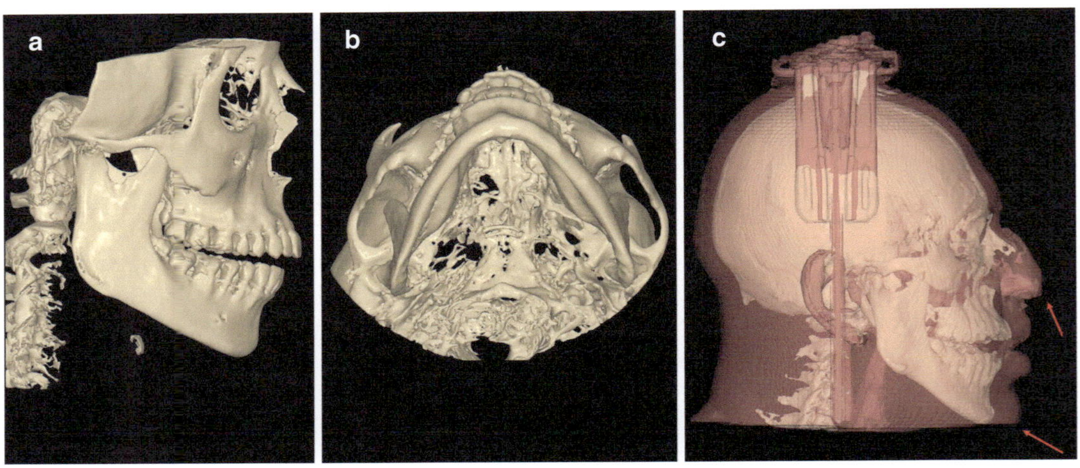

Fig. 11.1 The image is cropped (**a**, **b**) due to insufficient FOV range of the CBCT device. In the picture in (**c**), the nose tip and soft tissue chin tip could not be visualized. In addition, bone structures such as the anterior sinus wall and condyle could not be fully visualized due to thresholding

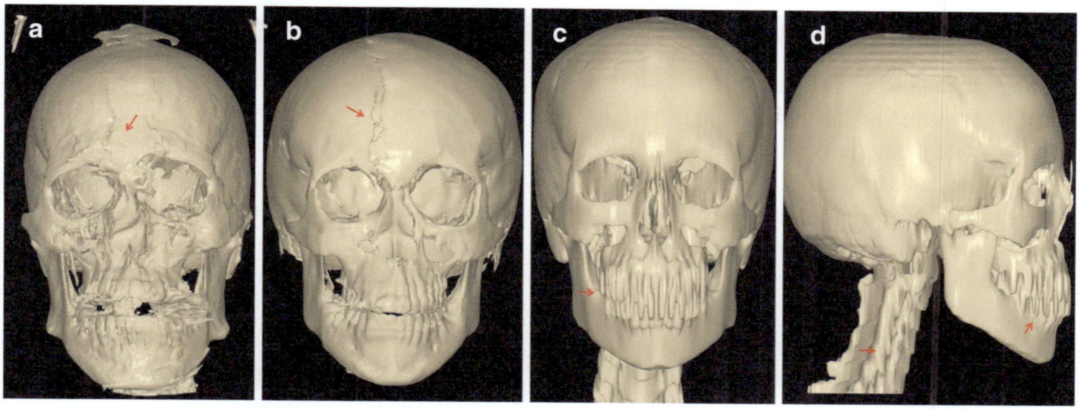

Fig. 11.2 Artifacts due to movement. Although the artifacts in (**a**, **b**) images are at a level that does not prevent virtual surgical planning, it is not possible to use the images in (**c**, **d**) for 3D surgery planning

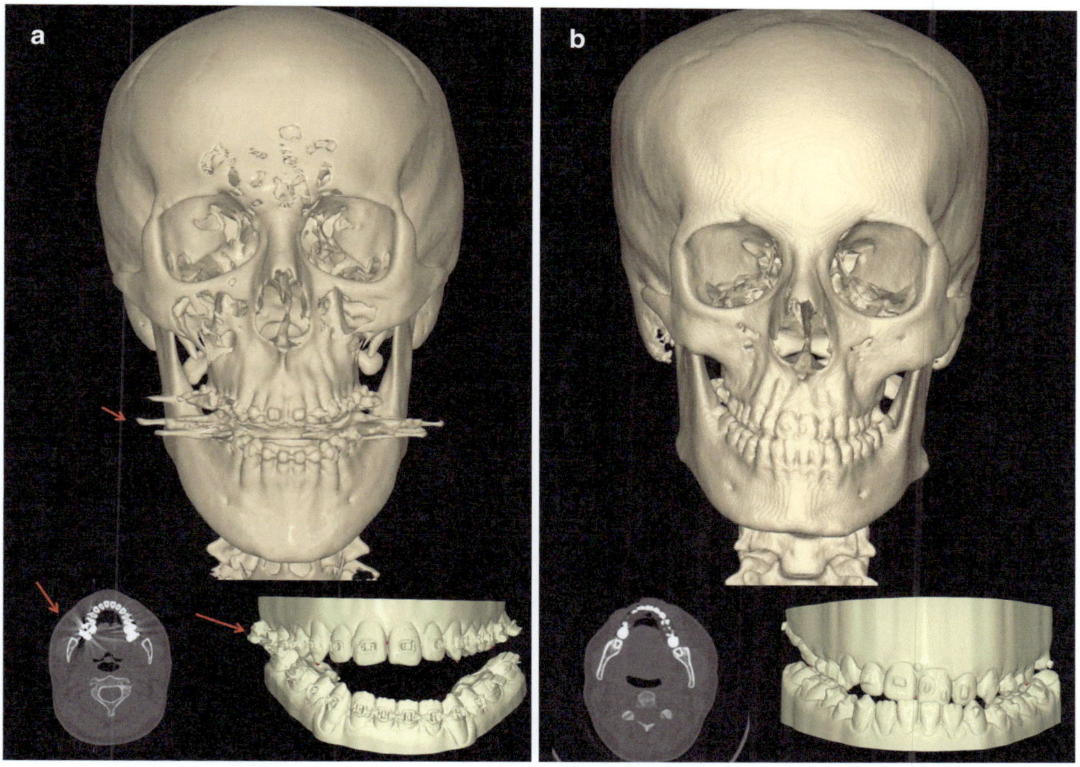

Fig. 11.3 The image in (**a**) has good image quality, but there are too many scatter images due to the bands and brackets. In contrast, in image (**b**), CBCT images obtained from a patient who received clear aligner treatment without brackets do not show any scatter-related artifacts

In routine practice, the patients are stabilized by the chin rest to minimize movement while CBCT images are acquired. These accessories used in the CBCT device to help stabilize the patient (e.g. chin rests, forehead supports) may distort the soft tissue surface anatomy recorded on the CBCT image [2]. Because, it causes deformations in the soft tissue due to the pressure applied. In addition, because of its radiopaque structure, the chin rest is included in the volumetric image and creates erroneous data. For this reason, while taking CBCT images for 3D orthognathic surgery planning, patients should be fixed with ear sticks in a way that does not press on the soft tissues of the patient instead of the chin rest (Fig. 11.4).

For proper imaging of the maxillofacial region, images should be acquired in the most reproducible position, with ideally in the "natural head position (NHP)," the mandible in the "centric relationship (CR)" position, and the lips in the resting position without forcing any closure, motionless, and the muscles of facial expression in repose [24]. This is of great importance in 3D surgical planning of cases characterized by dentofacial asymmetry, occlusal cant and/or vertical maxillary excess requiring impaction, especially when rotational jaw movements in the y and z axes are planned. The aim here is to accurately and reproducibly capture the centric relationship, to accurately preserve the exact relationship of the maxillary and mandibular teeth in both CT records and digital dental models, and to accurately combine digital dental models with the CT records.

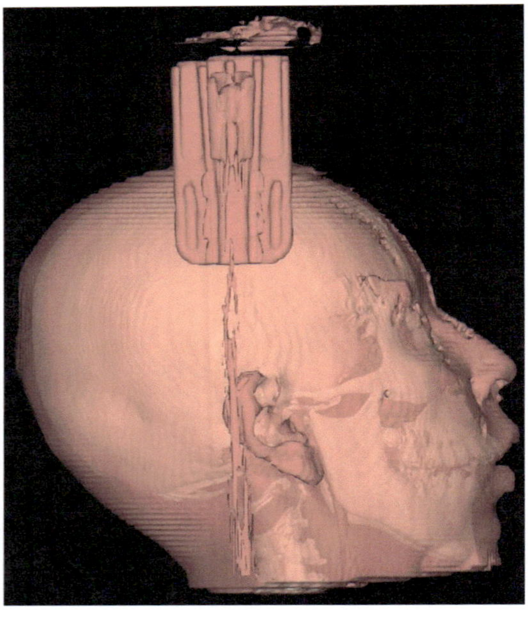

Fig. 11.4 The CBCT image of the patient has obtained with the chin rest. This situation both caused to deteriorate the appearance of the soft tissue pogonion area, which is a critical area during surgical planning, and caused the head position to deviate too much from the natural head posture by being unproperly adjusted

In order to keep the mandible in the desired "centric relationship" position in the CBCT image, bite registration should be taken using various waxes or impression-like materials before CBCT. Then CBCT images should be obtained with this bite registration material fixed in the upper and lower teeth. The bite registration should show directly the centric relationship of the mandible, neither thick enough to cause unnecessary autorotation nor thin enough to be in excessive contact with the teeth (Fig. 11.5). Also, the occlusal grooves (occluso-gingival thickness) in the bite registration should be deep enough to "lock" the teeth, but also shallow enough to prevent undercuts [23]. At the same time, the buccolingual wideness of the bite registration should be narrow enough not to affect the lip closure, but wide enough to cover the entire occlusal surface and overjet. The patient's soft tissues should not be deformed through the use of bite registration or head position stabilizing devices.

Accurate transfer of the centric relationship to CBCT is of greater importance in individuals with severe class II malocclusion or asymmetry, especially in maxillary first surgeries. Because the relaxed position of the muscles under general anesthesia in the operating room will allow the condyle to come to the centric position. However, in the preoperative CBCT records if the mandible is located in a different position (sagittally, transversally, or vertically) from the centric relationship for any reason, such as habit or improper tooth contact, all virtual planning will be designed through this location. Whereas during surgery -before osteotomies- the mandible will shift to the centric relationship position (different from its position at VSP) due to the relaxed muscles with the effect of general anesthesia. By

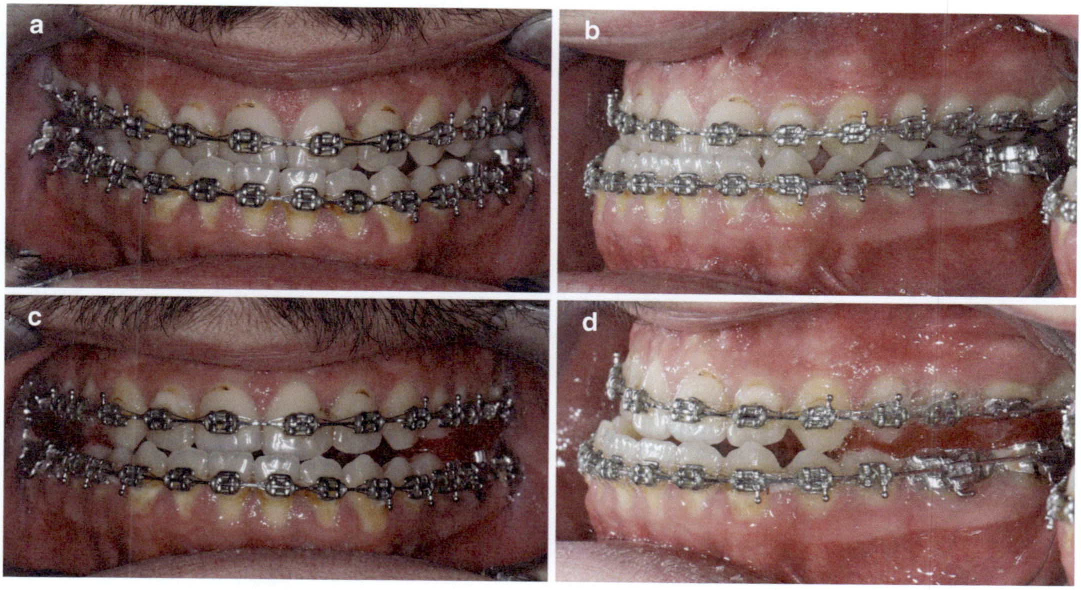

Fig. 11.5 View of occlusion with maximum intercuspidation (**a**, **b**) and with bite registration wax in centric relationship (**c**, **d**)

this way all maxillomandibular movements will be disrupted and an outcome beyond intended in virtual planning will occur [23].

These examples highlight the importance of recording a correct centric relationship when starting bimaxillary surgery with maxillary surgery. It also demonstrates the importance of executing each step of the protocol with precision, as the accuracy of each step builds on the accuracy of the previous one. Because an early error will be carried over to all subsequent steps [23]. In cases where it is impossible to accurately record the centric relationship, surgeons should start bimaxillary orthognathic surgery with the mandible [38].

11.2.2 Image Acquisition of the Dentition and Occlusion

Due to the limited spatial resolution of CBCT, a single scanning procedure of the patient's head does not allow accurate occlusal and intercuspation data, although CBCT imaging produces less artifacts at the occlusal level than MSCT imaging [39]. In CBCT imaging, the formation of scatter due to orthodontic metal brackets deteriorates the image quality and the interfering occlusal contacts create difficulties in isolating the maxilla and mandible separately during segmentation. The inability to scan teeth in detail with CBCT makes it impossible to precisely plan the postoperative occlusion and produces perfectly matched splints on 3D printers. For this reason, dental structures obtained in CBCT should be included in the system by matching directly or indirectly scanning 3D dental models.

Digital models used for 3D imaging of dental structures can be obtained indirectly (using extraoral 3D scanners) by scanning plaster models or by scanning the impression itself [40]. However, this method has various disadvantages such as the fact that the bracket undercuts do not allow detailed impression, the formation of tears or the separation of the impression material from the tray, the risk of bubbles, gaps, and fractures during model acquisition.

Another option is to directly scan the maxillary and mandibular dental arch and occlusion using a 3D intraoral scanner, instead of taking impressions or obtaining a plaster model. During this process, direct scanning of intraoral dental

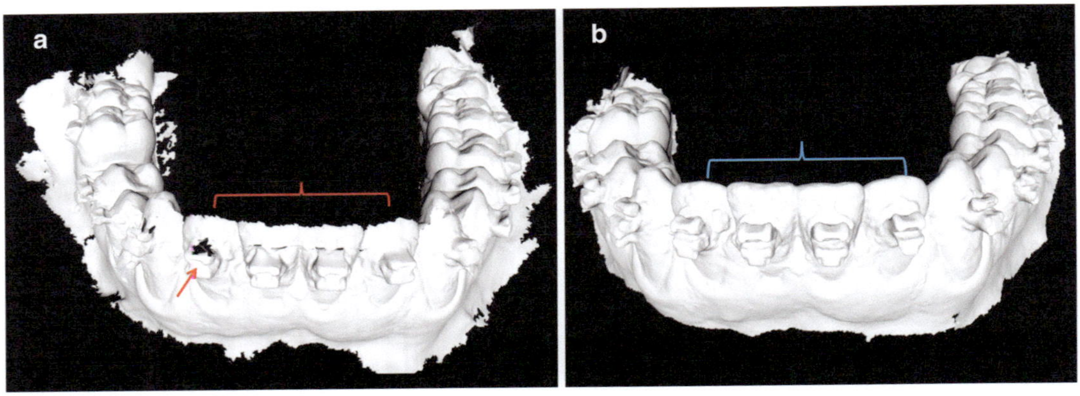

Fig. 11.6 Insufficient/poor quality scanned STL image (**a**) and appropriate scanned STL image (**b**) of the same patient

structures by removing the arch wires provides better results (Fig. 11.6). Direct intraoral scanning can give more accurate results since it does not contain impression-related errors that may occur in the indirect method, especially in patients wearing brackets. Although direct intraoral scanning is performed, special attention should be paid to the fact that the teeth and brackets (especially the surfaces where the splint will contact) are scanned in detail, include all borders, and that there are no gaps that will cause errors in the VSP program (Fig. 11.6) [41].

11.2.3 Image Acquisition of the Facial Tissue (Three Dimensional Scanning of the Face)

The CBCT examination is necessary to accurately visualize soft tissues. However, these do not have a photorealistic appearance, which is imperative in 3D virtual surgical planning (especially in asimetric cases), cleft lip and palate diagnosis, scarring assessment, and prediction of orthognathic surgery prognosis [42]. Structured light, laser triangulation, time-of-flight or stereophotogrammetry techniques can be used to acquire a triangulated facet model of the facial soft tissue surface; stereophotogrammetry also captures color and texture data [24]. Computer technologies have improved these techniques making the capture and building systems faster, simpler, and more precise. The photorealistic virtual face is a method that involves the overlaying and fusion of a CBCT soft tissue image with 3D stereophotographic images of the patient [43, 44].

Stereophotogrammetry has evolved in recent years, and these methods require two images one of each side of the patients' face to create a 3D model that can be observed and measured regardless of perspective. CBCT and 3D stereophotogrammetry (3D photographs) allow exploring the human face three-dimensionally with multiple useful applications that range from using the facial scans to measure all the aesthetic facial parameters to orthodontic diagnosis and evaluation of the craniofacial growth and development [45, 46].

With the introduction of 3D photographs, a 3D camera is used to capture the soft tissue surfaces of the face with correct geometry and texture information, with nonionizing image acquisition [46]. It is based on stereophotogrammetry, which is a method of obtaining an image by means of one or more stereo pairs of photographs being acquired simultaneously. The technique is based on the triangulation and fringe projection method. Image fusion (i.e., registration of a 3D photograph on a CBCT) results in an accurate and photorealistic digital 3D dataset of a patient's face [47, 48]. Augmenting 3D facial soft tissue texture provides improved patient assessment and communication and the production of an individualized 3D virtual treatment plan.

11.3 Processing of Acquired Image Data for 3D Virtual Augmented Model of Patient's Head

The accuracy of the computer simulation is strongly influenced by the way records are acquired, standardized, and augmented. Clinicians often obtain records from different methods and sources to establish treatment objectives and comprehensive management of patients. Usually, clinicians assess each of these records individually. Non-synchronized recordings can also lead to a less than ideal treatment process and thus might produce compromised patient assessment and treatment outcomes [2].

The first step of the planning process is to create a composite skull model, which reproduces both the bony structures and the dentition with a high degree of accuracy.

11.3.1 Transfer of CBCT Data

The purpose of 3D virtual imaging for orthognathic surgery is to create a single virtual anatomical model of the patient, including facial soft tissue structure, underlying bone structures and teeth [35]. To create a "3D virtual augmented/composite model" of the patient's head, "rigid registration" is necessary. Many types of "rigid registration" exist, including point-based, surface-based, and voxel-based rigid registration [49].

CBCT imaging is a 3D volume of Digital Imaging and Communications in Medicine (DICOM) data, consisting of a collection of "cubelike blocks" called "voxels." The CBCT DICOM data can be "rendered" to generate a 3D virtual image of the patient's head by "surface rendering" or [46] "volume rendering" [2].

"Surface rendering" is a reconstruction of 3D structure surfaces by segmentation based on gray scales, Hounsfield unit thresholds can be used to identify structure boundaries and to create a surface-rendered model. It allows digitization of 3D cephalometric landmarks, planning of 3D virtual osteotomies, definition of the 3D virtual occlusal relationship, maxillary and mandibular bony movements with additional soft tissue simulation, and 3D superimposition of datasets [50]. Moreover, it allows integration of 3D digital dental casts and 3D facial photographs into the CBCT scan [51, 52].

"Volume rendering" is a direct reconstruction of 3D structures by rendering a volume of voxels. With regard to each voxel, color and opacity are assigned based on various shading algorithms. Volume rendering allows more detailed anatomy of the teeth and interdental spaces. However, it does not allow user actions and interactions, such as 3D virtual osteotomies, bone fragment movements, or additional soft tissue simulation or 3D integration of datasets. For optimal 3D virtual treatment planning of orthognathic surgery, both "surface rendering" and "volume rendering" are usually used in combination.

To enable the 3D virtual treatment planning of orthognathic surgery, the obtained volumetric CBCT image data in the axial section are combined and processed with the help of the software and then segmented into hard and soft tissue. Surface representations of hard and soft tissues and teeth can be created and visualized in the software's 3D viewer. Threshold levels are set for creating a virtual volumetric rendering of the hard and soft tissues. It is adjusted separately for both soft tissue and hard tissue and must be handled with care. It should be neither dense enough to cause excessive scattering nor low enough that bone and soft tissue structures appear insufficient (Fig. 11.7).

Unlike MDCT data, thresholding of CBCT volumetric datasets currently leads to improper visualization of certain anatomic structures (e.g., soft tissue envelope, condyles, orbital walls) owing to the inherent inhomogeneity of the CBCT gray value data [35, 37]. This results in the unnatural appearance of the facial soft tissue mask obtained by CBCT. Advanced registration algorithms are available that further enrich the CBCT model of the patient's head with skin texture and color information to provide a more natural-looking rendering. Highly detailed tissue information can be added to the skin segmented from the CBCT scan by using 3D photographs or

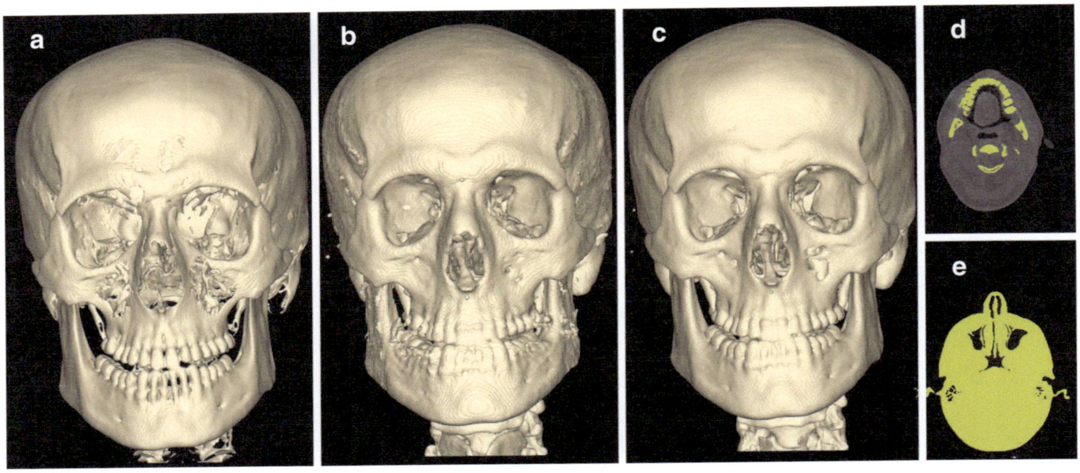

Fig. 11.7 As in view (**a**), when the threshold is lowered to increase the clarity of the teeth or to reduce the scattering, the appearance of structures such as the anterior sinus wall, orbit, and condyle is lost. When it is increased too much as in (**b**), although all the structures are visible, this time noises occur and artifacts increase. The most ideal is to keep the threshold at a level as in (**c**). The threshold settings are seen for tooth–bone tissues in (**d**) image and for soft tissues in (**e**)

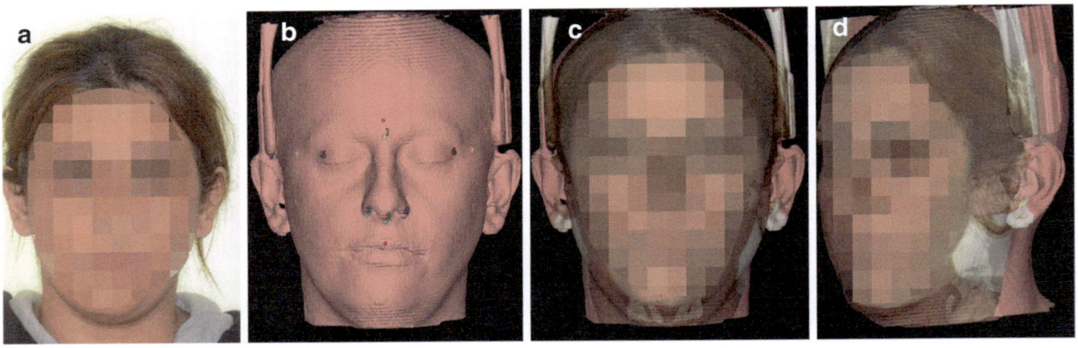

Fig. 11.8 A realistic soft tissue (**c**, **d**) image is obtained by overlaying the 2D photograph (**a**) on certain points on the CBCT soft tissue (**b**)

2D photographs with the same facial expression as the patient during the CBCT scan (Fig. 11.8) [27, 29, 48]. Registration algorithms incorporating photographic, laser, or optical surface scanning of facial features to augment the patient's CBCT surface with skin texture and color information may assist in providing realistic simulations [48, 53].

11.3.2 Integration of Digital Dental Casts in CBCT Scans to Augment the Patient's Dentition and Occlusion

Images derived from a single CBCT scan cannot provide accurate detailed information regarding the dentition or interocclusal relationships, which are mandatory for proper orthodontic preparation and surgical treatment planning and appropriate generation of surgical splints. Accordingly additional image acquisition of the patient's dentition in the form of 3D digital models is required in order to obtain accurate occlusal and intercuspation analysis [52]. These 3D digital models facilitate 3D measurement of tooth position, provide clear determination of the resulting occlusion, and allow 3D mapping of tooth movements in treatment plans [2].

For this purpose, these images obtained by direct or indirect 3D scanning and containing accurate interocclusal data should be integrated into the 3D CBCT model in order to improve 3D simulation algorithms and provide accurate planning. The resulting STL files were fused to the CBCT files using an integrated semiautomatic point-to-point reference algorithm [2]. The user indicates a number of dental landmarks (at anterior and bilaterally posterior side) on the virtual bony hard tissue rendering, with their corresponding points on the study model rendering and the software automatically fuses the STL file into the volumetric hard tissue model (Fig. 11.9) [26, 28].

After that, the compatibility of the CBCT slices and 3D dental model can be examined in detail, and if necessary the adaptation can be maximized by performing precise rotation and translation movements of 3D dental model in all three planes: sagittal, vertical, and transversal (Fig. 11.9). Thus, the low-resolution dental structures on the CBCT are replaced by the high-resolution 3D dental model [27, 29]. Through this procedure, the dental and skeletal anatomy is ultimately merged through superimposition of the Digital Imaging and Communications in Medicine (DICOM) data, yielding accurate occlusal topography for the establishment of occlusion and fabrication of splints.

11.3.3 Orientation of Three-Dimensional Virtual Augmented/Composite Model of the Patient's Head to Natural Head Position

Orientation of the head is the most important step in facial treatment planning. If this step does not receive adequate attention, the orthodontic and surgical results will be compromised from the outset [33]. For this reason, it is necessary to adjust the orientation of the head in the *X*, *Y*, *Z* plane after the intraoral model and volumetric CBCT data are merged. It is very important to have the clinical photographs and videos of the patient available at the planning session as they help to confirm the NHP, show the incisor expo-

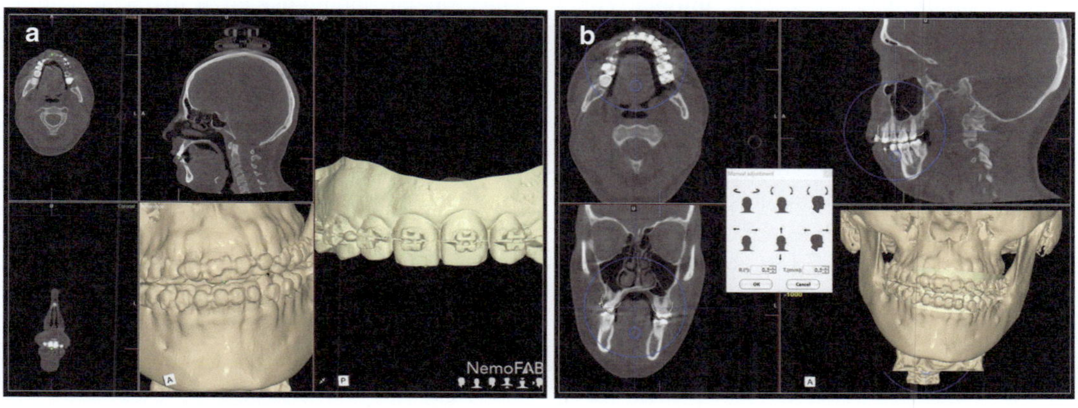

Fig. 11.9 3D STL dental models and CBCT images are superimposed by the algorithm which needs to determine three points at central incisor—right and left molars (**a**). Then, by performing translational and rotational movements on all three planes, maximum adaptation is achieved (**b**)

sure at rest and during animation, and help assess the position of the soft tissue facial midline in relation to the bony midline [24].

Positioning of the head is difficult in cone-beam computed tomography (CBCT), because the scanning time is relatively long (20–40 s) and this requires the patient's head to be fixed to avoid movement [54]. While obtaining tomographic images, although correct positioning is made, the natural head posture may deteriorate due to many factors such as the long irradiation time of the CBCT image, the inability to use the jaw tip apparatus used to fix the head, and the experience of the technician. For this reason, before starting the 3D analysis and surgical planning, the orientation of the head should be checked in terms of both soft tissue and hard tissue.

Because the images derived from CBCT are three-dimensional, the position of the head must be recorded in all three planes of space, as the pitch, roll, and yaw of the head accurately orientate the three-dimensional image [54].

The natural position of the head is stable and reproducible and indicates the true appearance of face [55]. The use of the NHP obviates internal landmarks and provides a reproducible reference framework [2]. Over the 10 years, different groups have published their experiences and recommendations regarding accurately representing the patient's natural head position. These techniques include data acquisition through cone-beam CT, use of a face-bow jig with an attached gyroscope, and patient-specific bite registration mounted to a fiducial facebow to generate numerical values for the pitch, roll, and yaw of the patient's head [4, 15, 56].

If the natural head position is disturbed while acquiring the CBCT image, the orientation of the head should be readjusted on the VSP software according to various references such as Frankfurt Horizontal plane, pupillary plane, facial midline. Using 3D software, the head should be moved through ranges of positions, along each planar axis, to reveal deviations from the desired corrected head posture. This part is one of the most important stages of 3D virtual planning as it will be a reference in terms of midline deviation, occlusal cant, asymmetry, and yaw movements during the virtual planning to be made later [33] (Fig. 11.10).

One of the most important advantages of 3D virtual planning is that yaw deviations in the axial plane, which are often overlooked in traditional 2D planning, can be evaluated and corrected. For orientation of head at axial plane, the best technique is to measure and observe multiple locations to best project of the face in a most forward position. Combining the observations of the foramen magnum, the position of the mid palatal suture, the outline of the frontal bones, and the forward projection of the lateral orbital rims will improve the accuracy of the axial orientation (Fig. 11.10) [33].

Especially in cases of asymmetry involving the orbit such as hemifacial microsomia, hemifacial hypertrophy, or in cases where the head-neck posture is severely impaired, the orientation of the head should be combined with clinical examination and head orientation should be provided as close to natural as possible [24]. Many techniques have been described for leveling the head in the frontal view, such as leveling the orbits, leveling the ears, leveling the globes, leveling the zygomatic arches, etc. All of these techniques are fraught with complicating factors as few humans have eyes, ears, or jaws which are parallel to the floor. The clinician needs to decide the facial level for each patient. The clinician should use all available structures of the face to decide the proper frontal plane orientation [33]. Also in patients with too much asymmetry, since the soft tissues will be affected, clinical evaluation of the upper midline will help give a more accurate idea after the mandible is shifted toward the midline as more symmetrical position.

For this reason, after the three-dimensional orientation of the head is adjusted, the obtained occlusal plane, bipupillary plane, maxillary inclination and rotation, axial orientation of the teeth, mandibular asymmetry, occlusal cant status, the position of the lips in relation to the teeth and jaws should be examined in detail and compared with the clinical findings and their overlap should be ensured [28].

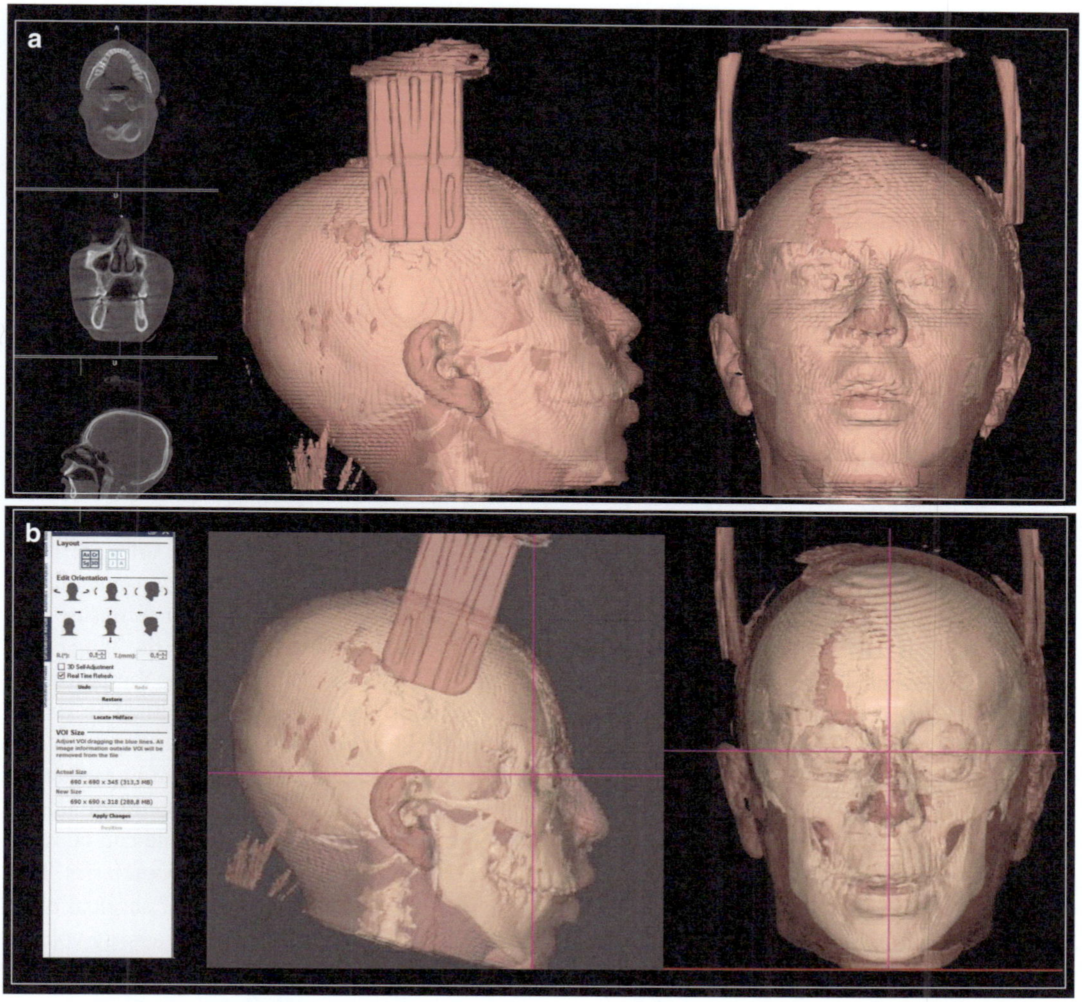

Fig. 11.10 (**a**) The position of the head is too distorted when acquiring the CBCT image. (**b**) The orientation of the head is adjusted in all three axes according to the natural head posture

11.4 Creation of Records and 3D Diagnosis for 3D Virtual Orthognathic Surgery

3D inspection of the virtual composite model of the patient's head is a great diagnostic tool for a maxillofacial deformity. Both "volume rendering" and "surface rendering" offer a thorough in-depth 3D virtual inspection [2]. The resulting images include original axial CBCT slices with coronal and sagittal reconstructions, allowing 2D examination of the patient's anatomy in three standard planes (axial, sagittal, coronal) and multiplane (Fig. 11.11). Thus, diagnostic lateral cephalometric, panoramic, anteroposterior radiographs can be obtained over CBCT images. By generating virtual lateral and frontal cephalograms from the patient's CBCT dataset, it bridges the gap between traditional cephalometry and three-dimensional cephalometry, including soft tissue and underlying bone-tooth structures [26, 28].

In this way, 3D analysis of hard and soft tissues and teeth is performed using traditional

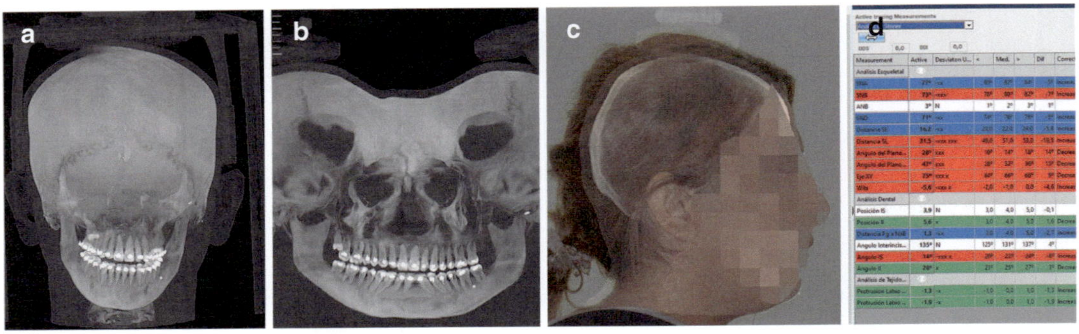

Fig. 11.11 From 3D CBCT data, 2D posteroanterior (**a**), panoramic (**b**), lateral cephalometric (**c**) radiographs can be obtained and detailed 2D/3D cephalometric analysis (**d**) can be performed

cephalometric analysis. Numerous measurements are made, such as sagittal and vertical positions of the maxilla and mandible, face heights, upper and lower incisors positions, maxillary-occlusal-mandibular plane angles, soft tissue profile, and nasolabial angle (Fig. 11.11).

Thus, except for clinical observation, the regions that deviate from the normal are determined with numerical data and a reference is created for the amount of movement to be applied in 3D planning [57].

Also apart from cephalometric analysis a large amount of clinical information can be obtained (e.g., condylar anatomy and location, maxillofacial bony and dental pathologic features, maxillary sinus pathologic features, nasal septum deviation, a restricted airway, dentoalveolar bone support to the teeth, and the pathway of the inferior alveolar nerve) [26, 28]. Also CBCT allows for systematic radiographic assessment of the temporomandibular joints, oro-, naso-, and hypopharynx, relative positions of the roots of the dentition within alveolar bone, fenestrations, and dehiscences [24].

In addition, depending on the software used, the center of rotation on the temporomandibular joints can be determined in order to ensure that the mandible autorotates around the hinge axis (Fig. 11.12). At the same time, the temporomandibular joint region can be examined in detail, and the position of the condyle in the fossa and the state of condylar resorption can be evaluated.

Besides, the minimum cross-sectional area of the airway and total airway volume can be measured by determining the airway boundaries. This provides an advantage in terms of surgical planning (Fig. 11.13). As it is known, airway volume is a factor that varies after orthognathic surgery and is a determining factor in planning. In patients with low airway volume, the amount of mandibular setback should be carefully evaluated.

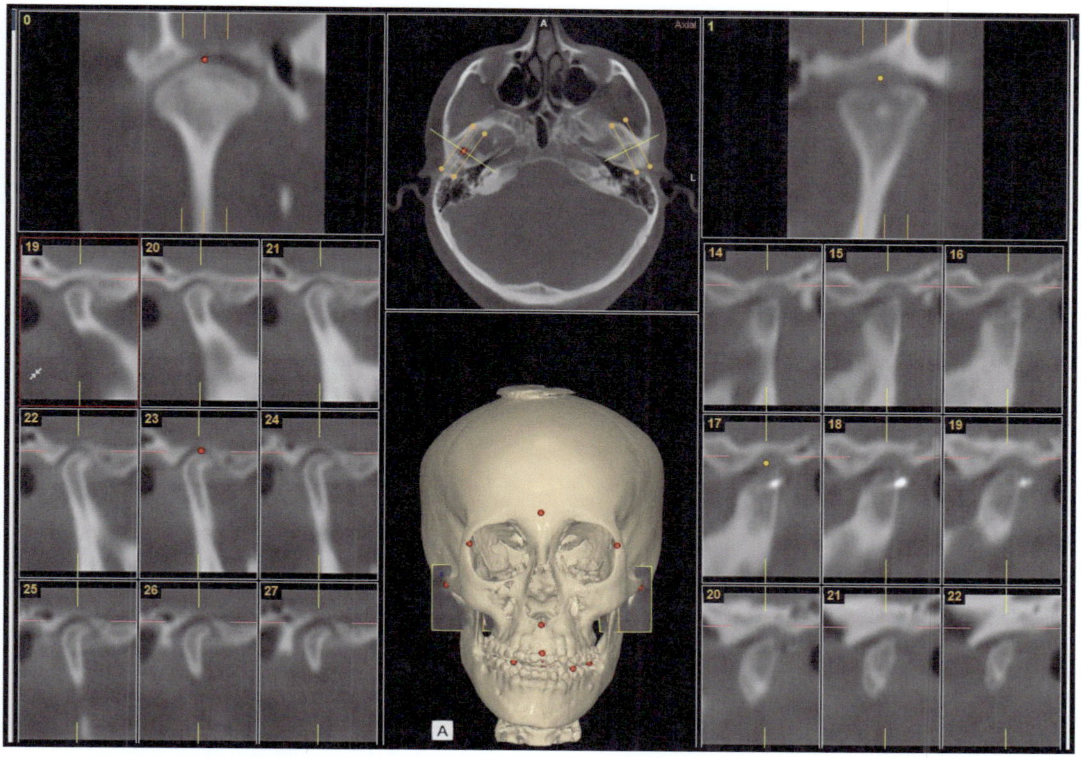

Fig. 11.12 Right and left temporomandibular joints can be examined structurally and spatially in axial, sagittal, and frontal sections. The image shows a difference due to condylectomy performed for condylar hyperplasia on the left side. In addition, the rotation center where the mandible autorotation will take place is determined at this stage and a correct autorotation axis for the mandible is determined

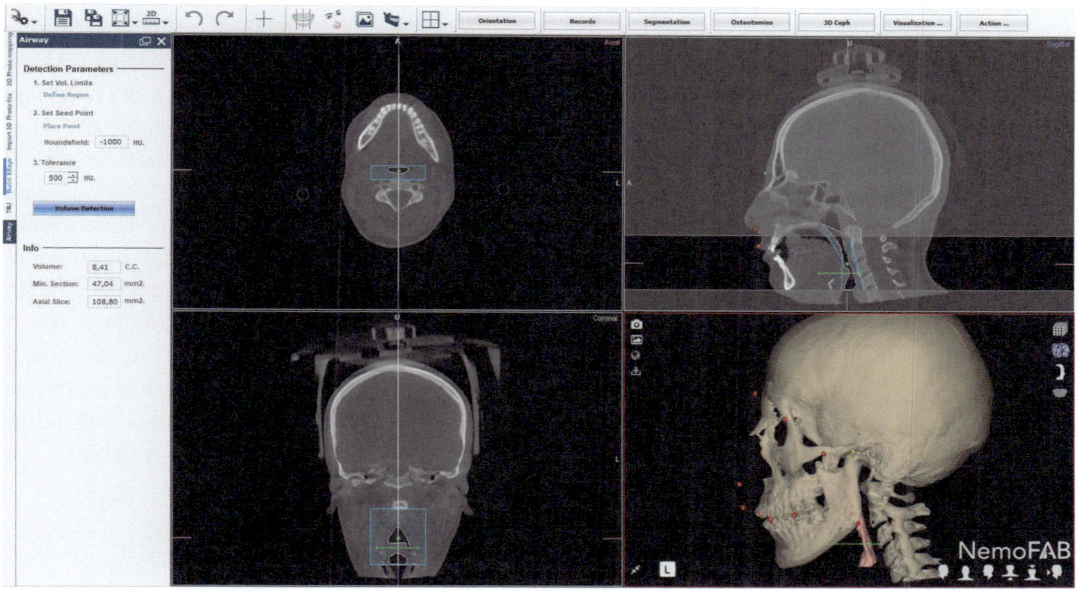

Fig. 11.13 Both the minimum cross-sectional area and the total volume can be measured by quickly determining the airway boundaries in axial, sagittal, and frontal sections with simple algorithms

11.5 Three-Dimensional Virtual Treatment Planning of Orthognathic Surgery

One of the most important advantages of 3D virtual surgery planning compared to traditional surgery planning is that the clinician has much more detailed information about the patient's anatomy in the course of planning. In addition, 3D virtual treatment planning allows the clinician to focus more on 3D facial harmony rather than just facial profile and/or dental occlusion. However, certain steps must be completed before the 3D virtual surgery planning stage.

11.5.1 Segmentation for 3D Virtual Orthognathic Surgery

Another important step for three-dimensional virtual surgical planning is to segment the maxilla and mandible as separate structures that allow independent surgical movements [2]. CBCT scan resolution is not high enough to define the surface of the condylar heads from the glenoid fossae surfaces and the maxillary dentition from the mandibular dentition. These structures can be "separated" through a process termed segmentation. Segmentation involves delineating and then color coding the structures manually or by using semi-automated or automated algorithms, normally using active contour-based segmentation methods [58].

While segmentation is done manually in some programs, automatic segmentation is provided in more recent programs. During this procedure, the maxilla and mandible must be completely independent. Therefore, it is very important that there are no continuous meshes between the maxilla and mandible on volume rendering. In such a case, the meshes connecting the maxilla and mandible should be cleaned and separated completely to ensure segmentation (Fig. 11.14). Again, a smooth surface should be created by removing impurities caused by various reasons such as scatter on the surface of the maxilla and mandible. Once the necessary images have been acquired, fused, rendered, and segmented, the 3D-VSP virtual model can be used for planning.

11.5.2 Creation of Osteotomy Lines for 3D Virtual Orthognathic Surgery

To develop a 3D simulation of surgery, the augmented/composite head model is initially prepared (precut) to simulate various osteotomies. Virtual osteotomy lines are determined for the maxilla, mandible and, if necessary, for the chin, passing the estimated locations of the osteotomy incisions planned for surgery such as LeFort I osteotomy, a sagittal split osteotomy, an intraoral vertical ramus osteotomy, an inverted "L" osteotomy, and/or a genioplasty (Fig. 11.15). Thereby the maxillary and mandibular structures that will be moved to the appropriate position during virtual surgical planning are isolated separately. This creates the potential to execute different surgical treatment plans virtually.

In this step, the clinician specifies the intended location and geometry of all osteotomies to be performed in the maxilla, proximal segments of the mandible, and anterior mandible. In the meantime, care should be taken not to damage any anatomical structures such as tooth roots and inferior alveolar canal while designing the osteotomy lines. In addition, the design of virtual osteotomy lines together with the surgical team that will perform the surgery will be beneficial in terms of ensuring that the jaw movements that will be planned in the next stage are transferred to the operating room correctly. In addition, determining the virtual osteotomy lines in the closest way to reality provides a great advantage in terms of seeing the bone interferences that will occur due to jaw movements correctly before the surgery.

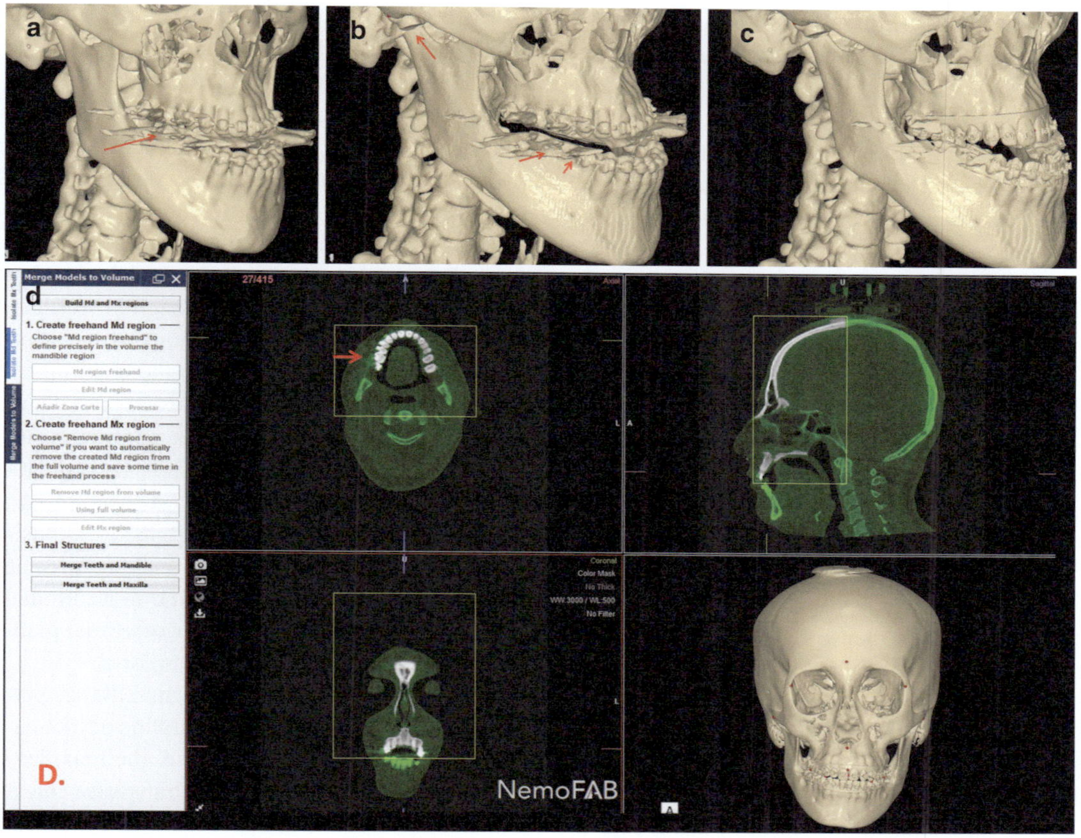

Fig. 11.14 Structures such as condyle or occlusal tooth contacts (**b**) that bridge the maxilla to mandible (**a**) should be removed on the CBCT surface rendering to enable segmentation. In this way, smooth segmentation can be achieved (**c**). In each section, it is tried to obtain a clean-perfect bone surface by removing the excess and image impurities separately (**d**)

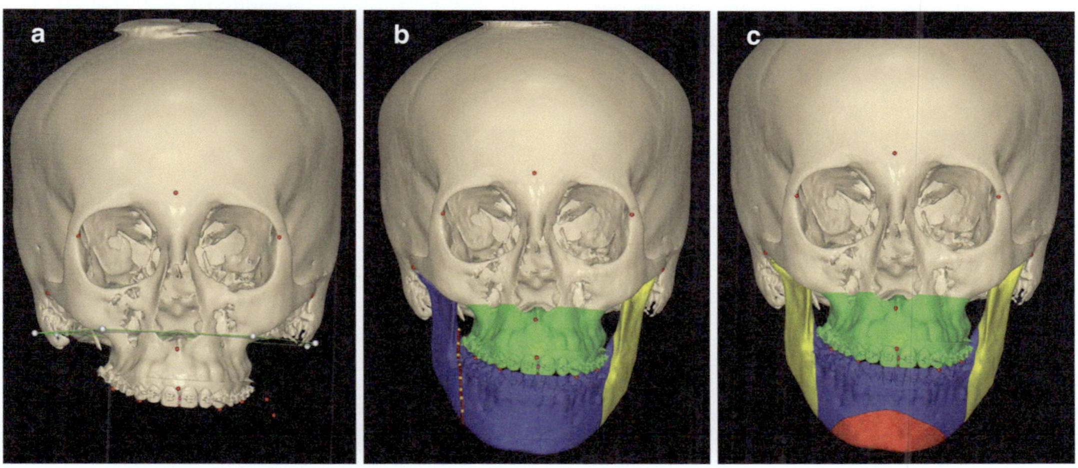

Fig. 11.15 *Virtual osteotomy lines* (**a**). LeFort 1 osteotomy (**b**). Sagittal split osteotomy (**c**). Genioplasty

11.5.3 Three-Dimensional Virtual Orthognathic Surgery

At this most critical stage, after the jaws are osteotomized, the bone segments are moved as desired, based on clinical examination and 3D analysis, in a way that both provide with ideal occlusion and obtain an ideal appearance in soft and hard tissues. So virtual planning, which provides translational and rotational freedom of movement in three different planes to the maxilla and mandible, provides simulation and visualization of the effects of different surgical techniques.

Virtual surgery planning usually starts with maxillary surgery. It has been stated that mandible-first surgery is more predictable in cases where the maxilla and mandible are both rotated counterclockwise. Apart from this, maxilla-first surgery has been generally thought to be more predictable [24, 59].

The virtual osteotomized maxillary segment(s) are repositioned three-dimensionally by making translational movements in relation to the three (x, y and z) spatial planes according to fascial planes and clinical analyses. Adjustments are then made using rotational movements around the x, y, and z axes, representing roll, pitch, and yaw, respectively [24].

Virtual simulation of bilateral sagittal split osteotomy of the mandible allows virtual repositioning and adjustment of the mandibular corpus for best dental occlusion while keeping the condyles in a centric position within the glenoid fossa [26, 28]. All movements can also be controlled using the milimetric measurements in the virtual volumetric analysis menu.

Bimaxillary surgery usually begins with maxillary repositioning first. A significant benefit of using 3D VSP in making these adjustments is that they can be made while referencing points and planes derived from the craniofacial bony structures. By adjusting the orientation of the head in the early stages of planning, the sagittal, vertical, and transversal direction deviations of the maxilla are determined according to the craniofacial structure. For this reason, while the maxilla is brought to the desired position as anterior–posterior and superoinferior as determined by cephalometric analysis and clinical measurements, however, the maxilla is brought to the ideal position according to the face by making precise yaw-roll-pitch movements. Similar to traditional model surgery, the primary focus of virtual planning is the position of the upper incisors.

Virtual manipulation of the maxilla is performed by first addressing any midline or inclination corrections. For this purpose, the maxillary dental midline is adjusted with transverse linear movements to coincide with the facial midline. It can also be corrected rotationally by selecting the upper dental midline or right/left canine tooth as rotation center (Fig. 11.16).

A submental and bird's-eye view is then used to assess and correct the maxillomandibular yaw by using a midsagittal plane through nasion and foramen magnum. This plane provides a visual comparison of the discrepancy between the right

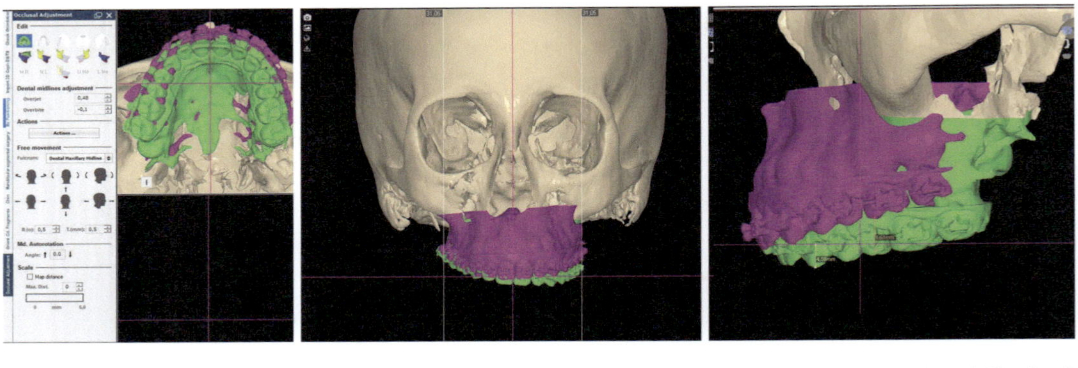

Fig. 11.16 The maxillary midline is moved rotationally and translationally and matched with the facial midline in all three planes

and left maxillary canines and mesiobuccal cusp of the maxillary first molars. Yaw correction (rotation round the vertical axis) allows for correction of the maxillary midline relative to the facial midline. Thanks to canine or midline axis rotations in this plane, maxillary yaw problems are corrected in a way that symmetry is provided both in the anterior canine region and posteriorly in the molar region (Fig. 11.16). This is especially valuable for facial asymmetry cases, where complex rotational corrections of the osteotomized bony segments in three dimensions are often required. In addition, the width discrepancy between the right and left gonial angles can be measured to the midsagittal plane and to the root of the zygomatic arches.

Although minor maxillary arch asymmetries may seem insignificant, it should be noted that once the maxilla is fixed in the planned position, it serves as a target for mandibular repositioning during bimaxillary surgery. Therefore, any asymmetry in the position of the maxilla will be magnified further away from the axis of asymmetry, creating even greater deviations in the mandible (especially in the gonial region). When Ellis et al. compared the maxillary position accuracy with the traditional method, they found that the posterior maxillary dental arch was calculated incorrectly by 1.9 mm in the mediolateral direction [10]. This may cause the patient to gain a more asymmetrical appearance after bimaxillary surgery to correct a symmetrical deformity. In such a case, although the dental midline coincides with the facial midline, it will cause an asymmetrical placement of the mandible due to the posterior maxillary asymmetry in the yaw axis. This will result in facial asymmetry by causing one side to appear longer than the other, especially in the ramus region [10].

The occlusal cant problem, which is frequently encountered especially in class III malocclusions and asymmetry cases, can also be corrected at this stage. Maxillary canting at the canine and mesiobuccal (MB) cusp tips of the first molars is assessed relative to the horizontal plane, which may or may not coincide with the infraorbital rims. The maxillary cant can be corrected by adjusting the roll of the osteotomized maxillary segment round the sagittal axis ("*x* axis") using the pupillary plane as a reference, providing no orbital dystopia is present. In accordance with the planning goal, the occlusal plane inclination can be corrected as parallel to the pupillary plane by impaction of the long/drooping side, or vice versa, by down fracture of short side. Correction of the maxillary cant is accomplished with simultaneous attention to mandibular symmetry at the inferior border.

Whether symmetry is achieved as a result of the movements obtained can be checked in detail with the drawn reference planes (Fig. 11.17).

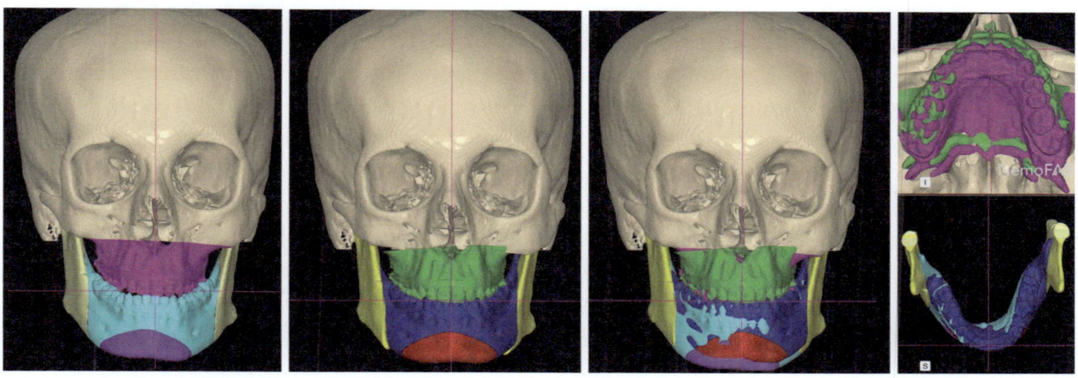

Fig. 11.17 In a patient with 3D asymmetry with Parry-Romberg syndrome, the right side was down fractured to correct the occlusal cant, though an asymmetric impaction was made on the left side. Thus, while the occlusal cant was corrected, the axial inclination of the upper incisors was also corrected. In addition, the maxilla was shifted to the left in a rotational and translational manner, ensuring symmetry of the maxillary dental midline with respect to the face, correcting the maxillary yaw deviation, and creating more space for mandibular asymmetry correction

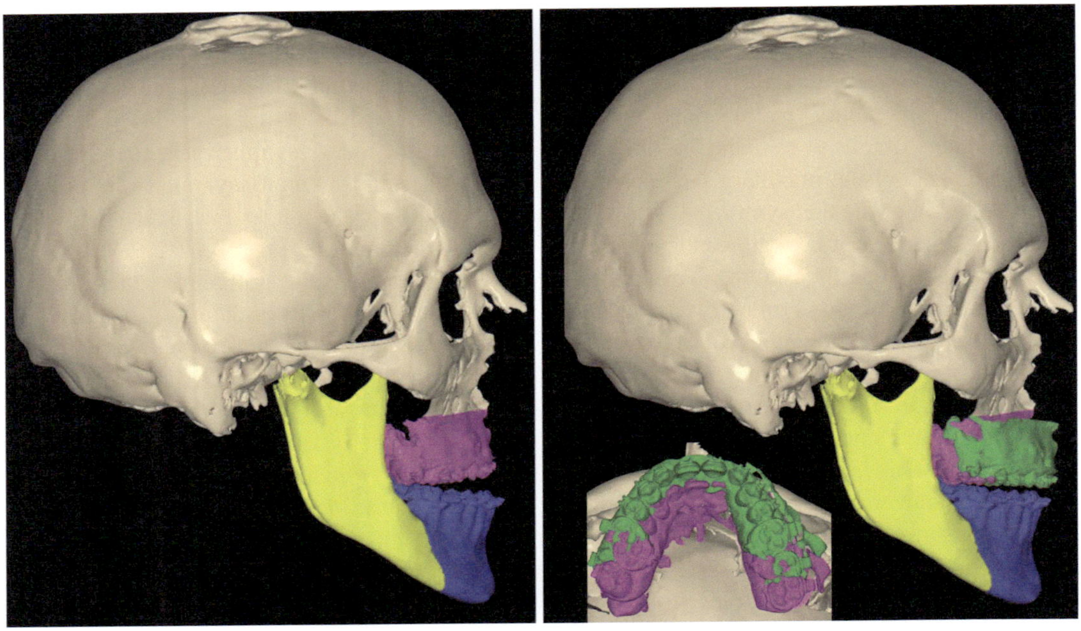

Fig. 11.18 In the patient characterized by class III-open bite and maxillary asymmetry, the maxilla was moved anteriorly and to the right side. At the same time, the anterior region of the maxilla was down fractured with clockwise rotation to correct the open bite and insufficient incisor display, and stabilization was achieved with iliac graft. Thus, the occlusal plane and smile line were corrected. For this purpose, mandible first surgery was performed

Then, based on clinical facial examination and 3D cephalometric analysis, the anterior–posterior and superior–inferior movements of the maxilla are performed, taking into account the ideal upper incisor position, incisors display, and the size of the desired soft tissue changes. Adjusting the pitch of the osteotomized maxillary segment (rotation round the transverse axis) allows for the upper incisor inclination to be corrected relative to the true vertical plane. Occlusal plane changes are completed by rotating clockwise or counterclockwise to improve facial balance and proportions (Fig. 11.18).

After the maxilla is placed in its final position, mandibular autorotation is performed until the mandible reaches the first tooth contact point with the proximal and distal segments. After that translational and rotational movements are made to the mandibular segment as determined by cephalometric analysis and clinical measurements to ensure maximum tooth contact at the targeted occlusion (Fig. 11.19).

While creating the targeted occlusion, the amount of occlusal contact on the teeth should be determined beforehand, and post-op premature contacts that may cause recurrence later should be avoided (Fig. 11.20).

Especially in bilateral sagittal split osteotomy (BSSO), the relationship of the proximal segments of the mandible with the distal segment is extremely important in terms of providing symmetry and predetermining the location and size of the bone interferences to be corrected during surgery. By 3D virtual surgery planning, the relationship of the proximal segments to the distal segment of the mandible can be visualized and any gaps or overlaps/interferences can be identified. This allows the surgeon to anticipate any required modification or bone grafting of the segments intraoperatively to ensure a stable fixation. In patients with facial asymmetry, the bones may be displaced asymmetrically, and there may be differences in size and shape from one side to the other (Fig. 11.21).

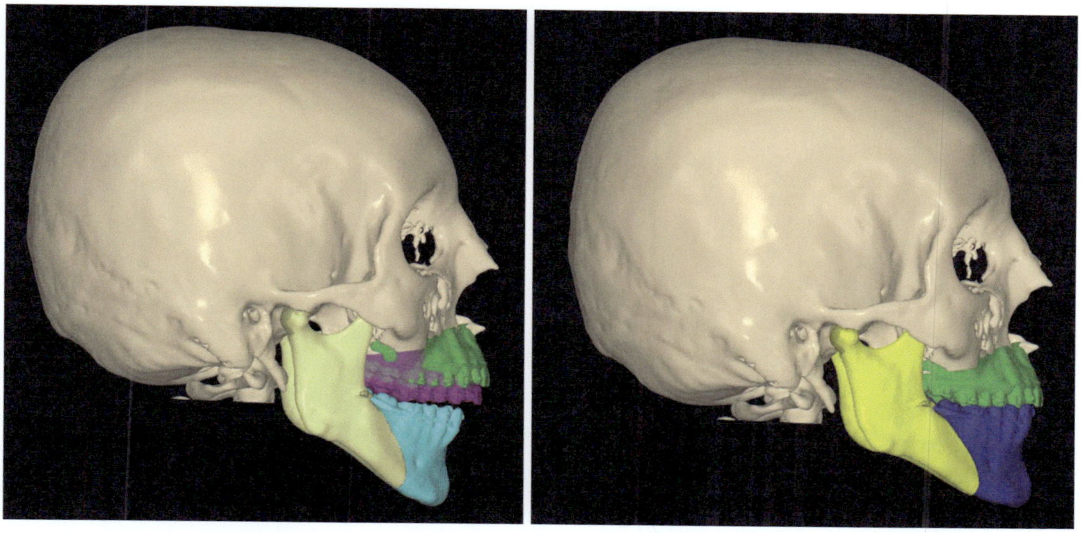

Fig. 11.19 Mandibular autorotation after maxillary impaction provides improvement in class II malocclusion and profile

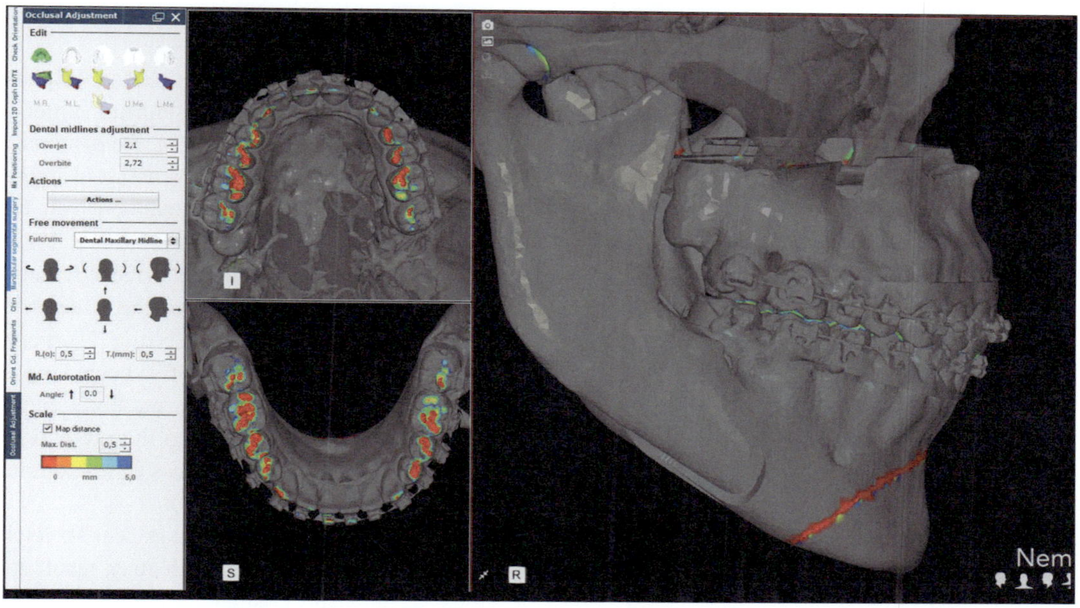

Fig. 11.20 While setting the final occlusion, the tooth contact points can be controlled with the help of a scale to ensure maximum intercuspidation without causing premature contacts

Although mostly double-jaw surgeries are started with maxillary surgery, for large advancement or cases where the condylar position is not ideal, a mandible-first surgical simulation can be viewed with the intermediate occlusal splint aimed to reposition the mandibula before the maxilla. Mandible-first surgery avoids the absolute need to achieve proper joint positioning during preoperative records. If the joints are not seated at correct position when initial records are

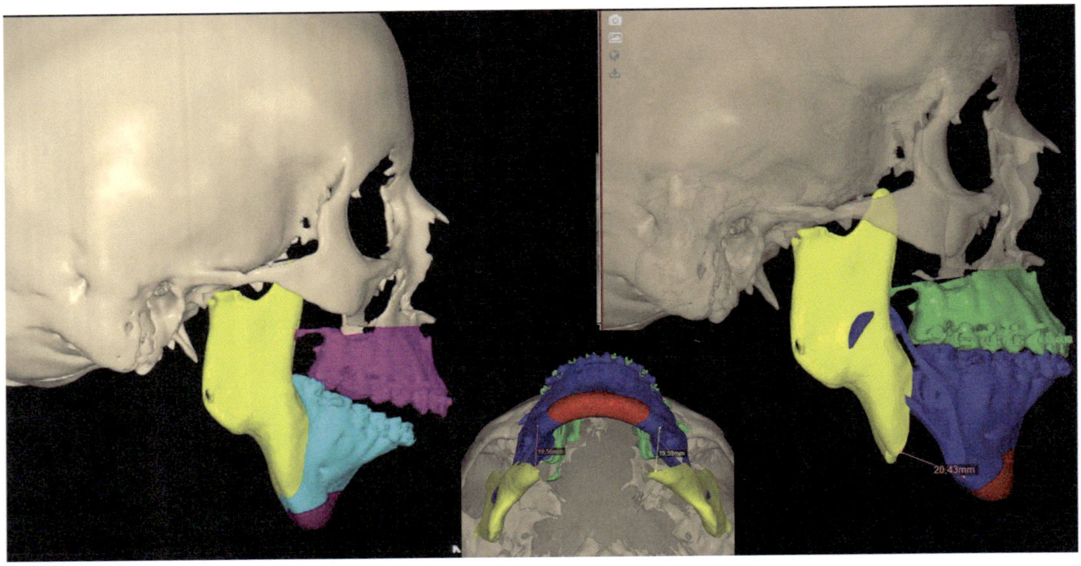

Fig. 11.21 The feasibility of bimaxillary surgery was evaluated in a patient with severe class II anomaly due to condylar hypoplasia, and it was clearly seen that the case was at the distraction limit due to the large gap between the bone segments in the mandible

obtained, the whole treatment plan will be flawed when seating the mandibular condyles at operation room [33] (Fig. 11.18). There are several indications that are suitable for mandible-first, surgery including cases with (1) counterclockwise rotation of the occlusal plane, (2) segmental maxillary osteotomies, (3) cleft maxilla, (4) downgrafting of the posterior maxilla, (5) large maxillomandibular advancement, (6) anterior open bite, and (7) inability to accurately register the bite [60].

Thanks to three-dimensional virtual assisted surgical planning, the perspective has expanded from isolated changes at the occlusal level to the assessment of tooth and skeletal movements. When the final occlusal position is established by computer-assisted surgical simulation, the expected skeletal changes can be fully evaluated and the resulting changes can be measured in millimeters on the *x-y-z* planes. Especially in complex asymmetry cases, significant cant and yaw deformities can be detected and measured sensitively, and necessary correction can be made by manipulation of virtual osteotomies (Fig. 11.22). Segment rotations and interferences can be identified to help predict skeletal movement and the need for reshaping during surgery. By using the 2D measurement tool, the distances between the bone segments, the amount of interference, the amount of local movement can be measured in detail (Fig. 11.23).

Thus, 3D virtual planning provides tremendous preoperative insight into the intended orthognathic correction. The virtual surgery allows anatomical evaluation of expected segment orientation and positioning and bony interventions. It greatly contributes to the prediction of possible grafting needs to assess rigid fixation and osteotomy space (Fig. 11.20).

Dentofacial deformities with a greater skeletal deviation than that seen in teeth may result in obvious skeletal and cosmetic asymmetry after correction with conventional orthognathic surgical planning where only the occlusion is targeted. Virtual planning provides the ability to evaluate these ongoing skeletal anomalies and it helps to contribute to treatment planning by taking additional precautions. For example, in patients with asymmetry such as hemimandibular hyperplasia, after occlusal correction, an asymmetrical image

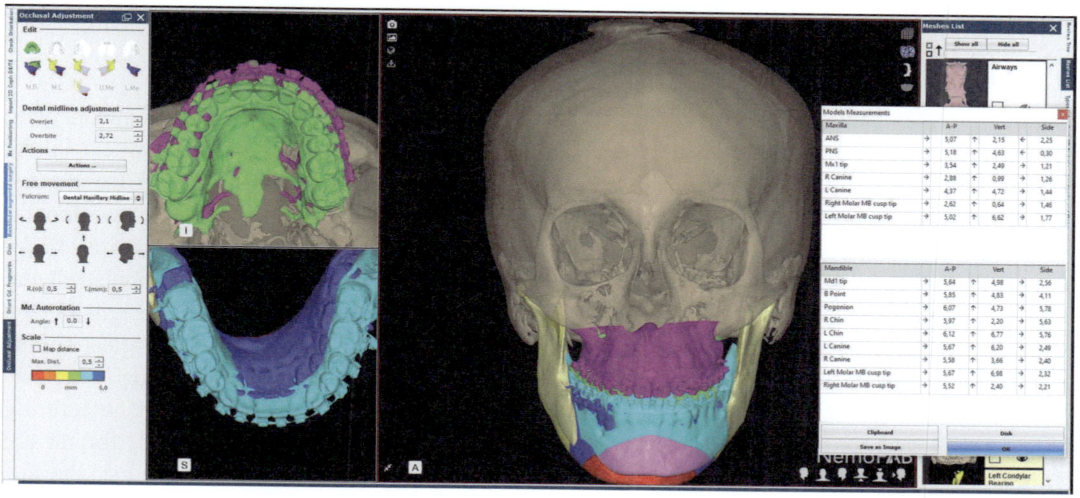

Fig. 11.22 In a patient with complex asymmetry, the movement occurring in each region can be determined in 3D with millimetric measurements

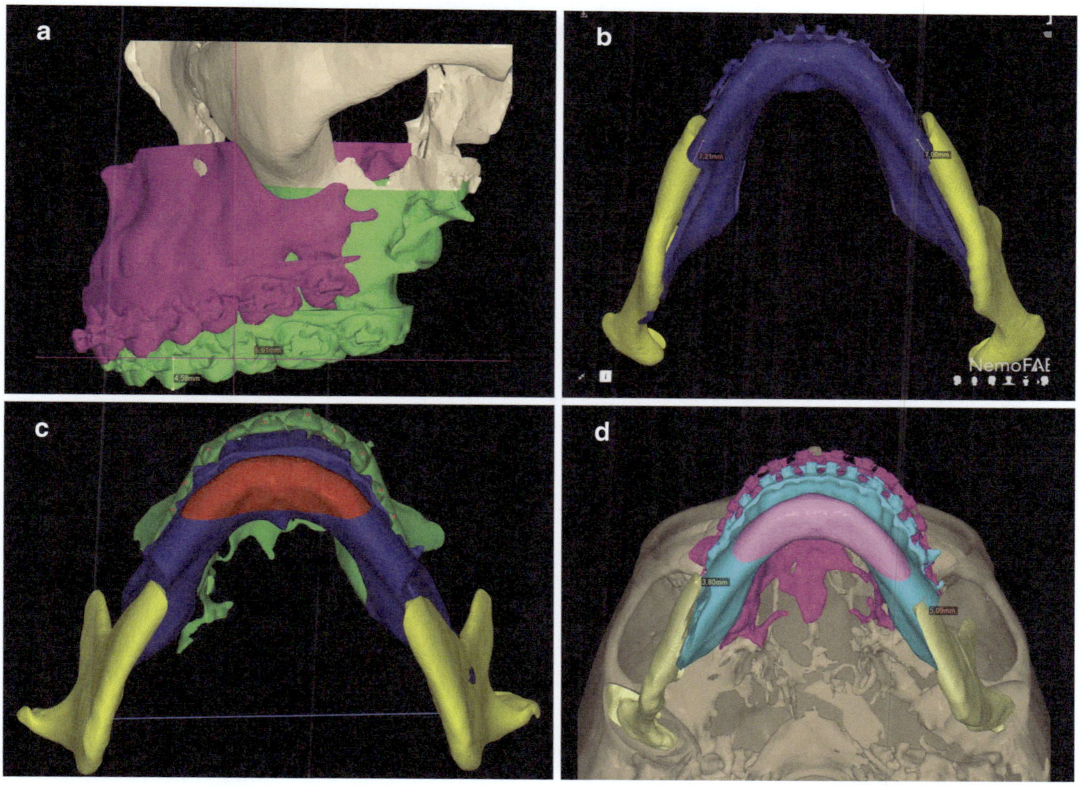

Fig. 11.23 Gap or interference areas between segments can be clearly seen in maxillary impaction (**a**), mandibular setback (**b**), mandibular advancement (**c**), and mandibular asymmetry (**d**) treatments

that still persists at the lower edge of the mandible can be detected and additional surgery can be planned for this region. Or similarly, in severe asymmetry cases genioplasty can be planned in the same session in addition to maxillomandibular correction [24].

Another important advantage of this virtual orthognathic planning is that different techniques (e.g., high and low osteotomy, segment osteotomy) can be simulated and the right decision can be taken more easily by creating a large number of different treatment plans [27, 29].

In the early stages of planning, the orthodontic and surgical treatment plan may be reviewed and presented to the patient, orthodontist, and the oral and maxillofacial surgeon. VSP provides various view options so that comparisons can be made between the preoperative state and the postoperative result. The 3D virtual surgical treatment plan can be easily transferred to the operating room in viewer format. Surgeons, anesthesiologists, and nurses can access a patient's personalized 3D virtual treatment plan at any time during surgery.

In the traditional method, errors and inaccuracies in model surgery (mounting, centric relationship recording, etc.) are often overlooked or undetected during presurgical laboratory work, but often manifest intraoperatively or postoperatively. 3D virtual planning can clearly show inaccuracies in data collection at the preoperative stage and provides an opportunity to address these inconsistencies before entering the operating room [3].

Soft tissue changes associated with movements of bone segments can be simulated using the software algorithm. Although this contributes to give patients and physicians an idea of the expected aesthetic changes, the actual estimation of soft tissue changes in 3D virtual planning is quite difficult and should not have diagnostic value [2]. The routine clinical use of 3D virtual surgery planning has shown that 3D soft tissue simulation still requires some improvement and cannot be trusted, especially in individuals with long faces and asymmetric individuals [35].

11.6 3D Surgical Splint Manufacturing

After the creation of an integrated treatment plan, intermediate and final 3D virtual surgical splints can be generated using CAD/CAM techniques. Surgical dental splints are created by a computational process after inserting a digital wafer between the maxillary and mandibular dental arches. 3D virtual surgical splints designed in the software are converted into real surgical splints that can be used during surgery using computer-aided design and computer-aided manufacturing techniques. Occlusal splints in STL format are designed and manufactured to reproduce the surgical plan in the operating room.

Splints are started to be designed on the software by choosing which jaw to start the operation with first. While designing the splint, special attention should be paid to ensure that it has sufficient depth/groove to grasp all the teeth and form a good guide. Since this can sometimes cause various seating problems in bracketed teeth, great attention should be paid to undercut areas (Fig. 11.24).

While the splint is being designed, adjusting the amount of offset in the buccal and lingual regions provides an advantage in terms of increasing splints rigidity and preventing fragility.

Stabilization of the splints to the dental arches during surgery is achieved by ligature wires. For this reason, it is necessary to create holes of appropriate width and frequency in the entire buccal region, through which the surgical wires can pass.

In this respect, the amount of buccal offset of the splint becomes even more important. For this reason, when determining the buccolingual width of the splints, the holes through which the wire ligatures will pass should also be taken into account (Fig. 11.24).

In some surgical plans, very tight occlusal contacts are obtained after surgery (which is what we want). However, in this case, the splint is also extremely thin. This causes to break the

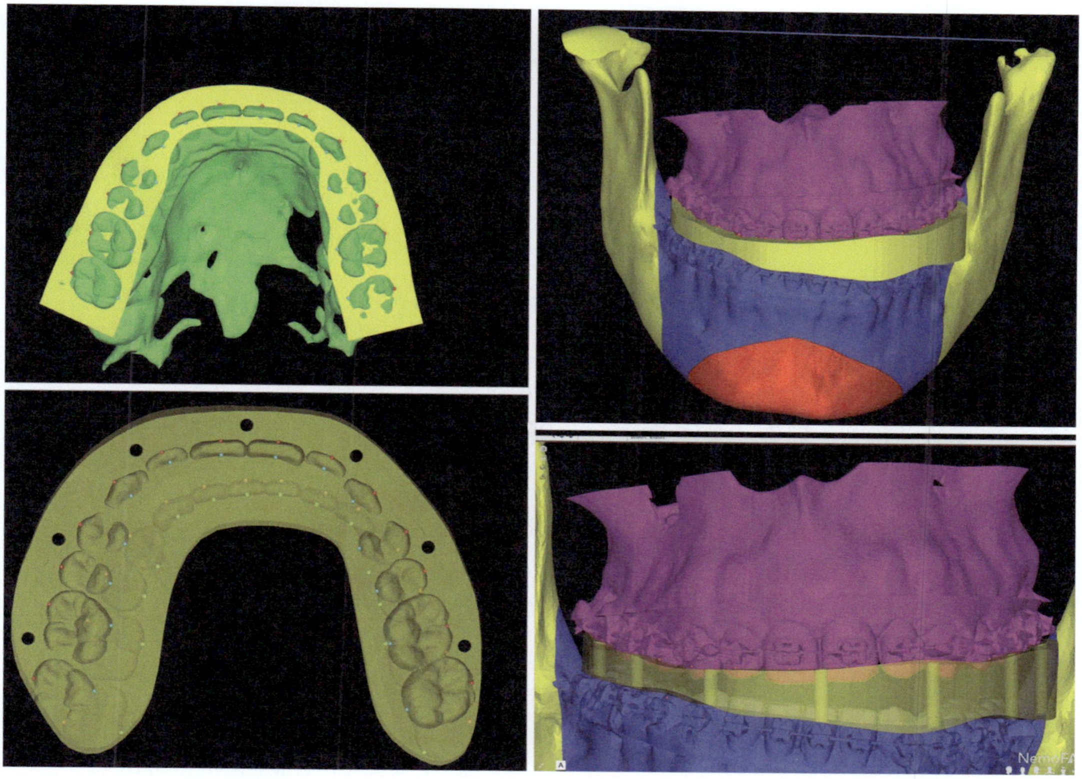

Fig. 11.24 The splint design should be prepared at a sufficient groove depth to grip the teeth tightly, with sufficient buccolingual width, with holes drilled for stabilization

splint as a result of the forces applied when removing it from the printer base, checking the adaptation in the clinic, or worse, during the surgical procedure. In order to prevent this situation, the interocclusal distance and thus the splint thickness can be increased by making a slight opening movement along the hinge axis without any extra sagittal or transversal movement of the mandible. Another alternative is to increase the depth of the groove by bringing the splint boundaries closer to the gingival or by inclining the splint boundaries buccally in the buccolingual direction to produce a thicker and rigid splint (Fig. 11.25).

In this way, 3D surgical splints designed virtually and produced in 3D printers can more accurately convey the surgical treatment plan, especially in complex cases where alignment, rotation, and translational movements of the jaw are combined. Gateno et al. showed that stereolithographic surgical splints have the same fit as conventional surgical splints [61]. In terms of splint fit, the method, device, and resin used for splint production is also extremely important. Our clinical observations are that digital splints can remain stable on the teeth until they do not need to be supported by any extra pressure in the mouth in almost any way (Fig. 11.26).

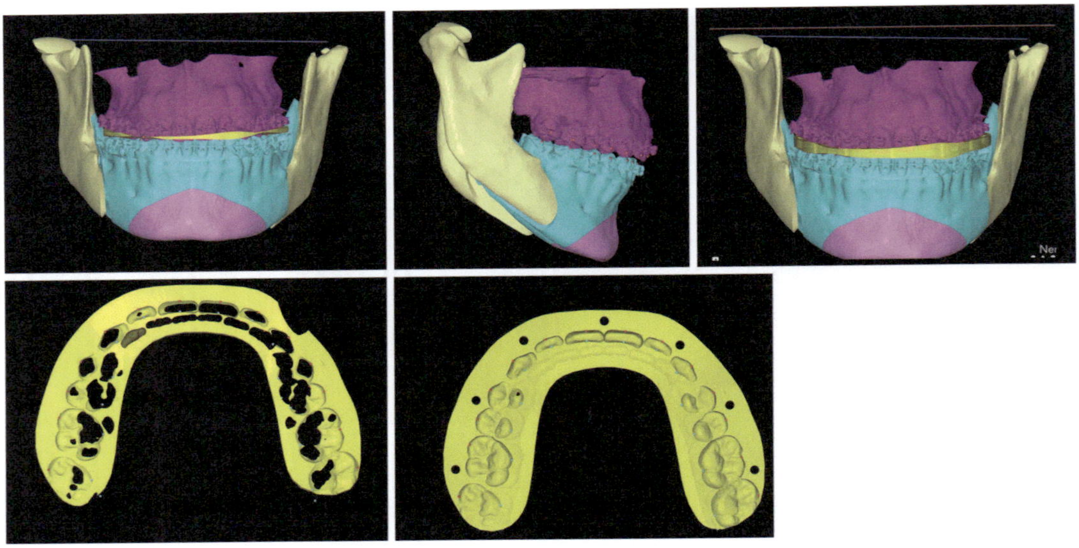

Fig. 11.25 In cases where the final occlusal contacts are too tight, the interocclusal space can be increased by slightly autorotating the mandible along the hinge axis to reduce fragility. Thus, a thicker and more rigid splint can be designed

11.7 Advantage and Disadvantage of Virtual Surgery Planning

Virtual surgical planning, which provides detailed 3D analysis of dentofacial deformities and treatment planning, has greatly increased the efficiency and accuracy of dentofacial deformity correction through orthognathic surgery in general. It can be said that virtual surgical planning increases the effectiveness of preoperative examination, provides an opportunity to demonstrate multidimensional correction at tooth and skeletal levels, provides insight into preoperative surgical intervention, and increases accuracy in transferring the virtual plan to the operating room [3].

The advantages of virtual surgery planning can be briefly summarized as follows:

- It provides a more accurate diagnosis and treatment planning by making detailed preoperative 3D analyses. It makes a great contribution to planning especially in asymmetry patients, occlusal cant, and yaw problems.

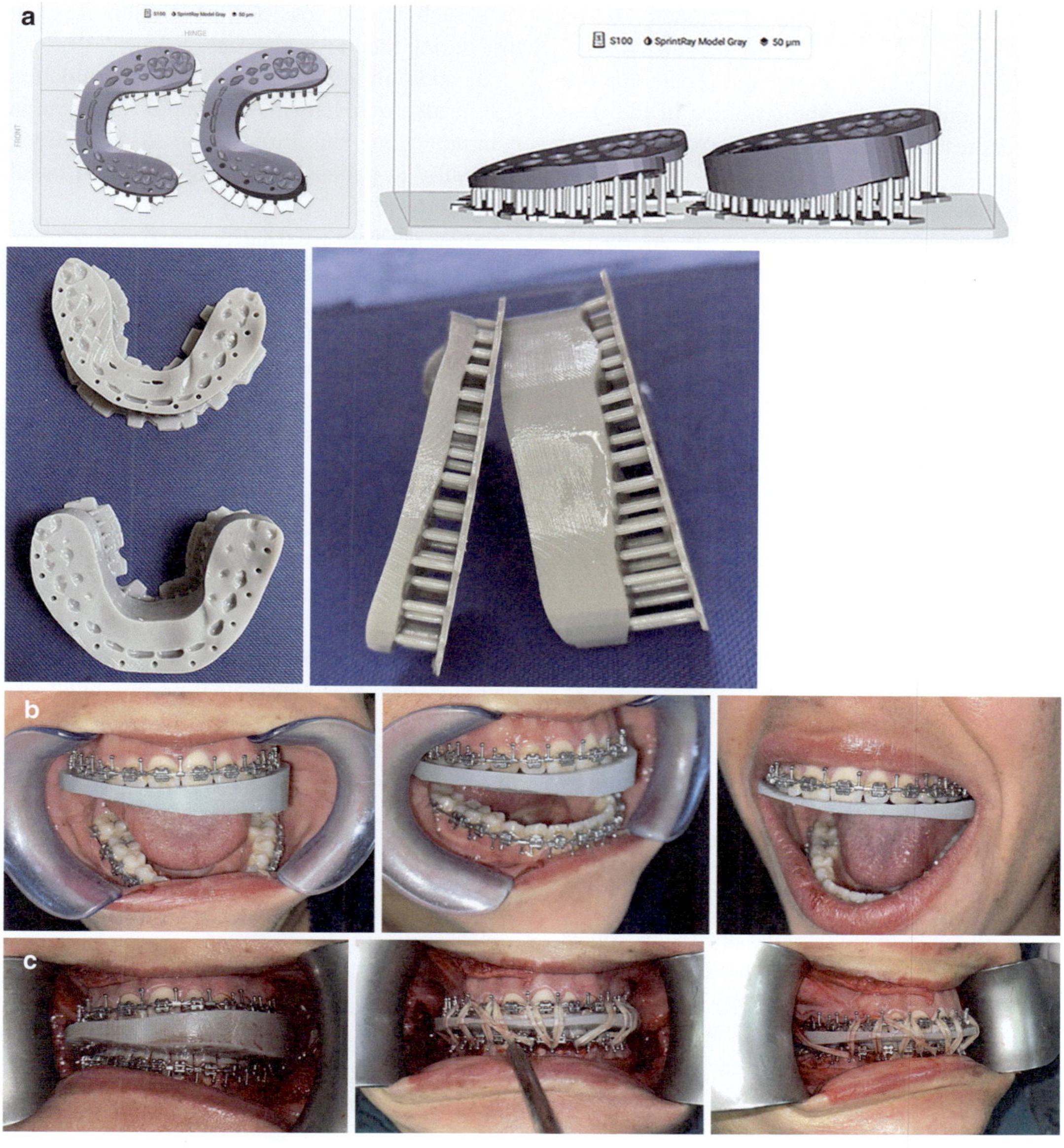

Fig. 11.26 Post-production (**a**), presurgical clinical rehearsal (**b**), and intraoperative use (**c**) of a 3D-printed splint

- The amount of three-dimensional movement is calculated detailly in all planes, and these are transfered more accurately to the operating room especially in complex cases where translation and rotation movements of the jaws are performed together.
- It allows the pre-determination of the interference areas that may occur in the bone segments during the surgery. Especially in asymmetric mandibular surgeries, it is important for surgeons to quantitatively calculate bone interferences and the amount of gap to occur before the operation.
- Repeatable simulation for alternative surgical plans using the same patient data can be done on the "virtual patient" and the most appropriate one can be selected by trying different planning alternatives.
- Perfectly compatible digital splints produced in 3D printers with CAD/CAM technology

provide more accurate placement during surgery.

- Precision in the planning and production process contributes to the accuracy of the treatment results and helps to shorten the operation time.
- Provides a strong communication between the entire orthognathic surgery team and can be used as an enlightening method to explain to trainees and explain the treatment plan to the patient.

Despite all these advantages, there are of course some disadvantages as well.

The first and biggest disadvantage of virtual surgery planning is the initial setup cost and familiarization process. Each virtual surgery planning software runs on a different system and requires a learning curve [35]. However, as the program is worked on and more cases are planned, this disadvantage becomes a great advantage in terms of preparation time and speed over time. Again, although the initial setup cost is high, it provides amortization in a short time in places such as universities where many orthognathic surgeries are performed [8, 62, 63].

Although there are advanced 3D imaging techniques for VSP that show the facial skeleton, dentition, and soft tissues separately, there is no single imaging technique that accurately reflects these three structures with optimal quality. Since the occlusal surface morphology cannot be displayed clearly with CBCT, the necessity of integrating digital dental models into CBCT creates a disadvantage.

Another disadvantage is that the production of 3D surgical splints on 3D printer is a time-consuming process. Although it varies according to the splint thickness and printer property, it may take 2–3 h to print the splints in a patient who will undergo bimaxillary surgery. After the print stage, it also includes other time-consuming steps such as removing the excess resin with an alcohol bath, cutting the connecting rods, light curing. All of this takes about half a day. It is really time-consuming for a surgeon or orthodontist to deal with these procedures without a technician.

As another option, out-of-office production services can be purchased, but this again involves risks such as cost, loss of time, and breakage or loss during the moving process [6].

In addition, since 3D soft tissue simulation still needs improvement, care should be taken in communicating this information to the patient, especially in patients with long faces and facial asymmetries [35].

Although VSP has transferred 2D imaging to 3D, a current disadvantage of the 3D virtual approach is that static diagnosis of the patient remains. In virtual surgery planning, virtual dynamic diagnosis of the patient by adding the fourth dimension such as smile aesthetics, habits, swallowing will probably be integrated in the future.

11.8 Traditional Surgery Planning vs. Virtual Surgery Planning

Although the newly developed 3D virtual surgery planning has advantages such as providing 3D detailed analysis, enabling different surgery plans, pre-detection of bone interferences or gaps that will occur during surgery, production of high precision splints in 3D printer, it is an issue that has been researched whether it is superior to the traditional method in terms of cost, time, and accuracy.

When the results of orthognathic surgery performed with TSP and VSP are compared in terms of accuracy, many studies have shown that VSP has higher accuracy than TSP [3, 64, 65]. Compared to conventional model surgery, VSP has been said to provide better clinical outcomes and allows "the average surgeon to achieve a good surgical outcome in an average day" [3].

In the multicenter study, it was determined that excellent accuracy was achieved in terms of maxillary and mandibular position and orientation with 3D virtual surgery planning (the maximum difference was 1 mm/1.8°). Finding similar results in different centers, despite different teams and different experiences, showed the reproducibility as well as the accuracy of this method [23].

When the accuracy of the 3D virtual planning at the condyle position was examined, it was found that the mean error on the *x*-*y*-*z* coordinates was less than 1 mm. The position of the condyles was found as the most accurate compared to the other landmarks after surgery. Agreement between the planned and actual outcome aided by virtual surgical planning was highest for the condyles, followed by the maxilla, and the distal segment of the mandible. Increasing error magnitudes were found for landmarks located further from the center of the body axis in the mandible [12].

When maxillary position accuracy is examined alone, both methods (traditional and virtual) demonstrated significant differences between the planned and actual outcome. The highest inaccuracies were observed in vertical impaction and midline correction. Considering clinical relevance, in vertical direction 73% in the TSP group and 46% in the VSP group achieved the desired maxillary position. No significant differences between TSP and VSP were observed in any dimension and as a result VSP and TSP were found to be as same clinical acceptable accuracy for maxillary positioning [66].

Similarly, the meta-analyses study showed that the VSP technique exhibited better accuracy in predicting SNA and SNB, although the difference was not statistically significant. Also the findings of this review showed that VSP and TSP are similar in surgical accuracy for hard tissue in the sagittal plane. Although VSP is significantly better at predicting certain reference areas, especially in the anterior area of the maxilla, the magnitude of these differences is not large enough to be clinically significant [6] as supported by previous findings [63, 67–69].

When compared in terms of time and cost, different results were found in different studies. The average times and costs for VSP were 194 ± 14.1 min and $2765.94 and for TSP were 540.9 ± 99.5 min and $3519.18. According to the results, VSP for bimaxillary orthognathic surgery takes significantly less time and is less expensive than TSP whether with or without asymmetry, or segmental surgery [70].

Not surprisingly, the VSP technique had a higher investment cost in the early stage than the TSP technique. After the initial cost investment, no advantage was found for TSP regarding cost [8, 62, 63].

The complexity of the surgery (single- or double-jaw surgery) has also been found to be effective in terms of time and cost. When TSP and VSP were compared in terms of time and cost in both double-jaw surgery and single-jaw mandibular surgery cases, it was determined that VSP provided an advantage of 62.8% in double-jaw surgery and 41.5% in single-jaw surgery in terms of time. In addition, it has been seen that virtual surgery planning is less costly except for splint production [8]. It is concluded that the more complex the surgery is, the more time-effective VSP is. Otherwise, in the case of relatively simple surgery, it can be concluded that TSP is more cost-effective than VSP. For this reason, it was thought that the traditional method would be more effective in single-jaw surgeries, as the preoperative preparation is easy, it takes less time, and it is less costly in traditional surgical planning [4, 8]. In double-jaw surgeries, it is stated that 3D virtual surgical planning will be more effective due to its potential advantage such as increasing the advantage level in terms of time and cost and providing accuracy [4].

A recent systematic review reported that virtual surgical planning has shown advantages over the traditional approach in shortening the surgical time and ischemia time for maxillofacial reconstruction and preoperative planning time for orthognathic surgery [71]. Thanks to surgical splints produced in 3D with CAD/CAM technology through virtual planning, it has been observed that the total operation time is shorter (40 min) due to faster and more accurate positioning of the jaws during surgery [63]. It has been stated that the operation time is shorter even in inexperienced surgeons because of the pre-determination of the interferences and the prevention of unstable contacts that may occur during the operation [5].

According to all these, it can be said that the new 3D virtual technology provides advantages not only in terms of accuracy but also in terms of ease of use, cost, time, and surgical time [62].

11.9 Conclusion

In particular, three-dimensional evaluation of facial morphology provides the diagnostic basis for making rational clinical decisions for the treatment of patients requiring combined orthodontic and surgical correction. Surgical and orthodontic treatment planning involving multiple procedures is now based on computer-assisted evaluation and virtual simulations using volumetric images, virtual models, and 3D printed splints, rather than two-dimensional (2D) radiographic images and plaster-based surgical simulations.

Although the outcome of orthognathic surgery depends on attention to intraoperative surgical technique, the creation of a precise presurgical plan is essential in the correction of dentofacial deformities. The ability to plan surgical correction at both the occlusal and skeletal levels has enormous benefits in treatment planning complex cases.

VSP is rapidly becoming the standard for correction of complex dentofacial deformities. VSP provides tremendous preoperative insight into the dental and skeletal movements anticipated, osteotomy orientation, and positioning and accurately transfers the virtual plan to correct the malocclusion and skeletal deformity. It improves the efficiency of the presurgical work-up, provides an opportunity to illustrate the multidimensional correction at the dental and skeletal levels, provides preoperative insight into the surgical intervention.

In a serious surgical operation such as orthognathic surgery, which individuals apply with great aesthetic-psychosocial hopes, the use of perfectly compatible splints designed with VSP instead of complex traditional surgery planning ensures that more accurate planning is transferred to the operating room and the accuracy of treatment results increases.

It is clear that the 3D approach represents a milestone in the development of orthognathic surgery. Also with rapid technological developments, image-navigation technology, augmented reality (AR), artificial intelligence (AI), and robotic-assisted orthognathic surgery have been applied in the field of orthognathic surgery. Robot-assisted orthognathic surgery is a combination of robotic technology and a navigation system in which robot-performed complete osteotomy following preoperative virtual surgical planning, with the plan transferred into actual surgery, showed good accuracy and feasibility. Augmented reality, which enables virtualization of the patient data directly at the operative site, could provide more accurate knowledge of the patient's internal anatomy and pathology. Artificial intelligence though still in the research process, 3D programs based on AI are being developed for 3D analysis and surgical planning, AI can be applied to imagery, planning, customized orthodontics, appliances, and follow-up patients soon will be provided more accurate and faster diagnosis. In future studies, technology-assisted orthognathic surgical methods will be applied to actual patients, and further research and analyses will continue.

References

1. Naini FB, Moss JP, Gill DS. The enigma of facial beauty: esthetics, proportions, deformity, and controversy. Am J Orthod Dentofac Orthop. 2006;130(3):277–82.
2. Elnagar MH, Aronovich S, Kusnoto B. Digital workflow for combined orthodontics and orthognathic surgery. Oral Maxillofac Surg Clin North Am. 2020;32(1):1–14. https://doi.org/10.1016/j.coms.2019.08.004. Epub 2019 Nov 4. PMID: 31699582.
3. Farrell BB, Franco PB, Tucker MR. Virtual surgical planning in orthognathic surgery. Oral Maxillofac Surg Clin North Am. 2014;26(4):459–73. https://doi.org/10.1016/j.coms.2014.08.011.
4. Hammoudeh JA, Howell LK, Boutros S, Scott MA, Urata MM. Current status of surgical planning for orthognathic surgery: traditional methods versus 3D surgical planning. Plast Reconstr Surg Glob Open. 2015;3(2):e307. https://doi.org/10.1097/GOX.0000000000000184. PMID: 25750846; PMCID: PMC4350313.
5. Hanafy M, Akoush Y, Abou-Elfetouh A, Mounir RM. Precision of orthognathic digital plan transfer using patient-specific cutting guides and osteosynthesis versus mixed analogue–digitally planned surgery: a randomized controlled clinical trial. Int J Oral Maxillofac Surg. 2020;49:62.

6. Chen Z, Mo S, Fan X, You Y, Ye G, Zhou N. A meta-analysis and systematic review comparing the effectiveness of traditional and virtual surgical planning for orthognathic surgery: based on randomized clinical trials. J Oral Maxillofac Surg. 2021;79(2):471.e1–471.e19. https://doi.org/10.1016/j.joms.2020.09.005. Epub 2020 Sep 9. PMID: 33031773.
7. Adolphs N, Liu W, Keeve E, Hoffmeister B. RapidSplint: virtual splint generation for orthognathic surgery—results of a pilot series. Comput Aided Surg. 2014;19:20.
8. Park SY, Hwang DS, Song JM, Kim UK. Comparison of time and cost between conventional surgical planning and virtual surgical planning in orthognathic surgery in Korea. Maxillofac Plast Reconstr Surg. 2019;41:35. https://doi.org/10.1186/s40902-019-0220-6.
9. Song KG, Baek SH. Comparison of the accuracy of the three-dimensional virtual method and the conventional manual method for model surgery and intermediate wafer fabrication. Oral Surg Oral Med Oral Pathol Oral Radiol Endod. 2009;107(1):13–21.
10. Ellis E III. Accuracy of model surgery: evaluation of an old technique and introduction of a new one. J Oral Maxillofac Surg. 1990;48(11):1161–7. https://doi.org/10.1016/0278-2391(90)90532-7. PMID: 1698956.
11. Park N, Posnick JC. Accuracy of analytic model planning in bimaxillary surgery. Int J Oral Maxillofac Surg. 2013;42:807–13.
12. Oh HJ, Moon JH, Ha H, Son IS, Lee YC, Lee SJ, Sohn HB, Seo BM. Virtually-planned orthognathic surgery achieves an accurate condylar position. J Oral Maxillofac Surg. 2021;79(5):1146.e1–1146.e25. https://doi.org/10.1016/j.joms.2020.12.048.
13. Barbenel JC, Paul PE, Khambay BS, et al. Errors in orthognathic surgery planning: the effect of inaccurate study model orientation. Int J Oral Maxillofac Surg. 2010;39:1103.
14. Sun Y, Luebbers HT, Agbaje JO, et al. Accuracy of upper jaw positioning with intermediate splint fabrication after virtual planning in bimaxillary orthognathic surgery. J Craniofac Surg. 2013;24:1871.
15. Xia J, Gateno J, Teichgraeber J. New clinical protocol to evaluate craniomaxillofacial deformity and plan surgical correction. J Oral Maxillofac Surg. 2009;67:2093.
16. Zizelmann C, Hammer B, Gellrich NC, et al. An evaluation of face-bow transfer for the planning of orthognathic surgery. J Oral Maxillofac Surg. 2012;70:1944.
17. Ellis E III, Tharanon W, Gambrell K. Accuracy of face-bow transfer: effect on surgical prediction and postsurgical result. J Oral Maxillofac Surg. 1992;50(6):562–7. https://doi.org/10.1016/0278-2391(92)90434-2. PMID: 1593315.
18. Gateno J, Forrest KK, Camp B. A comparison of 3 methods of face-bow transfer recording: implications for orthognathic surgery. J Oral Maxillofac Surg. 2001;59:635.
19. Macchi A, Carrafiello G, Cacciafesta V, et al. Three-dimensional digital modeling and setup. Am J Orthod Dentofac Orthop. 2006;129:605.
20. Whetten JL, Williamson PC, Heo G, et al. Variations in orthodontic treatment planning decisions of Class II patients between virtual 3-dimensional models and traditional plaster study models. Am J Orthod Dentofac Orthop. 2006;130:485.
21. Bamber MA, Firouzal R, Harris M, Linney A. A comparative study of two arbitrary face-bow transfer systems for orthognathic surgery planning. Int J Oral Maxillofac Surg. 1996;25:339.
22. Choi JY, Song KG, Baek SH. Virtual model surgery and wafer fabrication for orthognathic surgery. Int J Oral Maxillofac Surg. 2009;38:1306.
23. Hsu SS, Gateno J, Bell RB, et al. Accuracy of a computer-aided surgical simulation protocol for orthognathic surgery: a prospective multicenter study. J Oral Maxillofac Surg. 2013;71:128.
24. Donaldson CD, Manisali M, Naini FB. Three-dimensional virtual surgical planning (3D-VSP) in orthognathic surgery: advantages, disadvantages and pitfalls. J Orthod. 2021;48(1):52–63. https://doi.org/10.1177/1465312520954871.
25. Heiland M, Habermann CR, Schmelzle R. Indications and limitations of intraoperative navigation in maxillofacial surgery. J Oral Maxillofac Surg. 2004;62:1059.
26. Zinser MJ, Mischkowski RA, Sailer HF, et al. Computer-assisted orthognathic surgery: feasibility study using multiple CAD/CAM surgical splints. Oral Surg Oral Med Oral Pathol Oral Radiol. 2012a;113:673.
27. Zinser MJ, Mischkowski RA, Dreiseidler T, Thamm OC, Rothamel D, Zöller JE. Computer-assisted orthognathic surgery: waferless maxillary positioning, versatility, and accuracy of an image-guided visualisation display. Br J Oral Maxillofac Surg. 2013a;51(8):827–33. https://doi.org/10.1016/j.bjoms.2013.06.014. Epub 2013 Sep 14. PMID: 24045105.
28. Zinser MJ, Mischkowski RA, Sailer HF, Zöller JE. Computer-assisted orthognathic surgery: feasibility study using multiple CAD/CAM surgical splints. Oral Surg Oral Med Oral Pathol Oral Radiol. 2012b;113(5):673–87. https://doi.org/10.1016/j.oooo.2011.11.009.
29. Zinser MJ, Sailer HF, Ritter L, Braumann B, Maegele M, Zöller JE. A paradigm shift in orthognathic surgery? A comparison of navigation, computer-aided designed/computer-aided manufactured splints, and "classic" intermaxillary splints to surgical transfer of virtual orthognathic planning. J Oral Maxillofac Surg. 2013b;71(12):2151.e1–21. https://doi.org/10.1016/j.joms.2013.07.007. PMID: 24237776.
30. Cevidanes LH, Styner MA, Profitt WR. Image analysis and super-imposition of 3-dimensional cone-beam computer tomography models. Am J Orthod Dentofac Orthop. 2006;129:611.
31. Hwang DS. Practical utility of the three-dimensional approach in orthognathic surgery. J Korean Assoc

Oral Maxillofac Surg. 2021;47:337–8. https://doi.org/10.5125/jkaoms.2021.47.4.3376.
32. Uribe F, Janakiraman N, Shafer D, Nanda R. Three-dimensional cone-beam computed tomography-based virtual treatment planning and fabrication of a surgical splint for asymmetric patients: surgery first approach. Am J Orthod Dentofacial Orthop. 2013;144(5):748–58. https://doi.org/10.1016/j.ajodo.2012.10.029. PMID: 24182591.
33. Gunson MJ, Arnett GW. Orthognathic virtual treatment planning for functional esthetic results. Semin Orthod. 2019;25:230–47. https://doi.org/10.1053/j.sodo.2019.08.008.
34. Stokbro K, Aagaard E, Torkov P, et al. Virtual planning in orthognathic surgery. Int J Oral Maxillofac Surg. 2014;43:957.
35. Swennen GR, Mollemans W, Schutyser F. Three-dimensional treatment planning of orthognathic surgery in the era of virtual imaging. J Oral Maxillofac Surg. 2009;67(10):2080–92. https://doi.org/10.1016/j.joms.2009.06.007.
36. Kusnoto B, Kaur P, Salem A, et al. Implementation of ultra-low-dose CBCT for routine 2D orthodontic diagnostic radiographs: cephalometric landmark identification and image quality assessment. Semin Orthod. 2015;21(4):233–47.
37. De Vos W, Casselman J, Swennen G. Cone-beam computerized tomography (CBCT) imaging of the oral and maxillo-facial region: a systematic review of the literature. Int J Oral Maxillofac Surg. 2009;38:609.
38. Perez D, Ellis E III. Sequencing bimaxillary surgery: mandible first. J Oral Maxillofac Surg. 2011;69:2217.
39. Brüllmann D, Schulze RK. Spatial resolution in CBCT machines for dental/maxillofacial applications—what do we know today? Dentomaxillofac Radiol. 2015;44(1):20140204. https://doi.org/10.1259/dmfr.20140204.
40. Correia GD, Habib FA, Vogel CJ. Tooth-size discrepancy: a comparison between manual and digital methods. Dental Press J Orthod. 2014;19(4):107–13. https://doi.org/10.1590/2176-9451.19.4.107-113.oar. PMID: 25279529.
41. Kravitz ND, Groth C, Jones PE, Graham JW, Redmond WR. Intraoral digital scanners. J Clin Orthod. 2014;48(6):337–47. PMID: 25083754.
42. Francisco I, Ribeiro MP, Marques F, Travassos R, Nunes C, Pereira F, Caramelo F, Paula AB, Vale F. Application of three-dimensional digital technology in orthodontics: the state of the art. Biomimetics (Basel). 2022;7(1):23. https://doi.org/10.3390/biomimetics7010023. PMID: 35225915; PMCID: PMC8883890.
43. Lin C-Y, Hsung T-C, Khambay B. Reducing cone beam CT scan height as a method of radiation reduction for photorealistic three-dimensional orthognathic planning. J Craniomaxillofac Surg. 2015;43:907–12.
44. Plooij JM, Maal TJ, Haers P, Borstlap WA, Kuijpers-Jagtman AM, Bergé SJ. Digital three-dimensional image fusion processes for planning and evaluating orthodontics and orthognathic surgery. A systematic review. Int J Oral Maxillofac Surg. 2011;40:341–52.
45. Lane C, Harrell W. Completing the 3-dimensional picture. Am J Orthod Dentofac Orthop. 2008;133:612–20.
46. Ghoneima A, Allam E, Kula K, Windsor LJ. Three-dimensional imaging and software advances in orthodontics. In: Bourzgui F, editor. Orthodontics—basic aspects and clinical considerations. London: IntechOpen; 2012. p. 9500. https://doi.org/10.5772/32037. ISBN: 978-953-51-0143-7.
47. Kapila SD, Nervina JM. CBCT in orthodontics: assessment of treatment outcomes and indications for its use. Dentomaxillofac Radiol. 2015;44(1):20140282. https://doi.org/10.1259/dmfr.20140282.
48. Maal TJJ, Plooij JM, Rangel FA, et al. The accuracy of matching three-dimensional photographs with skin surfaces derived from cone-beam computed tomography. Int J Oral Maxillofac Surg. 2008;37(7):641–6.
49. Almukhtar A, Ju X, Khambay B, et al. Comparison of the accuracy of voxel based registration and surface based registration for 3D assessment of surgical change following orthognathic surgery. PLoS One. 2014;9(4):e93402.
50. Pauwels R, Araki K, Siewerdsen JH, Thongvigitmanee SS. Technical aspects of dental CBCT: state of the art. Dentomaxillofac Radiol. 2015;44(1):20140224. https://doi.org/10.1259/dmfr.20140224. PMID: 25263643; PMCID: PMC4277439.
51. Nahm K-Y, Kim Y, Choi Y-S, et al. Accurate registration of cone-beam computed tomography scans to 3-dimensional facial photographs. Am J Orthod Dentofac Orthop. 2014;145:256–64.
52. Rangel FA, Maal TJJ, de Koning MJJ, et al. Integration of digital dental casts in cone beam computed tomography scans—a clinical validation study. Clin Oral Investig. 2018;22(3):1215–22.
53. Xia J, Wang D, Samman N, Yeung RW, Tideman H. Computer-assisted three-dimensional surgical planning and simulation: 3D color facial model generation. Int J Oral Maxillofac Surg. 2000;29:2–10.
54. Damstra J, Fourie Z, Ren Y. Simple technique to achieve a natural position of the head for cone beam computed tomography. Br J Oral Maxillofac Surg. 2010;48(3):236–8. https://doi.org/10.1016/j.bjoms.2009.10.001.
55. Peng L, Cooke MS. Fifteen-year reproducibility of natural head posture: a longitudinal study. Am J Orthod Dentofac Orthop. 1999;116:82–5.
56. Polley JW, Figueroa AA. Orthognathic positioning system: intraoperative system to transfer virtual surgical plan to operating field during orthognathic surgery. J Oral Maxillofac Surg. 2013;71:911–20.
57. Zinser M, Zoeller J. Computer-designed splints for surgical transfer of 3D orthognathic planning. Facial Plast Surg. 2015;31(5):474–90. https://doi.org/10.1055/s-0035-1565010. Epub 2015 Nov 18. PMID: 26579863.
58. Yushkevich PA, Piven J, Hazlett HC, Smith RG, Ho S, Gee JC, et al. User-guided 3D active contour segmentation of anatomical structures: significantly improved efficiency and reliability. NeuroImage. 2006;31:1116–28.

59. Liebregts J, Baan F, de Koning M, Ongkosuwito E, Berge S, Maal T, et al. Achievability of 3D planned bimaxillary osteotomies: maxilla-first versus mandible-first surgery. Sci Rep. 2017;7:9314.
60. Borba AM, Borges AH, Ce PS, Venturi BA, Naclerio-Homem MG, Miloro M. Mandible-first sequence in bimaxillary orthognathic surgery: a systematic review. Int J Oral Maxillofac Surg. 2016;45:472–5.
61. Gateno J, Xia J, Teichgraeber JF, et al. The precision of computer-generated surgical splints. J Oral Maxillofac Surg. 2003;61:814.
62. Bengtsson M, Wall G, Becktor JP, Rasmusson L. A comparison of cost-effectiveness of computer-assisted 2- and 3-dimensional planning techniques in orthognathic surgery. Br J Oral Maxillofac Surg. 2019;57:352.
63. Schneider D, Kammerer PW, Hennig M, et al. Customized virtual surgical planning in bimaxillary orthognathic surgery: a prospective randomized trial. Clin Oral Investig. 2019;23:3115.
64. Ritto FG, Schmitt ARM, Pimentel T, Canellas JV, Medeiros PJ. Comparison of the accuracy of maxillary position between conventional model surgery and virtual surgical planning. Int J Oral Maxillofac Surg. 2018;47(2):160–6.
65. Zhang N, Liu S, Hu Z, Hu J, Zhu S, Li Y. Accuracy of virtual surgical planning in two-jaw orthognathic surgery: comparison of planned and actual results. Oral Surg Oral Med Oral Pathol Oral Radiol. 2016;122(2):143–51.
66. Quast A, Santander P, Kahlmeier T, Moser N, Schliephake H, Meyer-Marcotty P. Predictability of maxillary positioning: a 3D comparison of virtual and conventional orthognathic surgery planning. Head Face Med. 2021;17(1):27. https://doi.org/10.1186/s13005-021-00279-x.
67. Bengtsson M, Wall G, Greiff L, Rasmusson L. Treatment outcome in orthognathic surgery—a prospective randomized blinded case-controlled comparison of planning accuracy in computer-assisted two- and three-dimensional planning techniques (part II). J Cranio Maxillofac Surg. 2017;45:1419.
68. Gaber RM, Shaheen E, Falter B, et al. A systematic review to uncover a universal protocol for accuracy assessment of 3-dimensional virtually planned orthognathic surgery. J Oral Maxillofac Surg. 2017;75:2430.
69. Van Hemelen G, Van Genechten M, Renier L, Desmedt M, Verbruggen E, Nadjmi N. Three-dimensional virtual planning in orthognathic surgery enhances the accuracy of soft tissue prediction. J Craniomaxillofac Surg. 2015;43(6):918–25. https://doi.org/10.1016/j.jcms.2015.04.006.
70. Resnick CM, Inverso G, Wrzosek M, Padwa BL, Kaban LB, Peacock ZS. Is there a difference in cost between standard and virtual surgical planning for orthognathic surgery? J Oral Maxillofac Surg. 2016;74(9):1827–33. https://doi.org/10.1016/j.joms.2016.03.035.
71. Nilsson J, Hindocha N, Thor A. Time matters—differences between computer-assisted surgery and conventional planning in cranio-maxillofacial surgery: a systematic review and meta-analysis. J Oral Maxillofac Surg. 2020;48:132.

Digital Systems in Oral Pathology 12

Sofia Karachrysafi, Dimitrios Andreadis,
and Athanasios Poulopoulos

12.1 Introduction/General Information on Digital Pathology

Digital technology was firstly used in pathology in 1960s as remote diagnosis via real-time "television microscopy" [1]. A diagnostic field known as histopathology was developed on the visual interpretation of cellular biology depicted in pictures. The introduction of digital images to pathology has transformed this historical discipline into what is currently known as digital pathology (DP). Between nearby hospitals, colleges, teachers, and students, as well as between a person's home and place of employment, real-time digital image, and video sharing, can eliminate physical boundaries. Digital images seem to be well-suitable for computational pathology, which may be used for both complex machine learning, applications, and basic measurement and count. Most intriguingly, images can now be analyzed by machine learning for qualities other than traditional histopathological assessment (artificial intelligence), such as directly connecting images to clinical data (e.g., prognosis).

Digital pathology, also known as virtual microscopy, is a rapidly evolving field that involves the use of digital images of microscope slides for the viewing and analysis of tissue samples [2, 3]. This technology has the potential to revolutionize the field of pathology by enabling faster and more accurate diagnoses, as well as the ability to share images and collaborate with colleagues around the world [4]. It is currently used in a variety of settings, including academic medical centers, hospitals, and pharmaceutical companies [2, 3], significantly improving patient care conditions and enabling rapid information exchange between healthcare providers [5].

The evolution of digital pathology, or whole-slide imaging (WSI), has taken almost 20 years. It has progressed from attaching a camera to the lens of a microscope to the development of the first scanners to what we have today: technology that is quickly becoming indispensable in the anatomic laboratory. The first scanners were clunky instruments taking up large footprints—with long processing time (up to 6 min) expensive storage, and limited use cases. Scanners today can scan slides in as little as 30 s, be con-

The original version of the chapter has been revised. A correction to this chapter can be found at https://doi.org/https://doi.org/10.1007/978-3-031-52826-2_21

S. Karachrysafi
Laboratory of Histology-Embryology, Faculty of Health Sciences, Department of Medicine, Aristotle University of Thessaloniki, Thessaloniki, Greece
e-mail: skarachry@auth.gr

D. Andreadis (✉) · A. Poulopoulos
Department of Oral Medicine/Pathology, School of Dentistry, Aristotle University of Thessaloniki, Thessaloniki, Greece
e-mail: dandrea@dent.auth.gr; akpoul@dent.auth.gr

A. Delantoni, K. Orhan (eds.), *Digital Dentistry*, https://doi.org/10.1007/978-3-031-52826-2_12

figured at multiple magnifications, and handle up to 1000 slides at a time. Storage, now available in the cloud, is affordable, secure, and accessible.

Artificial intelligence (AI)-enhanced computational technologies provide the pathologist with a wide range of picture evaluation and presentation opportunities. Digital pathology has evolved in a way that is quite comparable to that of the mobile. Early iterations were excessively large, unusual, and constrained by availability, price, and demand. The mobile phone is being used in ways that no one could have predicted in the early 1980s and is as common as the watch. Similar to how the use of mobile phones has increased dramatically with more effective mobile devices, digital pathology as a field of study has grown with the development of whole-slide image scanners. Artificial intelligence (AI)-enhanced computational technologies provide the pathologist with a wide range of picture evaluation and presentation opportunities.

Today, digital pathology is applied mostly in three ways. First, research associations utilize digital pathology to create an effective research design, collect data, and manage databases for the millions of cases they presently manage and intend to use. These organizations include pharmaceutical corporations, CROs, and academic medical facilities. Second, for remote consultations, instruction, or quantitative analysis, clinical labs use digital pathology in a small number of cases.

Utilizing these digital pathology image systems and solutions has several significant results that would have a significant positive impact on translational and clinical research. One advantage of digital pathology is that it allows for the storage and easy retrieval of images, which can help maintain a record of a patient's history and the review of cases, for consultation with colleagues [4]. One of the main benefits of digital pathology is the ability to share images quickly and easily with colleagues for consultation or education [2, 3]. This can be especially useful in cases where a second opinion is needed or when working with a multidisciplinary team [4]. Digital pathology also has the potential to improve the training of medical students and residents by providing access to many slides and allowing for interactive learning [5].

Perhaps the most common application of DP to date is in medical education, which implementation is relatively simple. For training reasons, dedicated digital microscopes can stream live video of the slide-reviewing procedure to provide an understanding of the histological evaluation technique. Digital images can be utilized for tests, presentations, annotations, self- and remote study, and more. DP used in instruction is intended for illustration purposes and is free from medical and legal hazards. Because of this, many problems that arise when using DP for primary histopathological evaluation—such as precise color reproduction, resolution, scan completeness, out of focus areas, long-term data storage, etc. are of secondary relevance. As a result, pathologists and DP frequently first engage in the context of medical teaching.

Another area where digital pathology may have a significant impact is in the development of image analysis algorithms to assist in the interpretation of slides [6]. In clinical and research settings, digital pathology is used for the interpretation of slides for diagnostic purposes [6], or the analysis of tissue samples and for the identification of patterns and features that may not be visible to the human eye [5].

Computational pathology, involves the use of advanced image analysis algorithms to extract meaningful information from digital pathology images. These algorithms can be used to identify patterns and features that may not be visible to the human eye, which can aid in the diagnosis of diseases. In addition, computational pathology can be used to analyze large numbers of slides in a shorter period, which can be useful in research settings [7, 8].

One area where digital pathology is likely to have a significant impact in the development of personalized medicine. Digital pathology can be used to identify unique patterns and features in tissue samples that may be indicative of specific diseases or treatment responses. This information can be used to tailor treatment plans to the individual needs of each patient [8]. Another potential application of digital pathology is in drug development [7, 8]. Digital pathology can be used to analyze tissue samples from clinical trials to assess the efficacy of new drugs. This can help to improve the efficiency of the drug development process and ultimately lead to the development of more effective treatments.

The transition of clinical labs to an entirely digital process is the third and extremely fast use case. To assign cases to pathologists, manage workflow into worklists, provide quantitative image analysis for case types, integrate data into their current Lab Information System (LIS), and provide access to cases outside of the physical boundaries of the lab, these labs use computationally enabled digital pathology powered by AI. Diagnoses no longer need to be propped up by the practical transportation of tissue samples or the long delays that occur while pathologists are out of the office thanks to digital pathology.

The cost of AI-enabled digital pathology will certainly continue to decline, and there will be a wider range of applications available as the field develops. The need for more effective labs is driven by the shortage of pathologists and the increase in the volume of biopsies. Digital pathology technologies will be able to be used as part of integrated diagnostics and predictive decision-making thanks to crossover with other AI applications, such as those in radiology and MRI.

Some labs have already enabled their digital pathology system to automatically import a few images from their radiology PACS (Picture Archiving Communication System) upon case sign out, enabling treating physicians to examine and browse the very slide from which patient diagnosis is based. Radiologists can analyze radiographs, MRI and CT scans, and histology slides all in one view.

With so many labs using digital pathology successfully, the challenges of expanding server storage and reconfiguring infrastructure are suddenly less intimidating than previously. More and more laboratories will be reactivating their scanners and rejoining the discussion about the transition to digital pathology. As digital pathology and computational pathology become more widely used, labs will see more significant improvements in workflow efficiency and enter a new era of collaboration. The final result is that patients will receive diagnoses more quickly and accurately, and their doctors will have access to a larger volume of information.

Overall, digital pathology has the potential to significantly improve the accuracy and efficiency of pathology diagnoses and enhance the sharing of information between healthcare providers [6]. The technology will likely continue to evolve and be used in a variety of settings to improve the accuracy and efficiency of diagnoses and enhance the sharing of information between healthcare providers. Pathologists may receive extremely accurate, impartial, and reliable diagnostics remotely due to the development of digital pathology and AI-based methodologies, which provide significant advantages over conventional techniques [9]. As the use of digital pathology technology continues to grow, it is important to research to evaluate its effectiveness and explore its potential applications in various settings.

12.2 Applications-Advantages-Disadvantages

Overall digital technology in pathology helps in primary diagnosis, innate frozen section diagnosis, and in both real-time and delayed consultations by distance, providing an advantage over conventional glass slides [10]. Digital pathology also helps the undergraduates, postgraduates, and teachers to understand each slide with the help of image analysis software and encourages them for research work [11].

On the other hand, the expensive equipment also including secure platforms allowing exchange of images/documents as well as laboratory infrastructure and information systems for each pathology laboratories consist most important disadvantages [12].

12.2.1 Education

Glass slides have historically been the basis for education in the field of cell and tissue pathology, which has led to a reliance on double- or multiheaded conventional microscopes [13]. The multiheaded microscope, however, restricts the number of students who can use it. Presentations have traditionally used static visuals in the form of diapositives in addition to live viewing of glass slides. The next level was adding annotations to static digital images that could be added to instructional software. WSI eliminates the eventual variation between serial sections taken from tissue blocks and offers complete capacity for annotations, links, and incorporating questions, videos, and sound videos. It also provides the same image to the teacher and students and can be made available to an unlimited number of students at the same time (even remotely).

There are certain disadvantages to using digital images in education, including the fact that students no longer learn how to operate a microscope. A strong IT infrastructure is a requirement for digital education, and any software error or slow performance would have a negative impact on the education process. Last but not least, WSI from a competent scanner provides a resolution that is lower than when looking at glass slides under a good microscope but is still more than adequate for instructing students.

12.2.2 Digital Diagnostics

The limitations of the prior static and live systems (bias and error in identifying the data from microscopic fields in the static system and inadequate picture quality of the dynamic system) have been eliminated with the advent of WSI [14]. Digitalized slide-based diagnostics nowadays are available in some ways due to improvements in WSI visual resolution and scanning speed:

1. Digital consultation can be conducted within hours as opposed to days to weeks for complicated or rare issues received through normal mail.
2. Tele-revision and quality assurance (QA) is typical to update the essential pathology information for patients who have been diagnosed. Again, sending slides by conventional mail is slow and involves the risk of losing or damaging the slides. This can be done digitally, which eliminates the need to mail slides and significantly speeds up the revision process.
3. Image analysis: Image data analysis will improve histopathology's ability to diagnose. The implementation of programs for the identification of areas of interest will be effective and increase the speed of the process because WSI inspection takes slightly longer than traditional slides.
4. Panels and slide conferences, which are a particular kind of consultation. To discuss cases, specialized pathologists in particular fields of pathology typically get together physically regularly. With the help of the software, panel members can see and evaluate cases remotely by WSI or take part in a virtual panel, eliminating the need for them to physically travel to meet.

There are some disadvantages to using digital pathology in diagnosis, such as cost, training, limited cases, and quality control issues. Digital pathology technology and software can be expensive, which may make it difficult for some healthcare providers to adopt the technology. There may be a learning curve for healthcare providers in terms of using the technology and software, which can be time-consuming and challenging. Poor quality of digital images due to technical issues, like resolution, color balancing, and lighting, may lead to inaccuracies in diagnoses. This may also lead to a lack of trust in the technology which could hinder its adoption and usage.

12.2.3 Research

Digital slides can be viewed, annotated, and analyzed for scientific purposes (measuring areas and lengths). It is possible to apply image processing algorithms, and current concepts are constantly being produced. A significant benefit is the simplicity of (annotated) image exchange. TMAs may be simpler to evaluate since the grid of the cores can be evaluated, and each core may then be presented in a uniform grid and examined separately.

12.2.4 Digital Archiving

Glass slides have been used as the main method for storing microscopic data in pathology for a very long period. However, issues such as time, the necessity for huge storage facilities with reinforced floors, the fragility of transparency glass, the fading of the stain on top, and finally the labor and logistical challenges [15]. Fully digital slide archives would offer many benefits, including the ability to access the same case by several observers at once, permanent, high-quality storage of WSI, and simple case retrieval for teaching, research, clinicopathological conferences, and quality assurance.

12.3 Digital Pathology's Impact

1. Patients benefit from the ability to quickly send cases between organizations or across pathology networks, increasing access to expert assistance and opinion on diagnoses.
2. Improves laboratory productivity and connection, as well as workplace flexibility and efficiency, by assisting in the creation of digital training resources that promote the development of experts in training.
3. Sets the stage for the application of artificial intelligence to assist in the advancement of pathology services.

12.3.1 Digital Pathology Improvements: Quantitative Analysis of the WSI

Digital image analysis in pathology can quickly and precisely identify and quantify particular cell types as well as quantitatively assess histological characteristics, morphological patterns, and biologically significant regions of interest (such as tumoral or peritumoral regions, relationships between various immune cell populations, expression patterns, and metastasis presence, for example) [16, 17].

Additionally, quantitative image analysis methods make it possible to gather information from tissue slides that would not be accessible during manual evaluation using conventional microscopy. Additionally, manual labor can be time-consuming and subject to human error due to counting tiredness and other factors [18].

12.3.2 WSI

WSI are examined using an image viewer, which makes it possible to examine digital slides in a way that is similar to using a traditional microscope in three ways: (1) WSI can be analyzed at various magnifications, with the added benefit of in-between magnifications, if the viewer software provides it. (2) The slides may be navigated in both directions. (3) Certain scanners enable the scanning of multiple focus planes, enabling even up-and-down focusing [19].

12.3.3 AI and Machine Learning Are Two Developments in Computational Methods

The use of AI in pathology is a result of the demand for data repeatability and the developing complexity of the studies mentioned above [20, 21]. AI is a broad field of science that involves instructing machines to extract data or qualities that exceed what a human eye could see [21].

To train a machine classifier for a specific segmentation, diagnostic, or prognostic task, AI techniques are designed to first extract the necessary image representations [22]. The ability of AI to quickly evaluate massive amounts of data could significantly accelerate the discovery of novel histopathological characteristics that may improve the comprehension of our ability to anticipate how a patient's disease will progress and how the patient will likely respond to receiving treatment [23].

Despite the recent advances in AI, the translation of algorithms from pathology to clinical and prospective use remains problematic in terms of validation, interpretability, pathologist engagement, acceptance of patients and clinicians, and regulatory approval [24].

References

1. Weinstein RS. Prospects for telepathology. Hum Pathol. 1986;17:433–4.
2. Griffin J, Treanor D. Digital pathology in clinical use: where are we now and what is holding us back? Histopathology. 2017;70(1):134–45. https://doi.org/10.1111/his.12993.
3. Hanna MG, Pantanowitz L, Evans AJ. Overview of contemporary guidelines in digital pathology: what is available in 2015 and what still needs to be addressed? J Clin Pathol. 2015;68(7):499–505. https://doi.org/10.1136/jclinpath-2015-202914.
4. Al-Janabi S, Huisman A, Van Diest PJ. Digital pathology: current status and future perspectives: digital pathology. Histopathology. 2012;61(1):1–9. https://doi.org/10.1111/j.1365-2559.2011.03814.x.
5. Parwani AV, Amin MB. Convergence of digital pathology and artificial intelligence tools in anatomic pathology practice: current landscape and future directions. Adv Anat Pathol. 2020a;27(4):221–6. https://doi.org/10.1097/PAP.0000000000000271.
6. Hartman DJ, Pantanowitz L, McHugh JS, Piccoli AL, OLeary MJ, Lauro GR. Enterprise implementation of digital pathology: feasibility, challenges, and opportunities. J Digit Imaging. 2017;30(5):555–60.
7. Matsumoto T. Learning and practice of diagnostic pathology. Juntendo Med J. 2014;60(3):193–8. https://doi.org/10.14789/jmj.60.193.
8. Madabhushi A, Lee G. Image analysis and machine learning in digital pathology: challenges and opportunities. Med Image Anal. 2016;33:170–5. https://doi.org/10.1016/j.media.2016.06.037.
9. Mroz P, Parwani AV, Kulesza P. Central pathology review for phase III clinical trials: the enabling effect of virtual microscopy. Arch Pathol Lab Med. 2013;137(4):492–5.
10. Luo W, Hassell LA. Use cases for digital pathology. In: Digital pathology. Cham: Springer; 2016. p. 5–15.
11. Singhal I, Dave A, Arora M, Saluja P, Rai R. Oral pathology—the soul of dentistry. J Evolution Med Dent Sci. 2021;10(37):3283–8. eISSN - 2278-4802, pISSN - 2278-4748.
12. Soluk-Tekkesin M, Khurram SA. A new dawn: the impact of digital technologies in oral and maxillofacial pathology. J Exp Clin Med. 2021;38(S2):81–5. https://doi.org/10.52142/omujecm.38.si.dent.1.
13. Rocha R, Vassallo J, Soares F, Miller K, Gobbi H. Digital slides: present status of a tool for consultation, teaching, and quality control in pathology. Pathol Res Pract. 2009;205(11):735–41.
14. Teodorovic I, Isabelle M, Carbone A, Passioukov A, Lejeune S, Jaminé D, Therasse P, Gloghini A, Dinjens WNM, Lam KH, Oomen MHA, Spatz A, Ratcliffe C, Knox K, Mager R, Kerr D, Pezzella F, van Damme B, van de Vijver M, Riegman PHJ. TuBaFrost 6: virtual microscopy in virtual tumour banking. Eur J Cancer. 2006;42(18):3110–6. https://doi.org/10.1016/j.ejca.2006.04.033.
15. Gabril MY, Yousef GM. Informatics for practicing anatomical pathologists: marking a new era in pathology practice. Mod Pathol. 2010;23(3):349–58. https://doi.org/10.1038/modpathol.2009.190.
16. Barisoni L, Lafata KJ, Hewitt SM, Madabhushi A, Balis UG. Digital pathology and computational image analysis in nephropathology. Nat Rev Nephrol. 2020;16(11):669–85.
17. Tumeh PC, Hellmann MD, Hamid O, Tsai KK, Loo KL, Gubens MA, Rosenblum M, Harview CL, Taube JM, Handley N, Khurana N, Nosrati A, Krummel MF, Tucker A, Sosa EV, Sanchez PJ, Banayan N, Osorio JC, Nguyen-Kim DL, et al. Liver metastasis and treatment outcome with anti-pd-1 monoclonal antibody in patients with melanoma and NSCLC. Cancer Immunol Res. 2017;5(5):417–24. https://doi.org/10.1158/2326-6066.CIR-16-0325.
18. Dixon AR, Bathany C, Tsuei M, White J, Barald KF, Takayama S. Recent developments in multiplexing techniques for immunohistochemistry. Expert Rev Mol Diagn. 2015;15(9):1171–86. https://doi.org/10.1586/14737159.2015.1069182.
19. Glatz-Krieger K, Spornitz U, Spatz A, Mihatsch MJ, Glatz D. Factors to keep in mind when introducing virtual microscopy. Virchows Arch. 2006;448(3):248–55. https://doi.org/10.1007/s00428-005-0112-2.
20. Yuan J, Hegde PS, Clynes R, Foukas PG, Harari A, Kleen TO, Kvistborg P, Maccalli C, Maecker HT, Page DB, Robins H, Song W, Stack EC, Wang E, Whiteside TL, Zhao Y, Zwierzina H, Butterfield LH, Fox BA. Novel technologies and emerging biomarkers for personalized cancer immunotherapy. J Immunother Cancer. 2016;4(1):3. https://doi.org/10.1186/s40425-016-0107-3.
21. Aeffner F, Zarella MD, Buchbinder N, Bui MM, Goodman MR, Hartman DJ, Lujan GM, Molani MA, Parwani AV, Lillard K, Turner OC, Vemuri VNP, Yuil-Valdes AG, Bowman D. Introduction to digital image analysis in whole-slide imaging: a white paper from the digital pathology association. J Pathol Inform. 2019;10(1):9. https://doi.org/10.4103/jpi.jpi_82_18.
22. Vamathevan J, Clark D, Czodrowski P, Dunham I, Ferran E, Lee G, Li B, Madabhushi A, Shah P, Spitzer M, Zhao S. Applications of machine learning in drug discovery and development. Nat Rev Drug Discov. 2019;18(6):463–77. https://doi.org/10.1038/s41573-019-0024-5.
23. Barsoum I, Tawedrous E, Faragalla H, Yousef GM. Histo-genomics: digital pathology at the forefront of precision medicine. Diagnosis. 2019;6(3):203–12.
24. Jiang Y, Yang M, Wang S, Li X, Sun Y. Emerging role of deep learning-based artificial intelligence in tumor pathology. Cancer Commun (Lond). 2020;40:154–66.

Digital Dentistry Applications in Pediatric Dentistry

13

Ayşe Işıl Orhan, Tuğba Bezgin, and Kaan Orhan

13.1 Dental Educations

Dental education, which combines theoretical knowledge and clinical practice, is one of the areas impacted by these technological advancements [1, 2, 3]). To obtain the requisite competency skills, repeated training and practice are required [4]. Since most dental procedures such as cavity preparation, endodontic treatment, and oral surgical interventions are irreversible, it is not acceptable to learn these skills only on patients [5]. Preclinical and clinical education enables dental students to develop fine motor skills and hand–foot–eye coordination [6, 7]. Students repeat procedures till they demonstrate acceptable levels of skill, without putting actual patients at risk [5].

Traditionally, preclinical dental training was accomplished as bench-top exercise using hand-held dentiforms. More contemporary dental simulation systems were created in the late 1980s as an alternative to the conventional laboratory bench procedure labs. A clinic-like environment was provided where students prepared and restored removable plastic teeth (typodonts) on maxillary or mandibular plastic jaw models mounted on mannequin heads [2]. However, typodonts have physical features that are different from natural teeth, such as stiffness and friction [8].

Another possibility is using extracted natural teeth, but they are not always easy to attain. Finding natural primary teeth, however, is extremely difficult because children and their caregivers want to save the extracted teeth for the "tooth fairy" [7]. The simple versions of these simulators that have been used in dentistry for many years have been replaced by simulation laboratories with more advanced technology and realistic equipment. Most simulation laboratories have a simulated patient or manikin as well as computer-supported audiovisual systems to aid in the transfer of information from instructors, manuals, or reference material [9].

Virtual reality (VR) simulators, augmented reality (AR) simulators, and haptic simulators are currently employed in dentistry education as an alternative to conventional laboratory-based systems [1]. VR is an artificial computer-generated

A. I. Orhan (✉)
Faculty of Dentistry, Department of Pedodontics, Ankara Yıldırım Beyazıt University, Ankara, Turkey
e-mail: aiorhan@aybu.edu.tr

T. Bezgin
Faculty of Dentistry, Department of Pedodontics, Ankara University, Ankara, Turkey
e-mail: bezgin@dentistry.ankara.edu.tr

K. Orhan
Faculty of Dentistry, Department of Dento Maxillofacial Radiology, Ankara University, Ankara, Turkey

Ankara University Medical Design Application and Research Center (MEDITAM), Ankara, Turkey

Department of Oral Diagnostics, Faculty of Dentistry, Semmelweis University, Budapest, Hungary
e-mail: knorhan@dentistry.ankara.edu.tr

A. Delantoni, K. Orhan (eds.), *Digital Dentistry*, https://doi.org/10.1007/978-3-031-52826-2_13

simulation of a real-life environment or situation [10]. It uses software to create this immersive simulated environment. Users put on a head-mounted display that actively involves them in an experience in which they can interact with the environment and virtual characters in a realistic manner. So, they can pretend they are in a different environment and learn from their experiences, just like in real life [11]. Conversely, AR is the superimposition of a computer-generated virtual image on a user's view of the real world [1, 10, 12]. It is created as applications and utilized on mobile devices to combine virtual elements into the real world. A systematic review of clinical research on AR and VR in dental medicine revealed that these tools were mainly used for educational motor skill training in university settings [10].

The most recent improvement is the addition of haptic feedback to these computer-based simulations [13]. Haptic technology started to gain popularity in dentistry training once it was included into traditional VR-based dental simulators [6, 14]. With the use of haptic technology, surgeons may manipulate real-world things like surgical instruments and human organs virtually. They can also conduct tasks like pushing, pulling, and cutting soft or hard tissue with receiving realistic force feedback [6]. The use of haptic technology in dental education has made it feasible to design virtual teeth with different mechanical hardness properties and multiple layers for enhanced reality [14, 15]. Some advantages over traditional methods include reality, demonstration, automatic performance assessment, repeatable data usage, the ability to create a variety of scenarios, the possibility to repeat the same scenario, and cost-effectiveness [6, 14].

The first prototype dental haptic simulators were developed in the early 2000s [16]. Aside from prototypes developed in academic laboratories, commercially available dental simulators are also available today. They are mainly tailored to specific fields of dentistry [8]. Some are designed to detect caries lesions (The Iowa Dental Surgical Simulator) [17], others for periodontics (PerioSim) [18] or cavity preparation and restorative operations (HapTEL) [19]. There are also simulation systems that combine applications for several dental specialties on a single device [8]. Simodont [20], for example, offers cavity preparation and restoration, endodontic access preparation, and prosthodontics; VirTeaSy Dental [21] provides cavity preparation and restoration, endodontic access preparation, prosthodontics, and implantology; and iDental [8] offers cavity preparation, endodontic access preparation, and periodontics.

Pediatric dentistry is a branch of dentistry that provides complete care to children and adolescents, including restorative dentistry, pulp therapy, preventive and interceptive orthodontics, periodontics, prosthodontics, and oral surgical procedures. In short, pediatric dentistry is a discipline unto itself, but it also draws significantly from other disciplines [22]. Therefore, it is feasible to use existing simulators in the context of pediatric dentistry education. However, when it comes to treating primary teeth, the only systems featuring a pediatric dentition module at this moment are Simodont and VirTeaSy Dental.

Children frequently lack the self-control required to cope with the dental environment and may be unable to remain still during complex or lengthy dental procedures. Dental professionals who try to calm the child and use appropriate behavior management have a restricted amount of time to perform routine pediatric dental procedures. As a result, managing pediatric patients is difficult and causes high levels of stress in dental students. It is essential to give dental students preclinical training for pediatric restorative procedures in order to improve their clinical abilities [7].

Such technological developments might be a beneficial addition to the education of dental students, providing experience and patient management abilities earlier in the curriculum and before the provision of direct patient care [23]. So that they can perform these operations with greater assurance and in a timely manner when working with pediatric patients in a clinical setting [7]. The skills required to manage a distressed and disruptive child during dental treatment are as fundamental to successful treatment as are handpiece skills and knowledge of dental materials. The ability to manage distress and disruptive behavior has direct implications for the quality of dental care. In addition, disruptive child behavior increases delivery time and the risk of injury to the child [24].

Children are more challenging to simulate than adult patients because of their complex or unpredictable behavior during dental procedures [25]. The younger the child and the more threatening the procedure, the more often negative, disruptive behavior is observed [26]. Real child patients would be ideal for teaching behavioral management techniques; however, due to practical and ethical constraints, this may not be possible. To develop communication and behavioral skills in pediatric dentistry, interactive manikin models, multimedia software, virtual patients, or a combination of these three methods may be useful. Virtual clinics and patients are already used in case studies and role plays at the undergraduate and continuing education levels [25].

Only a small number of clinical research have investigated the effectiveness of VR in behavior management in pediatric dentistry education.

Boynton et al. [27] designed an internet-based instruction tool named "The Virtual Child" to increase predoctoral students' didactic knowledge of key concepts in pediatric behavior management through simulation. The effectiveness of this tool was assessed on two subsequent groups of junior dental students. The control group received two lectures of training within the scope of the traditional behavior management curriculum. The experimental group of dental students first received the two traditional lectures and then they were given behavior management simulation next. In the examination to evaluate each group's competency in behavior management, the simulation group performed significantly better.

Papadopoulos et al. [25] developed a virtual pediatric patient to support communication and behavior management training in pediatric dentistry. Dental students who were in their fourth year of study assessed the simulation. Both the experimental group which was exposed to the simulation and a control group were asked to complete a knowledge questionnaire at the end of the study. A statistically significant difference between the two groups was found, showing a positive learning effect from the VP.

These studies showed that using a simulation based on a virtual patient as an additional teaching tool improved students' knowledge of pediatric behavior management when compared to lecture alone [25, 27].

The influence of VR simulation on dental students' empathy levels was examined by Hu and Lai [28]. Dental students in their third year experienced a VR scenario as part of a seminar on behavior management. The scenario consisted of two parts: a negative example followed by a positive example. The Jefferson Scale of Empathy (JSE) was used to measure the level of empathy. Information on self-perceived ability, comfort, and impact of the intervention was collected via a self-administered questionnaire. JSE ratings significantly increased between pre- and post-intervention, indicating higher empathy. Following the intervention, dental students felt more comfortable communicating and interacting with children. The study discovered that using VR can improve dental students' empathy and confidence when communicating and interacting with children [28].

There are few studies investigating VR simulators in pediatric dentistry training.

In a 2020 study, Zafar et al. aimed to evaluate students' perceptions of the haptic Simodont dental trainer, their psychomotor skills, the effects of formal virtual skill training, and the transfer of pediatric dentistry restorative skills learned in Simodont to the traditional simulation. Dental students enrolled in a Doctor of Dental Medicine program who had completed their training in Simodont and traditional preclinical simulation laboratories for pulpotomies and stainless-steel crowns (SSC) were administered a questionnaire. Fifty-one percent of students thought that Simodont helped their learning, and 56% of students reported that Simodont training made it easier for them to understand activities related to pediatric dentistry. In general, for both practical tasks, participants preferred simulation training to Simodont. Eighty-eight percent of the participants disagreed that Simodont should replace traditional simulation. According to the authors, Simodont might be utilized as a supplement to help dental students prepare for preclinical pediatric dentistry restorative exercises. However, it is still insufficient to replace traditional simulation training [7].

Zafar et al. [3] carried out a study to investigate dentistry students' perceptions of local anesthesia (LA) VR simulation on a pediatric patient and see whether it can improve their learning. A self-administered survey was completed by second-year dental students both before and after using the dentistry LA VR simulator. Following the use of dental LA VR, 89.9% of study participants thought that their LA skills would improve; 83.1% reported feeling more engaged in the learning activity; 55.0% said it improved their understanding of anatomical landmarks; and 56.4% agreed that it added value compared with traditional LA teaching methods. The authors came to the conclusion that the use of VR provided an additional method of LA training in pediatric dentistry; however, it cannot be used in place of traditional phantom head training techniques [3].

The only clinical study using AR in pediatric dentistry evaluated the effect of an AR simulator on learning perception and acute stress level in students administering the first LA to pediatric patients in comparison to traditional teaching techniques. Fourth- and fifth-year students took part in the study. Students in the study group used an AR simulator in a dental office for 2 h each for 2 weeks in addition to the traditional training. Students who used the AR approach had a statistically significant shorter time to complete the infiltrative anesthesia technique for the anterior superior alveolar nerve. Salivary cortisol level measured to assess acute stress was statistically significant in all subjects before and after anesthesia; however, there was no statistically significant difference between the groups. Although AR practice cannot reduce acute stress in students administering LA to pediatric patients for the first time, it can improve syringe manipulation and be very useful for students transitioning from preclinical to clinical skills [5].

A systematic review reported that studies reporting AR and VR technology in dentistry are scarce, and scientifically proven recommendations for clinical protocols cannot be made at this time.

However, AR/VR technologies that offer interactive learning concepts with 24/7 access and objective evaluation are gaining popularity and significance in dentistry education. The near future will reveal the full potential of AR/VR technology in dentistry as a result of the ongoing advancements in information technology [10].

13.2 Oral Health Promotion

Oral diseases are an important global public health problem due to their high prevalence and significant socioeconomic impact [29, 30]. Dental caries and periodontal diseases constitute the most important part of the global burden of oral diseases [31]. In the Global Burden of Disease (GBD) 2010 Study, untreated caries in permanent teeth was the most prevalent condition, with a global prevalence of 35% for all ages combined. Severe periodontitis and untreated caries in deciduous teeth were the 6th and 10th most prevalent conditions, respectively, affecting 11% and 9% of the global population [32]. Since 1990, when the first year for which statistics on oral diseases were available from the GBD dataset, oral diseases have continued to be the most prevalent conditions worldwide [33]. In 2017, there were 3.5 billion cases of oral diseases worldwide, of which 2.3 billion involved untreated caries in permanent teeth, 796 million severe periodontitis, 532 million untreated caries in deciduous teeth, 267 million total tooth loss, and 139 million other conditions [34].

Oral diseases are caused by a number of modifiable risk factors common to many noncommunicable diseases (NCDs), including high intake of free sugars, tobacco use, harmful use of alcohol and poor hygiene, and their underlying social and commercial determinants [30, 35, 36]. Oral diseases are chronic and progressive. They start in early childhood and continue throughout life, negatively affecting individuals' well-being and quality of life. In addition to causing persistent pain, sepsis, and discomfort, poor oral health also causes absence from work and school, which impairs learning and reduces productivity. They disproportionately affect people in low- and middle-income countries and also poorer and marginalized groups in society [30].

The costs of treating oral diseases impose heavy financial burdens to individuals and healthcare systems [30, 33]. The treatment-oriented, interventionist, technical, increasingly high-tech and specialized approach adopted in dentistry has failed to address the global burden of oral diseases [35]. The currently dominant tradition of dentistry needs to be changed to incorporate more oral health promotion strategies [37].

In fact, most oral diseases are largely preventable through simple and cost-effective methods that include reducing or eliminating these risks and strengthening healthy behaviors [38]. But interventions that focus only on changing oral health behaviors and lifestyle choices have limited success. A comprehensive integrative strategy that takes account of the common risk factors and the key determinants of health will result in fair and equitable approaches to promoting better oral health and general health [38, 39]. The burden of oral diseases and other noncommunicable diseases can be reduced through public health interventions by addressing common risk factors, such as reducing free sugar intake and promoting a healthy diet, quitting tobacco use, reduction of alcohol consumption, reduction of traumatic dental injuries, and adequate fluoride exposure [36].

Oral health promotion is defined as any combination of oral health education and legal, fiscal, economic, environmental, organizational, and technical interventions designed to facilitate the achievement of oral health and the prevention of disease [40]. Systematic reviews have demonstrated that oral health promotion programs targeting children and adolescents enhance clinical oral health outcomes [41–43]. Interventions for oral health promotion programs that are often employed include community-based oral health education and training programs, screening of children's teeth, toothbrushing under supervision with an appropriate amount of fluoride toothpaste, and dietary management recommendations [41].

Oral health education is an essential component of oral health promotion [40]. The purpose of oral health education is to enhance knowledge, which may result in the adoption of favorable oral health practices that promote better oral health. It has been provided to individuals and groups in places like dental offices, schools, workplaces, daycare centers, senior living facilities, etc. as an important and essential component of dental health services. Oral health promotion information has been traditionally delivered in the form of instructions, written materials, videos, demonstrations of oral hygiene practices, group discussions, campaigns, and lectures. There have been many different educational interventions utilized, ranging from the simple dissemination of information to the use of programs involving psychological and behavior change strategies [44].

With the increasing accessibility of mobile devices, oral health promotion projects have been further supported by mobile technology [45]. According to figures from the International Telecommunication Union (ITU), in 2022, 73% of people aged 10 and older worldwide will own a mobile phone, which is 7% points greater than the proportion of people who use the Internet [46]. The systematic review, which aimed to determine the effect of teledentistry-based (telematic) strategies on oral health prevention and promotion, showed that mHealth (messages and apps) is a promising clinical tool [47].

mHealth or mobile health is defined as medical and public health practice supported by mobile devices, such as mobile phones, patient monitoring devices, personal digital assistants (PDAs), and other wireless devices. It involves the use of and capitalization on a mobile phone's core utility of voice and short messaging service (SMS) as well as more complex functionalities and applications, including general packet radio service (GPRS), third- and fourth-generation mobile telecommunications (3G and 4G systems), global positioning systems (GPS), and Bluetooth technology [48].

The most popular mHealth strategies for promoting oral health were mobile apps and mobile messages [45]. A systematic review examining the effectiveness of text messages and mobile apps in improving oral health knowledge and/or reducing gingival inflammation found that the adjunct use of mHealth to improve the understanding of conventional oral hygiene instructions significantly improved plaque removal and gingivitis and increased knowledge of oral self-care. Text messaging was found to be the most popular mHealth tool used in the studies [49].

Text messaging is useful for promoting numerous health-related behaviors. The Text2Floss Study examined the feasibility and utility of a 7-day text messaging intervention (2-way SMS service) to improve oral health knowledge and behavior in mothers of young children. Mothers who brought their children aged 5 years or younger for dental care were included in the study. Text group received text messages for 7 days, asking about flossing and presenting oral health information. Oral health behaviors and knowledge were surveyed pre- and post-intervention. Mothers receiving text messages flossed more, had higher total and specific knowledge, and tried to improve their child's oral health behaviors and decrease their soda and sugary snacks more than control mothers. Using text messages to encourage flossing and to deliver oral health information was considered acceptable [50].

Mobile app-based interventions have been found to be helpful in enhancing a variety of health promotion habits, such as diet and physical activity [51]. There is also some evidence to suggest that mobile phones are effective in improving adherence to oral hygiene advice in orthodontic patients [52]. A comprehensive survey of app stores in 2019 found 612 oral health-related apps [53]. As apps are easily accessed by the majority, this makes them ideal for delivering oral health information, especially in situations where face-to-face dental care is limited [54]. The majority of dental caries prevention apps focused on dental hygiene, according to a systematic review; however, many of them were not of high quality. It was also found that there is a lack of apps targeting parents of children under the age of six, with most apps aimed at young adults or adolescents. Among the 40 apps examined, the Brush DJ app had the highest overall MARS (Mobile App Rating Scale) rating of 4.4 [55].

The Brush DJ app was developed to use the opportunity mobile apps offer to motivate an evidence-based oral hygiene routine. The app plays music, either from a playlist or at random from the user's device and cloud, in an effort to encourage users to brush for 2 min. The app instructs users to spit after brushing rather than rinsing to maintain fluoride levels. Users of the app can set reminders to brush twice daily, use mouthwash at a different time of the day than toothbrushing, change their toothbrushes every 3 months, and schedule appointments with their dentist, hygienist, therapist, and orthodontist. The app also contains the patient information included in "Public Health England's Delivering Better Oral Health: An Evidence-Based Toolkit for Prevention" document. Additionally, it provides links to animated YouTube videos that demonstrate the correct way to use a manual toothbrush, floss, and interdental brushes. In a preliminary study, user perception of the app was evaluated and found to be a promising tool to motivate an evidence-based oral hygiene routine [56].

Behavioral change is an important aspect of oral health promotion [57]. Mobile phones are an excellent choice for delivering behavioral interventions since they are highly valued portable devices that owners keep with them throughout the day. They present a chance to bring behavioral interventions into crucial real-world situations when people make decisions about their health and encounter barriers to behavior change [58]. It is necessary to ensure that health promotion apps provide accurate and safe information and ideally using effective and multiple behavior change techniques [54]. Popular health and lifestyle apps found to have low amounts of theory-based behavior change techniques (BCTs) in a study. The authors suggest that BCTs could be used more frequently to improve interventions and increase user engagement [59].

A theory-based mobile app named "WhiteTeeth" was created to promote oral health behaviors (i.e., increasing exposure to fluoride and improving dental plaque levels) in addition to usual care for adolescent orthodontic patients. The app used a variety of behavior change techniques, targeting not only oral health behavior but also the psychosocial factors that are associated with this behavior and had been identified through the Health Action Process Approach (HAPA) theory. The incorporated behavior change techniques were coaching to set goals, action plans, and reminders; self-monitoring of oral health behaviors and dental plaque; providing feedback and practical support; reviewing behavioral goals; and creating coping plans. Results of a randomized controlled trial showed that the WhiteTeeth app was effective in reducing dental plaque in adolescents with fixed orthodontic appliances [60, 61].

Through the use of technology, patients should have more control of their care in the future, allowing clinicians to more efficiently use their time and resources [54]. The increasing use of mHealth apps driven by increasing public use of mobile devices presents a call for dental researchers, health system managers, policy makers, and health professionals to engage with and provide more rigorous scientific recommendations around oral health apps [55].

13.3 Digital Caries Detection

In dentistry, a successful treatment requires first and foremost a timely, precise, and correct diagnosis. In 1997, Pitts defined the ideal caries diagnosis method as a simple, reliable, non-invasive, sensitive, and specific procedure that can directly measure the activity and size of the lesion, can base the dynamic process of caries on a biological basis, can be accepted by the patient and dentist, and can be applied quickly [62]. This topic is covered in detail in Chap. 6. However, its use in pediatric dentistry will be briefly reviewed here.

Diagnosis of caries lesions is basically a visual method based on the evaluation of clinical examination and radiographs, as well as tactile data using a dental probe [63]. The traditional method in caries diagnosis is primarily a combination of visual examination and subjective evaluation of the sense of touch, and it is supported by radiographs. For many years, examining color, surface roughness, and location with the help of dental probe and bitewing radiographs have been the subjective evaluation method for the clinician in determining the presence or absence of caries [64]. These methods generally show low sensitivity and high specificity, which causes the majority of lesions to be overlooked [65].

Radiographic imaging is based on the principle that the loss of minerals in enamel and dentin with the progression of caries allows the passage of X-rays (reduction of attenuation) [66]. The radiographic imaging of initial occlusal caries requires approximately 30–40% mineral loss for the lesions to be detected. Therefore, initial caries lesions cannot be detected radiographically [67]. However, the radiographic method is susceptible to certain drawbacks such as X-ray exposure, subjective evaluation of the images, and optical illusions that can be mistaken for caries. Bitewing radiography (BW) is reportedly a better performing detection method with higher sensitivity in interproximal caries in dentin than in enamel [68, 69]. It is shown to have a sensitivity range of 0.54–0.66 and a specificity of 0.83–0.95 for dentinal caries [63, 70]. BW is a less reliable technique for the detection of enamel caries, with a reported sensitivity range of 0.3–0.41 and a specificity of 0.76–0.78 [63, 70, 71]. The American Academy of Pediatric Dentistry recommends posterior radiographs at 6- to 12-month intervals to detect interproximal caries when it cannot be examined visually or with a probe for patients who are at increased risk for caries and with clinical caries, versus 12- to 24-month intervals for patients without clinical caries [72].

Introducing alternative methods for detecting incipient caries that use less or no radiation would be beneficial to the contemporary practice of pediatric dentistry. The development of new methods and devices with technological progress offered to the use of dentists is aimed at reducing the amount of invasive restoration and provide better preventive treatments by ensuring that even the slightest deformities in dental hard tissues are eliminated [73]. The ideal caries detection method should be accurate, precise, easy to use, and applicable for every surface of the tooth.

13.3.1 Fiber Optic Transillumination (FOTI) Method

In this method, high-intensity white light from the light source is applied to the buccal or lingual surface of the tooth with the help of a fiber optic tip with a diameter of 0.5 mm. The FOTI system uses the different refractive properties of intact dental tissue and carious lesions with altered mineral density. When the surface is examined occlusally, dark shadows due to demineralization in enamel and dentin allow the detection of early enamel and dentin lesions [74].

It has been reported that this method, which is particularly effective in the diagnosis of interface caries, can also be used successfully in the evaluation of enamel cracks [75]. FOTI was proposed as a valid, efficient alternative to bitewing radiographs in clinical trials of caries-prophylactic agents with a sensitivity of 0.73 and specificity of 0.99 [76].

The advantages of the method are that patients are not exposed to ionizing radiation, it is a minimally invasive diagnostic method, it allows painless diagnosis, and the device can be used repeatedly [77].

13.3.2 Digital Fiber Optic Transillumination (DIFOTI) Method

Although FOTI is a simple method, the DIFOTI method, which is applied together with digital imaging, has been developed due to its disadvantages such as being subjective, not being able to save the image, not being able to print out data, and requiring experience and careful examination. In this method, which is based on the same principle as FOTI, demineralized areas are observed as dark shadows due to the differences in the scattering and absorption of light photons between healthy and demineralized tissues. In the DIFOTI system, images are provided by a digital CCD camera, while visible light is used to transilluminate the tooth. The use of CCD allows the comparison of changes in different exams over time as it provides the projection of snapshots. In addition, the non-invasive nature of the method allows the device to be used repeatedly [78, 79].

This method aids visual inspection; however, since there is no software that analyzes images in this system, the evaluation is made subjectively by the examiner. In addition, correlation between DIFOTI and bitewing radiographs in diagnosing approximal carious lesions was found to be low for lesions in enamel [80, 81].

13.3.3 Quantitative Light Effected Fluorescence (QLF) Method

In the QLF method, caries is diagnosed by using the fluorescence characteristic that changes due to the demineralization of dental hard tissues. It is a device that is used in the measurement of caries lesion by using the relationship of light scattering and scattering with mineral loss and provides quantitative evaluation of dental plaque, bacterial activity, tartar, and discoloration [82, 83]. Dental hard tissue has its own natural fluorescence called autofluorescence. With QLF, green fluorescence originating from the hard tissues of the tooth and red fluorescence originating from external origin occur. With the changes in the mineral structure of the tooth, a decrease in the amount of natural fluorescence is observed [84].

In the method, the tooth surface is illuminated by using an optical filtering system that produces blue light at a wavelength of 404 nm or an argon laser that produces blue-green light at a wavelength of 488 nm [85]. The fluorescence of the enamel, which corresponds to the yellow region in the light spectrum, is passed through a high-pass yellow filter and a digital image is created by transferring the obtained data to the computer. Fluorescence differences between intact and demineralized tissues are evaluated in the computer program. The fluorescence in the tooth structure decreases with demineralization and the fluorescence of the carious lesion seen with QLF is lower than the values in the intact tissues of the tooth. Therefore, demineralized areas appear as dark areas with QLF [84]. While QLF can only distinguish enamel demineralizations, it cannot distinguish between caries, hypoplasia, or anatomical features [86].

Lenzi et al. [87] used this technique for secondary caries diagnosis of primary molar occlusal restorations and concluded the performance of the fluorescence-based methods is good, but similar to that obtained with visual and radiographic methods.

13.3.4 Laser Fluorescence Method

In order to eliminate the deficiencies of traditional methods, many caries diagnosis methods working on different principles have been developed. The most used method among current and non-invasive caries diagnosis methods is the fluorescence method [88]. The working principle of this method is that the carious lesion absorbs and scatters the laser beam differently than the surrounding healthy tissue [89]. With the DIAGNOdent device, a red diode laser beam with a wavelength of 655 nm is applied to the occlusal surface of the tooth with a special tip, passing through the fiber bundle. The beam absorbed by the tooth is reflected back as fluorescence photons. A filter is placed around the main fiber that can absorb the scattered light. The fluorescence signals passing through the filter are collected and digitally measured by a photodiode and transmitted to the monitor. The intensity of the recovered fluorescence beam is directly proportional to the lesion depth. This system has been calibrated considering healthy standard enamel. As the numerical value increases, the probability of caries increases. The measurement scale produced by the manufacturer is as follows: values between 5 and 25 indicate initial lesion, values between 26 and 35 indicate early dentin caries, values greater than 35 indicate advanced dentin caries [83, 89].

One of the widely used clinically used devices working with laser fluorescence principle is DIAGNOdent (KaVo, Biberach, Germany). The advantages of the system are that it does not contain X-rays, allows early caries detection in the fissure area, which is difficult to diagnose clinically and radiographically, is non-invasive and can be repeated, and painless diagnosis increases the patient's confidence in the physician [89].

However, it is expensive, cannot make a differential diagnosis in advanced dentin caries with exposed pulp, fails in the diagnosis of secondary caries in the restoration and adjacent teeth, and is very sensitive to the presence of plaque or calculus and can give a signal as if there is a change in the enamel or dentin structure if attention is not paid (i.e., false positive value). In addition, the fact that coloration other than carious tissue causes fluorescent signal is still a problem that needs a solution [90–92].

In a study with DIAGNOdent, only hypomineralization was reported in the teeth, although a high value was measured in two of the seven teeth used. For this reason, the inability to distinguish the difference between hypomineralization and the presence of carious tissue with this device has been reported as a disadvantage [92]. However, in a recent study, it was reported that it was successfully used to measure the remineralization difference in hypomineralized teeth [93].

Some features of the DIAGNOdent device were developed and the DIAGNOdent Pen device (KaVo, Biberach, Germany) with the same working principle was produced. Unlike the DIAGNOdent device, it is aimed to provide easier access to the fissures and interfaces of the device head by reducing the diameter of the head applied to the tooth and enabling it to rotate. In addition, the DIAGNOdent Pen is lighter than the DIAGNOdent device and is easier to use clinically, thanks to its reduced size [94–96]. An in vivo study by Subka [97] examined clinically 1030 proximal surfaces by using meticulous visual examination (ICDAS), bitewing radiographs, and a DIAGNOdent pen in pediatric patients. The result of the study showed that for D_1 (enamel and dentine caries) lesions diagnostic threshold, the sensitivity of ICDAS visual examination with temporary tooth separation, radiographic examination, and LF pen examination was 0.52, 0.75, 0.14, 0.58, and the specificity at this threshold was 0.89, 0.88, 0.97, and 0.85, respectively.

Recently developed systems use fluorescence method and intraoral camera together. One of them is the Soprolife intraoral camera (Acteon,

France). It has 450 nm wavelength emission and 20 nm bandwidth, which illuminates tooth surfaces using 2 types of LEDs. By combining the autofluorescent image and the anatomical image, Soprolife can detect the differences in the density, structure, and/or chemical composition of biological tissues [98].

13.3.5 Light Emitting Diode (LED) Caries Diagnostic Method

LED-based caries ID device is one of the newest developed caries diagnostic devices. The working principle of the device is based on the reflection and refraction of the LED (light emitting diode) light in the tooth tissue. The advantages of the device are that it is easy to use, gives objective findings, and is portable. It is used in the evaluation of occlusal and approximal caries [99].

As a result of the loss of mineral in the enamel tissue, the translucent structure deteriorates and this deteriorated structure shows different optical properties compared to the intact tooth tissue. The LED-based device captures the moment when the tooth tissue reflects and refracts light through its fiber optic tip and converts it into electrical signals, and these values are analyzed to determine the presence or absence of caries. The change of light from green to red and the increase in the number of signal sounds suggest the presence of caries [99, 100].

13.3.6 Electrical Conductivity Measurement Method (ECM)

The ECM method is a diagnostic method that works on the basis of measuring the conductivity change in the tissues due to demineralization caused by caries. Robust tooth tissue shows very good insulating properties. However, although no deterioration is observed on the tooth surface, the electrical conductivity of the tooth tissue changes with demineralization. Electrical conductivity measurements are made using the increase in conductivity of enamel caries in pits and fissures [101].

In the study of Longbottom et al. [102], although ECM was found to be successful on the occlusal surface, it was reported that it had limited working capacity on occlusal surfaces, while it was observed that ECM was more successful on flat surfaces and approximal surfaces.

13.3.7 Alternative Current Impedance Spectroscopy Method

One of the non-invasive methods developed for caries detection is the measurement method known as alternating current impedance spectroscopy. The conductivity of the tissue, whose mineral structure changes with the formation of caries, differs from the intact tissue. This method is based on the evaluation of the change in mineral density with the direct application of low voltage current to the tooth surface [103]. CarieScan Pro (CarieScan Ltd., Dundee, Scotland) is a device that works with this method. There are very few clinical studies on this device, which was developed for the detection of dentin lesions on posterior occlusal surfaces. However, there are also disadvantages such as not being able to detect root caries at interfaces and not distinguishing secondary caries [103, 104].

13.3.8 Optical Coherence Tomography (OCT) Method

Optical coherence tomography is a non-invasive imaging technique that provides cross-sectional examination of biological structures. Its use in dentistry is the evaluation of the remineralization–demineralization degrees of the dental tissue [105, 106]. In this technique, a broadband, near-infrared light source with a wavelength of 840–1310 nm is used, which has high tissue penetration and no biological harm reported so far. With this method, an image of 0.6–2 mm is obtained in dentin, while a deeper imaging is obtained in enamel, which is a more transparent tissue [107, 108].

The most important advantage it provides in terms of intraoral diagnosis is that it can provide information about both the structural features and surface contours of hard and soft tissues. Other advantages include using non-ionizing radiation close to infrared, having high axial resolution, being a small and practical appliance, allowing instantaneous images and simultaneous Doppler (flow velocity) measurements [109].

Thomas et al. [110] used this technique to evaluate remineralization activity in primary molars and correlate it with stereomicroscopic histologic images. The authors revealed that OCT images correlated to histology and concluded that OCT could monitor surface/subsurface in situ de/remineralization activity non-invasively.

13.3.9 Near-Infrared Light Transillumination (NILT)

The past two decades have seen the development of the near-infrared light transillumination (NILT), a caries detection method that has come as a further advancement of the digital imaging fiber optic transillumination method (DIFOTI). The two systems primarily differed in such aspects that the DiFOTI system functions using visible light, whereas the NILT system operates in long-wave light. Using longer wavelengths is advantageous in that it reduces scattering that allows near-infrared light to pass through objects more deeply. The clinical application may secure reduced radiation exposure. Furthermore, the intraoral camera might be better tolerated than intraoral sensors, offering ease of use and time efficacy [111]. KaVo®, DIAGNOcam® (KaVo Dental, Lake Zurich, IL, USA) is a new device using the NILT technology.

In an in vivo study on permanent teeth, it was determined that DIAGNOcam showed superior sensitivity than conventional bitewing radiographs in the diagnosis of initial interproximal caries [112]. Alamoudi et al. [113] found that DIAGNOcam showed higher sensitivity as a result of their in vivo study, in which they compared the efficacy of bitewing radiographs and DIAGNOcam in the diagnosis of cavitated interproximal caries of primary molar teeth, and suggested that this device, which does not contain ionizing radiation, be used for caries diagnosis especially in pediatric patients. However, a recent study evaluating the specificity and sensitivity of a NILT device (DEXIS CariVu DEXIS, LLC, Hatfield, PA, USA) for detection of interproximal caries lesions of primary molars revealed the system had limitations as a stand-alone method [114].

The iTero Element 5D imaging system (Align Technology, California, USA) and TRIOS 4 (3Shape A/S, Copenhagen, Denmark) systems produced with similar technologies are also currently available in the market. There is no research on primary teeth in the literature yet with these systems.

13.3.10 Ultrasonic Imaging

The modus operandi for ultrasonic imaging is that high-frequency waves (1–20 MHz) are applied through a probe to the material or biological tissue, and the returning waves are absorbed by the probe and converted into electrical impulses and detected as echoes [115, 116].

Ultrasonic system in dentistry: It is routinely used for calculus removal, irrigation of root canals, and mechanical cleaning of instruments. However, unlike the use of diagnostic ultrasound in medicine, it has received little attention in dentistry in terms of diagnosis, and studies on this subject have been increasing in recent years. In the light of these studies, it is accepted that solid and demineralized enamel tissues can be easily distinguished in the diagnosis of non-cavitated enamel caries, since sound waves have different travel times in two different environments. In addition, if ultrasonic waves are applied perpendicular to the surface, the defect in the tissue can be detected more easily [115, 117].

13.4 Three-Dimensional (3D) Printing in Pediatric Dentistry

With the developing science and technology, the innovations in printing technologies not only leave the traditional methods behind but also create an infrastructure for the changes in the world. While the functions and capabilities of 2D printers continue to increase, a new perspective was brought to printing technology by the announcement of three-dimensional (3D) technology known as additive manufacturing or rapid prototyping in the 1980s. In 1987, 3D printing became commercial and has been used in various fields from biomedical science to space science and continues to be used [118]. The use of 3D printing in the field of medicine and dentistry allows for customization and personalization of medical and dental products. The most important disadvantage of this technology is the price, so accessibility is still low [119, 120]. In pediatric dentistry, 3D printing technology is a current topic of research and has gained its way by its child friendly practice tool with the help of intraoral scanners [121].

13.4.1 Digital Impressions Intraoral Scanner

Today, there is a digital change in the field of impression taking in dentistry. With the development of systems in this area, it is expected that the impression taking procedure, which is an uncomfortable procedure for both adult and pediatric patients, will be more tolerable. Intraoral scanners are devices that provide three-dimensional images of teeth and oral tissues. Scanning of arches can be done with pauses and breaks and this is an important advantage over the conventional impression technique for pediatric patients [121, 122]. In a study by Yılmaz and Aydın [123], the digital impression method compared with the conventional impression method was found to be both more comfortable and preferable by the children. These systems have other advantages such as low storage space, rapid access to three-dimensional (3D) records, and facilitating communication with professionals and patients. However, the daily use of digital applications is not yet routine. The risk of corruption in electronic storage, data loss in case of dependency on third parties, high cost of operating system and equipment prevent it from getting into routine [124]. In addition, in pediatric patients the chair time during intraoral scanning may increase due to the clinician's experience, scanner probe size, shallow depth of the vestibular sulcus, and the presence of missing or erupting teeth [125].

However, it is a fact the sensitivity of the intraoral scanners is higher than the conventional method. In the scans, real tissue anatomy with a low margin of error can be obtained. In the study of Garino and Garino [126] evaluating the efficacy of intraoral scanners, 16 different measurements were made by the same investigator at different times on both digital and plaster models, and the digital models were found to be more sensitive for all measurements.

One of the most recent of these systems is the Trios System (3 Shape A/S, Copenhagen, Denmark). It takes image recording with the principle of ultra-fast optical section and confocal microscopy. The system has the capability of acquiring 3000 images per second [127]. The system can perform intraoral scanning in about 5 min. Scanning of teeth and soft tissues in the lower and upper dental arch can be performed simultaneously. The data obtained includes tooth and gingiva color [128].

13.4.2 3D Printing in Fabrication of Space Maintainers and Crowns

A common problem in pediatric patients is the premature loss of primary teeth that results in the disruption of the arch integrity, and space maintainers (SM) are used to prevent such problems. Some disadvantages, such as corrosion and appliance breakage of conventional space maintainers have led to the development of more aesthetic and metal-free space maintainers, such as a fiber-inserted composite space maintainer and a CAD/CAM-supported ceramic band-loop space maintainer. Space maintainers that use CAD-CAM or 3D print technology with modern and biocompatible materials are called "Digital Space Maintainers" [129, 130].

Intraoral scanners promote the quick fabrication of customized chair side space maintainers [131, 132]. Digital impressions combined with CAD/CAM technology allow a completely digital workflow. In addition, it was reported the band fit of metallic band–loop space maintainers fabricated by conventional and 3D printing technologies had no difference [133]. With this technique, the requirement of laboratory procedures, human-based errors, and the need for additional dental visits are prevented. Zirconia or polyether ether ketone (PEEK) materials can also be preferred for fixed or removable space maintainers fabrication using CAD/CAM technology [130, 134]. Polyether ether ketone-based materials have a unique mix of strong mechanical properties and are rigid, opaque, and biocompatible. They are chemically resistant, stable against high-temperatures, have dimensional stability, and they offer a wide array of processing possibilities. These materials are suitable for patients with metal allergy or metallic distaste [129]. PEEK polymer was evaluated by Kun et al. [135] in children with unilateral loss of either the first or second molars and were found to be 75% lighter than conventional SMs.

Custom crowns can also be printed using rapid prototyping. The same digital dentition data can be used to design the custom crown and 3D print the crown. These crowns are 3D printed and wrapped up to the thickness of 1 mm [119]. CAD/CAM technology offers a restoration method that reduces risk of human error and it provides highly aesthetic outcomes; however, its costs are relatively high [136]. New materials such as resin nanoceramics rather than ceramic blocks are recommended as they offer optimized mechanical properties and higher degrees of monomer polymerization, and less abrasion of the opposing dental arch when compared to ceramic restorations; they are also easily repaired using composite resin, if necessary [136, 137]. CAD/CAM resin restorations overcome the disadvantages of direct composites by avoiding the negative effects of polymerization shrinkage and allowing for proper dental anatomy, interproximal contact points, occlusal relationships, and reconfiguration of aesthetics [138]. Nanoceramics are composed of 80% nanoceramic particles (zirconium and silico nano-particles bound together) and 20% resin. Although nanoceramic blocks have high durability, the elasticity modulus being close to dentin provides flexibility to the ceramic. Thanks to this flexibility feature, the amount of stress in the restoration is reduced, and the amount of wear caused by the restoration on the antagonist tooth enamel is minimized. When adaptation and fracture resistance of these crowns were evaluated in in vitro conditions, their performance was better than prefabricated crowns in the market [139, 139].

Onlays produced by CAD/CAM can be preferred for the treatment of primary molar teeth with extended caries. Minimal invasive procedure; high strength, biocompatibility, and aesthetic success; no gingival trauma; easy execution; and patient and parent satisfaction are major benefits of this technique [141, 142]. Endocrown restorations produced with CAD/CAM offer pediatric dentists an effective and perfectly compatible conservative treatment option for the restoration of endodontically treated teeth instead of using prefabricated crowns [143].

CAD/CAM restorations can also be performed on teeth with developmental defects such as molar incisor hypomineralization, amelogenesis imperfecta, and dentinogenesis imperfecta. Aesthetic and restorations with long-term good prognosis are provided in young patients with CAD/CAM restorations, which is an innovative treatment approach for these teeth [144–146].

It has been reported that restorations produced by CAD/CAM for patients with special needs are the best solution in terms of both acceptable clinical steps and longevity, aesthetics, and prevention of caries. It has been emphasized that it can provide a good aesthetic, functional, and permanent restoration in a single session and without the need for general anesthesia for these patients [147].

However, custom made CAD/CAM crowns are expensive, fabrication expertise and expensive equipment are required [121].

13.4.3 3D Printing Application in Autotransplantation: Autogenous Transplantation of Teeth

In autogenous tooth transplantation, a recipient socket should be prepared for the placement of the donor tooth. 3D printing technology could be useful in terms of guide preparation in this treatment method. With conventional technique, the transplanted tooth is under the risk of periodontal ligament injury, especially during the testing of its fit inside the new alveolar bed. Instead, surgical templates can be produced for optimal placement of the donor tooth. For this purpose, a model of the tooth to be donated can be created with three-dimensional printers using computerized tomography or cone-beam tomography. With this new technology, minimizing extra-oral time and limiting possible damage to the donor tooth's periodontal tissue is possible [121, 148, 149].

Reshaping of autotransplanted teeth is usually delayed for 3–4 months after the procedure so as not to interfere with the natural healing process. This period requires the use of temporary aesthetic restorations for autotransplanted teeth. Ali Al-Rimawi et al. [150] stated that temporary restorations designed and produced with CAD/CAM technology are ideally compatible with the gingiva and are a suitable temporary restoration option for autotransplanted teeth.

13.4.4 3D Printing in Regenerative Endodontics

Regenerative endodontics have seen groundbreaking advancements, thanks to the shift to digital workflow [151, 152]. In endodontics, the notion of additive manufacturing can be used to provide stem cells, pulp scaffolds, injectable calcium phosphates, growth hormones, and gene therapy. Manufacturing dental tissue is bolstered by 3D Ca-P porous granules by providing favorable 3D substrate conditions for human dental pulp stem cell growth and odontogenic differentiation [151].

In regenerative endodontics the use of a scaffold is vital to ensure a setting for the growth and development of cells and vasculature. The suggested protocol for providing a scaffold is the introduction of a sterile file 2 mm past the apical foramen to allow the entire canal to fill with blood to the level of the cemento-enamel junction. However, this technique has limitations in that both the concentration and the composition of cells trapped in the clot are unpredictable, as restoring function in tissue engineering requires effective concentrations and composition of cells. In addition, in certain circumstances it may not be possible to produce bleeding in a canal [153, 154]. These setbacks have led researchers to search for better 3D scaffolds that can be constructed regardless of whether bleeding can be induced. Use of synthetic polysaccharide hydrogels such as VitroGel 3D as a scaffold is a promising method for promoting intracanal hard tissue deposition and continued root growth in regenerative endodontic treatments. It can mimic the extracellular matrix in the pulp, adapts to canal morphology, shows low cytotoxicity, and is a biodegradable material. However, as with other injectable scaffolds, production difficulties and cost hinder its clinical feasibility in Vitrogel 3D [155].

Osteogenic activity, according to research, is improved in vitro by applying 3D printed polycaprolactone covered with freeze-dried platelet-rich plasma to dental pulp cells. Also, anatomically formed tooth-like tissue was created utilizing 3D printed polyepsilon-caprolactone and hydroxyapatite scaffolds [156].

The ideal scaffold for regenerative endodontics has yet to be found. Further research—both in vitro and in vivo—is required. Advanced computer-aided design and 3D printing can provide scaffolds like polymers which have the potential to contribute to the growth of specific cell types such as pulpal cells. The future of regenerative endodontics bodes well owing to the discoveries and advancements in scaffold technology [151].

13.5 Artificial Intelligence in Pediatric Dentistry

Among the diseases seen during childhood, dental caries is one of the most common and presents as a major public health issue affecting children of all ages in the developing and developed countries. Early detection and control of these diseases is important for a child's oral health and general well-being [157]. Artificial intelligence models have been used for the detection of plaque on primary teeth [158] as well as for the prediction of children's oral health status and treatment needs [159]; detection, classification, and prediction of dental caries [160, 161]; detection and categorization of fissure sealants [162]; and the determination of the chronological age [163].

With an eye to identifying risk factors for oral diseases, such as dental caries, caries risk prediction models have been deployed, which would eventually contribute to improving patient care by leading to the development of preventive measures [164]. Caries management by risk assessment (CAMBRA) and the Cariogram are the most commonly used caries risk assessment models [157].

Cariogram is a free Swedish software program that compiles a multitude of caries risk factors such as caries experience, amount of plaque, mutans streptococci (MS), saliva secretion, buffer capacity, systemic diseases, diet content, diet frequency, fluoride usage, and the clinical judgment of the dentist. Cariogram provides the patient with graphical data which present a risk profile by identifying predominant caries risk factors [157]. Cariogram presented moderate to good performance in elderly patients. However, for preschool and schoolchildren/adolescents, the quality of evidence was limited [165].

CAMBRA is another caries risk assessment approach. Two different forms are used according to the patients' age. The forms differ regarding risk factors, disease indicators, and protective factors. However, both forms consider caries experience – carious lesions and/or new restorations within the last 3 years – as the strongest future caries predictor [157, 165].

References

1. Moussa R, Alghazaly A, Althagafi N, Eshky R, Borzangy S. Effectiveness of virtual reality and interactive simulators on dental education outcomes: systematic review. Eur J Dent. 2022;16(1):14–31. https://doi.org/10.1055/s--0041-1731837. Epub 2021 Aug 24. PMID: 34428851; PMCID: PMC8890935.
2. Jasinevicius TR, Landers M, Nelson S, Urbankova A. An evaluation of two dental simulation systems: virtual reality versus contemporary non-computer-assisted. J Dent Educ. 2004;68(11):1151–62. PMID: 15520234.
3. Zafar S, Siddiqi A, Yasir M, Zachar JJ. Pedagogical development in local anaesthetic training in paediatric dentistry using virtual reality simulator. Eur Arch Paediatr Dent. 2021;22(4):667–74. https://doi.org/10.1007/s40368-021-00604-7. Epub 2021 Feb 10. PMID: 33566287; PMCID: PMC7874567.
4. Dixon J, Towers A, Martin N, Field J. Re-defining the virtual reality dental simulator: demonstrating concurrent validity of clinically relevant assessment and feedback. Eur J Dent Educ. 2021;25(1):108–16. https://doi.org/10.1111/eje.12581. Epub 2020 Aug 28. PMID: 32780500.
5. Mladenovic R, Dakovic D, Pereira L, Matvijenko V, Mladenovic K. Effect of augmented reality simulation on administration of local anaesthesia in paediatric patients. Eur J Dent Educ. 2020;24(3):507–12. https://doi.org/10.1111/eje.12529. Epub 2020 Apr 13. PMID: 32243051.
6. Xia P, Lopes AM, Restivo MT. Virtual reality and haptics for dental surgery: a personal review. Vis Comput. 2013;29:433–47.
7. Zafar S, Lai Y, Sexton C, Siddiqi A. Virtual reality as a novel educational tool in pre-clinical paediatric dentistry training: students' perceptions. Int J Paediatr Dent. 2020;30(6):791–7. https://doi.org/10.1111/ipd.12648. Epub 2020 May 4. PMID: 32274838.
8. Wang D, Li T, Zhang Y, Hou J. Survey on multisensory feedback virtual reality dental training systems. Eur J Dent Educ. 2016;20(4):248–60. https://doi.org/10.1111/eje.12173. Epub 2015 Nov 7. PMID: 26547278.
9. Buchanan JA. Use of simulation technology in dental education. J Dent Educ. 2001;65(11):1225–31. PMID: 11765868.
10. Joda T, Gallucci GO, Wismeijer D, Zitzmann NU. Augmented and virtual reality in dental medicine: a systematic review. Comput Biol Med. 2019;108:93–100. https://doi.org/10.1016/j.compbiomed.2019.03.012. Epub 2019 Mar 15. PMID: 31003184.

11. Pottle J. Virtual reality and the transformation of medical education. Future Healthc J. 2019;6(3):181–5. https://doi.org/10.7861/fhj.2019-0036. PMID: 31660522; PMCID: PMC6798020.
12. Farronato M, Maspero C, Lanteri V, Fama A, Ferrati F, Pettenuzzo A, Farronato D. Current state of the art in the use of augmented reality in dentistry: a systematic review of the literature. BMC Oral Health. 2019;19(1):135. https://doi.org/10.1186/s12903-019-0808-3. PMID: 31286904; PMCID: PMC6613250.
13. Leleve A, Mcdaniel T, Rossa C. Haptic training simulation. Front Virtual Real. 2020;1(3):1–6. https://doi.org/10.3389/frvir.2020.00003.
14. Konukseven EI, Onder ME, Mumcuoglu E, Kisnisci RS. Development of a visio-haptic integrated dental training simulation system. J Dent Educ. 2010;74(8):880–91. PMID: 20679458.
15. Yoshida Y, Yamaguchi S, Kawamoto Y, Noborio H, Murakami S, Sohmura T. Development of a multi-layered virtual tooth model for the haptic dental training system. Dent Mater J. 2011;30(1):1–6. https://doi.org/10.4012/dmj.2010-082. Epub 2011 Jan 26. PMID: 21282895.
16. Ranta JF, Aviles WA. The virtual reality dental training system—simulating dental procedures for the purpose of training dental students using haptics. Presentation at the Fourth Phantom Users Group Workshop, November 1999.
17. Thomas G, Johnson L, Dow S, Stanford C. The design and testing of a force feedback dental simulator. Comput Methods Prog Biomed. 2001;64(1):53–64. https://doi.org/10.1016/s0169-2607(00)00089-4. PMID: 11084233.
18. Luciano C, Banerjee P, DeFanti T. Haptics-based virtual reality periodontal training simulator. Virtual Reality. 2009;13:69–85.
19. Tse B, Harwin W, Barrow A, Quinn B, San Diego JP, Cox M. Design and development of a haptic dental training system—HapTEL. In: Presentation at EuroHaptics international conference on generating and perceiving tangible sensations 2010, Amsterdam, July 8–10, 2010.
20. Simodont. n.d. https://www.simodontdentaltrainer.com/. Accessed 20 Dec 2022.
21. Virteasy Dental Haptic Simulator. n.d. https://virteasy.com/dental/. Accessed 20 Dec 2022.
22. Pinkham JR, Berg JH. The practical importance of pediatric dentistry. In: Pinkham JR, Casamassimo PS, Fields HW, McTigue D, Nowak A, editors. Pediatric dentistry: infancy through adolescence. 4th ed. Amsterdam: Elsevier; 2005. p. 2–8.
23. Perry S, Bridges SM, Burrow MF. A review of the use of simulation in dental education. Simul Healthc. 2015;10(1):31–7. https://doi.org/10.1097/SIH.0000000000000059. PMID: 25574865.
24. Allen KD, Wallace DP. Management of children's distress and disruptions during dental treatment I. In: Mostofsky DI, Fortune F, editors. Behavioral dentistry. 2nd ed. Hoboken: Wiley Blackwell; 2013. p. 209–28.
25. Papadopoulos L, Pentzou A, Louloudiadis K, Tsiatsos T. Design and evaluation of a simulation for pediatric dentistry in virtual worlds. J Med Internet Res. 2013;15(10):e240. https://doi.org/10.2196/jmir.2651.
26. Brill WA. Child behavior in a private pediatric dental practice associated with types of visits, age and socio-economic factors. J Clin Pediatr Dent. 2000;25(1):1–7. https://doi.org/10.17796/jcpd.25.1.545025p1g72x730q. PMID: 11314346.
27. Boynton JR, Green TG, Johnson LA, Nainar SM, Straffon LH. The virtual child: evaluation of an internet-based pediatric behavior management simulation. J Dent Educ. 2007;71(9):1187–93. PMID: 17761625.
28. Hu S, Lai BWP. Increasing empathy for children in dental students using virtual reality. Int J Paediatr Dent. 2022;32(6):793–800. https://doi.org/10.1111/ipd.12957. Epub 2022 May 5. PMID: 35146818.
29. Dye BA. The global burden of oral disease: research and public health significance. J Dent Res. 2017;96(4):361–3. https://doi.org/10.1177/0022034517693567. Epub 2017 Feb 1. PMID: 28318392; PMCID: PMC6728669.
30. Peres MA, Macpherson LMD, Weyant RJ, Daly B, Venturelli R, Mathur MR, Listl S, Celeste RK, Guarnizo-Herreño CC, Kearns C, Benzian H, Allison P, Watt RG. Oral diseases: a global public health challenge. Lancet. 2019;394(10194):249–60. https://doi.org/10.1016/S0140-6736(19)31146-8. Erratum in: Lancet 2019 Sep 21;394(10203):1010. PMID: 31327369.
31. Petersen PE. The burden of oral disease: challenges to improving oral health in the 21st century. Bull World Health Organ. 2005;83(1):3. Epub 2005 Jan 21. PMID: 15682238; PMCID: PMC2623460.
32. Marcenes W, Kassebaum NJ, Bernabé E, Flaxman A, Naghavi M, Lopez A, Murray CJ. Global burden of oral conditions in 1990–2010: a systematic analysis. J Dent Res. 2013;92(7):592–7. https://doi.org/10.1177/0022034513490168. Epub 2013 May 29. PMID: 23720570; PMCID: PMC4484374.
33. World Health Organization. Global oral health status report: towards universal health coverage for oral health by 2030. Geneva. Licence: CC BY-NC-SA 3.0 IGO. 2022. https://www.who.int/publications/i/item/9789240061484. Accessed 20 Dec 2022.
34. GBD 2017 Oral Disorders Collaborators, Bernabe E, Marcenes W, Hernandez CR, Bailey J, Abreu LG, Alipour V, Amini S, Arabloo J, Arefi Z, Arora A, Ayanore MA, Bärnighausen TW, Bijani A, Cho DY, Chu DT, Crowe CS, Demoz GT, Demsie DG, Dibaji Forooshani ZS, Du M, El Tantawi M, Fischer F, Folayan MO, Futran ND, Geramo YCD, Haj-Mirzaian A, Hariyani N, Hasanzadeh A, Hassanipour S, Hay SI, Hole MK, Hostiuc S, Ilic MD, James SL, Kalhor R, Kemmer L, Keramati M, Khader YS, Kisa S, Kisa

A, Koyanagi A, Lalloo R, Le Nguyen Q, London SD, Manohar ND, Massenburg BB, Mathur MR, Meles HG, Mestrovic T, Mohammadian-Hafshejani A, Mohammadpourhodki R, Mokdad AH, Morrison SD, Nazari J, Nguyen TH, Nguyen CT, Nixon MR, Olagunju TO, Pakshir K, Pathak M, Rabiee N, Rafiei A, Ramezanzadeh K, Rios-Blancas MJ, Roro EM, Sabour S, Samy AM, Sawhney M, Schwendicke F, Shaahmadi F, Shaikh MA, Stein C, Tovani-Palone MR, Tran BX, Unnikrishnan B, Vu GT, Vukovic A, Warouw TSS, Zaidi Z, Zhang ZJ, Kassebaum NJ. Global, regional, and national levels and trends in burden of oral conditions from 1990 to 2017: a systematic analysis for the global burden of disease 2017 study. J Dent Res. 2020;99(4):362–73. https://doi.org/10.1177/0022034520908533. Epub 2020 Mar 2. PMID: 32122215; PMCID: PMC7088322.

35. Watt RG, Daly B, Allison P, Macpherson LMD, Venturelli R, Listl S, Weyant RJ, Mathur MR, Guarnizo-Herreño CC, Celeste RK, Peres MA, Kearns C, Benzian H. Ending the neglect of global oral health: time for radical action. Lancet. 2019;394(10194):261–72. https://doi.org/10.1016/S0140-6736(19)31133-X. PMID: 31327370.
36. World Health Organization. Oral health. Key facts. 2022. https://www.who.int/news-room/fact-sheets/detail/oral-health. Accessed 20 Dec 2022.
37. Bracksley-O'Grady S, Anderson K, Masood M. Oral health academics' conceptualisation of health promotion and perceived barriers and opportunities in dental practice: a qualitative study. BMC Oral Health. 2021;21(1):165. https://doi.org/10.1186/s12903-021-01508-0. PMID: 33771160; PMCID: PMC8004464.
38. World Dental Federation. The challenge of oral disease—a call for global action. The oral health atlas. 2nd ed. Geneva. 2015. https://www.fdiworlddental.org/sites/default/files/2021-03/complete_oh_atlas-2_0.pdf. Accessed 20 Dec 2022.
39. Watt RG, Sheiham A. Integrating the common risk factor approach into a social determinants framework. Community Dent Oral Epidemiol. 2012;40(4):289–96. https://doi.org/10.1111/j.1600--0528.2012.00680.x. Epub 2012 Mar 20. PMID: 22429083.
40. Strippel H. Oral health promotion. In: Kirch W, editor. Encyclopedia of public health. Dordrecht: Springer; 2008. p. 1049–52.
41. Fraihat N, Madae'en S, Bencze Z, Herczeg A, Varga O. Clinical effectiveness and cost-effectiveness of oral-health promotion in dental caries prevention among children: systematic review and meta-analysis. Int J Environ Res Public Health. 2019;16(15):2668. https://doi.org/10.3390/ijerph16152668. PMID: 31349691; PMCID: PMC6696287.
42. Ghaffari M, Rakhshanderou S, Ramezankhani A, Noroozi M, Armoon B. Oral health education and promotion programmes: meta-analysis of 17-year intervention. Int J Dent Hyg. 2018;16(1):59–67. https://doi.org/10.1111/idh.12304. Epub 2017 Aug 24. PMID: 28836347.
43. Tsai C, Raphael S, Agnew C, McDonald G, Irving M. Health promotion interventions to improve oral health of adolescents: a systematic review and meta-analysis. Community Dent Oral Epidemiol. 2020;48(6):549–60. https://doi.org/10.1111/cdoe.12567. Epub 2020 Aug 7. PMID: 32767825.
44. Nakre PD, Harikiran AG. Effectiveness of oral health education programs: a systematic review. J Int Soc Prev Community Dent. 2013;3(2):103–15. https://doi.org/10.4103/2231-0762.127810.
45. Wang K, Yu KF, Liu P, Lee GHM, Wong MCM. Can mHealth promotion for parents help to improve their children's oral health? A systematic review. J Dent. 2022;123:104185. https://doi.org/10.1016/j.jdent.2022.104185. Epub 2022 Jun 9. PMID: 35691452.
46. International Telecommunication Union (ITU). Facts and figures 2022. 2022. https://www.itu.int/itu-d/reports/statistics/facts-figures-2022/. Accessed 20 Dec 2022.
47. Fernández CE, Maturana CA, Coloma SI, Carrasco-Labra A, Giacaman RA. Teledentistry and mHealth for promotion and prevention of oral health: a systematic review and meta-analysis. J Dent Res. 2021;100(9):914–27. https://doi.org/10.1177/00220345211003828. Epub 2021 Mar 26. PMID: 33769123.
48. World Health Organization. WHO Global Observatory for eHealth. mHealth: new horizons for health through mobile technologies: second global survey on eHealth. Geneva. 2011. https://apps.who.int/iris/handle/10665/44607. Accessed 20 Dec 2022.
49. Toniazzo MP, Nodari D, Muniz FWMG, Weidlich P. Effect of mHealth in improving oral hygiene: a systematic review with meta-analysis. J Clin Periodontol. 2019;46(3):297–309. https://doi.org/10.1111/jcpe.13083. PMID: 30761580.
50. Hashemian TS, Kritz-Silverstein D, Baker R. Text2Floss: the feasibility and acceptability of a text messaging intervention to improve oral health behavior and knowledge. J Public Health Dent. 2015;75(1):34–41. https://doi.org/10.1111/jphd.12068. Epub 2014 Aug 4. PMID: 25091471.
51. Lee M, Lee H, Kim Y, Kim J, Cho M, Jang J, Jang H. Mobile app-based health promotion programs: a systematic review of the literature. Int J Environ Res Public Health. 2018;15(12):2838. https://doi.org/10.3390/ijerph15122838. PMID: 30551555; PMCID: PMC6313530.
52. Sharif MO, Newton T, Cunningham SJ. A systematic review to assess interventions delivered by mobile phones in improving adherence to oral hygiene advice for children and adolescents. Br Dent J. 2019;227(5):375–82. https://doi.org/10.1038/s41415-019-0660-5. PMID: 31520040.
53. Fijačko N, Gosak L, Cilar L, Novšak A, Creber RM, Skok P, Štiglic G. The effects of gamification and

oral self-care on oral hygiene in children: systematic search in app stores and evaluation of apps. JMIR Mhealth Uhealth. 2020;8(7):e16365. https://doi.org/10.2196/16365. PMID: 32673235; PMCID: PMC7381071.

54. Kaczmarczyk KH, Gray-Burrows KA, Vinall-Collier K, Day PF. Oral health promotion apps: an assessment of message and behaviour change potential. Int J Qual Health Care. 2021;33(1):mzaa112. https://doi.org/10.1093/intqhc/mzaa112. PMID: 32909613.
55. Chen R, Santo K, Wong G, Sohn W, Spallek H, Chow C, Irving M. Mobile apps for dental caries prevention: systematic search and quality evaluation. JMIR Mhealth Uhealth. 2021;9(1):e19958. https://doi.org/10.2196/19958. PMID: 33439141; PMCID: PMC7840287.
56. Underwood B, Birdsall J, Kay E. The use of a mobile app to motivate evidence-based oral hygiene behaviour. Br Dent J. 2015;219(4):E2. https://doi.org/10.1038/sj.bdj.2015.660. PMID: 26315196.
57. McGrath C. Behavioral sciences in the promotion of oral health. J Dent Res. 2019;98(13):1418–24. https://doi.org/10.1177/0022034519873842. PMID: 31746683.
58. Dennison L, Morrison L, Conway G, Yardley L. Opportunities and challenges for smartphone applications in supporting health behavior change: qualitative study. J Med Internet Res. 2013;15(4):e86. https://doi.org/10.2196/jmir.2583. PMID: 23598614; PMCID: PMC3636318.
59. Antezana G, Venning A, Blake V, Smith D, Winsall M, Orlowski S, Bidargaddi N. An evaluation of behaviour change techniques in health and lifestyle mobile applications. Health Informatics J. 2020;26(1):104–13. https://doi.org/10.1177/1460458218813726. Epub 2018 Nov 30. PMID: 30501364.
60. Scheerman JFM, van Empelen P, van Loveren C, van Meijel B. A mobile app (whiteteeth) to promote good oral health behavior among Dutch adolescents with fixed orthodontic appliances: intervention mapping approach. JMIR Mhealth Uhealth. 2018;6(8):e163. https://doi.org/10.2196/mhealth.9626. PMID: 30120085; PMCID: PMC6119215.
61. Scheerman JFM, van Meijel B, van Empelen P, Verrips GHW, van Loveren C, Twisk JWR, Pakpour AH, van den Braak MCT, Kramer GJC. The effect of using a mobile application ("WhiteTeeth") on improving oral hygiene: a randomized controlled trial. Int J Dent Hyg. 2020;18(1):73–83. https://doi.org/10.1111/idh.12415. Epub 2019 Aug 9. PMID: 31291683; PMCID: PMC7004072.
62. Pitts NB. Diagnostic tools and measurements—impact on appropriate care. Community Dent Oral Epidemiol. 1997;25(1):24–35. https://doi.org/10.1111/j.1600-0528.1997.tb00896.x. PMID: 9088689.
63. Bader JD, Shugars DA, Bonito AJ. Systematic reviews of selected dental caries diagnostic and management methods. J Dent Educ. 2001;65(10):960–8. PMID: 11699997.
64. Selwitz RH, Ismail AI, Pitts NB. Dental caries. Lancet. 2007;369(9555):51–9. https://doi.org/10.1016/S0140-6736(07)60031-2. PMID: 17208642.
65. Bader JD, Shugars DA, Bonito AJ. A systematic review of the performance of methods for identifying carious lesions. J Public Health Dent. 2002;62(4):201–13. https://doi.org/10.1111/j.1752-7325.2002.tb03446.x. PMID: 12474624.
66. Kühnisch J, Bücher K, Hickel R. The intra/inter-examiner reproducibility of the new DIAGNOdent Pen on occlusal sites. J Dent. 2007;35(6):509–12. https://doi.org/10.1016/j.jdent.2007.02.001. Epub 2007 Mar 28. PMID: 17395355.
67. White SC, Pharoah MJ. Oral radiology: principles and interpretation. 5th ed. Toronto: Mosby; 2004. p. 297–313.
68. Abdelaziz M, Krejci I, Perneger T, Feilzer A, & Vazquez L. Near infrared transillumination compared with radiography to detect and monitor proximal caries: a clinical retrospective study. J Dent, 2018;70:40–45.
69. Russotto F, Tirone F, Salzano S, Borga FC, Paolino D, Ferraro A, & Botasso S. Clinical evaluation of near-infrared light transillumination (NIRT) as an interproximal caries detection tool in a large sample of patients in a private practice. J Radiol Imaging, 2016;1(1):1-5.
70. Schwendicke F, Tzschoppe M, Paris S. Radiographic caries detection: a systematic review and meta-analysis. J Dent. 2015;43(8):924–33. https://doi.org/10.1016/j.jdent.2015.02.009. Epub 2015 Feb 24. Erratum in: J Dent. 2021 Nov;114:103783. PMID: 25724114.
71. Zandoná AF, Zero DT. Diagnostic tools for early caries detection. J Am Dent Assoc. 2006;137(12):1675–84. https://doi.org/10.14219/jada.archive.2006.0113; quiz 1730. Erratum in: J Am Dent Assoc. 2007 Mar;138(3):298. PMID: 17138712.
72. AAPD. Prescribing dental radiographs for infants, children, adolescents, and individuals with special health care needs. Pediatr Dent. 2017;39(6):205–7. PMID: 29179358.
73. Gündüz K, Çelenk P. Çürük anısında kullanılan yeni yöntemler. Cumhuriyet Üniversitesi Diş Hekimliği Fakültesi Dergisi. 2003;6:1.
74. Mialhe FL, Pereira AC, Meneghim Mde C, Ambrosano GM, Pardi V. The relative diagnostic yields of clinical, FOTI and radiographic examinations for the detection of approximal caries in youngsters. Indian J Dent Res. 2009;20(2):136–40. https://doi.org/10.4103/0970-9290.52881. PMID: 19553711.
75. Angmar-Månsson B, ten Bosch JJ. Advances in methods for diagnosing coronal caries—a review. Adv Dent Res. 1993;7(2):70–9. https://doi.org/10.1177/08959374930070021801. PMID: 8260014.
76. Peers A, Hill FJ, Mitropoulos CM, Holloway PJ. Validity and reproducibility of clinical examination, fibre-optic transillumination, and

bite-wing radiology for the diagnosis of small approximal carious lesions: an in vitro study. Caries Res. 1993;27(4):307–11. https://doi.org/10.1159/000261556. PMID: 8402807.
77. Rankovic JM, Kapor S, Khazaei Y, Crispin A, Schüler I, Krause F, Ekstrand K, Michou S, Eggmann F, Lussi A, Huysmans MC, Neuhaus K, Kühnisch J. Systematic review and meta-analysis of diagnostic studies of proximal surface caries. Clin Oral Investig. 2021;25(11):6069–79. https://doi.org/10.1007/s00784-021-04113-1. Epub 2021 Sep 4. PMID: 34480645; PMCID: PMC8531083.
78. Astvaldsdóttir A, Ahlund K, Holbrook WP, de Verdier B, Tranæus S. Approximal caries detection by DIFOTI: in vitro comparison of diagnostic accuracy/efficacy with film and digital radiography. Int J Dent. 2012;2012:326401. https://doi.org/10.1155/2012/326401. Epub 2012 Nov 4. PMID: 23213335; PMCID: PMC3508587.
79. Bin-Shuwaish M, et al. Estimation of clinical axial extension of Class II caries lesions with ultraspeed and digital radiographs: an in-vivo study. Oper Dent. 2008;33(6):613–21.
80. Antipoviene A, Girijotaite M, Bendoraitiene EA. Assessment of the depth of clinically detected approximal caries lesions using digital imaging fiber-optic transillumination in comparison to periapical radiographs. J Oral Maxillofac Res. 2020;11(1):e3. https://doi.org/10.5037/jomr.2020.11103. PMID: 32377327; PMCID: PMC7191380.
81. Lara-Capi C, Cagetti MG, Lingström P, Lai G, Cocco F, Simark-Mattsson C, Campus G. Digital transillumination in caries detection versus radiographic and clinical methods: an in-vivo study. Dentomaxillofac Radiol. 2017;46(4):20160417.
82. Gürses M, Ünlü N. Okluzal çürük teşhis yöntemlerine güncel bakış. Selcuk Dent J. 2017;4(3):153–61.
83. Korkut B, Tağtekin DA, Yanıkoğlu FÇ. Diş çürüklerinin erken teşhisi ve teşhiste yeni yöntemler: QLF, Diagnodent, Elektriksel İletkenlik ve Ultrasonik Sistem. Ege Üniversitesi Diş Hekimliği Fakültesi Dergisi. 2011;32(2):55–67.
84. Sailer R, Paulus R, Hibst R. Analysis of carious lesions and subgingival calculi by fluorescence spectroscopy. Caries Res. 2001;35(4):267.
85. Choo-Smith LP, Dong CC, Cleghorn B, Hewko M. Shedding new light on early caries detection. J Can Dent Assoc. 2008;74(10):913–8. PMID: 19126361; PMCID: PMC2700544.
86. Tam LE, McComb D. Diagnosis of occlusal caries: part II. Recent diagnostic technologies. J Can Dent Assoc. 2001;67(8):459–64.
87. Lenzi TL, Piovesan C, Mendes FM, Braga MM, Raggio DP. In vitro performance of QLF system and conventional methods for detection of occlusal caries around tooth-colored restorations in primary molars. Int J Paediatr Dent. 2016;26(1):26–34. https://doi.org/10.1111/ipd.12154. Epub 2015 Jan 21. PMID: 25604208.
88. Jablonski-Momeni A, Heinzel-Gutenbrunner M, Klein SM. In vivo performance of the VistaProof fluorescence-based camera for detection of occlusal lesions. Clin Oral Investig. 2014;18:1757–62.
89. Lussi A, Hibst R, Paulus R. DIAGNOdent: an optical method for caries detection. J Dent Res. 2004;83 Spec No C:C80–3. https://doi.org/10.1177/154405910408301s16. PMID: 15286128.
90. Lussi A, Imwinkelried S, Pitts N, Longbottom C, Reich E. Performance and reproducibility of a laser fluorescence system for detection of occlusal caries in vitro. Caries Res. 1999;33(4):261–6. https://doi.org/10.1159/000016527. PMID: 10343088.
91. Lussi A, Megert B, Longbottom C, Reich E, Francescut P. Clinical performance of a laser fluorescence device for detection of occlusal caries lesions. Eur J Oral Sci. 2001;109(1):14–9. https://doi.org/10.1034/j.1600-0722.2001.109001014.x. PMID: 11330928.
92. Shi XQ, Welander U, Angmar-Månsson B. Occlusal caries detection with KaVo DIAGNOdent and radiography: an in vitro comparison. Caries Res. 2000;34(2):151–8. https://doi.org/10.1159/000016583. PMID: 10773633.
93. Olgen IC, Sonmez H, Bezgin T. Effects of different remineralization agents on MIH defects: a randomized clinical study. Clin Oral Investig. 2022;26(3):3227–38. https://doi.org/10.1007/s00784-021-04305-9. Epub 2021 Nov 25. PMID: 34821978.
94. De Benedetto MS, Morais CC, Novaes TF, de Almeida Rodrigues J, Braga MM, Mendes FM. Comparing the reliability of a new fluorescence camera with conventional laser fluorescence devices in detecting caries lesions in occlusal and smooth surfaces of primary teeth. Lasers Med Sci. 2011;26(2):157–62. https://doi.org/10.1007/s10103-010-0757-1. Epub 2010 Feb 16. PMID: 20157753.
95. Huth KC, Neuhaus KW, Gygax M, Bücher K, Crispin A, Paschos E, Hickel R, Lussi A. Clinical performance of a new laser fluorescence device for detection of occlusal caries lesions in permanent molars. J Dent. 2008;36(12):1033–40. https://doi.org/10.1016/j.jdent.2008.08.013. Epub 2008 Oct 18. PMID: 18930575.
96. Rodrigues JA, Hug I, Diniz MB, Lussi A. Performance of fluorescence methods, radiographic examination and ICDAS II on occlusal surfaces in vitro. Caries Res. 2008;42(4):297–304. https://doi.org/10.1159/000148162. Epub 2008 Jul 29. PMID: 18663299.
97. Subka S, Rodd H, Nugent Z, & Deery C. In vivo validity of proximal caries detection in primary teeth, with histological validation. International journal of paediatric dentistry, 2019;29(4):429–38.
98. Akyıldız E, Özalp N. Diagnosis of early dental caries by traditional, contemporary and developing imaging methods. EADS. 2022;49(1):38–45.

99. Strassler HE, Sensi LG. Technology-enhanced caries detection and diagnosis. Compend Contin Educ Dent. 2008;29(8):464–5, 468, 470 passim. PMID: 18935786.
100. Aktan AM, Cebe ME, Ciftci Me, Sirin Karaarslan E. A novel LED based device for occlusal caries detection. Lasers Med Sci. 2012;27:1157–63.
101. Ricketts DN, Kidd EA, Liepins PJ, Wilson RF. Histological validation of electrical resistance measurements in the diagnosis of occlusal caries. Caries Res. 1996;30(2):148–55. https://doi.org/10.1159/000262152. PMID: 8833140.
102. Longbottom C, Huysmans MC. Electrical measurements for use in caries clinical trials. J Dent Res. 2004;83 Spec No C:C76–9. https://doi.org/10.1177/154405910408301s15. PMID: 15286127.
103. Huysmans MC, Longbottom C, Pitts NB, Los P, Bruce PG. Impedance spectroscopy of teeth with and without approximal caries lesions—an in vitro study. J Dent Res. 1996;75(11):1871–8. https://doi.org/10.1177/00220345960750110901. PMID: 9003234.
104. Akgul S, Bala O, Yikilgan I. Performance of different methods for detection of incipient occlusal caries lesions: an in vitro study. Photomed Laser Surg. 2018;36(4):191–7.
105. Mandurah MM, Sadr A, Shimada Y, Kitasako Y, Nakashima S, Bakhsh TA, Tagami J, Sumi Y. Monitoring remineralization of enamel subsurface lesions by optical coherence tomography. J Biomed Opt. 2013;18(4):046006. https://doi.org/10.1117/1.JBO.18.4.046006. PMID: 23563920.
106. Tezuka H, Shimada Y, Matin K, Ikeda M, Sadr A, Sumi Y, Tagami J. Assessment of cervical demineralization induced by Streptococcus mutans using swept-source optical coherence tomography. J Med Imaging (Bellingham). 2016;3(1):014504. https://doi.org/10.1117/1.JMI.3.1.014504. Epub 2016 Mar 8. PMID: 27014718; PMCID: PMC4782037.
107. Amaechi BT, Podoleanu AG, Komarov G, Higham SM, Jackson DA. Quantification of root caries using optical coherence tomography and microradiography: a correlational study. Oral Health Prev Dent. 2004;2(4):377–82. PMID: 16296256.
108. Ergücü Z, Türkün LŞ. Çürükle ilgili klinik çalışmalarda kurgulama, yürütme ve analiz yöntemleri. Hacettepe Dişhekimliği Fakültesi Derg. 2007;31(1):25–35.
109. Otis LL, Everett MJ, Sathyam US, Colston BW Jr. Optical coherence tomography: a new imaging technology for dentistry. J Am Dent Assoc. 2000;131(4):511–4. https://doi.org/10.14219/jada.archive.2000.0210. PMID: 10770016.
110. Thomas CS, Sharma DS, Sheet D, Mukhopadhyay A, Sharma S. Cross-sectional visual comparison of remineralization efficacy of various agents on early smooth surface caries of primary teeth with swept source optical coherence tomography. J Oral Biol Craniofac Res. 2021;11(4):628–37. https://doi.org/10.1016/j.jobcr.2021.09.006. Epub 2021 Sep 20. PMID: 34603951; PMCID: PMC8473773.
111. Lederer A, Kunzelmann KH, Heck K, Hickel R, Litzenburger F. In vitro validation of near-infrared transillumination at 780 nm for the detection of caries on proximal surfaces. Clin Oral Investig. 2019;23(11):3933–40. https://doi.org/10.1007/s00784-019-02824-0. Epub 2019 Jan 28. PMID: 30693402.
112. Baltacıoğlı IH, Orhan K. Comparison of diagnostic methods for early interproximal caries detection with near-infrared light transillumination: an in vivo study. BMC Oral Health. 2017;17(1):130.
113. Alamoudi NM, Khan JA, El-Ashiry EA, Felemban OM, Bagher SM, Al-Tuwirqi AA. Accuracy of the DIAGNOcam and bite-wing radiographs in the diagnosis of cavitated proximal carious lesions in primary molars. Niger J Clin Pract. 2019;22:1576–82.
114. Alrayyes S, Horn A, Kratunova E, Koerber A. Evaluation of a near-infrared light transillumination device for caries detection in interproximal primary molar surfaces. J Dent Child (Chic). 2021;88(3):180–6. PMID: 34937628.
115. Ng SY, Ferguson MW, Payne PA, Slater P. Ultrasonic studies of unblemished and artificially demineralized enamel in extracted human teeth: a new method for detecting early caries. J Dent. 1988;16(5):201–9. https://doi.org/10.1016/0300-5712(88)90070-x. PMID: 3063732.
116. Yanikoglu FC, Ozturk F, Hayran O, Analoui M, Stookey GK. Detection of natural white spot caries lesions by an ultrasonic system. Caries Res. 2000;34(3):225.
117. Fontana M, Yanıkoğlu FÇ, Özturk F. Comparison of QLF, ultrasound and confocal microscopy in the measurement of remineralization. Caries Res. 1999;33:357–65.
118. Zhou W, Qiao Z, Nazarzadeh Zare E, Huang J, Zheng X, Sun X, Shao M, Wang H, Wang X, Chen D, Zheng J, Fang S, Li YM, Zhang X, Yang L, Makvandi P, Wu A. 4D-printed dynamic materials in biomedical applications: chemistry, challenges, and their future perspectives in the clinical sector. J Med Chem. 2020;63(15):8003–24. https://doi.org/10.1021/acs.jmedchem.9b02115. Epub 2020 Apr 17. PMID: 32255358.
119. Hazra Y, Rao A, Suprabha BS. 3-D printing: its applications in pediatric dental practice: a review of literature. Indian J Contemp Dent. 2022;10(2):17–23.
120. Tian Y, Chen C, Xu X, Wang J, Hou X, Li K, Lu X, Shi H, Lee ES, Jiang HB. A review of 3D printing in dentistry: technologies, affecting factors, and applications. Scanning. 2021;2021:9950131. https://doi.org/10.1155/2021/9950131. PMID: 34367410; PMCID: PMC8313360.
121. Kalaivanan D, Kalimreddy P, Kodical SR, Ramasetty AP. Three dimensional printing—from a pediatric dentist's perspective: 3D printing in pediatric dentistry—a literature review. Int J Pedod Rehabil. 2022;7(1):42–9.

122. Burhardt L, Livas C, Kerdijk W, van der Meer WJ, Ren Y. Treatment comfort, time perception, and preference for conventional and digital impression techniques: a comparative study in young patients. Am J Orthod Dentofac Orthop. 2016;150(2):261–7.
123. Yılmaz H, Aydın MN. Digital versus conventional impression method in children: Comfort, preference and time. International J Pediatr Dent. 2019;29(6):728-735.
124. Fleming PS, Marinho V, Johal A. Orthodontic measurements on digital study models compared with plaster models: a systematic review. Orthod Craniofac Res. 2011;14(1):1–16. https://doi.org/10.1111/j.1601-6343.2010.01503.x. Epub 2010 Nov 22. PMID: 21205164.
125. Grünheid T, McCarthy SD, Larson BE. Clinical use of a direct chairside oral scanner: an assessment of accuracy, time, and patient acceptance. Am J Orthod Dentofac Orthop. 2014;146(5):673–82. https://doi.org/10.1016/j.ajodo.2014.07.023. Epub 2014 Oct 28. PMID: 25439218.
126. Garino F, Garino GB. Comparison of dental arch measurements between stone and digital casts. World J Orthod. 2002;3(3):250–4.
127. Logozzo S, Franceschini G, Kilpelä A, Caponi M, Governi L, Blois L. A comparative analysis of intraoral 3D digital scanners for restorative dentistry. Internet J Med Technol. 2011;5(1):1–2.
128. Patzelt SB, Lamprinos C, Stampf S, Att W. The time efficiency of intraoral scanners: an in vitro comparative study. J Am Dent Assoc. 2014;145(6):542–51. https://doi.org/10.14219/jada.2014.23. PMID: 24878708.
129. Dhanotra KG, Bhatıa R. Digitainers—digital space maintainers: a review. Int J Clin Pediatr Dent. 2021;14(Suppl 1):S69.
130. Soni HK. Application of CAD-CAM for fabrication of metal-free band and loop space maintainer. J Clin Diagn Res. 2017;11(2):ZD14–6. https://doi.org/10.7860/JCDR/2017/23459.9246. Epub 2017 Feb 1. PMID: 28384989; PMCID: PMC5376843.
131. Khanna S, Rao D, Panwar S, Pawar BA, Ameen S. 3D printed band and loop space maintainer: a digital game changer in preventive orthodontics. J Clin Pediatr Dent. 2021;45(3):147–51. https://doi.org/10.17796/1053-4625-45.3.1. PMID: 34192758.
132. Pawar BA. Maintenance of space by innovative three-dimensional-printed band and loop space maintainer. J Indian Soc Pedod Prev Dent. 2019;37(2):205–8. https://doi.org/10.4103/JISPPD.JISPPD_9_19. PMID: 31249187.
133. Tokuc M, Yilmaz H. Comparison of fit accuracy between conventional and CAD/CAM-fabricated band-loop space maintainers. Int J Paediatr Dent. 2022;32(5):764–71. https://doi.org/10.1111/ipd.12955. Epub 2022 May 20. PMID: 35122341.
134. Ierardo G, Luzzi V, Lesti M, Vozza I, Brugnoletti O, Polimeni A, Bossù M. Peek polymer in orthodontics: a pilot study on children. J Clin Exp Dent. 2017;9(10):e1271–5. https://doi.org/10.4317/jced.54010. PMID: 29167720; PMCID: PMC5694159.
135. Kun J, Dinggui Z, Wei L, Li D, Wang X, Jing JL, Wu G. Clinical application of digital space maintainer fabricated by polyetherketoneketone for premature loss of deciduous teeth [J/CD]. Chin J Stomatol. 2019;13:368–72.
136. Demirel A, Bezgin T, Akaltan F, Sarı Ş. Resin nanoceramic CAD/CAM restoration of the primary molar: 3-year follow-up study. Case Rep Dent. 2017;2017:3517187. https://doi.org/10.1155/2017/3517187. Epub 2017 Jun 20. PMID: 28713601; PMCID: PMC5496112.
137. Ruse ND, Sadoun MJ. Resin-composite blocks for dental CAD/CAM applications. J Dent Res. 2014;93(12):1232–4. https://doi.org/10.1177/0022034514553976. Epub 2014 Oct 24. PMID: 25344335; PMCID: PMC4462808.
138. Güzel KU, Akarçay Ç. İntraoral Tarayıcı ve Cad/Cam Sistemlerinin Çocuk Diş Hekimliğinde Kullanım Alanları. ADO Klinik Bilimler Dergisi. 2022;11(1):78–84.
139. Oguz EI, Bezgin T, Orhan AI, Orhan K. Comparative evaluation of adaptation of esthetic prefabricated fiberglass and CAD/CAM crowns for primary teeth: microcomputed tomography analysis. Biomed Res Int. 2021;2021:1011661. https://doi.org/10.1155/2021/1011661. PMID: 34616841; PMCID: PMC8487845.
140. Oğuz EI, Bezgin T, Işil Orhan A, Buyuksungur A, Orhan K. Fracture resistance of esthetic prefabricated and custom-made crowns for primary molars after artificial aging. Pediatr Dent. 2022;44(5):368–74. PMID: 36309781.
141. Dursun E, Monnier-Da Costa A, Moussally C. Chairside CAD/CAM composite onlays for the restoration of primary molars. J Clin Pediatr Dent. 2018;42(5):349–54. https://doi.org/10.17796/1053-4625-42.5.5. Epub 2018 May 15. PMID: 29763356.
142. Mittal HC, Goyal A, Gauba K, Kapur A. Clinical performance of indirect composite onlays as esthetic alternative to stainless steel crowns for rehabilitation of a large carious primary molar. J Clin Pediatr Dent. 2016;40(5):345–52. https://doi.org/10.17796/1053-4628-40.5.345. PMID: 27617373.
143. Bilgin MS, Erdem A, Tanrıver M. CAD/CAM endocrown fabrication from a polymer-infiltrated ceramic network block for primary molar: a case report. J Clin Pediatr Dent. 2016;40(4):264–8. https://doi.org/10.17796/1053-4628-40.4.264. PMID: 27471802.
144. Davidovich E, Dagon S, Tamari I, Etinger M, Mijiritsky E. An innovative treatment approach using digital workflow and CAD-CAM part 2: the restoration of molar incisor hypomineralization in children. Int J Environ Res Public Health. 2020;17(5):1499. https://doi.org/10.3390/ijerph17051499. PMID: 32110963; PMCID: PMC7084897.
145. Halal R, Nohra J, Akel H. Conservative anterior treatment with CAD-CAM technology and polymer-infiltrated ceramic for a child with amelo-

genesis imperfecta: a 2-year follow-up. J Prosthet Dent. 2018;119(5):710–2. https://doi.org/10.1016/j.prosdent.2017.07.018. Epub 2017 Sep 27. PMID: 28967409.
146. Moussally C, Fron-Chabouis H, Charrière A, Maladry L, Dursun E. Full-mouth rehabilitation of hypocalcified-type amelogenesis imperfecta with chairside computer-aided design and computer-aided manufacturing: a case report. Oper Dent. 2019;44(3):E145–58. https://doi.org/10.2341/17--241-T. Epub 2019 Mar 8. PMID: 30849013.
147. Noirrit E, Chabreron O, Nasr K, Esclassan R. A contribution of CAD/CAM treatment of a dental trauma in a special care patient. Spec Care Dentist. 2018;38(1):55–7. https://doi.org/10.1111/scd.12261. Epub 2017 Dec 18. PMID: 29251793.
148. Anssari Moin D, Derksen W, Verweij JP, van Merkesteyn R, Wismeijer D. A novel approach for computer-assisted template-guided autotransplantation of teeth with custom 3D designed/printed surgical tooling. An ex vivo proof of concept. J Oral Maxillofac Surg. 2016;74(5):895–902. https://doi.org/10.1016/j.joms.2016.01.033. Epub 2016 Jan 29. PMID: 26907556.
149. Cahuana-Bartra P, Cahuana-Cárdenas A, Brunet-Llobet L, Ayats-Soler M, Miranda-Rius J, Rivera-Baró A. The use of 3D additive manufacturing technology in autogenous dental transplantation. 3D Print Med. 2020;6(1):16. https://doi.org/10.1186/s41205-020-00070-9. PMID: 32710145; PMCID: PMC7379801.
150. Al-Rimawi A, EzEldeen M, Schneider D, Politis C, Jacobs R. 3D printed temporary veneer restoring autotransplanted teeth in children: design and concept validation ex vivo. Int J Environ Res Public Health. 2019;16(3):496. https://doi.org/10.3390/ijerph16030496. PMID: 30754648; PMCID: PMC6388193.
151. Gathani KM, Raghavendra SS. Scaffolds in regenerative endodontics: a review. Dent Res J (Isfahan). 2016;13(5):379–86. https://doi.org/10.4103/1735-3327.192266. PMID: 27857762; PMCID: PMC5090995.
152. Murray PE, Garcia-Godoy F, Hargreaves KM. Regenerative endodontics: a review of current status and a call for action. J Endod. 2007;33(4):377–90. https://doi.org/10.1016/j.joen.2006.09.013. Epub 2007 Feb 20. PMID: 17368324.
153. Bezgin T, Sönmez H. Review of current concepts of revascularization/revitalization. Dent Traumatol. 2015;31(4):267–73. https://doi.org/10.1111/edt.12177. Epub 2015 May 6. PMID: 25950886.
154. Bezgin T, Yilmaz AD, Celik BN, Kolsuz ME, Sonmez H. Efficacy of platelet-rich plasma as a scaffold in regenerative endodontic treatment. J Endod. 2015;41(1):36–44. https://doi.org/10.1016/j.joen.2014.10.004. Epub 2014 Nov 12. PMID: 25459571.
155. Raddall G, Mello I, Leung BM. Biomaterials and scaffold design strategies for regenerative endodontic therapy. Front Bioeng Biotechnol. 2019;7:317. https://doi.org/10.3389/fbioe.2019.00317. PMID: 31803727; PMCID: PMC6874017.
156. Li S, Xu Y, Yu J, Becker ML. Enhanced osteogenic activity of poly (ester urea) scaffolds using facile post-3D printing peptide functionalization strategies. Biomaterials. 2017;141:176–87.
157. Eden E, editor. Evidence-based caries prevention. Berlin: Springer; 2016.
158. You W, Hao A, Li S, Wang Y, Xia B. Deep learning-based dental plaque detection on primary teeth: a comparison with clinical assessments. BMC Oral Health. 2020;20(1):1–7.
159. Wang Y, Hays RD, Marcus M, Maida CA, Shen J, Xiong D, et al. Developing children's oral health assessment toolkits using machine learning algorithm. JDR Clin Transl Res. 2020;5(3):233–43.
160. Karhade DS, Roach J, Shrestha P, Simancas-Pallares MA, Ginnis J, Burk ZJ, et al. An automated machine learning classifier for early childhood caries. Pediatr Dent. 2021;43(3):191–7.
161. Ramos-Gomez F, Marcus M, Maida CA, Wang Y, Kinsler JJ, Xiong D, et al. Using a machine learning algorithm to predict the likelihood of presence of dental caries among children aged 2 to 7. Dent J. 2021;9(12):141.
162. Schlickenrieder A, Meyer O, Schönewolf J, Engels P, Hickel R, Gruhn V, et al. Automatized detection and categorization of fissure sealants from intraoral digital photographs using artificial intelligence. Diagnostics. 2021;11(9):1608.
163. Zaborowicz K, Biedziak B, Olszewska A, Zaborowicz M. Tooth and bone parameters in the assessment of the chronological age of children and adolescents using neural modelling methods. Sensors. 2021;21(18):6008.
164. Doméjean S, Banerjee A, Featherstone JD. Caries risk/susceptibility assessment: its value in minimum intervention oral healthcare. Br Dent J. 2017;223(3):191–7.
165. Mejàre I, Axelsson S, Dahlën GA, Espelid I, Norlund A, Tranæus S, Twetman S. Caries risk assessment. A systematic review. Acta Odontol Scand. 2014;72(2):81–91.

14 Digital Dentistry Applications in Periodontics

Revan Birke Koca and Kaan Orhan

14.1 Digital Periodontal Indices

14.1.1 Conventional Periodontal Probing

Periodontal diseases are common multifactorial and chronic inflammations. They affect both the soft tissues and the hard tissues surrounding the teeth. There are various periodontal diseases and some concepts have emerged to distinguish them from each other. The most practical and cost-effective of these are periodontal indices. Around the mid-twentieth century, Löe et al. published some parameters that can be evaluated in intraoral examination to distinguish between gingival and periodontal conditions and to observe the effectiveness of the periodontal treatment [1, 2]. While the gingival index (GI) included gingival inflammation, the periodontal index (PI) included the level of clinical attachment loss, the plaque index (PI) the presence/absence of microbial dental plaque at the gingival margin, and the bleeding on probing index (BOP) also included the presence/absence of bleeding in the periodontal pocket [3]. Although many researchers have stated different types of indices over the years, their purpose and basic principles were the same. Values measured by the periodontal probe in the indices are plotted on a standardized periodontal chart (Fig. 14.1). Periodontal values of each patient for each session should be entered on the periodontal chart and the progress between sessions should be followed.

14.1.2 Periodontal Probing on Digital Images

Periodontal pocket depth index is most commonly measured by probing as it is a simple, easily accessible, and economical technique. However, it is invasive although minimally causes temporary bacteremia, takes time, and varies according to the clinician, the measured angle, and the type of probe, has been increased the need for digitalization.

The probing depth (periodontal pocket measurement) and the keratinized tissue width can be measured with the intraoral scanner, which is used in many applications of digital dentistry [4]. The images resulting from an intraoral scan are compared with CBCT sections and the distance between the marginal gingiva and the alveolar crest is measured digitally (Fig. 14.2) [5]. Chung

R. B. Koca (✉)
Department of Periodontology, Faculty of Dentistry, University of Kyrenia, Kyrenia, Cyprus

K. Orhan
Faculty of Dentistry, Ankara University, Ankara, Turkey

Ankara University Medical Design Application and Research Center (MEDITAM), Ankara, Turkey

Department of Oral Diagnostics, Faculty of Dentistry, Semmelweis University, Budapest, Hungary
e-mail: knorhan@dentistry.ankara.edu.tr

A. Delantoni, K. Orhan (eds.), *Digital Dentistry*, https://doi.org/10.1007/978-3-031-52826-2_14

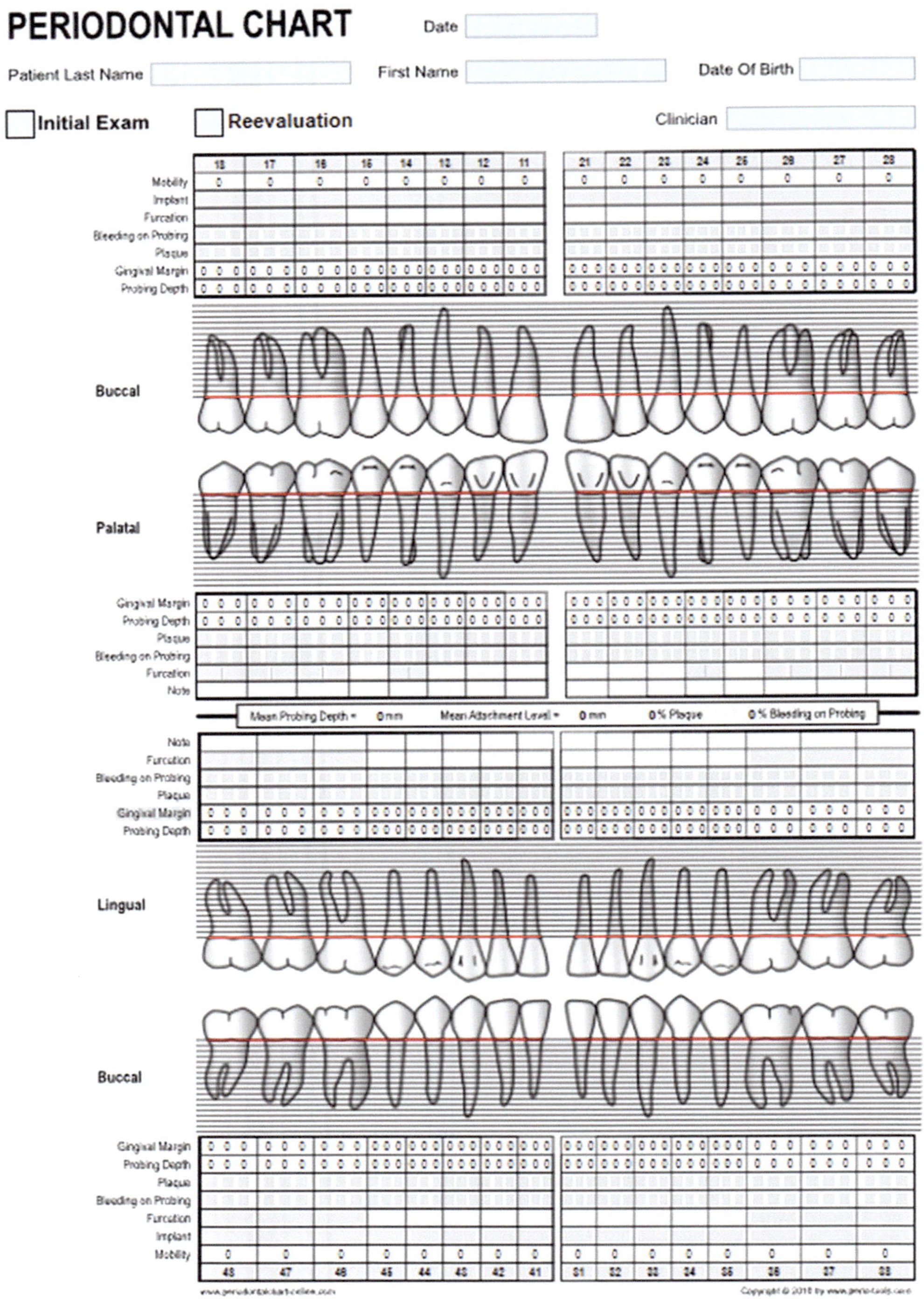

Fig. 14.1 Periodontal chart by the University of Bern

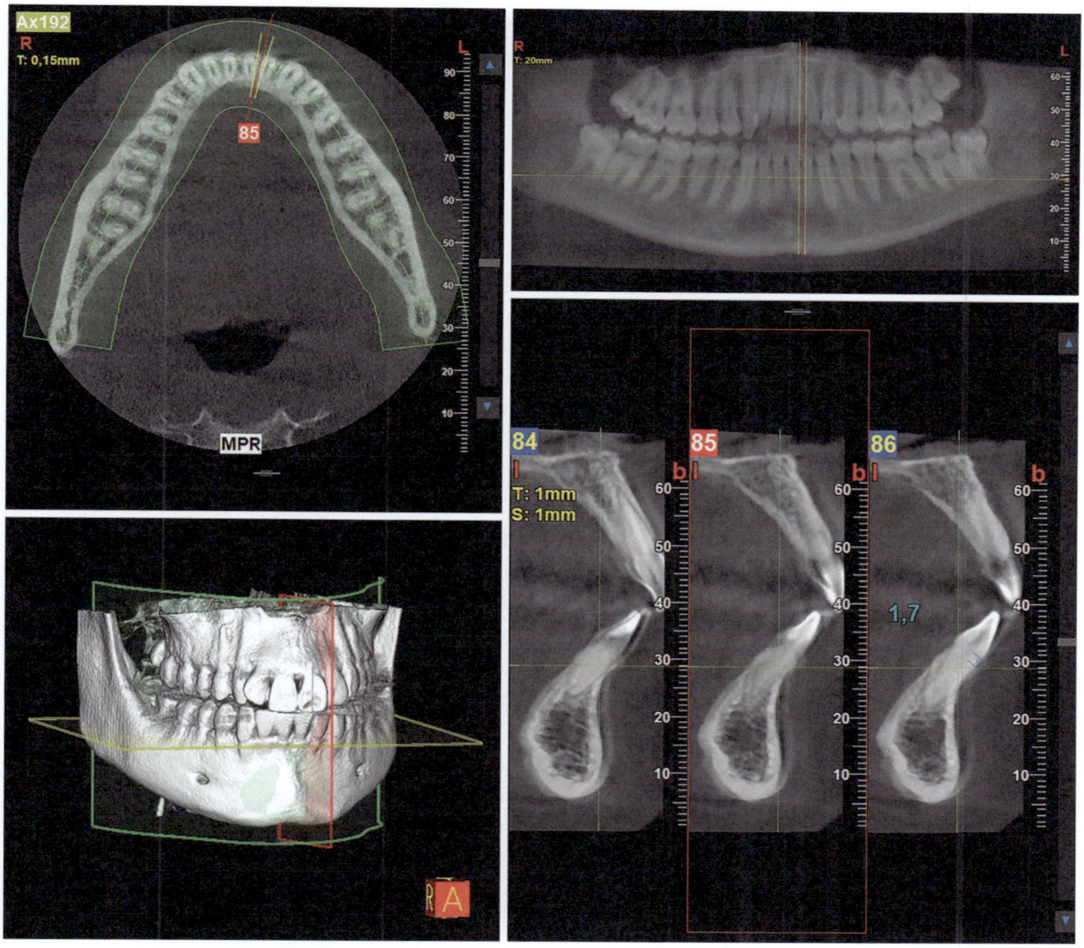

Fig. 14.2 Measurement of keratinized gingival width from a CBCT section

et al. indicated that digital measurement correlated with the clinical application regarding probing depth index [6]. However, digital probing depth measurement is not used frequently due to CBCT radiation dose, also the advantages of conventional probing such as application multiple times, ease of administration, and low cost [7].

14.1.3 Digital Periodontal Probe

In a healthy pocket, the probe cannot penetrate the connective tissue attachment, even when applied with a relatively high force, while in the presence of inflammation it stops at the level of intact connective tissue [8]. However, the measured values may differ depending on the type of probe used, the angle of the probe, the applied force, and the clinician's experience. The automatic periodontal probes, which were developed to compensate for the errors from the differences in probing, have recently become an innovative method.

14.1.3.1 Advantages of Digital Probes Over Manual

- The applied force is controlled.
- Pocket depth does not change according to the user.
- Pocket depth does not change depending on the probe type.
- Pocket depth value can be read from the digital display.
- Reduces chair time.

Today, there are many different types of digital probe systems. Florida Probe® (Florida Probe Corp, Gainesville, FL, USA), Inter-Probe™ (The Dental Probe Inc., VA, USA), and Probe One™ (The Dental Probe Inc., VA, USA), PA-ON probe (Orange Dental, Biberach, Germany) are the most widely used automatic probes.

Florida Probe® is a digital periodontal measurement system developed in 1988, consisting of a handpiece, a foot pedal, and a monitor. Its sensitivity is 0.2 mm (it increases the accuracy of measurements) and a constant probing pressure of 15 g due to the coil springs inside [9]. This probe can record probing depth (PD), gingival plaque, recession, hyperplasia, bleeding, calculus, suppuration, tooth mobility, furcation involvement, mucogingival junction, and missing teeth [10]. In addition, the values are saved in the system without the need for an assistant to write them down, saving a significant amount of time. Inter-Probe is a digital probing system that uses a stand-alone computer system to record data, while Probe One does data transfer via a USB. Both systems use a constant probing pressure of 15 g. The handpiece automatically measures the pocket depth and records it on the periodontal chart. The PA-ON probe always applies limited pressure into the pocket, ensuring a standard measurement (20 g ~ 0.25 N) (Fig. 14.3). The results measured with the probe are transferred to the software of the clinic and data entry is made into the digital periodontal chart without the need for manual recording.

Despite all these advantages, the lack of tactile sensation of digital periodontal probes can be considered a disadvantage [11].

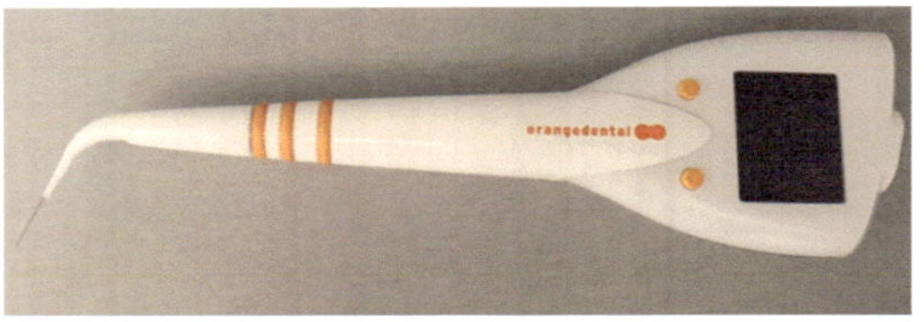

Fig. 14.3 Digital periodontal probe

14.1.4 Ultrasonic Periodontal Probe

Ultrasound (US) is concerned with frequencies above the range that the human ear can hear. In US imaging, high-frequency (2–20 MHz) sound waves are sent to the human body and the sounds returning from the tissues are converted into electronic impulses with the help of a transducer to create an image [12]. Ultrasonography, as a real-time, dynamic, non-invasive, and diagnostic tool that does not use ionizing radiation, has an important role in soft tissue evaluation [13]. This device consists of a computer, monitor, keyboard, footswitch, handpiece, probe, and a transducer at the tip. At the tip of the probe, there is a gentle stream of water to ensure good binding of the ultrasonic energy to the tissues [14]. The ultrasound probe tip is gently placed on the gingival margin and then swept across the gingival sulcus to measure pocket depth. The data is transferred to the computer by an artificial intelligence program that converts electronic impulses to millimeters [15].

Periodontal pockets can often be difficult to identify with the US probe. In this case, the frequency can be increased. Studies show that the gingival groove, enamel-cementum junction, and marginal gingiva can be identified in high-frequency gingival US examinations, and the measurements correlate with the microscopic analysis which is the gold standard [16].

14.2 Keratinized Tissue Measurement

Keratinized mucosa, located in the vestibule of teeth and implants, is considered the key to maintaining periodontium or peri-implanter health. According to many researchers, keratinized tissue less than 2 mm is considered sufficient for the inflammatory process to occur [17]. Increasing the height and width of the keratinized tissue reduces plaque index, bleeding on probing, inflammation and marginal bone loss around teeth and implants [18]. Keratinized mucosa may be distinguished from the alveolar mucosa being firmer and pinker due to the keratin layer and less vascularization, and its width is measured with a periodontal probe conventionally [19].

Intraoral scanners provide information about the oral cavity, gingiva, teeth, and dentures [20]. Keratinized tissue can be distinguished from the alveolar mucosa due to the lighter color in the scanned image. The researchers measured the width of the keratinized gingiva on histological sections to test this and found a high positive correlation with the value they measured from the scanned image [19]. The gingival keratinized width measured from the scanner is reliable to eliminate the limitations of periodontal probes.

14.3 Ultrasound Applications

The imaging techniques containing ionizing radiation demonstrate jawbones and teeth, yet they have been insufficient in soft tissue imaging in dentistry. The gingiva and periodontal ligament, which are the elements of the periodontium, are soft tissues and different imaging techniques were needed to image them. Ultrasonography, which is frequently used in the medical field, has become increasingly widespread in dentistry after Baum et al. used it for the first time in 1963 [21]. The superiorities of ultrasound are that it is a real-time, dynamic, ionizing radiation-free, and non-invasive technique [22]. In this way, information about the gingival thickness and vascularization or rigidity, depth, and borders of a gingival lesion was obtained before the biopsy or pre- and postoperation (Fig. 14.4) [23]. Ultrasound also eliminated the limitations of other imaging techniques, such as using ionizing radiation or being two-dimensional [24].

In addition to the imaging and periodontal pocket depth measurement described above, ultrasound also can be used in clinical applications such as calculus detection, scaling and root planning, root detoxification, and bone surgery [14]. Ultrasound detects calculus by distinguishing hard tissues such as calculus and tooth surface in the subgingival area with its specialized tips [25]. The cavitation action has a negative effect on bacteria in the microbial plaque. The US tip vibrates and produces mechanical energy with the cavitation, and it can disrupt bacteria and remove plaque and calculus [26, 27]. Piezosurgery® (Mectron Medical Technology, Carasco, Italy), which has become increasingly popular in recent years, uses ultrasonic vibrations to provide safe and precise osteotomies. It consists of a piezoelectric handpiece, a foot pedal and a main powered unit [28]. Its superiority to

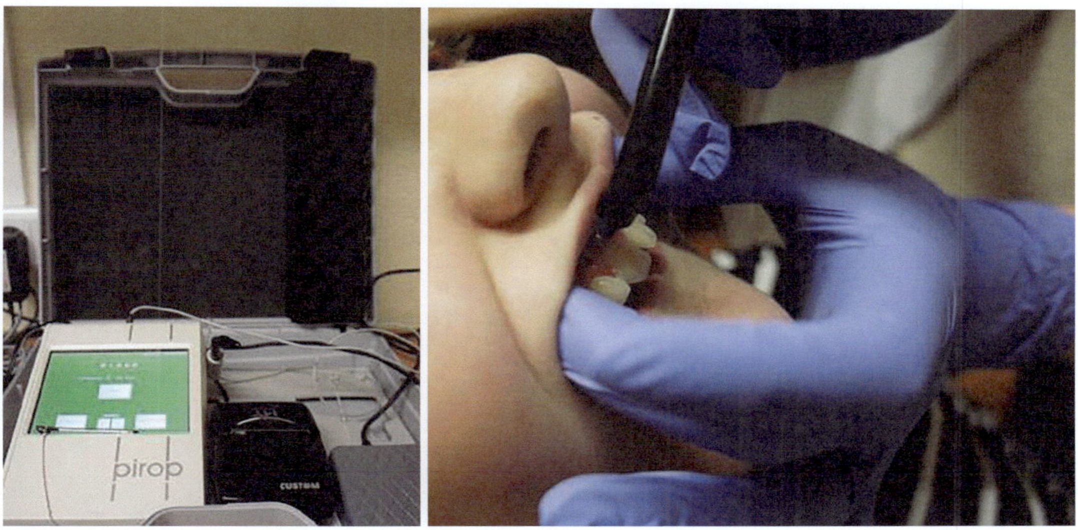

Fig. 14.4 Gingival thickness measured using US

other techniques used in osteotomy is that it stops working in soft tissues. It targets only mineralized tissue; thus the anatomical structures are not damaged [29]. Another advantage is the patient comfort provided by the absence of high-speed handpiece sound and vibrating movement [30]. Compared to others, the incision is slower yet safer.

CBCT has long been the gold standard for the examination of bone underlying the implant-planned mucosa. However, one of the limitations of CBCT is its inability to visualize soft tissues. The thickness of the mucosa can also be measured by ultrasound before the implant operation (Fig. 14.5). Moreover, ultrasound can be used to evaluate gingival tissue and vascularization in

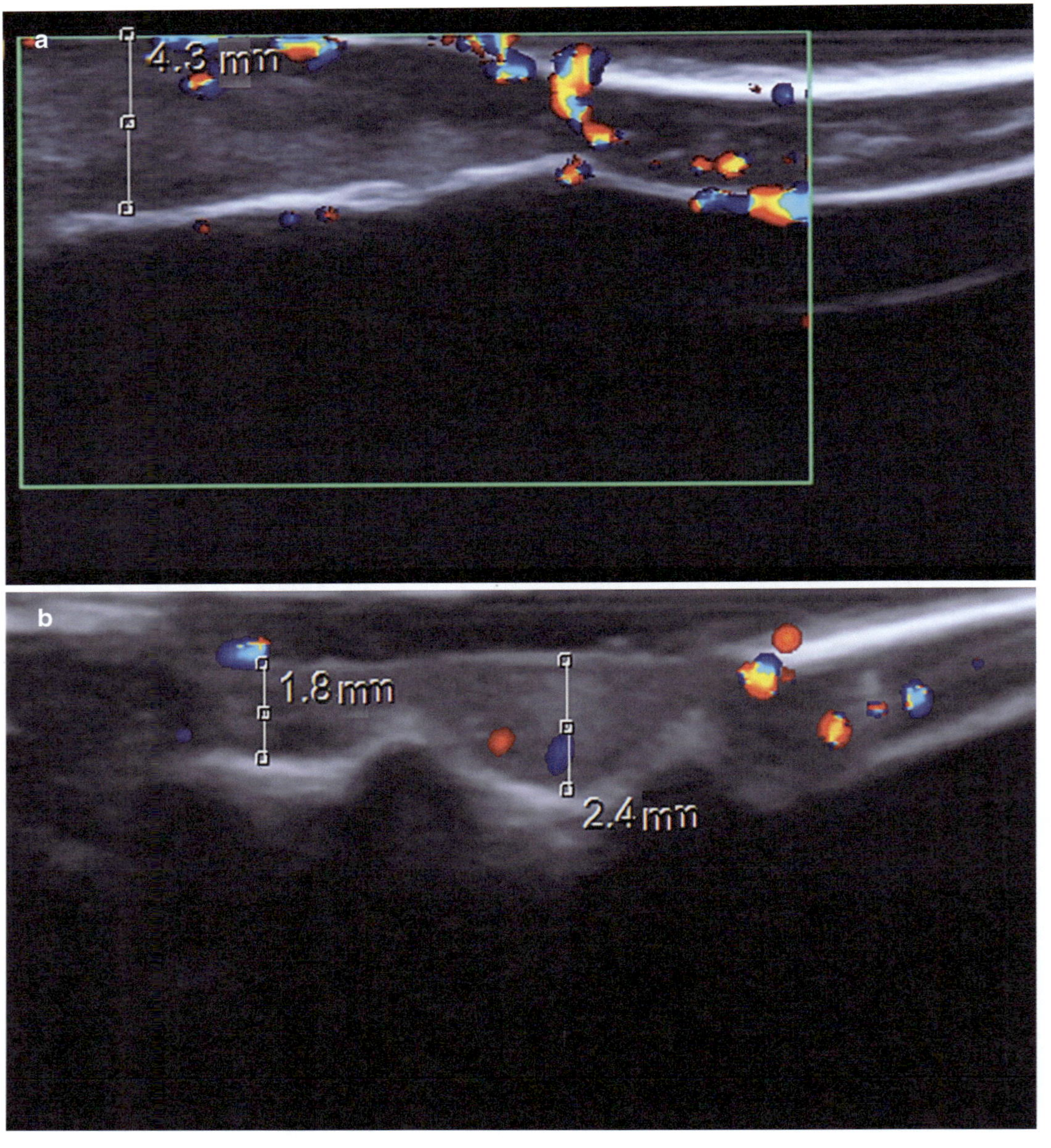

Fig. 14.5 US image of the thickness of the implant-planned mucosa of two different phenotypes

donor and recipient areas in mucogingival surgery. Choosing the donor site from the more vascularized and thicker side can increase the success and healing of the graft. The pathway of the greater palatine artery can be determined to prevent hemorrhagic complications while grafting as well [31].

14.3.1 Photoacoustic Imaging (PAI)

Photoacoustic imaging is a hybrid imaging method that combines visible and near-infrared light stimulation with acoustic sensing [32]. Extends the utility of ultrasound by activating optical absorption-based contrast. In conventional ultrasound, an electronic impulse created by sound waves is converted into images, whereas in photoacoustic imaging, light produces acoustic waves that can be detected by ultrasound transducers for image production [33]. The superiority of ultrasound over other imaging techniques is also in photoacoustic imaging. In addition to ultrasound, it can also image hard tissues such as teeth and bone [34].

The image is obtained with a contrast agent in this method. For instance, the periodontal pocket depth can be measured, the gingival groove is irrigated with the contrast agent and an image is taken [32]. Thus, the pocket depth is measured without affecting the penetration depth with the probe. It is especially ideal where probing would be invasive, such as in areas of augmentation or around implants.

14.4 Digital Smile Design (DSD)

People pay more attention to their appearance day by day, and an aesthetic smile is an important part of looking pleasant. Clinicians need to identify the causes of dissatisfaction or anxiety in patients' smiles and make treatment analyses accordingly. An aesthetic smile is a harmony in which the face, teeth, and gingiva are with each other. A change in any of these factors will affect the other. There are several different methods of providing smile aesthetics according to the etiological factor. Important steps including appropriate pretreatment examination, diagnosis, and treatment planning should be considered to achieve an optimum aesthetic result and an ideal smile [35].

Recently, many software that ensure smile design have been released such as Microsoft PowerPoint (Microsoft Office, Microsoft, Albuquerque, New Mexico, US), Smile Designer Pro (SDP) (Tasty Tech Ltd., Toronto, Ontario, Canada), DSD App by Coachman (DSDApp LLC, Florida, US), Photoshop (Adobe, Mountain View, California, US), Cerec SW 4.2 (Sirona Dental Systems Inc., Long Island City, New York, US), Planmeca Romexis Smile Design (PRSD, Helsinki-Uusimaa, Finland), etc. They evaluate the factors affecting the smile through the patient's photographs and analyze a treatment plan [36]. Digital smile design (DSD) programs can determine the etiological factor, provide predictable treatment results, and increase communication between the patient and the clinician [37].

DSD software is discussed in generations in Coachman's report. Accordingly, in the first generation, reference lines are placed on the photographs as analog, and in the second generation, digital 2D drawings and photo integration take place. Drawings can be placed on photographs in this generation. In the third generation, digital 2D drawings and connections with the analog model are available. This generation is the beginning of the digital-analog connection, which combines a 2D digital smile design with a 3D wax-up. In the fourth generation, full integration into digital dentistry was achieved with the removal of 3D wax-up models from the scanner [36].

Some references should be taken into account when performing a smile analysis. These include the smile arc, smile line, upper lip curvature, smile design, labiodental relationship, teeth appearance when smiling, buccal corridor, incisal edge, and zenith points of teeth [38]. *The smile arc* is the relationship between the curvature of the maxillary anterior teeth and the upper border of the lower lip. It is defined as an imaginary line from the zenith point of the central teeth to that of the canines [39]. *The smile line* is the rate of appearance of the maxillary anterior teeth during smiling. It can be high, medium, or low [40]. *The upper lip curvature* is evaluated by drawing a horizontal line on the lower edge of the upper lip and checking its relationship with the commissures. Commissures are classified as "up" if they are above the line, "straight" if they are within 1 mm of the line, and "down" if they are below the line [41]. Three patterns have been identified in *smile design*. The commissure smile is a typical pattern of a Cupid bow in which the maxillary first molars lie a few millimeters above the incisal edges of the central incisors. The second of them is a cuspid smile in which the lips look like a diamond when maxillary first molars lie at the same level with incisal edges of the central teeth. The last smile type is the complex smile. The lips are shaped to show both the upper and lower jaw teeth while smiling [42]. *The number of teeth visible when smiling* is categorized as visible teeth up to the canines, first premolars, second premolars, or first molars [38]. *The labiodental relationship between the lower lip and maxillary central teeth* is the distance between the upper border of the lower lip and the lower border of the maxillary central teeth when smiling. The lower lip may "slightly touch," "not touch" the incisal edge of the maxillary teeth, or "cover" the anterior teeth [43].

14.5 Gingivectomy/Crown Lengthening Procedures

Many etiological factors can cause aesthetic problems while smiling. One of these, and the most common, is the insufficient gingival-crown ratio. Although it does not cause any pathological problems, the person may feel aesthetic concern since the gingival appears excessively during smiling. This problem can be eliminated with the smile design by gingivectomy in case of the indication. With the developing technology, software have been developed that ensures the postoperative potential smile design is shown to the patient before the operation.

Digital smile design makes results more predictable and facilitates communication with the patient from precreated face photos and digital drawings. In addition, planning in the first session and the patient's participation in the planning are the advantages of this technique. However, despite its innovative potential, the use of DSD requires clinician training and skill to ensure its effective use.

A photograph of the patient smiling or a photograph to be taken with the camera at that moment is uploaded to the software. Horizontal and vertical reference lines are superimposed on the photograph according to the facial, tooth, and gingival analysis. The evaluation criteria described under the title of digital smile design are also valid in gingivectomy cases. The tooth proportion suitable for the patient's profile is determined and the appropriate tooth set is selected from the software database. These proportions can be in different shapes such as oval, square, triangle, or rectangular (Fig. 14.6). According to the new design, a wax-up model can be created and transferred to the patient's mouth to guide gingival surgery, or a mock-up model can be produced from 3D printers. Gingivectomy is performed by taking the created model as a guide.

There are an increasing number of papers on gummy smile treatment or gingivectomy with digital smile design in the literature [44, 45]. Gingivectomy planned with a digital smile design gives an idea about the predictability of the treatment, reduces errors, and enables risk factors to be controlled. It provides a better understanding of the procedures required to achieve the final result acceptable to the patient [46].

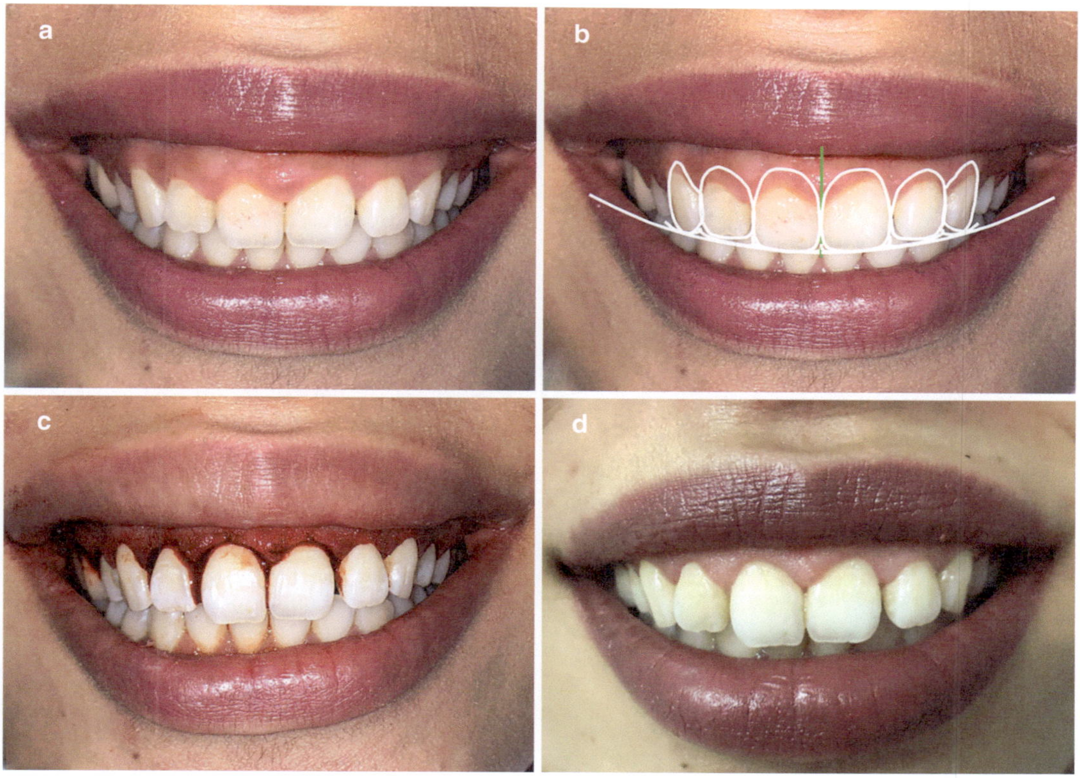

Fig. 14.6 (**a**) Initial intraoral image of the patient. (**b**) Gingivectomy planned in the digital smile design program. (**c**) Postop image of gingivectomy. (**d**) Intraoral image of seventh postoperative day

14.6 Mucogingival Operations

Gingival recessions are mucogingival deformities that can occur due to many etiological factors, with the apical displacement of the marginal gingiva. Insufficient attached gingival width, involvement of the frenulum, periodontal infections, iatrogenic factors, parafunctional habits such as nail biting or irritant factors such as piercing may be involved in their etiology [47]. Depending on the causes and clinical conditions, they are usually treated with soft tissue augmentations. Which soft tissue augmentation technique will be used in the treatment of gingival recession depends on the type of recession and the remaining periodontal tissue support.

Procedures such as free gingival graft containing only epithelium or subepithelial connective tissue grafting containing epithelium and underlying connective tissue can be used to cover the root surfaces and increase the width of the keratinized gingiva. Connective tissue grafting can be performed with many flap techniques such as coronally positioned, laterally positioned or tunnel techniques [48]. However, these methods may lead to many complications or technical difficulties such as papilla laceration, necrosis of the graft, re-recession of the gingiva, postoperative scar tissue formation, hemorrhagic complications, or mobilization of the flap in especially thin biotypes [49, 50].

Although a few are in the literature, several digital mucogingival surgical guided publications have been released to help to reduce these difficulties and complications. In a recent study, the mucogingival junction was designated independently in digital models obtained by an intraoral scanner and conventional models with impression material and the two groups were similar statistically [51]. Fons-Badal et al. digitally measured the patients' tissue gains after soft tissue grafting. The researchers took a digital impression with intraoral scanners before and after mucogingival surgery. They created a 3D transform matrix from adjacent teeth of the augmented area and compared the volume gains [52]. Marques et al. compared two tunnel techniques with connective tissue grafts performed on denuded roots. They scanned the pre and postoperative sites with an intraoral scanner and evaluated them in various regards [48].

Pre- and postoperative digital evaluation of the mucogingival site is an easy, painless, reproducible, and non-invasive technique. In addition, it is satisfactory since the patients can see the effects of the operations, and an objective measurement method for the scientific studies.

14.7 Summary

The applications that have been made in periodontology for years, keep up with the digital age and now offer more technological and more predictable opportunities. Although the definition and clinical picture of the diseases do not change, it is now possible to diagnose the diseases faster and to foresee the post-treatment situations. Digitization in periodontology is emerging and there are few studies in the literature. However, many technological developments are waiting to be discovered and evidence-based studies can be done. Increasing digitalization will also bring about increasing globalization in the scientific world. Just as radiographs used to be printed, but are now digital and transferable. Digital dentistry is expected to grow and become more involved in clinical, laboratory and student education.

References

1. Kononen E, Gursoy M, Gursoy UK. Periodontitis: a multifaceted disease of tooth-supporting tissues. J Clin Med. 2019;8(8):1135.
2. Loe H. The gingival index, the plaque index and the retention index systems. J Periodontol. 1967;38(6):610–6.
3. Hujoel PP. Definitive vs. exploratory periodontal trials: a survey of published studies. J Dent Res. 1995;74(8):1453–8.
4. Celeghin G, Franceschetti G, Mobilio N, Fasiol A, Catapano S, Corsalini M, et al. Complete-arch accuracy of four intraoral scanners: an in vitro study. Healthcare (Basel). 2021;9(3):246.
5. Patcas R, Markic G, Muller L, Ullrich O, Peltomaki T, Kellenberger CJ, et al. Accuracy of linear intraoral measurements using cone beam CT and multidetector CT: a tale of two CTs. Dentomaxillofac Radiol. 2012;41(8):637–44.
6. Chung HM, Park JY, Ko KA, Kim CS, Choi SH, Lee JS. Periodontal probing on digital images compared to clinical measurements in periodontitis patients. Sci Rep. 2022;12(1):1616.
7. Greenstein G. Current interpretations of periodontal probing evaluations: diagnostic and therapeutic implications. Compend Contin Educ Dent. 2005;26(6):381–2; 384, 387–90 passim; quiz 98-9.
8. Barendregt DS, Van der Velden U, Timmerman MF, van der Weijden GA. Comparison of two automated periodontal probes and two probes with a conventional readout in periodontal maintenance patients. J Clin Periodontol. 2006;33(4):276–82.
9. Kour A, Kumar A, Puri K, Khatri M, Bansal M, Gupta G. Comparative evaluation of probing depth and clinical attachment level using a manual probe and Florida probe. J Indian Soc Periodontol. 2016;20(3):299–306.
10. Osborn JB, Stoltenberg JL, Huso BA, Aeppli DM, Pihlstrom BL. Comparison of measurement variability in subjects with moderate periodontitis using a conventional and constant force periodontal probe. J Periodontol. 1992;63(4):283–9.
11. Renatus A, Trentzsch L, Schonfelder A, Schwarzenberger F, Jentsch H. Evaluation of an electronic periodontal probe versus a manual probe. J Clin Diagn Res. 2016;10(11):ZH03–ZH7.
12. Koca RB, Unsal G, Soluk Tekkesin M, Kasnak G, Orhan K, Ozcan I, et al. A review with an additional case: amelanotic malignant melanoma at mandibular gingiva. Int Cancer Conf J. 2020;9(4):175–81.
13. Sculean A, Gruber R, Bosshardt DD. Soft tissue wound healing around teeth and dental implants. J Clin Periodontol. 2014;41(Suppl 15):S6–22.
14. Bains VK, Mohan R, Bains R. Application of ultrasound in periodontics: part II. J Indian Soc Periodontol. 2008;12(3):55–61.
15. Farr C. Ultrasonic probing: the wave of the future in dentistry. Dent Today. 2000;19(3):86–91.
16. Chifor R, Badea ME, Mitrea DA, Badea IC, Crisan M, Chifor I, et al. Computer-assisted identification of the gingival sulcus and periodontal epithelial junction on high-frequency ultrasound images. Med Ultrason. 2015;17(3):273–9.

17. Wang Q, Tang Z, Han J, Meng H. The width of keratinized mucosa around dental implants and its influencing factors. Clin Implant Dent Relat Res. 2020;22(3):359–65.
18. Souza AB, Tormena M, Matarazzo F, Araujo MG. The influence of peri-implant keratinized mucosa on brushing discomfort and peri-implant tissue health. Clin Oral Implants Res. 2016;27(6):650–5.
19. Lee JS, Jeon YS, Strauss FJ, Jung HI, Gruber R. Digital scanning is more accurate than using a periodontal probe to measure the keratinized tissue width. Sci Rep. 2020;10(1):3665.
20. Deferm JT, Schreurs R, Baan F, Bruggink R, Merkx MAW, Xi T, et al. Validation of 3D documentation of palatal soft tissue shape, color, and irregularity with intraoral scanning. Clin Oral Investig. 2018;22(3):1303–9.
21. Shah N, Bansal N, Logani A. Recent advances in imaging technologies in dentistry. World J Radiol. 2014;6(10):794–807.
22. Tsiolis FI, Needleman IG, Griffiths GS. Periodontal ultrasonography. J Clin Periodontol. 2003;30(10):849–54.
23. Natori T, Koga M, Anegawa E, Nakashima Y, Tetsuka M, Yoh J, et al. Usefulness of intra-oral ultrasonography to predict neck metastasis in patients with tongue carcinoma. Oral Dis. 2008;14(7):591–9.
24. Jeffcoat MK, Wang IC, Reddy MS. Radiographic diagnosis in periodontics. Periodontol. 2000;1995(7):54–68.
25. Meissner G, Oehme B, Strackeljan J, Kuhr A, Kocher T. A method for the validation of a new calculus detection system. J Clin Periodontol. 2005;32(6):659–64.
26. Clark SM. The ultrasonic dental unit: a guide for the clinical application of ultrasonics in dentistry and in dental hygiene. J Periodontol. 1969;40(11):621–9.
27. Walmsley AD, Laird WR, Williams AR. Dental plaque removal by cavitational activity during ultrasonic scaling. J Clin Periodontol. 1988;15(9):539–43.
28. Eggers G, Klein J, Blank J, Hassfeld S. Piezosurgery: an ultrasound device for cutting bone and its use and limitations in maxillofacial surgery. Br J Oral Maxillofac Surg. 2004;42(5):451–3.
29. Stubinger S, Kuttenberger J, Filippi A, Sader R, Zeilhofer HF. Intraoral piezosurgery: preliminary results of a new technique. J Oral Maxillofac Surg. 2005;63(9):1283–7.
30. Vercellotti T, Nevins ML, Kim DM, Nevins M, Wada K, Schenk RK, et al. Osseous response following resective therapy with piezosurgery. Int J Periodontics Restorative Dent. 2005;25(6):543–9.
31. Koca-Unsal RB, Unsal G, Kasnak G, Firatli Y, Ozcan I, Orhan K, et al. Ultrasonographic evaluation of the titanium-prepared platelet-rich fibrin effect in free gingival graft procedures. J Periodontol. 2022;93(2):187–94.
32. Moore C, Bai Y, Hariri A, Sanchez JB, Lin CY, Koka S, et al. Photoacoustic imaging for monitoring periodontal health: a first human study. Photo-Dermatology. 2018;12:67–74.
33. Zackrisson S, van de Ven S, Gambhir SS. Light in and sound out: emerging translational strategies for photoacoustic imaging. Cancer Res. 2014;74(4):979–1004.
34. Chuembou Pekam F, Marotti J, Wolfart S, Tinschert J, Radermacher K, Heger S. High-frequency ultrasound as an option for scanning of prepared teeth: an in vitro study. Ultrasound Med Biol. 2015;41(1):309–16.
35. Nold SL, Horvath SD, Stampf S, Blatz MB. Analysis of select facial and dental esthetic parameters. Int J Periodontics Restorative Dent. 2014;34(5):623–9.
36. Coachman C, Calamita MA, Sesma N. Dynamic documentation of the smile and the 2D/3D digital smile design process. Int J Periodontics Restorative Dent. 2017;37(2):183–93.
37. Stanley M, Paz AG, Miguel I, Coachman C. Fully digital workflow, integrating dental scan, smile design and CAD-CAM: case report. BMC Oral Health. 2018;18(1):134.
38. Khan M, Kazmi SMR, Khan FR, Samejo I. Analysis of different characteristics of smile. BDJ Open. 2020;6:6.
39. Sarver DM, Ackerman MB. Dynamic smile visualization and quantification: part 2. Smile analysis and treatment strategies. Am J Orthod Dentofac Orthop. 2003;124(2):116–27.
40. Sabri R. The eight components of a balanced smile. J Clin Orthod. 2005;39(3):155–67; quiz 4.
41. Al-Johany SS, Alqahtani AS, Alqahtani FY, Alzahrani AH. Evaluation of different esthetic smile criteria. Int J Prosthodont. 2011;24(1):64–70.
42. Rubin LR. The anatomy of a smile: its importance in the treatment of facial paralysis. Plast Reconstr Surg. 1974;53(4):384–7.
43. Tjan AH, Miller GD, The JG. Some esthetic factors in a smile. J Prosthet Dent. 1984;51(1):24–8.
44. Cervino G, Fiorillo L, Arzukanyan AV, Spagnuolo G, Cicciu M. Dental restorative digital workflow: digital smile design from aesthetic to function. Dent J (Basel). 2019;7(2):30.
45. do Vale Voigt M, Espindola-Castro LF, de Melo Monteiro GQ, Ortigoza LS, Dos Santos Torreao A, Georg R. DSDapp use for multidisciplinary esthetic planning. J Esthet Restor Dent. 2020;32(8):738–46.
46. Arias DM, Trushkowsky RD, Brea LM, David SB. Treatment of the patient with gummy smile in conjunction with digital smile approach. Dent Clin N Am. 2015;59(3):703–16.
47. Zucchelli G, Mounssif I. Periodontal plastic surgery. Periodontol 2000. 2015;68(1):333–68.
48. Marques T, Santos NM, Fialho J, Montero J, Correia A. A new digital evaluation protocol applied in a retrospective analysis of periodontal plastic surgery of gingival recessions. Sci Rep. 2021;11(1):20399.
49. Cortellini P, Bissada NF. Mucogingival conditions in the natural dentition: narrative review, case definitions, and diagnostic considerations. J Periodontol. 2018;89(Suppl 1):S204–S13.
50. Zuhr O, Rebele SF, Cheung SL, Hurzeler MB, Research Group on Oral Soft Tissue B, Wound H. Surgery without papilla incision: tunneling flap

procedures in plastic periodontal and implant surgery. Periodontol 2000. 2018;77(1):123–49.
51. Brandenburg LS, Schlager S, Harzig LS, Steybe D, Rothweiler RM, Burkhardt F, et al. A novel method for digital reconstruction of the Mucogingival borderline in optical scans of dental plaster casts. J Clin Med. 2022;11(9):2383.
52. Fons-Badal C, Alonso Perez-Barquero J, Martinez-Martinez N, Faus-Lopez J, Fons-Font A, Agustin-Panadero R. A novel, fully digital approach to quantifying volume gain after soft tissue graft surgery. A pilot study. J Clin Periodontol. 2020;47(5):614–20.

Digital Dental Applications in Endodontics

15

Georgios Mikrogeorgis and Antigoni Delantoni

15.1 Part I

15.1.1 Advanced Radiographic Systems: Cone Beam Computed Tomography in Diagnosis

15.1.1.1 Detection of Periapical Lesions

With the advances in radiographic systems and particularly the introduction of CBCT in endodontics, various imaging features of the third dimension of teeth have been added to help dentists visualize what was often missed in images.

The most common periapical pathologies are viewed in the following figure (Fig. 15.1).

CBCT imaging has the ability to detect small areas of periapical pathosis prior to being apparent on 2D radiographs [1]. Furthermore, there are clinical studies in which periapical periodontitis detected in intraoral radiographs and CBCT was 20% and 48%, respectively [2]. Also, in a 1-year post-treatment study, the absence of a periapical radiolucency was found in 93% of the cases when evaluated by 2D radiographs, but only 74% when using CBCT [3]. Similar results have found in ex vivo studies, in which simulated periapical lesions were created [4, 5].

However, there are some limitations in the interpretation of CBCT periapical findings, whereas the CBCT-PAI score is commonly greater than the 2D PAI score, and some teeth with healthy pulps may demonstrate a widened apical PDL space on CBCT [6].

To better understand the use of CBCT in small periapical lesions the following comparison of a 2D radiograph and the corresponding 3D CBCT section are shown (Fig. 15.2).

15.1.1.2 Detection of Cracked Teeth and Root Fractures

Two-dimensional radiographs (2D) are of limited value for the diagnosis of vertical root fractures (VRF) and usually only provide indirect evidence of the presence of a VRF. The three-dimensional nature of complex tooth anatomy and surrounding structures can make interpretation of 2D images challenging and unreliable. Several studies have demonstrated the value of CBCT as an aid in the detection of VRF. In a comparative study evaluating the sensitivity and specificity of CBCT and periapical radiographs in detecting VRF, sensitivity and specificity for VRF detection of CBCT were 79.4% and 92.5% and for PR were 37.1% and 95%, respectively. In the same

G. Mikrogeorgis (✉)
Department of Endodontology, Dental School, Aristotle University of Thessaloniki, Thessaloniki, Greece
e-mail: gmicro@dent.auth.gr

A. Delantoni
Faculty of Dentistry, Aristotle University of Thessaloniki, Thessaloniki, Greece
e-mail: andelant@dent.auth.gr

A. Delantoni, K. Orhan (eds.), *Digital Dentistry*, https://doi.org/10.1007/978-3-031-52826-2_15

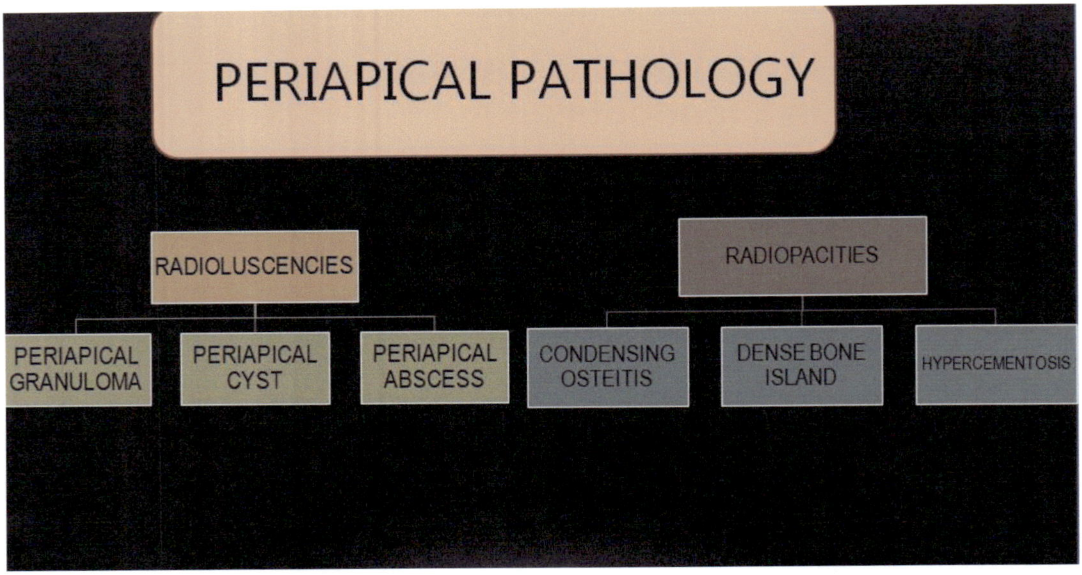

Fig. 15.1 A schematic diagram of all major periapical pathologies, both of radiolucencies and radiopacities

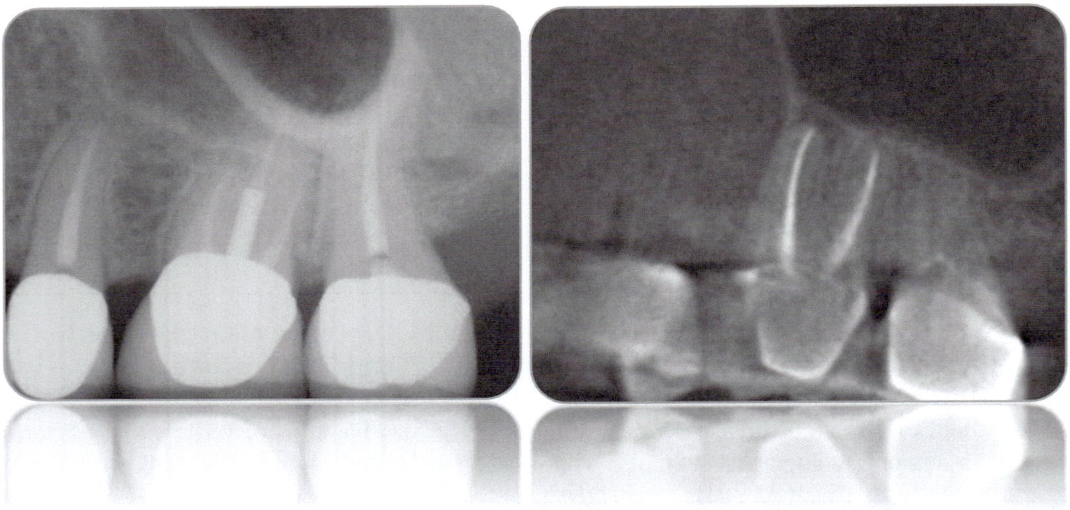

Fig. 15.2 The typical periapical radiograph does not show the small periapical lesion of the distal root of the first molar which is clearly seen on the CBCT section of the patient

study, it was reported that the specificity of CBCT was reduced in the presence of root canal filling material [7]. Higher sensitivity and specificity were observed in a clinical study where the definitive diagnosis of vertical root fracture was confirmed at the time of surgery to validate CBCT findings, with sensitivity being 88% and specificity 75% [8]. Several case series studies have concluded that CBCT is a useful tool for the diagnosis of vertical root fractures. In vivo studies [9, 10] evaluating CBCT in the detection of vertical root fractures agreed that sensitivity, specificity, and accuracy of CBCT were generally higher and reproducible. The detection of fractures was significantly higher for all CBCT systems when compared to intraoral radiographs. However,

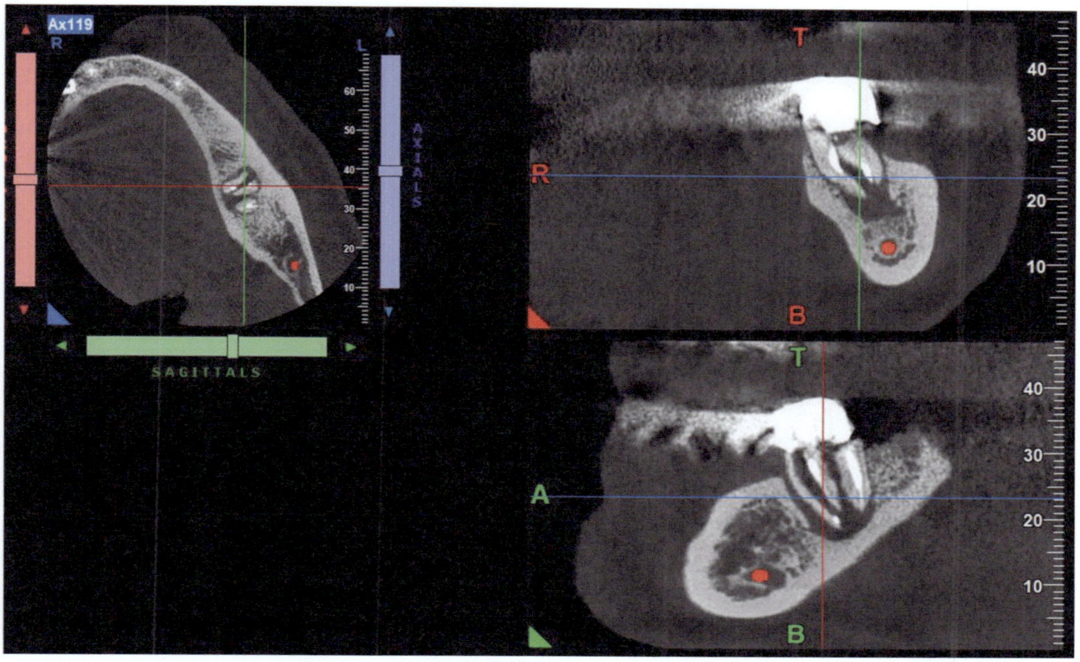

Fig. 15.3 A vertical root fracture on a molar tooth as seen in all levels on the CBCT images

these results should be interpreted with caution because the detection of vertical root fracture is dependent on the size of the fracture, presence of artifacts caused by obturation materials and posts, and the spatial resolution of the CBCT. The diagnostic ability of CBCT to assess longitudinal root fractures in endodontically treated and restored teeth was evaluated, in a recent study [11]. An example of a vertical fracture with the use of CBCT can be seen in the following figure in all three levels (Fig. 15.3).

The presence of gutta-percha or cast-gold posts reduced the overall sensitivity and specificity. This was attributed to star-shaped streak artifacts that mimic fractured lines in the axial spatial view. One significant problem, which can affect the image diagnostic quality and accuracy of CBCT images, is the scatter and beam hardening caused by high-density neighboring structures, such as enamel, metal posts, and restorations. If this scatter and beam hardening is associated with or close to the tooth being assessed, the overall sensitivity and specificity are dramatically reduced. Due in part to the common presence of imaging artifacts, several investigators have questioned the superiority of CBCT in the diagnosis of VRF and urge caution in relying solely on CBCT for diagnosis of VRF [12, 13]. While we agree that caution may be warranted when using only one diagnostic test or finding, we believe that the preponderance of the evidence currently available supports the value of CBCT as an aid in the diagnosis of VFR [14, 15], and CBCT may be particularly useful in the diagnosis of horizontal and oblique fractures commonly associated with dental trauma [16]. In particular, the CBCT sagittal view provides diagnostic information for traumatized anterior teeth that is not available with 2D periapical imaging as can be seen in the following image (Fig. 15.4):

15.1.1.3 Detection of Inflammatory Resorptive Defects

Definitive diagnosis root resorption and treatment planning is ultimately dependent on the radiographic representation of the disease. 2D imaging offers limited diagnostic potential when compared to 3D imaging [17, 18] (Fig. 15.5).

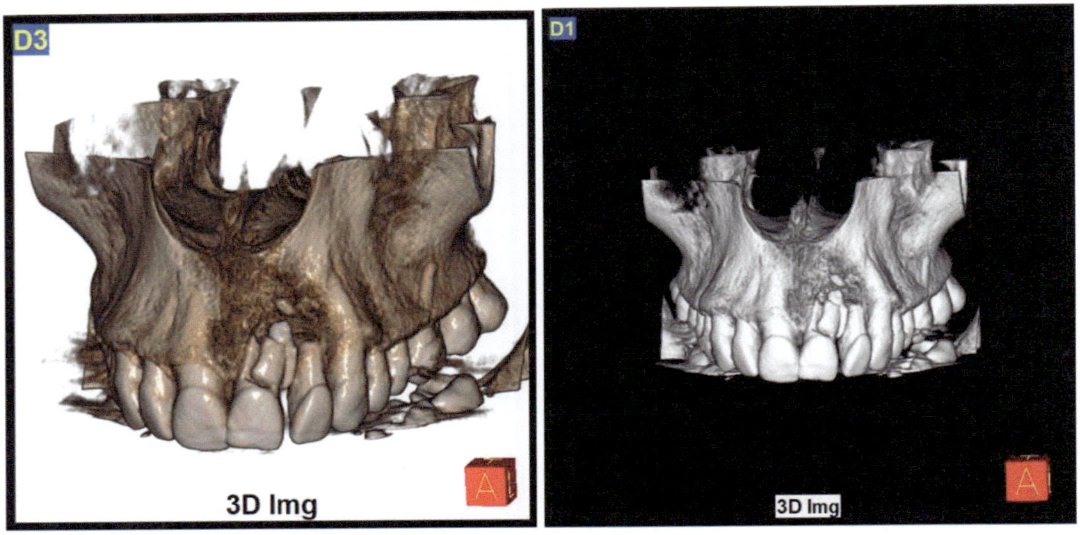

Fig. 15.4 3D reconstruction of a broken anterior central incisor after a facial trauma, where the multiple fragments of the tooth are easily seen

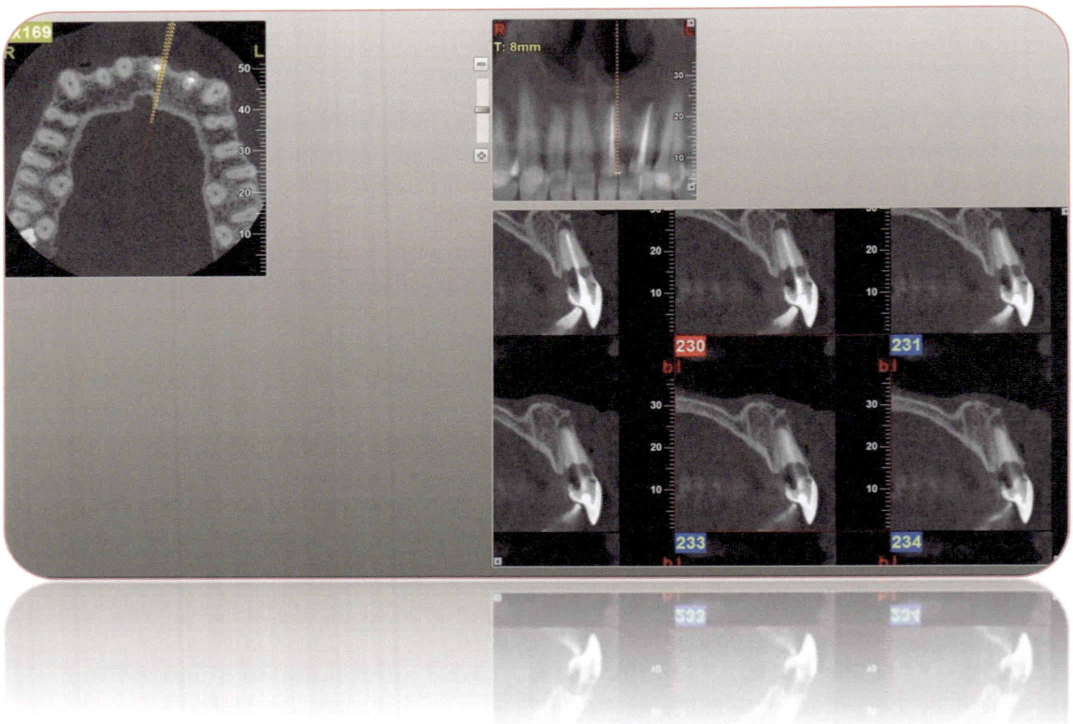

Fig. 15.5 In the panoramic section we see the 2D panoramic image limitation while the sections clearly show the internal root resorption of the tooth

15.1.1.4 Traumatic Dental Injuries

Traumatic dental injuries (TDI) present a clinical challenge with regard to diagnosis, treatment planning, and prognosis. Radiographic assessment is important to identify the location, type, and severity of TDI. According to the 2012

International Association of Dental Traumatology guidelines [19], a series of periapical radiographs from different angulations and an occlusal film are recommended for evaluation of TDI. CBCT was recommended as well for the visualization of TDI, particularly root fractures and lateral luxation, monitoring of healing, and complications. Unfortunately, 2D imaging has limitations in the diagnosis and detection of TDI due to projection geometry, magnification, superimposition of anatomic structures, distortion, and processing errors. In the diagnosis of horizontal root fractures (HRF) utilizing 2D imaging, the fracture line will only be detected if the X-ray beam passes directly through it. The 2D nature limits the accuracy in the diagnosis of the location, severity, and extent of HRF. The risk of misdiagnosis of the location and extent of the fracture by using only 2D intraoral radiography could lead to improper treatment and an unfavorable outcome. Because of the limitations of intraoral radiography, CBCT was suggested as the preferred imaging modality for diagnosis of HRF [20]. CBCT overcomes several of the limitations of 2D imaging by providing a considerable amount of 3D information about the nature and extent of the HRF. The significant difference in the nature of HRF when assessed with 2D radiographs compared to CBCT has been reported [21]. Limited FOV CBCT imaging seems to be generally advantageous in the diagnosis, assessment of prognosis, treatment planning, and treatment follow-up of HRF cases.

15.1.2 Conclusion

CBCT is a valuable adjunct to assist in the diagnosis of periapical hard tissue changes, root fractures, traumatic dental injuries and inflammatory root resorption. Conventional 2D radiography and CBCT both record structural changes in the bone. However, CBCT imaging has the ability to detect periapical pathosis prior to being apparent on 2D radiographs. Preoperative factors such as the presence and true size of a periapical lesion play an important role in endodontic treatment outcome. Success, when measured by radiographic criteria, is higher when teeth are endodontically treated before radiographic signs of periapical disease are detected. According to the 2015 joint statement from the American Association of Endodontists and American Academy of Oral and Maxillofacial Radiology, CBCT is the imaging modality of choice for the following diagnostic situations [22]:

1. Patients presenting with contradictory or nonspecific clinical signs and symptoms associated with untreated or previously endodontically treated teeth.
2. Diagnosis and management of limited dento-alveolar trauma, root fractures, luxation, and/or displacement of teeth and localized alveolar fractures, in the absence of other maxillofacial or soft tissue injury that require other advanced imaging modalities.
3. Localization and differentiation of external and internal resorptive defects and the determination of appropriate treatment and prognosis.
4. If clinical examination and 2D intraoral radiography are inconclusive in the detection of vertical root fracture (VRF).

15.1.2.1 The Impact of Cone Beam Computed Tomography in Nonsurgical and Surgical Treatment Planning

Cone beam computed tomography (CBCT) is a diagnostic imaging modality which provides a three-dimensional image of the maxillofacial region and is capable of providing images at a relatively low radiation dose and with sufficient spatial resolution for applications in endodontic diagnosis and treatment planning. CBCT overcomes many limitations with conventional radiography such as early detection of invasive cervical resorption lesions, vertical root fractures, and three-dimensional evaluation of the root canal space and surrounding anatomy [7, 8 17, 23–26]. Diagnostic information directly influences treatment planning and clinical decisions. Accurate data leads to better treatment decisions and potentially more predictable outcomes [27]. While conventional periapical radiography has been used for many years as a diagnostic aid in endodontics, some studies now demonstrate the inferiority of periapical radiographs in detecting periradicular pathosis when compared to CBCT

[1, 28–31]. CBCT has been successfully used in endodontics and several recent studies have demonstrated the advantages of CBCT over periapical radiographs [32–36]. The effective radiation dose when using CBCT is higher than conventional two-dimensional radiography, and the benefit to the patient must therefore outweigh any potential risks of the additional radiation exposure. Radiation dose should be kept as low as reasonably achievable (ALARA) [37, 38]. The value of CBCT for endodontic diagnosis and treatment planning should be determined on an individual basis to assure that the benefit/risk assessment supports the use of CBCT.

Ee et al. (2014) compared differences in endodontic treatment planning decisions using either CBCT or periapical radiographs [39]. Thirty endodontic cases completed in a private endodontic practice were randomly selected to be included in this study. Each case was required to have a preoperative digital periapical radiograph and a CBCT scan. Three board-certified endodontists reviewed the 30 preoperative periapical radiographs. The evaluators were not involved in the initial diagnosis or treatment of these 30 cases. Two weeks later, the CBCT volumes were reviewed in random order by the same evaluators. The evaluators were asked to select a preliminary diagnosis and treatment plan based solely on interpretation of the periapical and CBCT images. Diagnosis and treatment planning choices were then compared to determine if there was a change in decision-making from viewing just the periapical radiograph to the CBCT scan. In addition, both decisions were compared to the reference standard (known diagnosis confirmed during nonsurgical treatment and/or surgical exploration or extraction). A difference in treatment plan between the two imaging modalities was recorded in 19 out of 30 cases (63.3%) ($P = 0.001$) for examiner #1, 17 out of 30 cases (56.6%) ($P = 0.012$) for examiner #2, and 20 out of 30 cases (66.7%) ($P = 0.008$) for examiner #3. The problem of incorrect, delayed, or inadequate endodontic diagnosis and treatment planning places the patient at risk and could result in unnecessary or inappropriate treatment.

Under the conditions of the previous study [39], CBCT was a more accurate imaging modality for diagnosis of tooth anatomy and periradicular pathosis when compared to diagnosis using only periapical radiographs. An accurate diagnosis was reached in 36.6–40% of the cases when using periapical radiographs compared to an accurate diagnosis in 76.6–83.3% of the cases when using CBCT. This high level of misdiagnosis is potentially clinically relevant, especially in cases of invasive cervical root resorption and vertical root fracture where a lack of early detection could lead to unsuccessful treatment and tooth loss. The previous study also demonstrates that the treatment plan may be directly influenced by information gained from a CBCT scan as the examiners altered their treatment plan after viewing the CBCT scan in 62.2% of the cases overall (range from 56.6 to 66.7%). This high number indicates that CBCT had a significant influence on the treatment plan (Fig. 15.6).

It can be concluded that a preoperative CBCT scan provides more diagnostic information than a preoperative periapical radiograph and that this information can directly influence a treatment plan. Although imaging is a very important diagnostic tool in endodontics, it should always be used as an adjunct to the clinical examination. The addition of subjective and objective clinical findings to CBCT should allow for an even more accurate clinical diagnosis and appropriate treatment plan.

15.1.2.2 Conclusion

Cone beam computed tomography overcomes many of the limitations of periapical radiography. The increased diagnostic information provided by the CBCT scan should result in more accurate diagnosis and improved decision-making for the management of complex endodontic problems.

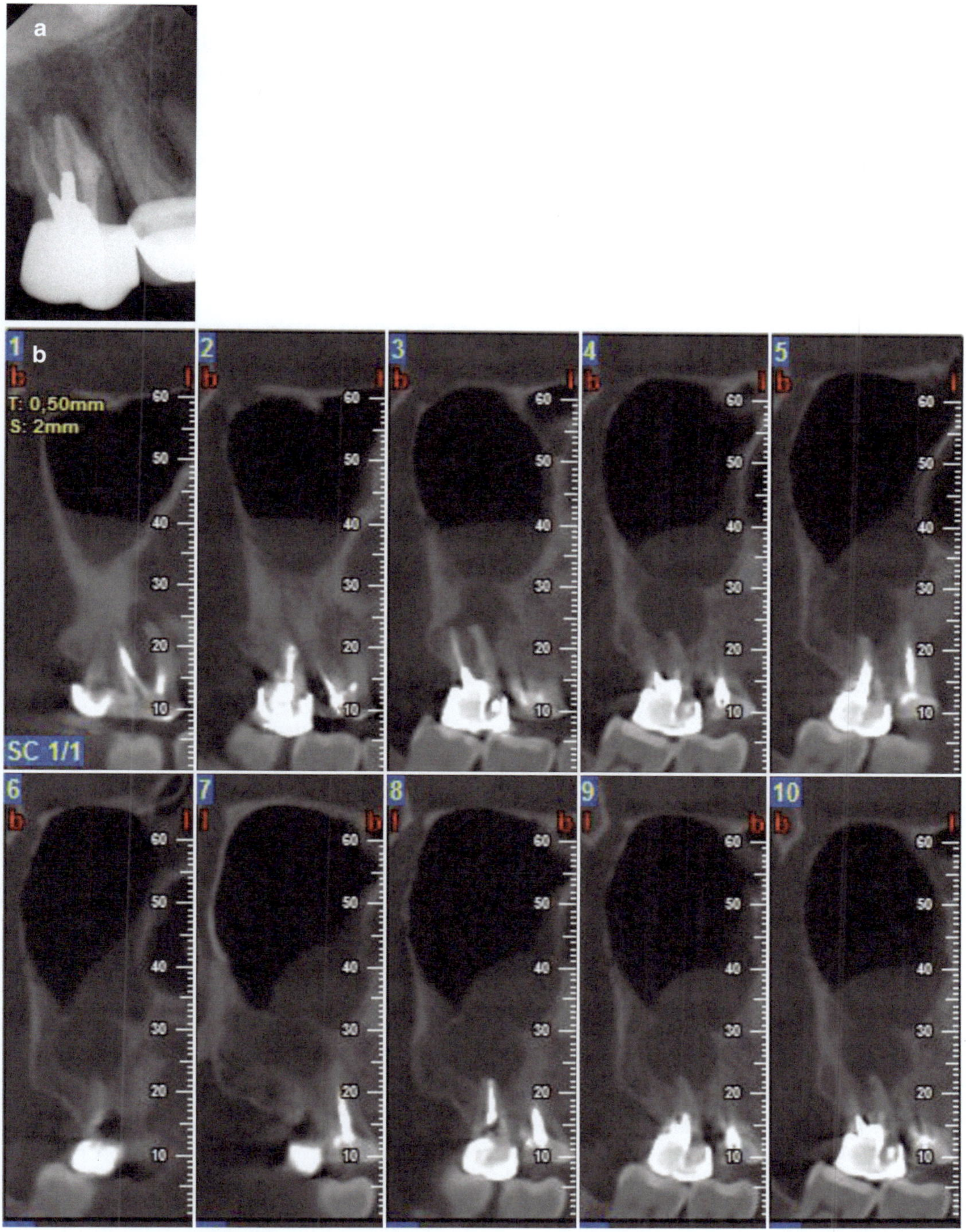

Fig. 15.6 (**a**) A typical recall periapical radiograph of a maxillary right second molar (#17). The root canal treatment was completed approximately 5 years ago and the tooth is currently asymptomatic, negative to percussion, palpation, and bite stress testing. The periapical radiograph shows possible widening of the apical periodontal ligament space on the mesial buccal root but the extent, or even the definitive presence, of apical pathosis is uncertain. (**b**) CBCT reveals an extended periapical lesion with perforation of the sinus floor and inflammatory sinus mucositis

15.2 Part II Other Digital Endodontic Applications and Systems

15.2.1 Three-Dimensional Evaluation of Internal Tooth Anatomy

A thorough knowledge of the root canals anatomy and morphology is essential in clinical endodontics and a requirement for a successful endodontic outcome. Improper working knowledge of the root canals anatomy has been referred as second only to errors in diagnosis and treatment planning as a cause of persistent apical pathology [40]. The clinical application of CBCT imaging has impacted virtually every aspect of endodontics.

15.2.2 Endodontic Access Design

Gaining access to the pulp chamber to facilitate the identification of all canal orifices represents the first technical step in root canal treatment that irreversibly alters tooth structure. Traditional access designs tend to be somewhat standardized per tooth type and are typically depicted in most texts with easily identifiable canal orifices at the base of a large pulpal floor. Many teeth requiring endodontic treatment present with pulp chambers that have significant alterations in volumetric space and shape due to excess deposits of tertiary dentin in response caries, bacterial ingress, dental procedures, and/or surface tooth loss over time. The integration of modern endodontic techniques and technology can assist in shaping the endodontic access based on the specific pulp chamber morphology of the tooth being treated.

Traditional access designs are treatment planned from parallel periapical and bitewing radiographs as well as clinical anatomic landmarks. This limits radiographic access design to a single plane and creates reliance upon the suggested access design standardizations. A more conservative and customized endodontic access can be designed from the anatomical information available on the CBCT volume. Precision vertical depth measurements can be determined from the occlusal plane to multiple levels within the pulp chamber in both the coronal and sagittal planes. Additionally, the lateral extension of the access as it relates to the occlusal surface can be determined from measurements available in the axial plane. Maintaining a conservative endodontic access minimizes the unnecessary removal of tooth structure and may improve overall fracture resistance [41].

15.2.3 Evaluation of Complex Roots and Root Canal Variations

Many anatomic and morphologic variations in tooth anatomy exist within the global population. In vivo identification of more complex anatomical root forms and root canal configurations can be best observed using CBCT imaging. Multiple published case reports demonstrate the significant advantages of CBCT over traditional radiographic imaging for the detection and management of a wide variety of anatomic and morphologic tooth and root variations [42].

15.2.3.1 Maxillary Molar Teeth

The Mesiobuccal Root Complex

The mesiobuccal root complex of the maxillary first permanent molar is one of the most well-documented and studied root canal systems in the endodontic literature. It is generally broad buccolingually with prominent depressions on the mesial and distal surfaces and usually contains two canals. One ex vivo study reported the presence of two mesiobuccal canals in the coronal half of maxillary first molars to be as high as 95.2% with 71% having separate apical portals of exit [43]. Similar variations occur in the maxillary second molars, although with less reported frequency [44]. The clinical detection and treatment of second mesiobuccal canals (MB2) can be enhanced with the acquisition of a CBCT scan [45]. The presence of an additional root and/or root canal can often be detected by studying the buccopalatal extent of the mesiobuccal root complex in the axial and coronal planes (Fig. 15.7).

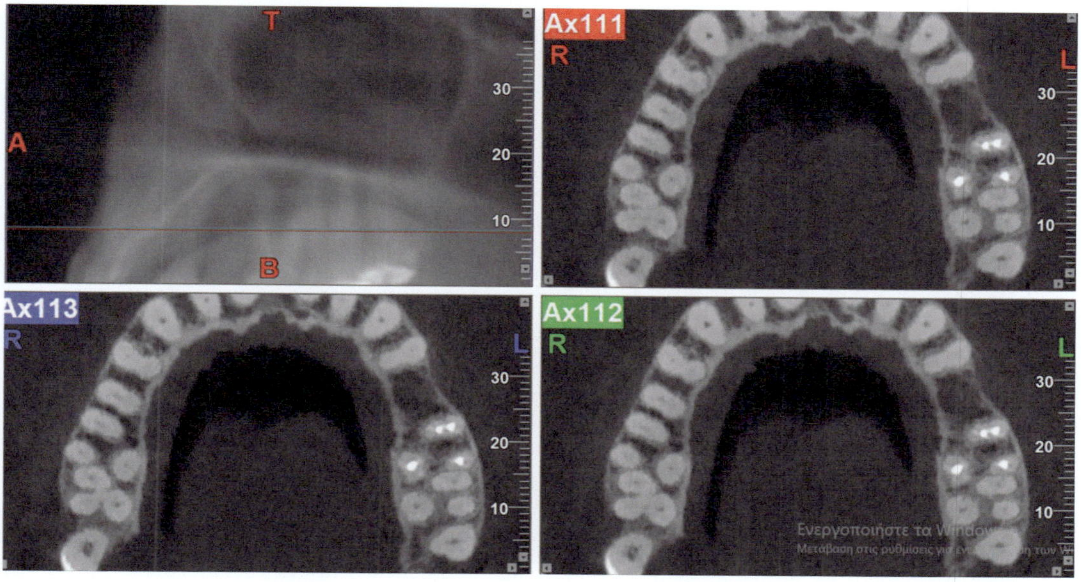

Fig. 15.7 CBCT images of an endodontically treated maxillary left first molar (#26) with two mesiobuccal root canals

Multiple Palatal Roots and Canals

A maxillary permanent molar with four roots and/or four root canals is not unusual when the additional root or root canal is located within the mesiobuccal root complex, but occasionally an additional root or root canal can be associated with the palatal root. This morphologic variation has been suggested to occur more frequently in maxillary second molars with a reported frequency of 0.4–1.4% [46, 47]. A CBCT scan can aid in the recognition of this rare anatomical variation as well as determine the exact location of the additional canal orifice for maximum conservation of tooth structure during endodontic access preparation.

15.2.3.2 Mandibular Molar Teeth

Radix Entomolaris and Radix Paramolaris

Mandibular permanent molars will occasionally present with an additional separate root located either to the lingual (radix entomolaris) or to the buccal (radix paramolaris). The literature suggests that the highest incidence of these morphologic variations is present in populations with Mongoloid ancestry (such as Chinese, Eskimo, and Native Americans) and occurs at a frequency of 5–40% [48]. Although traditional two-dimensional imaging at various angles can reveal clues as to the presence of these additional roots, exposing the anatomic location of the additional canal orifice during endodontic access can pose a clinical challenge. A CBCT scan will not only confirm the presence of these additional roots but also assist in determining the exact location of the canal orifice so that a proper access design can be planned.

C-Shaped Canal

A “C-shaped” root canal system is considered to be a variation in root morphology that causes the root to take on the shape of the letter “C” when viewed in cross section. The canals may or may not be separate. C-shaped canal configurations vary greatly among different ethnicities and have been reported to be as high as 30% among individuals of Asian descent. This variation occurs most often in mandibular second molars, but has also been documented in maxillary first molars, mandibular first and third molars, and mandibular premolars [49].

Isthmus Canals

An isthmus is often present between the buccal and lingual canals in mesial and/or distal roots of mandibular permanent molar teeth. Occasionally, an additional canal can be identified and treated within this isthmus space. When present, these canals are referred to as middle mesial and/or middle distal canals. Middle mesial canals have been reported to occur at rate as high as 15%, with 6.7% being identified as independent. The incidence of a middle distal canal is reported to be much less, with the highest frequency reported at 3%. The usefulness of CBCT imaging to identify and manage such canals has been reported in the literature [50, 51].

15.2.3.3 Maxillary Premolar Teeth

Maxillary permanent premolar teeth are generally broad buccolingually and narrow mesiodistally. They can present with two separate roots containing one canal per root or one broad root containing one or multiple canals. When one broad root is present, the corresponding internal anatomy can consist of a single ribbon-shaped canal or one of several documented multiple canal classifications with various levels of canal division and separate apical foramina. On occasion these teeth can present with a third root and/or third root canal. The frequency for this anatomic variation has been reported to be as high as 6% for maxillary permanent first premolars and 3% for maxillary permanent second premolars [46]. The addition of a CBCT scan can help determine the class of canal division, the presence of bifidity or trifurcation, and the exact level at which the canal division(s) occurs.

15.2.3.4 Mandibular Premolar Teeth

Mandibular permanent first premolar teeth are reported to have one canal 74% of the time, two canals 25.5% of the time, and three canals 0.5% of the time, whereas mandibular permanent second premolar teeth are reported to have one canal 88% of the time and a second or third canal only 12% of the time [47]. Just as in maxillary permanent premolar teeth, the traditional radiographic presence of a "fast break" generally indicates a canal division. CBCT imaging can help further determine the presence of multiple canals at the level of the suspected canal division.

15.2.3.5 Mandibular Anterior Teeth

Mandibular permanent central and lateral incisors are narrow mesiodistally and broad buccolingually with corresponding ribbon-shaped root canal systems. Although most mandibular incisors are reported to have only one canal, the incidence of two canals has been reported to range from 12.4 to 53%. A more recent publication reported that the frequency of two canals in mandibular incisors is 36.25%, with 1.3% of these canals having separate foramina [52]. Mandibular canines are commonly presented as having a single root canal, but the presence of a second canal cannot be ignored. Its prevalence has been shown to vary from 10.3% to 31.8%, while the percentage frequency of a two-rooted configuration has been reported to range from 0.7% to 11.7% [52]. The anatomic positioning of these teeth in the dental arch makes access to the lingual extent of the root canal system challenging. A cone beam scan can be studied in the sagittal and axial plane to determine the presence or absence of an additional root canal or root, as well as aid in the creation of an endodontic access designed for maximum visualization and minimal removal of tooth structure (Fig. 15.8).

15.2.3.6 Additional Morphological Considerations

Dens Invaginatus

Dens invaginatus is a developmental anomaly resulting from infolding of the enamel organ during tooth development. It is most commonly observed on maxillary lateral incisors and presents with varying degrees of severity and complexity [53]. CBCT imaging demonstrates the unique internal features of this anomaly as well as the challenges associated with endodontic treatment (Fig. 15.9).

Accessory Canals

Multiple communications exist between the dental pulp and the surrounding periodontium via the

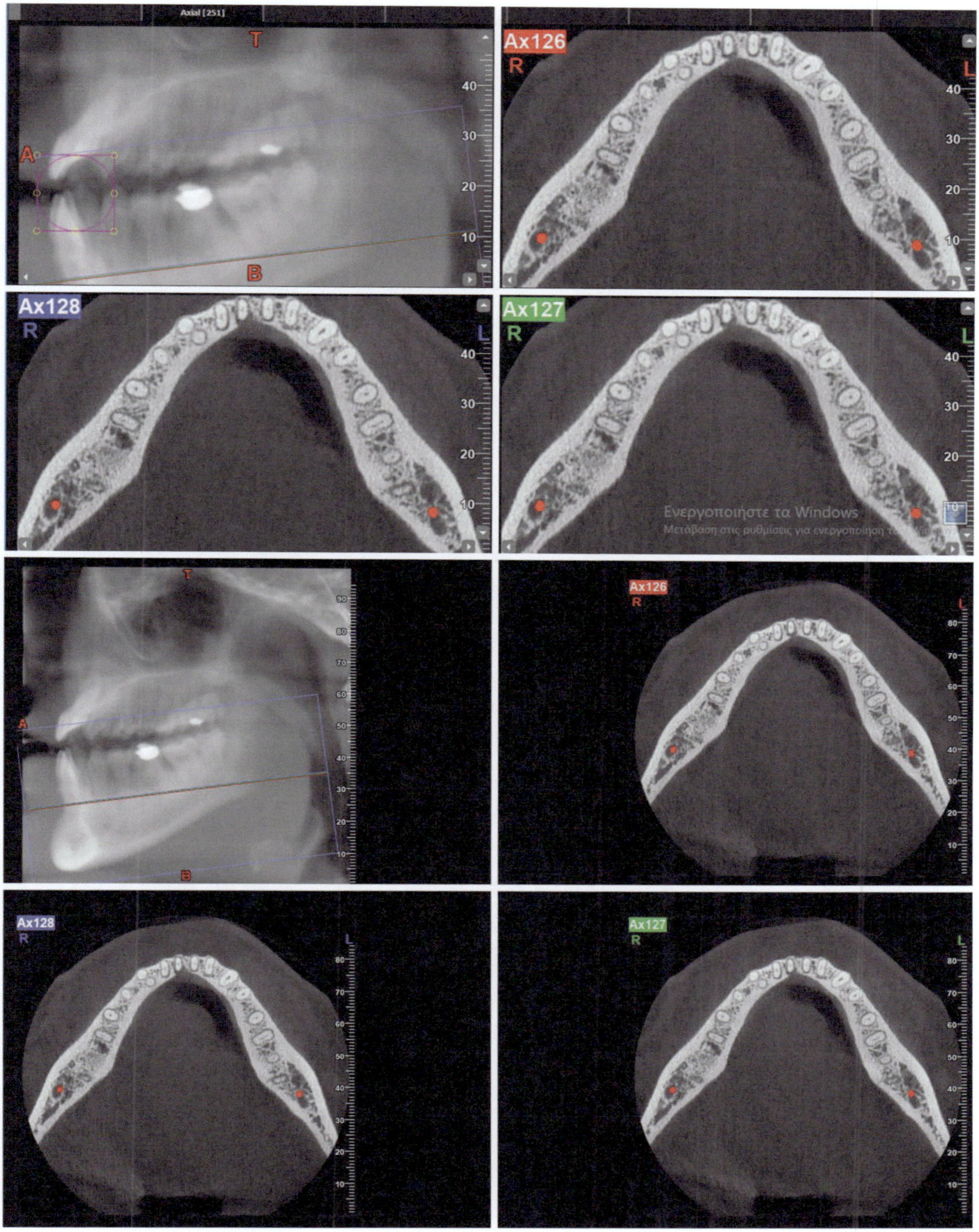

Fig. 15.8 CBCT images of a mandibular left canine (#33) with two roots (buccal and lingual)

apical foramen and accessory (lateral) canals. The distribution of accessory canals has been documented to occur at various levels throughout the root canal system as well as the floor of the pulp chamber, with the greatest number of accessory canals concentrated in the apical third of the

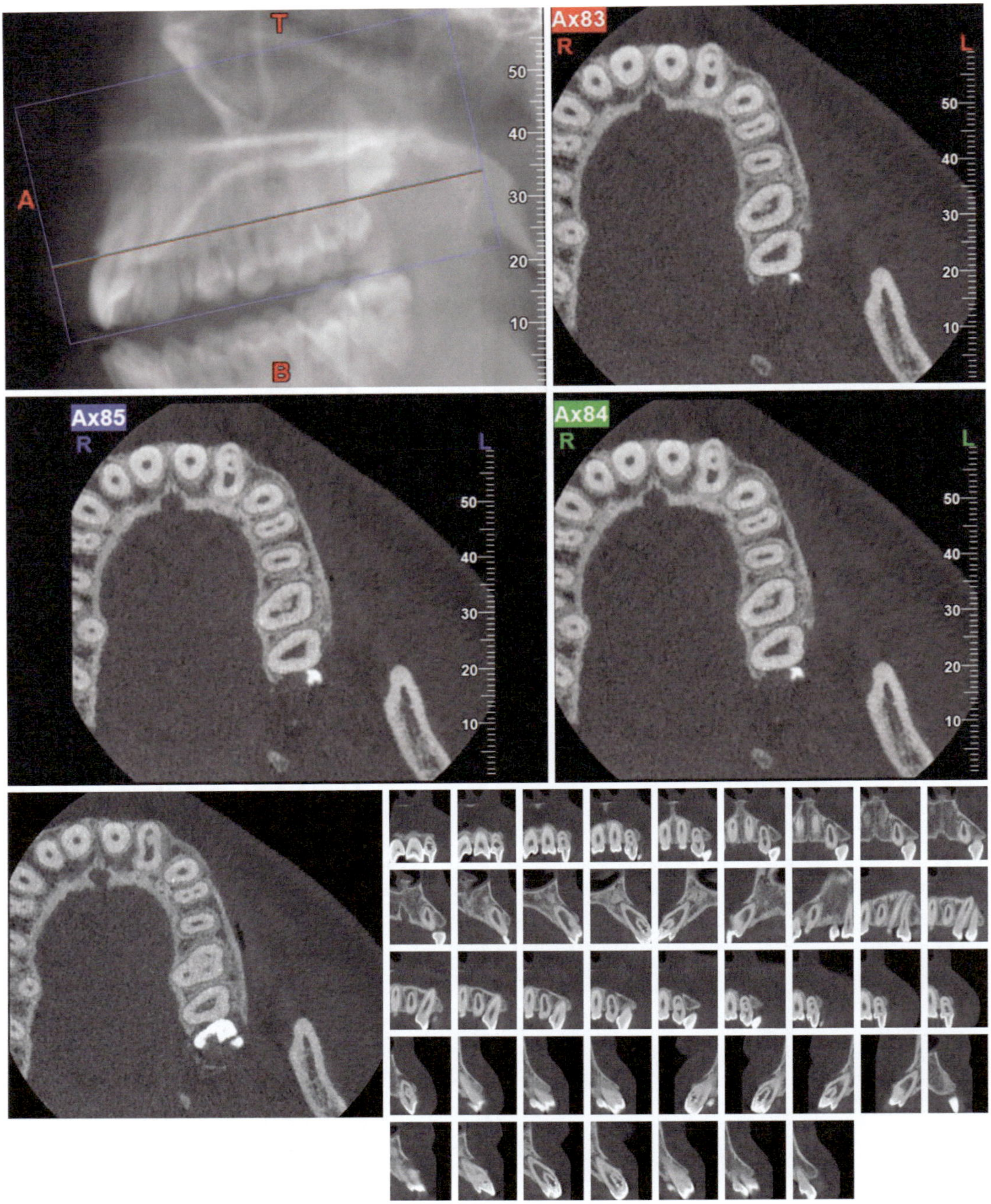

Fig. 15.9 CBCT images of a dens invaginatus maxillary left lateral incisor (#22) with periapical lesion and destruction of buccal cortical bone

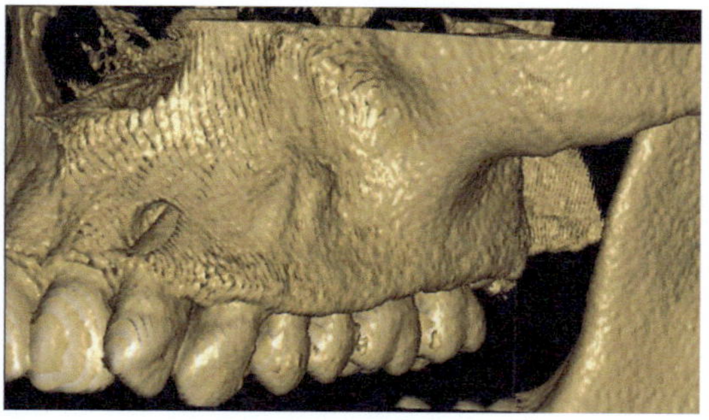

Fig. 15.9 (continued)

root canal system [54]. Occasionally, accessory canals can be identified on a CBCT scan. The verifiable presence of these canals as well as the ability to determine their exact location can facilitate successful treatment of such intricate ancillary anatomy.

Position of the Apical Foramen

The anatomical opening at the apex of the root through which nerves and blood vessels pass is often referred to as the apical foramen. This anatomic landmark represents the recommended apical termination of root canal instrumentation and obturation. The apical foramen can often present coronally in relation to the radiographic apex [55]. When the relationship between a coronally positioned apical foramen and the radiographic apex is exaggerated, two-dimensional endodontic radiographs create the illusion of clinically inadequate, incomplete, and/or inappropriate canal management. CBCT imaging can often confirm accurate management of these root canal systems by visually demonstrating the true position of the apical foramen as it relates to the anatomic root apex.

Canal Confluence

When two canals leave the pulp chamber and merge to form a single canal short of the apical foramen, the canals are considered to be confluent. With the exception of severely rotated teeth, it is impossible to view canal confluence on a two-dimensional radiograph. Canal confluence can only be viewed in the coronal plane of posterior teeth or the sagittal plane of anterior teeth. Therefore, a CBCT scan may be the only opportunity to identify the presence of canal confluence as well as the level at which the canal confluence occurs.

15.2.3.7 Conclusion

Variety of number and morphology of root canals may occur at any level within a single root. Two-dimensional radiographs tend to make the root canal system appear uniform and consistent in shape, and aberrant root canal configurations are not generally visible. The more we view CBCTs, the more we realize that unconventional anatomy should be considered the norm rather than the exception. Proper knowledge of root canal anatomy and morphology will cue the astute clinician to look for canal orifices in locations where they are typically observed. However, canals are not always readily apparent or easily identified. Cone beam imaging has introduced an accurate, nondestructive, real-time method for clinical chair side evaluation of tooth anatomy and morphology, comparable to that of the histological gold standard. The decision to incorporate CBCT imaging as a preoperative method to evaluate tooth anatomy can complex root anatomy.

15.3 Part III

15.3.1 Digital Guided Endodontics

The primary aim of endodontic treatment is the negotiation, debridement, and disinfection of the affected and infected root canal spaces. Therefore, the root canal's anatomy complexity represents one of the eminent challenges facing endodontists in clinical practice [56]. Advances in instrumentation notwithstanding, successful outcomes have been enhanced through the widespread utilization, at the specialist level, of the surgical operating microscope (SOM). It has proven itself indispensable in locating canals, identifying the location of MB2, removing separated instruments, perforation repair, and generally enhancing the delivery of quality care [57].

Furthermore, digital dentistry has become a reality of clinical procedures and has been widely explored by oral rehabilitation, implantology, orthodontics, oral surgery, among others [58]. The possibility of faithfully copying the dental or facial anatomy and transferring this model to the virtual environment stimulated a new moment, the era of digital planning. The development of specific software for this purpose made it possible to virtually plan many clinical procedures, evaluating possible errors or accurately predicting the amount of tooth preparation. Thus, treatment by trial and operative procedures error may be avoided, and it is planned more efficiently and with less clinical time with the patient.

Digital endodontics incorporated different tools and developed its own, further advancing in resolving complex cases [59]. The faithful copy of the internal anatomy provided by the advancement of CBCT devices and software, associated with the digital resources of 3D planning and printing, enabled the advent of guided endodontics. This technique is used at different stages of root canal treatment, with specific indications and greater results predictability.

15.3.1.1 Digital Resources in Endodontics

CBCT is the basis of digital planning in endodontics. Endodontics bases its planning on information obtained from meticulous navigation through CBCT images, which provide details of the internal anatomy of the teeth and adjacent structures. On the other hand, digital planning applied to oral rehabilitation is primarily based on the images obtained by intraoral scanners, which copy the external surface of teeth and adjacent periodontal tissues. The structures of interest for endodontics have tiny dimensions, representing a significant challenge for the endodontist in detecting root ramifications, fractures, perforations and determining different levels of obliteration and thickness of root canal walls. This complex condition in visualizing the endodontic microanatomy requires high-resolution imaging exams.

The CBCT image's quality is determined by the characteristics of the tomographic device, acquisition settings, patient stability and by the software for acquiring and running the images. In diagnosing endodontic microanatomy, it is more important to prioritize image acquisition using high-resolution CT scanners with a better focal point than the equipment capable of acquiring large volumes and recording larger areas. The quantity and density of materials present in the patient's mouth can also influence image quality, as dense materials can produce artifacts that overlay essential details. This inconvenience caused by artifacts can be minimized by using an advanced image software, that increase the quality of the CBCT image, improve the diagnostic capacity and consequently positively impact clinical decision-making [27, 39].

Digital planning software was also fundamental for advancing digital endodontics toward developing guides applied to endodontic area. Digital planning software imports DICOM files from CBCT exams and uses them as parameters to outline guides with computer-aided design (CAD—computer-aided design) tools. In modeling the guides, current digital planning software needs to synchronize the DICOM file with the digital file of a model of the patient's arch in STL (Standard Tessellation Language) format. The digital model is obtained with intraoral scanning equipment [58].

The 3D printing technology (stereolithography technique) allows the production of endodontic guides. The three-dimensional design of the guide developed by the digital planning software is also exported in STL format. Before 3D printing, the planned STL needs to be prepared to transform the guide's STL file into a sequence of numerous layers or slices. The smaller the thickness of the slices, the greater the reliability of the printed guide, but the more time will be spent in the printing process. Currently, endodontic guides are printed in light-curing liquid resin with direct light processing technology (DLP—direct light processing) due to the better cost–benefit ratio [60].

15.3.1.2 Guided Endodontics Indications

Guided endodontics has been indicated in different clinical situations. A better understanding of its characteristics and the exploration of digital resources in endodontics provided greater clinical applicability. Indications should not be interpreted as a specific convenience resource and facilitator for professionals with less clinical experience and/or who do not use the appropriate technology for complex endodontic treatments but rather as an additional tool for the endodontists [61].

The initial indication of guided access is related to calcified root canals [62–64]. Root canal calcification may reach only the cervical third of the root canal or extend to the middle or apical third. The cause may be associated with several factors, such as a consequence of traumatic dental injury, an orthodontic treatment, response to pulp injuries such as caries or restorative materials, or even in older patients [65]. In these cases, root canal treatment becomes necessary when calcification is related to periapical pathologies [59, 62, 63] (Fig. 15.10).

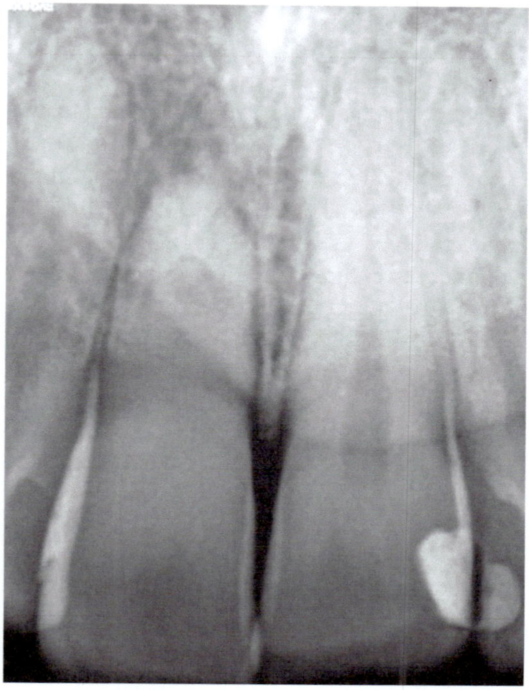

Fig. 15.10 A periapical radiograph of a maxillary right central incisor (#11) with calcified root canal and periapical lesion, indicated for guided endodontics

Coronary access represents the most challenging operative step in teeth with calcified root canals, making it difficult to maintain the correct trepanation direction when it extends mainly to the middle and apical thirds. Even for experienced endodontists, it can result in deviations or perforations, increasing the chances of failure [59]. In this sense, using the guided technique provides greater safety, greater predictability, less volume of dental tissue removed, and shorter clinical time with the patient [66–68].

Guided endodontics has also been indicated in cases of endodontic surgery [69, 70]. A guide for surgical access is necessary, with less removal of bone tissue and better location of the lesion region and dental apex [70]. Furthermore, these guided procedures reduce the risk of trans and post-surgical complications, such as bleeding or damage to neighboring anatomical structures. In addition to these factors, it leads to a shorter healing time and a better prognosis [69].

Challenging cases related to surgical access and proximity to sensitive anatomical structures can be better performed using prototype guides. Benjamin et al. [70] reported three cases with surgical guides used in a targeted endodontic microsurgery approach, illustrating the diagnostic value of CBCT imaging for detecting neurovascular bundles and the use of the guides to mitigate the risk of injury to these important structures. Giacomo et al. [71] demonstrated the use of guided access in surgeries related to the palatal root of maxillary second molar, fused roots of a maxillary first molar, and a mandibular second premolar with apical proximity to the mental foramen. In all reported cases, guides promoted an accurate osteotomy and apicectomy related to angulation, diameter, and extension.

The use of fiberglass posts in oral rehabilitation has become a reality in recent years. However, when necessary, its removal represents a great challenge for dentists and may lead to root deviations or perforations, cracks, or even fractures [72]. Thus, virtual planning and printing of guides have contributed to greater safety in this procedure and reduced clinical time, bringing greater patient comfort and reducing professional stress [72–75].

Access in teeth with developmental anomalies has also been one of the indications for using endodontic guides [76–78]. Dental malformations, such as *dens invaginatus,* can represent a complicating issue when endodontic treatment is required. Thus, the association of a correct diagnosis with three-dimensional imaging exams leads to more assertive treatments. However, these anomalies make proper access difficult, increasing the possibility of excessive tooth wear, error in the access direction, or even root perforations. In this sense, guided access has been a viable and predictable alternative.

An important topic to be raised refers to teeth with cracks, root fractures or resorptions. For accurate planning, a CBCT with high spatial resolution must be carefully analyzed by a well-trained professional, tracking the tooth thoroughly to verify the viability of the tooth for the application of the guided technique.

15.3.1.3 Planning and Digital Flow of Guided Endodontics

The guided endodontics technique can be divided into:

1. A laboratory phase for production of the endodontic guide, in which most processes are performed in the absence of the patient, with the aid of digital tools;
2. A clinical phase of application of the guide in operative procedures.

The digital flow of guided endodontics follows the same sequence of processes performed in the digital flow of implantology for guided surgical procedures in implant installation. Once the indication for the use of an endodontic guide is stated, the professional must check if the patient has both the CBCT exam in the region of interest and the patient's arch model in digital format. Since the Digital Flow starts with the acquisition of DICOM and STL files, and if the patient has performed this acquisition recently, without further dental interventions that may have changed the internal dental anatomy or the surface of the oral tissues (teeth/periodontium), these files can be assessed. If the patient does not have them, or has any of these files in poor quality, a new request must be made. The DICOM file will be obtained by requesting the CBCT exam, and the STL file will be obtained by scanning the intra-oral arch of the patient.

After acquiring the DICOM and STL files, the planning of the endodontic guide is carried out by digital planning centers (planning centers) or trained professionals, using specific software for planning surgical guides. These planning tools were developed to guide the installation of implants and not wear and tear on the internal part of the tooth. Therefore, sometimes, the guided endodontics technique may be contraindicated during the planning phase due to the scarcity of resources applied to the reduced dimensions of the endodontics area of operation. In addition to the dimensions of wear length and diameter, the direction and region to be worn by the drill must be carefully planned. Trajectories that promote wear of critical anatomical structures for tooth longevity, such as incisal edge, enamel bridges, and cusp tips, should be avoided. Once the wear length and trajectory planning have been defined, it is essential to estimate the thickness of tooth tissue after the guided procedure has been performed. Plans should not project wear at a distance of less than 1 mm from the root surface in contact with the periodontal ligament to avoid perforation accidents. Although guided wear is predictable, it is considered an average of deviations of up to 0.4 mm at the end of the drill in guided wear to the apical third of the root [79]. Deviations are minimized by rigorous planning and guide printing. The more adapted the occlusal surface of the teeth, the greater the stability of the guide and the lesser the risk of deviation during the wearing procedure. Inspection windows are planned in different parts of the guide to verify adaptation in the operative phase.

Clinical situations unfavorable to the stability of the guides require the planning of resources that limit their mobility. For example, guides supported by a reduced number of teeth or the absence of teeth adjacent to the region of the guided procedure are unfavorable factors for its stability. In these situations, we must plan the stabilization of the guide with fixation pins. The use of metal rings is also a feature that helps in the stability of guided wear. According to the planned path, the metal ring can restrict the drill's movement in a linear direction in the crown/apex direction.

Once the endodontic guide project is completed, a detailed virtual planning report must be sent to the dentist responsible for the case, for analysis and approval. Only after approval, the STL file of the guide design is sent for 3D printing. Finally, endodontic guides are printed on resins that can be autoclaved.

15.3.1.4 Clinical Operative Steps

To be successful in guided endodontic accesses, it is essential that all previous laboratory steps have been fulfilled. Furthermore, the technological resources for the diagnosis and planning of the digital flow are of fundamental importance to provide a correct indication of the use of guides, as well as the materialization of this resource. Therefore, the approach will be step-by-step to facilitate understanding, what the clinician must establish from the arrival of the printed guide to the guided access through a clinical case of root canal obliteration with previous nonsuccess access associated with apical periodontitis.

Endodontic guides are designed and printed in digital planning centers and delivered to the clinician ready to use. However, in addition to participating in the guide planning, the endodontist is responsible for checking various aspects that may interfere with the final result of the treatment. A virtual planning report is sent by the Planning Centers with information about the intraoral scan, the drill trajectory, guide length on adjacent teeth, and also about the presence and position of visual inspection windows. Thus, possible distortions or failures in printing the guide should be verified through the final report, such as incorrect positioning of the visual inspection windows, presence or absence of a metal ring, and the extension and support of the guide different from what was planned (Fig. 15.11).

After confirming the quality of the printed guide, the tests are carried out in the mouth to verify its perfect adaptation and stability. Planning can be carried out for guides with support only on adjacent teeth or guides with support on adjacent teeth and fixed in bone [59, 62]. However, regardless of the choice of fixation on bone or not, the visual inspection windows are an essential indicator of the perfect adaptation of the guide. They indicate that the planning and printing were carried out correctly.

Currently, endodontics uses instruments and software for planning guided surgery for implant dentistry and, therefore, the drill used for the vast majority of guided approaches is 1.3 mm in diameter. Unfortunately, this drill does not have cutting power in enamel. Therefore, it is necessary to perform slight prior wear with diamond drills in the enamel region so that the implant drill works primarily on dentin. Then, a marking is made with the guide already positioned to carry out the initial wear, seeking the point of choice.

Following operative stages, the next step is to perform the guided endodontic approach. For this, an electric motor in continuous rotation with a speed set at 800 RPM and a torque of 4.0 Ncm is required. After re-verifying the perfect position of the guide, it must be stabilized with manual support and constant irrigation. Finally, the drill must go in until it taps the ring's base, which is the depth reference, and it must go through until reaching the planned point (Fig. 15.12).

The irrigation process must be continuous and carried out toward the inside of the guide. At each advancement of 3 mm, the path's interior is created, and the end of the drill is washed, removing all the excess of adhered dentin. As soon as the drill touches the ring base, the guided access is completed, and the next step should be taken, which is the mapping and location of the calcified canal with small-caliber files.

In the clinical case in question, absolute isolation was performed, and access to the calcified root canal was reached with a #10 K-file. Then, the root canal treatment was carried out following the entire protocol of root canal preparation, enhancement of the irrigating solution, use of

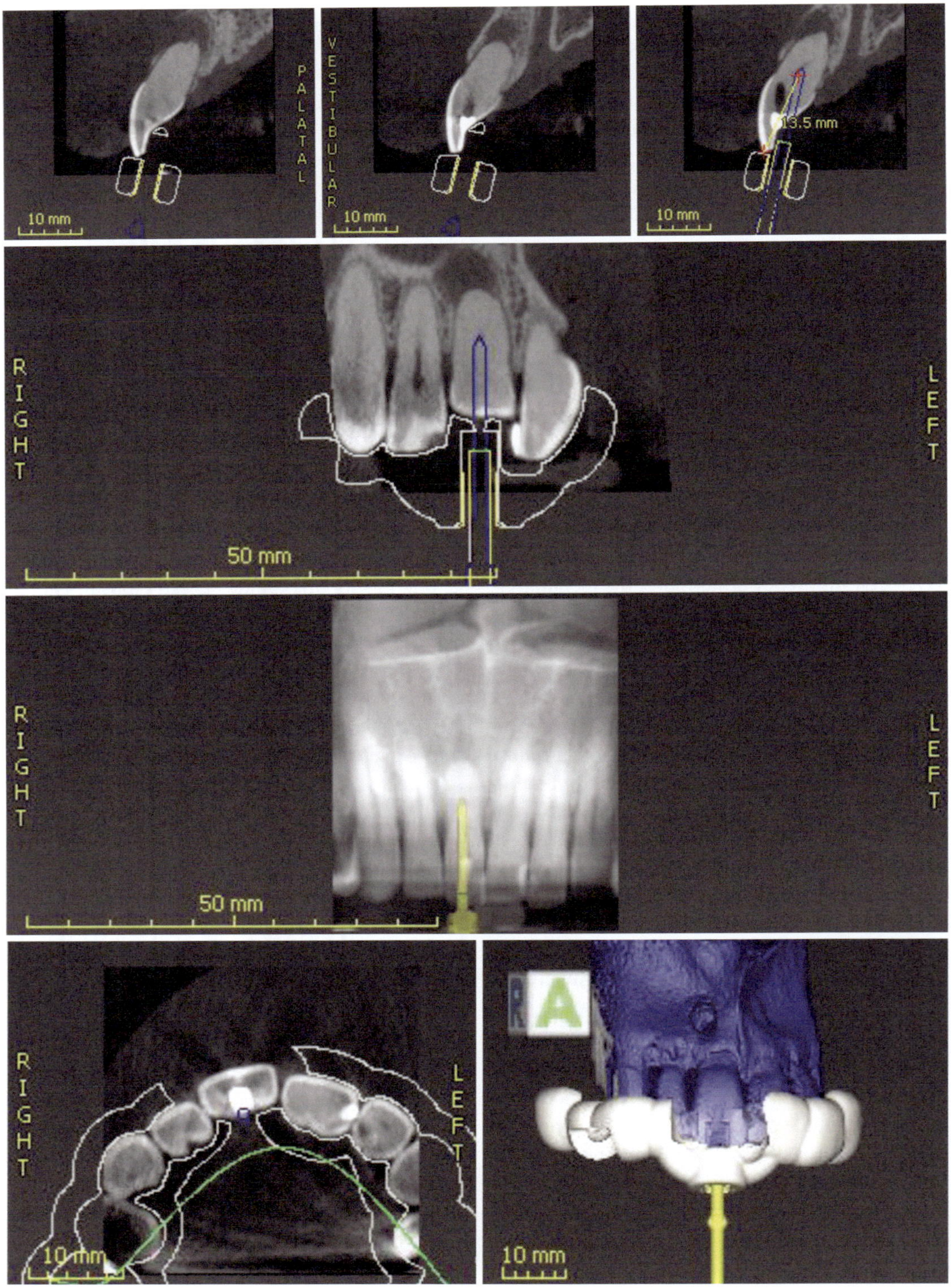

Fig. 15.11 CBCT images of tooth #11, which is shown in Fig. 15.10, show root canal calcification and the incorrect course of the first attempt at endodontic access, starting at the center of the palatal surface and toward the buccal surface. Also, the access path and guide outlined by the digital planning can be seen

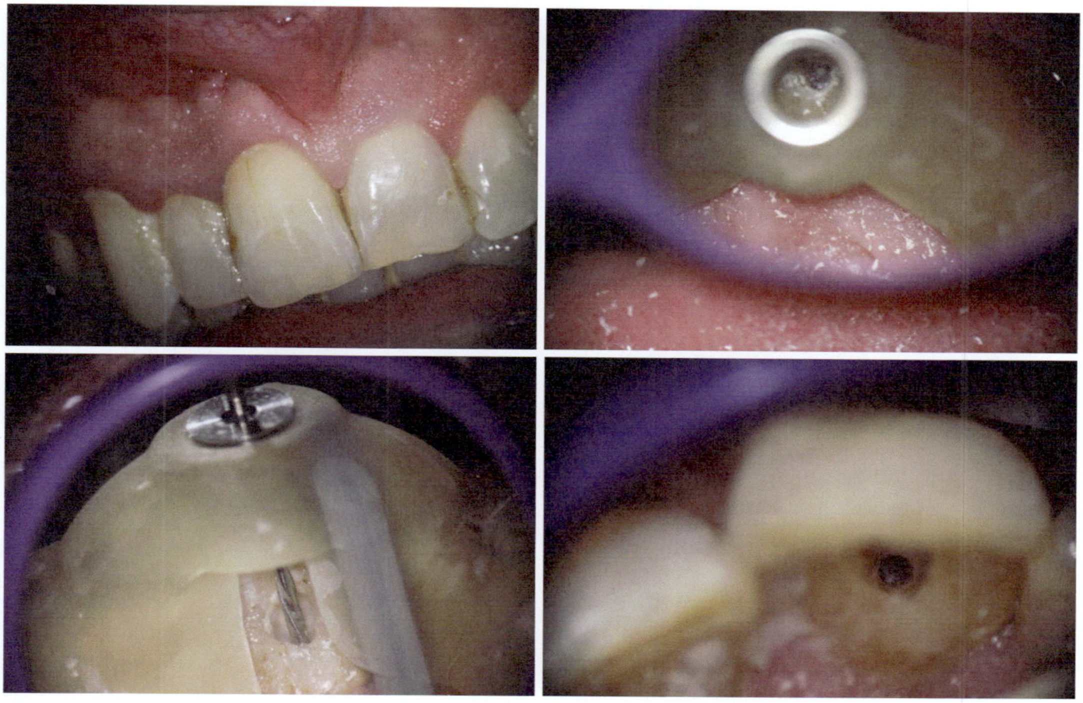

Fig. 15.12 Initial clinical appearance of tooth #11, which is shown in Figs. 15.10 and 15.11, and clinical operative steps of guided endodontic access

intracanal medication based on calcium hydroxide paste, and subsequently filled. After the case report conclusion, a new CBCT acquisition was performed, which showed the correct path of the drill in the guided endodontic access, without excessive wear and deviation, which provided free access to the root canal. This illustrative clinical case aimed to demonstrate the application protocol and the accuracy of guided endodontics in solving calcified canals, providing greater safety to the operator.

15.3.1.5 Discussion

Guided endodontics is a technique in constant evolution. Technological advances provide tools that are increasingly more adequate and precise for endodontics, evolving toward a more accurate technique with lower cost and greater reach to the clinician. Even so, it has limitations, and these must be evaluated before planning and executing it.

The complex anatomy of root canals, despite involving the main indications for guided planning, may also represent some limitations of the technique. Guided access is only possible in the straight region of the root canal and becomes imprecise in curvature areas. In this sense, the planning must be evaluated well, directing the wear and the drills only to the straight portion and avoiding bending. Another aspect related to dental anatomy refers to the root diameter. The different root and root canals configurations [56] in the various teeth groups may reflect in roots with minimal thickness in the mesiodistal and/or buccolingual direction, making the use of burs in this region incompatible (e.g., lower incisors or mesiobuccal roots of the upper molars).

Other limitations can be added [80–82]. Patients with restricted mouth opening may hinder or even contraindicate guided access, especially in posterior teeth. CBCT exams that present image artifacts in the region can also limit the virtual planning and accuracy of the prototype guides for the technique.

However, the evolution of the technological tools used leads to expanding its indications and greater exploration of digital endodontics. A significant advance experienced in recent years refers to CBCT images. More modern appliances, and more innovative software with a greater number of resources [80, 81], have enabled a more faithful copy of the internal anatomy of the teeth, avoiding distortions that lead to inaccuracy and access errors. Thus, with the elimination of image artifacts arising from high-density materials, guided access can be efficiently planned in the vast majority of indicated cases.

In this sense, technological advances open up other possibilities, such as the reduction of operative steps. With software capable of faithfully and accurately reconstructing anatomical structures without distortions, intraoral scanning may soon be eliminated. The 3D reconstructions will be used as three-dimensional models of the arcade and converted into STL files. This reduction in operative steps is advantageous to both the patient (lower cost in preparing the guide) and the dentist (lesser chance of distortions due to the elimination of steps).

Another aspect that has been evolving is also the tools used in the clinical stage of guided endodontics. The adaptation of drills from Implantology characterizes a significant limitation of the technique, which has been overcome with the development of instruments for endodontics. The ultrasonic inserts developed for this purpose will represent a considerable advance in guided endodontics, with even more controlled wear (due to the smaller diameters of these inserts) and the possibility of more efficient irrigation during its use. However, the action of the ultrasonic insert can be restricted in guides with metal rings. Therefore, ultrasonic requires planning non-restrictive guides, with greater relief (offset) in the space the insert passes through the guide. In addition, non-restrictive guides require greater attention to perform the technique, allowing greater deviation from the worn path. It is currently indicating this type of guide for the following clinical situations: teeth with fragile roots that need a small amount of wear; or delimit osteotomy and apicectomy in endodontic surgeries.

Guided endodontics technology represents a new perspective for complex endodontic cases, which could lead to errors in surgical procedures using the conventional technique. It is a precise, effective and easy clinical application technique [80–83]. It represents the incorporation of technological resources and digital planning in the life of the endodontist, giving greater predictability to cases in which it is applied in clinical practice.

Furthermore, it requires minimal financial investment in the office since image capture equipment, virtual planning, and guides printing are part of the equipment of digital planning centers. In addition, it takes a shorter number of clinical sessions, increasing patient comfort and reducing professional stress.

References

1. De Paula-Silva FW, Wu MK, Leonardo MR, da Silva LA, Wesselink PR. Accuracy of periapical radiography and cone-beam computed tomography scans in diagnosing apical periodontitis using histopathological findings as a gold standard. J Endod. 2009;35(7):1009–12.
2. Patel S, Wilson R, Dawood A, Mannocci F. The detection of periapical pathosis using periapical radiography and cone beam computed tomography—part 1: preoperative status. Int Endod J. 2012;45(8):702–10.
3. Patel S, Wilson R, Dawood A, Mannocci F. The detection of periapical pathosis using periapical radiography and cone beam computed tomography—part 2: a 1-year post-treatment followup. Int Endod J. 2012;45(8):711–23.
4. Sogur E, Grondahl H, Bakst G, Mert A. Does a combination of two radiographs increase accuracy in detecting acid-induced periapical lesions and does it approach the accuracy of conebeam computed tomography scanning. J Endod. 2012;38(2):131–6.
5. Patel S, Dawood A, Mannocci F, Wilson R, Pitt FT. Detection of periapical bone defects in human jaws using cone beam computed tomography and intraoral radiography. Int Endod J. 2009;42(6):507–15.
6. Pope O, Sathorn C, Parashos P. A comparative investigation of cone-beam computed tomography and periapical radiography in the diagnosis of a healthy periapex. J Endod. 2014;40(3):360–5.
7. Hassan B, Metska ME, Ozok AR, van der Stelt P, Wesselink PR. Detection of vertical root fractures in endodontically treated teeth by a cone beam computed tomography scan. J Endod. 2009;35:719–22.

8. Edlund M, Nair MK, Nair UP. Detection of vertical root fractures by using cone-beam computed tomography: a clinical study. J Endod. 2011;37(6):768–72.
9. Metska ME, Aartman IH, Wesselink PR, Özok AR. Detection of vertical root fracture in vivo in endodontically treated teeth by cone-beam computed tomography scans. J Endod. 2012;38(10):1344–7.
10. Brady E, Mannocci F, Wilson R, Brown J, Patel S. A comparison of CBCT and periapical radiography for the detection of vertical root fractures in non-endodontically treated teeth. Int Endod J. 2014;47(8):735–46.
11. Melo SLS, Bortoluzzi EA, Abreu M, Correa LR, Correa M. Diagnostic ability of a cone-beam computed tomography scan to assess longitudinal root fractures in prosthetically treated teeth. J Endod. 2010;36:1879–82.
12. Corbella S, Del Fabbro M, Tamse A, Rosen E, Tsesis I, Taschieri S. Cone beam computed tomography for the diagnosis of vertical root fractures: a systematic review of the literature and meta-analysis. Oral Surg Oral Med Oral Pathol Oral Radiol. 2014;118(5):593–602.
13. Rosen E, Taschieri S, Del Fabbro M, Beitlitum I, Tsesis I. The diagnostic efficacy of cone beam computed tomography in endodontics: a systematic review and analysis by a hierarchical model of efficacy. J Endod. 2015;41(7):1008–14.
14. Long H, Zhou Y, Ye N, Liao L, Jian F, Wang Y, Lai W. Diagnostic accuracy of CBCT for tooth fractures: a meta-analysis. J Dent. 2014;42(3):240–8.
15. Ma RH, Ge ZP, Li G. Detection accuracy of root fractures in cone-beam computed tomography images: a systematic review and meta-analysis. Int Endod J. 2016;49(7):646–54.
16. Avsever H, Gunduz K, Orhan K, Uzun I, Ozmen B, Egrioglu E, Midilli M. Comparison of intraoral radiography and cone-beam computed tomography for the detection of horizontal root fractures: an in vitro study. Clin Oral Investig. 2014;18(1):285–92.
17. Estrela C, Bueno MR, De Alencar AH, Mattar R, Valladares Neto J, Azevedo BC, De Araújo Estrela CR. Method to evaluate inflammatory root resorption by using cone beam computed tomography. J Endod. 2009;35(11):1491–7.
18. Durack C, Patel S, Davies J, Wilson R, Mannocci F. Diagnostic accuracy of small volume cone beam computed tomography and intraoral periapical radiography for the detection of simulated external inflammatory root resorption. Int Endod J. 2011;44(2):136–47.
19. Diangelis AJ, Andreasen JO, Ebeleseder KA, et al. International Association of Dental Traumatology guidelines for the management of traumatic dental injuries: 1—fractures and luxations of permanent teeth. Dent Traumatol. 2012;28:2–12.
20. May JJ, Cohenca N, Peters OA. Contemporary management of horizontal root fractures to the permanent dentition: diagnosis—radiologic assessment to include cone-beam computed tomography. J Endod. 2013;39(3 Suppl):S20–5.
21. Iikubo M, Kobayashi K, Mishima A, et al. Accuracy of intraoral radiography, multidetector helical CT, and limited cone-beam CT for the detection of horizontal tooth root fracture. Oral Surg Oral Med Oral Pathol Oral Radiol Endod. 2009;108:e70–4.
22. AAE and AAOMR Joint Position Statement. Use of cone beam computed tomography in endodontics. J Endod. 2015;41(9):1393–6.
23. Maini A, Durning P, Drage N. Resorption: within or without? The benefit of cone-beam computed tomography when diagnosing a case of an internal/external resorption defect. Br Dent J. 2008;9:135–7.
24. Bernardes RA, de Moraes IG, Húngaro Duarte MA, et al. Use of cone-beam volumetric tomography in the diagnosis of root fractures. Oral Surg Oral Med Oral Pathol Oral Radiol Endod. 2009;108:270–7.
25. Fayad MI, Ashkenaz PJ, Johnson BR. Different representations of vertical root fractures detected by cone-beam volumetric tomography: a case series report. J Endod. 2012;38:1435–42.
26. Michetti J, Maret D, Mallet JP, Diemer F. Validation of cone beam computed tomography as a tool to explore root canal anatomy. J Endod. 2010;36:1187–90.
27. Liang YH, Li G, Wesselink PR, Wu MK. Endodontic outcome predictors identified with periapical radiographs and cone-beam computed tomography scans. J Endod. 2011;37:326–31.
28. Velvart P, Hecker H, Tillinger G. Detection of the apical lesion and the mandibular canal in conventional radiography and computed tomography. Oral Surg Oral Med Oral Pathol Oral Radiol Endod. 2001;92:682–8.
29. Stavropoulos A, Wenzel A. Accuracy of cone beam dental CT, intraoral digital and conventional film radiography for the detection of periapical lesions: an ex vivo study in pig jaws. Clin Oral Investig. 2007;11:101–6.
30. Nakata K, Naitoh M, Izumi M, et al. Effectiveness of dental computed tomography in diagnostic imaging of periradicular lesion of each root of a multirooted tooth: a case report. J Endod. 2006;32:583–7.
31. Lofthag-Hansen S, Huumonen S, Grondahl K, Grondahl HG. Limited cone-bean CT and intraoral radiography for the diagnosis of periapical pathology. Oral Surg Oral Med Oral Pathol Oral Radiol Endod. 2007;103:114–9.
32. Cotton TP, Geisler TM, Holden DT, et al. Endodontic applications of cone-beam volumetric tomography. J Endod. 2007;33:1121–32.
33. Patel S, Dawood A, Whaites E, Pitt FT. New dimensions in endodontic imaging: part 1. Conventional and alternative radiographic systems. Int Endod J. 2009;42:447–62.
34. Patel S. New dimensions in endodontic imaging: part 2. Cone beam computed tomography. Int Endod J. 2009;42:463–75.

35. Scarfe WC, Farman AG, Sukovic P. Clinical applications of cone-beam computed tomography in dental practice. J Can Dent Assoc. 2006;72:75–80.
36. Nair MK, Nair UP. Digital and advanced imaging in endodontics: a review. J Endod. 2007;33:1–6.
37. Farman AG, Farman TT. A comparison of 18 different x-ray detectors currently used in dentistry. Oral Surg Oral Med Oral Pathol Oral Radiol Endod. 2005;99:66–71.
38. Farman AG. ALARA still applies. Oral Surg Oral Med Oral Pathol Oral Radiol Endod. 2005;100:395–7.
39. Ee J, Fayad MI, Johnson BR. Comparison of endodontic diagnosis and treatment planning decisions using cone-beam volumetric tomography versus periapical radiography. J Endod. 2014;40:910–6.
40. Walton WE, Vertucci FJ. Internal anatomy. In: Walton WE, Torabinejad M, editors. Principles and practice of endodontics. 3rd ed. Philadelphia, PA: Saunders; 2002. p. 176–81.
41. Krishan R, Paque F, Ossareh A, Kishen A, Dao T, Friedman S. Impacts of conservative endodontic cavity on root canal instrumentation efficacy and resistance to fracture assessed in incisor, premolar and molars. J Endod. 2014;40:1160–6.
42. Kfir A, Telishevsky-Strauss Y, Leitner A, Metzger Z. The diagnosis and conservative treatment of a complex type 3 dens invaginatus using cone beam computed tomography (CBCT) and 3D plastic models. Int Endod J. 2013;46:275–88.
43. Kulild JC, Peters DD. Incidence and configuration of canal systems in the mesiobuccal root of maxillary first and second molars. J Endod. 1990;16:311.
44. Peikoff MD, Christie WH, Fogel HM. The maxillary second molar: variations in the number of roots and canals. Int Endod J. 1996;29:365–9.
45. Vizzotto MB, Silveira PF, Arus NA, Montagner F, Gomes BO, da Silveira HE. CBCT for the assessment of second mesiobuccal (MB2) canals in maxillary molar teeth: effect of voxel size and presence of root filling. Int Endod J. 2013;46:870–6.
46. Vertucci FJ, Seelig A, Gillis R. Root canal morphology of the human maxillary second premolar. Oral Surg Oral Med Oral Pathol Oral Radiol Endod. 1974;38:456–64.
47. Vertucci FJ. Root canal morphology of mandibular premolars. J Am Dent Assoc. 1978;97(1):47–50.
48. De Moor R, Deroose C, Calberson F. The radix entomolaris in mandibular first molars: an endodontic challenge. Int Endod J. 2004;37:789–99.
49. Chai WL, Thong YL. Cross sectional morphology and minimum canal wall widths in c-shaped roots of mandibular molars. J Endod. 2004;30:509–12.
50. Ahmed HA, Abu-bakr NH, Yahia NA, Ibrahim YE. Root and canal morphology of permanent mandibular molars in a Sudanese population. Int Endod J. 2007;40:766–71.
51. La SH, Jung DH, Kim EC, Min KS. Identification of independent middle mesial canal in mandibular first molar using cone-beam computed tomography imaging. J Endod. 2010;237:1–4.
52. Martins RN, Versiani MA. CBCT and micro-CT on the study of root canal anatomy. In: Versiani MA, Basrani BR, Sousa-Neto MD, editors. The root canal anatomy in permanent dentition. Cham: Springer International Publishing AG; 2019. p. 94–100.
53. Hulsman M, Dens invaginatus. Aetiology, classification, prevalence, diagnosis and treatment considerations. Int Endod J. 1997;30:79.
54. Gutmann JL, Fan B. Tooth morphology, isolation, and access. In: Hargreaves KM, Berman LH, editors. Cohen's pathways of the pulp. 11th ed. St. Louis, MI: Elsevier; 2016. p. 130–208.
55. Souza RA, Figueiredo JAP, Colombo S, Dantas JCP, Lago M, Pecora JD. Location of the apical foramen and its relationship with foramina file size. Dental Press Endod. 2011;1:64–8.
56. Vertucci FJ. Root canal morphology and its relationship to endodontic procedure. Endod Topics. 2005;10:3–29.
57. Decurcio DA, Rossi-Fedele G, Estrela C, Pulikkotil SJ, Nagendrababu V. Machine-assisted agitation reduces postoperative pain during root canal treatment: a systematic review and meta-analysis from randomized clinical trials. J Endod. 2019;45:387–93.
58. Alauddin MS, Baharuddin AS, Ml MG. The modern and digital transformation of oral health care: a mini review. Healthcare (Basel). 2021;9:118.
59. Loureiro MAZ, Silva JA, Chaves GS, Capeletti LR, Estrela C, Decurcio DA. Guided endodontics: the impact of new technologies on complex case solution. Aust Endod J. 2021;47(3):664–71.
60. Park ME, Shin SY. Three-dimensional comparative study on the accuracy and reproducibility of dental casts fabricated by 3D printers. J Prosthet Dent. 2018;119:861.
61. Connert T, Weiger R, Krastl G. Present status and future directions—guided endodontics. Int Endod J. 2022;55 Suppl 4(Suppl 4):995–1002.
62. Krastl G, Zehnder MS, Connert T, Weiger R, Kühl S. Guided endodontics: a novel treatment approach for teeth with pulp canal calcification and apical pathology. Dent Traumatol. 2016;32:240–6.
63. Connert T, Zehnder MS, Amato M, Weiger R, Kijhl S, Krastl G. Microguided endodontics: a method to achieve minimally invasive access cavity preparation and root canal location in mandibular incisors using a novel computer-guided technique. Int Endod J. 2018;51:247–55.
64. Lara-Mendes STO, Barbosa CFM, Santa-Rosa CC, Machado VC. Guided endodontic access in maxillary molars using cone-beam computed tomography and computer-aided design/computer-aided manufacturing system: a case report. J Endod. 2018;44:875–9.
65. Moreno-Rabie C, Torres A, Lambrechts P, Jacobs R. Clinical applications, accuracy and limitations of guided endodontics: a systematic review. Int Endod J. 2020;53:214–31.
66. Connert T, Zehnder MS, Weiger R, Kijhl S, Krastl G. Microguided endodontics: accuracy of a min-

iaturized technique for apically extended access cavity preparation in anterior teeth. J Endod. 2017;43:787–90.
67. Connert T, Krug R, Eggmann F, Emsermann I, ElAyouti A, Weiger R, Kijhl S, Krastl G. Guided endodontics versus conventional access cavity preparation: a comparative study on substance loss using 3-dimensional-printed teeth. J Endod. 2019;45:327–31.
68. Loureiro MAZ, Elias MRA, Capeletti LR, Silva JA, Siqueira PC, Chaves GS, Decurcio DA. Guided endodontics: volume of dental tissue removed by guided access cavity preparation-an ex vivo study. J Endod. 2020;46:1907–12.
69. Ahn SY, Kim NH, Kim S, Karabucak B, Kim E. Computer-aided design/computer-aided manufacturing-guided endodontic surgery: guided osteotomy and apex localization in a mandibular molar with a thick buccal bone plate. J Endod. 2018;44:665–70.
70. Benjamin G, Ather A, Bueno MR, Estrela C, Diogenes A. Preserving the neurovascular bundle in targeted endodontic microsurgery: a case series. J Endod. 2021;47:509–19.
71. Giacomino CM, Ray JJ, Wealleans JA. Targeted endodontic microsurgery: a novel approach to anatomically challenging scenarios using 3-dimensional-printed guides and trephine burs-a report of cases. J Endod. 2018;44:671–7.
72. Maia LM, Bambirra J, Cinior W, Toubes KM, Moreira J, Cinior G, de Carvalho Machado V, Parpinelli BC, Ribeiro Sobrinho AP. Endodontic guide for the conservative removal of a fiber-reinforced composite resin post. J Prosthet Dent. 2021;128:4; in press.
73. Maia LM, Moreira Jiinior G, Albuquerque RC, de Carvalho MV, da Silva NRFA, Hauss DD, da Silveira RR. Three-dimensional endodontic guide for adhesive fiber post removal: a dental technique. J Prosthet Dent. 2019;121:387–90.
74. Perez C, Finelle G, Couvrechel C. Optimisation of a guided endodontics protocol for removal of fibre-reinforced posts. Aust Endod J. 2020;46:107–14.
75. Schwindling FS, Tasaka A, Hilgenfeld T, Rammelsberg P, Zenthofer A. Three-dimensional-guided removal and preparation of dental root posts-concept and feasibility. J Prosthodont Res. 2020;64:104–8.
76. Mena-Alvarez J, Rico-Romano C, Lobo-Galindo AB, Zubizarreta-Macho A. Endodontic treatment of dens evaginatus by performing a splint guided access cavity. J Esthet Restor Dent. 2017;29:396–402.
77. Ali A, Arslan H, Jethani B. Conservative management of type II dens invaginatus with guided endodontic approach: a case series. J Conserv Dent. 2019;22:503–8.
78. Zubizarreta-Macho A, Valle Castano S, Montiel-Company JM, Mena-Alvarez J. Effect of computer-aided navigation techniques on the accuracy of endodontic access cavities: a systematic review and meta-analysis. Biology. 2021;10:212.
79. Zehnder MS, Connert T, Weiger R, Krastl G, Kiihl S. Guided endodontics: accuracy of a novel method for guided access cavity preparation and root canal location. Int Endod J. 2016;49:966–72.
80. Buchgreitz J, Buchgreitz M, Mortensen D, Bjorndal L. Guided access cavity preparation using cone-beam computed tomography and optical surface scans—an ex vivo study. Int Endod J. 2016;49:790–5.
81. Buchgreitz J, Buchgreitz M, Bjorndal L. Guided endodontics modified for treating molars by using an intracoronal guide technique. J Endod. 2019;45:818–23.
82. Kostunov J, Rammelsberg P, Klotz AL, Zenthofer A, Schwindling FS. Minimization of tooth substance removal in normally calcified teeth using guided endodontics: an in vitro pilot study. J Endod. 2021;47:286–90.
83. Torres A, Lerut K, Lambrechts P, Jacobs R. Guided endodontics: use of a sleeveless guide system on an upper premolar with pulp canal obliteration and apical periodontitis. J Endod. 2021;47:133–9.

Part III

The Future of Digital Dentistry and Applications

Digital Applications in Dental and Craniofacial Tissue Engineering

16

Foteini Machla, Ioannis Angelopoulos, Maria Kokoti, and Athina Bakopoulou

Abbreviations

3DBP	Three-dimensional bioprinting
4DP	Four-dimensional printing
AI	Artificial intelligence
AM	Additive manufacturing
BCP	Biphasic calcium phosphate
CAD/CAM	Computer-aided design and manufacturing
CLSM	Confocal laser scanning microscopy
DT	Digital twins
ECM	Extracellular matrix
ELISA	Enzyme-linked immunosorbent assay
EMA	European medicines agency
FDA	Food and drug administration
FDM	Fused deposition modeling
FEA	Finite element analysis
GBR	Guided bone regeneration
GTR	Guided tissue regeneration
Hap	Hydroxyapatite
HT	High-throughput
iPSC	Induced pluripotent stem cell
IR	Infrared
LOC	Lab-on-chip
MCT	Microcomputed tomography
ML	Machine learning
MRI	Magnetic resonance imaging
NMR	Nuclear magnetic resonance
OOC	Organ-on-chip
PCL	Polycaprolactone
PCR	Polymerase chain reaction
PDL	Periodontal ligament
PGA	Polyglycolic acid
PLA	Polylactic acid
SEM	Scanning electron microscopy
SHED	Human exfoliated stem cells
SLA	Stereolithography
SLS	Selective laser sintering
STEM	Science, technology, engineering, and mathematics
TEM	Transmission electron microscopy
TERM/D	Tissue engineering and regenerative medicine/dentistry
UV-vis	Ultraviolet visible

F. Machla · I. Angelopoulos · M. Kokoti
A. Bakopoulou (✉)
Tissue Engineering Core Unit, Department of Prosthodontics, School of Dentistry, Aristotle University of Thessaloniki, Thessaloniki, Greece
e-mail: fcmachla@dent.auth.gr, iangelopoulos@dent.auth.gr; mkokoti@dent.auth.gr; abakopoulou@dent.auth.gr

16.1 Introduction: Tissue Engineering and Regenerative Dentistry

Tooth loss is a condition that affects a significant part of the population. It causes major problems in terms of oral functions, as it disrupts mastica-

A. Delantoni, K. Orhan (eds.), *Digital Dentistry*, https://doi.org/10.1007/978-3-031-52826-2_16

tory muscle activity and causes temporomandibular joint dysfunction [1]. The main causes of tooth loss include dental caries, periodontal diseases, and tooth injury [2]. With aging, the number of people who lose their teeth increases; in the USA, 35% of the population is edentulous by the age of 65. Current treatments to restore tooth loos involve tooth replacement with prosthetic restorations, such as fixed partial dentures, removable dentures, and dental implants [3]. Although these therapies have been extensively used to restore tooth loss, further technological improvements to generate biological teeth from autologous human tissues would be a valuable clinical tool [4].

Tissue engineering (TE) is a multidisciplinary field, which involves aspects of cellular/molecular/developmental biology, genetics, and engineering [5]. The goal of tissue engineering is to develop fully functioning bioengineered organs using three-dimensional technologies, involving biodegradable materials and various cell types to replace damaged organs following diseases, injury, or aging [6]. However, further technological developments are required to create such artificial organs, which can immediately function [7].

Recently, tissue engineering (TE) and regenerative medicine/dentistry (RM/D) are gathering a lot of research attention. Over the years a research shift regarding tissue reconstruction has been observed leading to the wider application of regenerative over conventional tissue replacement approaches [8]. In previous decades medical devices, such as metal implants or other materials, were applied to replace the defected area of interest. Later, more biocompatible and bioinert materials were used for the same purpose, while gradually bioactive materials were investigated for their biological properties (biocompatibility, biodegradability, differentiation inducing capacity). The latest trend for tissue/organ reconstruction is based on the combination of the so-called TE triad; stem cells, signaling molecules, and scaffolds aiming at the regeneration of fully functional systems [9]. Over the years, the TE of whole organs, including heart, lung, and liver have been approached, along with smaller scale models, such as quasi-tissues or organoids [10]. Approaches for tissue engineering and regeneration of oral tissues, including enamel [11], dentin [12], pulp [13], periodontal ligament (PDL) [14], cementum [15], oral mucosa [16], orofacial bone [17], and cartilage [18] tissues have been made, along with whole bioengineered tooth [19], or partial bio-roots engineering concepts [20], with various progress on each case.

Tissue engineering, as well as most disciplines of the so-called STEM family (science, technology, engineering, and mathematics), is closely associated with and directly dependent on the digital world. The biological, chemical, and physical properties of the subcellular, cellular, and tissue level need to be translated to humanly compatible signals and, vice versa a human-originated manipulation has sometimes to be detailed/fine-tuned to cellular language. Digital technologies often through extensive programming codes are called to help to bridge this gap. Data from the cellular level are translated into digits, and through software are interpretable by humans to lead to conclusions (output). Less often signals can be sent from humans translated to interpretable-by-tissues/cells signals (input). TERM/D is strongly attached to the digital world, from computational biology to in silico clinical trials.

16.2 Aim: Digital Twins

The need for TERM/D has led to a tremendously advanced research methodology. Until now, mostly trial-and-error procedures are being established, though the demands for quality and quantity control and outcome prediction are increased. More standardized protocols for easier reproducibility and focused expectations are required by global institutions, such as the Food and Drug Administration (FDA) and European Medicines Agency (EMA). Furthermore, the recent 3R (replacement, reduction, and refinement) principal guidelines for research on animals, make the term digital twins (DT) extremely relevant [21].

In a nutshell, a digital twin is a digital representation of a physical object; the virtual twin reflects the physical object, interacts with it, and eventually can self-evolve [22]. In medicine, in the framework of the Physiome Project, the European Commission initiated the "Virtual Physiological Human-VPH" project, a global effort to concentrate the knowledge on human physiology and create relevant digital models [23]. The goal of VPH is the development of diagnostic, prognostic, probabilistic, and therapeutic models targeting personalized healthcare [24]. Among others, the digestive, musculoskeletical, nervous, and immune systems are being investigated; firstly, extracting information on the physiological anatomy and function of these systems, and secondly, providing the retrieved knowledge for the in silico composition [24]. Even though in TERM/D the concept of DT is still at an early stage, many steps are being made toward this aim, starting with simple cell cultures to more complex tissue constructs [25].

16.3 Digitalization of Physiology: Extracting and Translating Biological Data

16.3.1 Basic Biological Computer-Aided Experimental Methodologies

Information from in vitro/in vivo and clinical studies require to be interpretable by humans. One of the most widely used pieces of information is imaging. Cell attachment, morphology, proliferation, viability, migration/invasion, uptake, transfection, and differentiation can be illustrated to different extents through **qualitative imaging**. The scaffold's structure, chemical composition, biodegradation, ECM, and tissue formation can be perceived also by imaging. Scanning electron microscopy (SEM), transmission electron microscopy (TEM), and confocal laser scanning microscopy (CLSM) are some of the daily used techniques for interpreting the different types of data. Microcomputed tomography (μCT), immuno-fluorescence, and cyto−/histo-chemistry also provide new knowledge about the biological state of the investigated TE triad. **Quantitative imaging** can give information for size, area, profile, distance, and direction of the displayed compartments, while pixel values and intensity-thresholded items can be translated to other types of information, like cellular viability, uptake, transfection, or differentiation ability [26].

Spectroscopy (infrared—IR, ultraviolet-visible—UV-vis, nuclear magnetic resonance—NMR, Raman, and X-ray) is also a useful tool for characterizing biological and physical properties [27]. Counting, sorting, and characterizing cells, detecting microorganisms, biomarkers, and proteins, and measuring genome size are some of the useful properties that can be interpreted by flow cytometry [28]. A plate reader is also frequently used, translating optical (light or fluorescent) alterations to biological behavior. For instance, an enzyme-linked immunosorbent assay (ELISA) reader quantifies the fluorescent, chemiluminescent, or chromogenic response of the tested sample [29].

In cell research, well-established cell **viability assays** provide an easy and quick way to interpret biological processes, such as cell metabolic and proliferation activity. The tetrazolium reduction, resazurin reduction, and protease activity assays measure some aspect of general metabolism or an enzymatic activity as a marker of viable cells [30]. An incubated reagent is associated with the conversion of a substrate to a colored or fluorescent product that can be detected with a plate reader, generating a signal that is proportional to the number of viable cells present. Similarly, in TE research, the **expression of biomolecules,** such as proteins, cellular **differentiation,** and **ECM formation** are among the mostly evaluated biological endpoints for assessing the regenerative behavior of the engineered constructs. Among other properties of the final stages of the regenerated tissues are the barrier formation ability and the functional response.

16.3.2 Advanced Translational Models

Biosensors are appliances that track via receptors the biological, physical, or chemical properties of a substance (analyte) and translate them into electronic signals via transducers so that they can be displayed on a computer [31]. Among other molecules, cells, antibodies, and nanoparticles can be bioreceptors, while heat, light, electromagnetic irradiation, and pH are some of the signals that can be detected [32]. In TERM, some of the applications of biosensors are the detection of small molecules, such as glucose, hydrogen peroxide, and some proteins, that can depict in real time the differential state of the TE constructs [33]. Furthermore, cell behavior, such as polarity, proliferation, and differentiation can be investigated by biosensors [34].

High-throughput (HT) systems are scaled-up procedures using advanced degrees of automation, such as **HT screening** for drug discovery, **HT cell biology** for rapid robotized experimental techniques, and **HT sequencing** for massively parallel sequencing of DNA [35, 36]. The ultimate goal of HT models is to minimize the handling steps and the duration of the procedure. Among others, microengineered 3D tissue models have been used for HT screening [37]. In TERM, HT systems can accelerate the discovery of potentially suitable constructs for organ/tissue regeneration [38]. Innovative biomaterials and suitable signaling biomolecules from large libraries with specific differentiation induction properties can be used for TE [38].

Lab-on-chips (LOC) are mini analytical devices integrating laboratory procedures such as polymerase chain reaction (PCR), on a single chip. These devices improve the ergonomics, speed, and cost—by reducing the number of reagents—of conventional techniques [39]. Regarding stem cell research, LOCs have been used for controlling the culturing conditions, and for cell characterization and differentiation using miniature biosensors on-a-chip [40]. Neural TE has been approached using LOCs [41].

Following similar technologies, **organ-on-chips (OOC)** are miniature devices containing TE tissues/organs and are considered to be the next-generation laboratory platforms [42]. One of the special characteristics of these chips is the **microfluidic system** that they facilitate [43]. These microfluidic systems can be precisely controlled regarding fluidic pressure and velocity, by electronic devices [44].

Many tissues, organs, and systems have been tissued engineered via OOCs, such as the liver, lung, kidney, heart, and intestine [45]. Compartments of the craniofacial area have been also approached using OOCs, such as the skin [46], vessels [47], nerves [48], bones [49], and muscles [50]. Regarding TERD, Franca et al. in 2020 developed a two-chambered tooth-on-chip model, where stem cells from the apical papilla were seeded on a dentin mini scaffold, recapitulating the dentin-pulp interface [51].

16.4 In Silico Tissue Engineering: Designing, Optimizing, and Manufacturing Engineered Organs

16.4.1 Finite Element Analysis

Computational modeling is a useful tool for comprehending tissue development but also for predicting the outcome related to specific mechanical and physical stimuli. In particular, finite element analysis (FEA), a mathematical modeling method, is used in mechanical analysis in health-related problem solving [52]. FEA has been utilized to model complex anatomical structures, analyze their physical properties, and study and predict their response to applied specific mechanical stimuli [53]. Some of the advantages of this method are that FEA reduces the cost and duration of the study, while minimizing the use of animals [54]. Recent advances in digital imaging techniques, including μCT, and magnetic resonance imaging (MRI), favored the geometric modeling of organs and tissues, providing the digitalized physiological anatomy of the developed virtual elemental grids [55]. The physical and mechanical properties of many tissues have been investigated in the literature, and thus digital libraries are being created to provide the most suitable parameters [56, 57]. In dentistry, the finite element method has been applied to various fields, such as implantology, orthodontics, and prosthodontics [58].

In the craniofacial area, FEA has been utilized to model soft and hard tissues of the face, where models for predicting the outcome of a surgical reconstruction seem to gather the highest research interest [59–62]. Dental tissues have also been studied using the finite element method: enamel [63, 64], dentin [65, 66], cementum [67], pulp [68], and PDL [69–71], along with craniofacial tissues, including alveolar bone [72–74], temporomandibular joint [75–77], and oral mucosa [78–80]. Among other properties, the elastic modulus, and Poisson's ratio of dental and craniofacial tissues, along with the computational parameters of the number of elements and nodes have been described [81, 82]. The above-mentioned studies approach the biomechanical properties of each tissue as closely as possible, connecting them with the mathematical models that mimic them best. These properties are later applied to the desired tissue engineering constructs, aiming for the most suitable biomimetic tissue fabrication [83].

16.4.2 Digital Scaffold Manufacturing; Computer-Aided Design and Fabrication

Current approaches to tissue engineering include the use of materials biodegradable synthetics, as a scaffold to maintain tissue cells ex vivo. The properties of the ideal biomimetic scaffold have rigorously been described regarding the desired tissue to be regenerated. The material to be used has to be of certain characteristics depending on the target tissue, including biocompatibility, degradation period, mechanical properties, and morphology. The digitalization of the physical and mechanical properties of the physiological tissue has allowed these parameters to be integrated, providing a custom-made scaffolds.

The hydrophilicity, mechanical strength, roughness, surface topography, nanotopography, porosity (pore size and interconnectivity), degradation rate, and bioactivity play an important role in bone tissue engineering. The above-mentioned parameters can be digitally designed and manipulated in favor of optimal bone scaffold fabrication in cases of guided bone regeneration (GBR). Hard (enamel, dentin, and cementum) and soft (PDL and pulp) dental tissues have unique histological characteristics, requiring the customization of the relevant scaffold biofabrication process and mechanical, chemical, and physical properties.

Computer-aided design and manufacturing (CAD/CAM) raise new tools to be used for TERM/D applications. CAD/CAM has been utilized for creating the perfect-fitting scaffold in cases of tissue defects but also is widely used for fabricating the optimal extracellular matrix (ECM) of the targeted tissue [84]. Compartmentalization has been utilized to achieve the regeneration of multiple neighboring tissues; different properties can be adapted in the specific tissue areas and interfaces. For instance, in guided tissue regeneration (GTR) the scaffold can consist of a mechanically strong drafting material for the GBR, and a soft membrane for the PDL tissue engineering [85]. Computational methods have been applied to characterize, design, and improve TE scaffolds, aiming for a 3D printing fabrication [86].

Additive manufacturing has been widely used for fabricating tissue engineering scaffolds [87]. Among the available biofabrication methods, the most described ones are stereolithography (**SLA**), selective laser sintering (**SLS**), and fused deposition modeling (**FDM**). Nowadays, 3D printing (**3DP**), has gained a lot of research interest in biomedical engineering. Three-dimensional (3D) bioprinters (**3DBP**), combine biological elements, such as cells and growth factors in their bioink, while in 4D printing (**4DP**), biomaterials' final form is affected by external stimuli, such as temperature, humidity, and pH [88, 89].

Regarding periodontal regeneration, many membranes and scaffolds have been designed and 3D-printed [90, 91]. Park et al. designed a parallel- and obliquely-oriented fiber system for approaching the engineering of the periodontal complex [92]. In another study, a perpendicularly oriented micro-tubular scaffold design resulted in a cellular anchoring between the tissues, and oriented formation of fibers [93]. Interestingly, a clinical case study by Rasperini et al. proposed a 3D-printed biodegradable scaffold with promising results [94]. The periodontal complex TE, including the PDL, cementum, and bone tissues, has been approached by 3D-printing different microarchitectures of a polycaprolactone (PCL)-hydroxyapatite (HAp) bioink, in combination with a spatial and time-dependent delivery of growth factors [95].

Three-dimensionally (3D) printed scaffolds for alveolar bone TE have also been investigated in the literature with promising results [85]. In a randomized clinical trial, PCL scaffolds were 3D-printed for the preservation of the alveolar ridge [96]. Various materials have been utilized for craniofacial in vivo bone tissue engineering and regeneration, such as biphasic calcium phosphate (BCP) ceramics for sinus augmentation applications [97], and HAp scaffolds after mandibular condyle resection [84].

Several efforts also aimed to regenerate the dentin/pulp complex by means of customized scaffolds. Dentin has a similar chemical composition to bone tissue, however, the architecture of dentin, with the dentinal tubules, is quite different. Alginate-containing 3D-bioprinted hydrogel scaffolds showed odontogenic differentiation in vitro [98]. Nejad et al. suggested the combination of PCL/45S5 Bioglass and PCL/hyaluronic acid for TE of the dentin-pulp complex [99]. A patient-specific dentin-pulp complex bioprinting approach using fibrin and PCL revealed the odontogenic differentiation of dental stem cells and mineralized tissue formation [100]. Three-dimensional bioprinting was used to fabricate carboxymethyl chitosan and alginate—containing scaffolds for enamel tissue regeneration [101]. Mooney et al., aiming at the regeneration of the pulp, seeded cells in a synthetic polymer of polyglycolic acid (PGA) and performed in vitro and in vivo analysis [102]. Their approaches are basically a proof-of-concept to test whether pulp cultured cells can grow well and produce the PGA matrix, and whether the bioengineered pulp can be vascularized using in vivo study models. Other groups have reported the regeneration of pulp and dentin with the use of "tooth disc" model in which a poly L-lactic acid (PLA) scaffold seeded with cells from human exfoliated deciduous teeth (SHED) [103].

The main limitation of the current research models is the cell source, the appropriate biomaterial, and the cellular interactions between the different types of cells. Irrespective to the cell source, delivering stem cells for dental tissue regeneration may encounter translational obstacles. Up to date, the disproportionate costs of marketing and struggles with regulatory approval have inhibited any profound clinical translation in the dental tissue engineering. 3D bioprinting could be an alternative approach to focus on the limitations mentioned above as it permits to biofabricate tissues with better precision. Additive manufacturing (AM) is crucial for the biofabrication of bioengineered implants/scaffolds with specified architecture mimicking the in vivo analog modifying it accordingly depending on the necessity of each patient. The combination of various biomaterials such poly (ε-caprolactone) (PCL) [104] as to mimic the hard part of the dental tissue or collagen [105] and alginate [106] to mimic the soft part of dental tissue and the addition of biological factors (cells, growth factors) could enhance the regeneration capacity and repair damaged tissues [107]. Besides the advantage of high seeding efficiency and uniform distribution, embedding of cells during seeding fabrication of the scaffold by means of rapid prototyping opens the possibility of positioning spatially controlled by one or more cell types. This is an important prerequisite for the manufacture of complex tissue-engineered constructs to regenerate damaged or lost tissue in interfaces, such as osteochondral tissue, and an essential requirement for the novel approach to organ impression [108], as shown in Fig. 16.1.

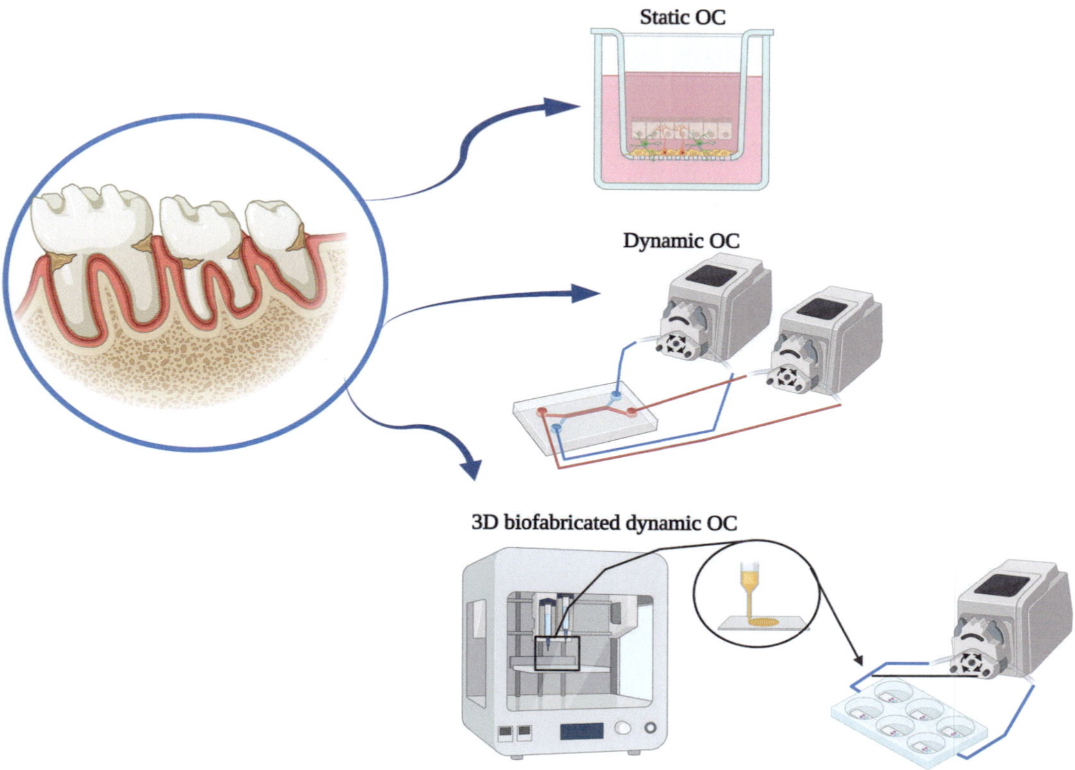

Fig. 16.1 Diagrammatic representation of the different dental biofabrication approaches to build 3D organotypic culture models, as analogues to recapitulate the in vivo tissues

16.5 Future Perspectives: Artificial Intelligence and Machine Learning in TERM/D

More advanced technologies are already finding applications in the TERM/D field, and it is expected to minimize the use of laboratory animals and reduce the time and cost of laboratory research, providing accurate predictions for the most efficient experimental design. **Artificial intelligence (AI)**, the ability of a computer to perform tasks that in other terms would require human intelligence, is receiving tremendous attention in medicine [109]. In clinical dentistry, the application of **machine learning (ML)** is also progressing [110]. The virtual branch of AI is connected to ML expressed as mathematical models that enhance machine training [111]. ML is conventionally divided into three categories: unsupervised (by identifying patterns), supervised (by classifying data and making predictions), and reinforcement learning (by positive or negative external feedback) [109].

While the availability of TE data is significant, the efficiencies to extract these data are still growing [112]. AI provides the ability for the optimization of biomaterial design, the prediction of scaffold modeling and fabrication, and spatiotemporal analysis of cell and tissue systems [113]. Barrera et al. employed virtual tomography and artificial neural networks to predict the mechanical properties of innovative scaffolds [114]. AI-assisted the imaging, detection, and prediction of the differentiation induction of organoids [115]. Even though AI and ML applications in dental tissue regeneration are still at the initial stage, other tissues, such as bone and cartilage have received more attention [112, 116].

AI can reduce the use or even replace the conventional experimental methodologies. Pillar and Ozcan studied AI-guided virtual histological tissue staining [117], while Wang and Fernandez-

Gonzalez reviewed the ability of a supervised ML model to analyze in vivo microscopy [118]. Xu et al. implemented artificial neural networks to predict the development of vasculature [119]. Brain and cardiac tissue characterization were approached via ML-assisted quantitative ultrasound techniques and light-scattering spectroscopy, respectively [120, 121]. Cardiovascular tissue biomechanics modeling [122] and bone mechanics after damage have also been assessed [123]. The prediction of electromagnetic properties of tissues in vivo has also been approached [124].

Stem cell research is also receiving a lot of machine-assisted attention. Specifically, the reprogramming, culturing, and differentiation abilities of induced pluripotent stem cells (iPSCs) have been assisted by AI and ML [125]. Both methods have been utilized for the comprehension of cellular procedures, viability prediction, and characterization of stemness [126]. Furthermore, these techniques have been applied to investigate the effect of spatial cues, the immunologic reaction, as well as the differentiation potential of stem cells [116].

AI and ML applications in TERM/D, as with any other cutting-edge technology, have many emerging constraints and capacities for optimization, however, their potential is of great significance [127].

The pipeline of workflow can be summarized in Fig. 16.2.

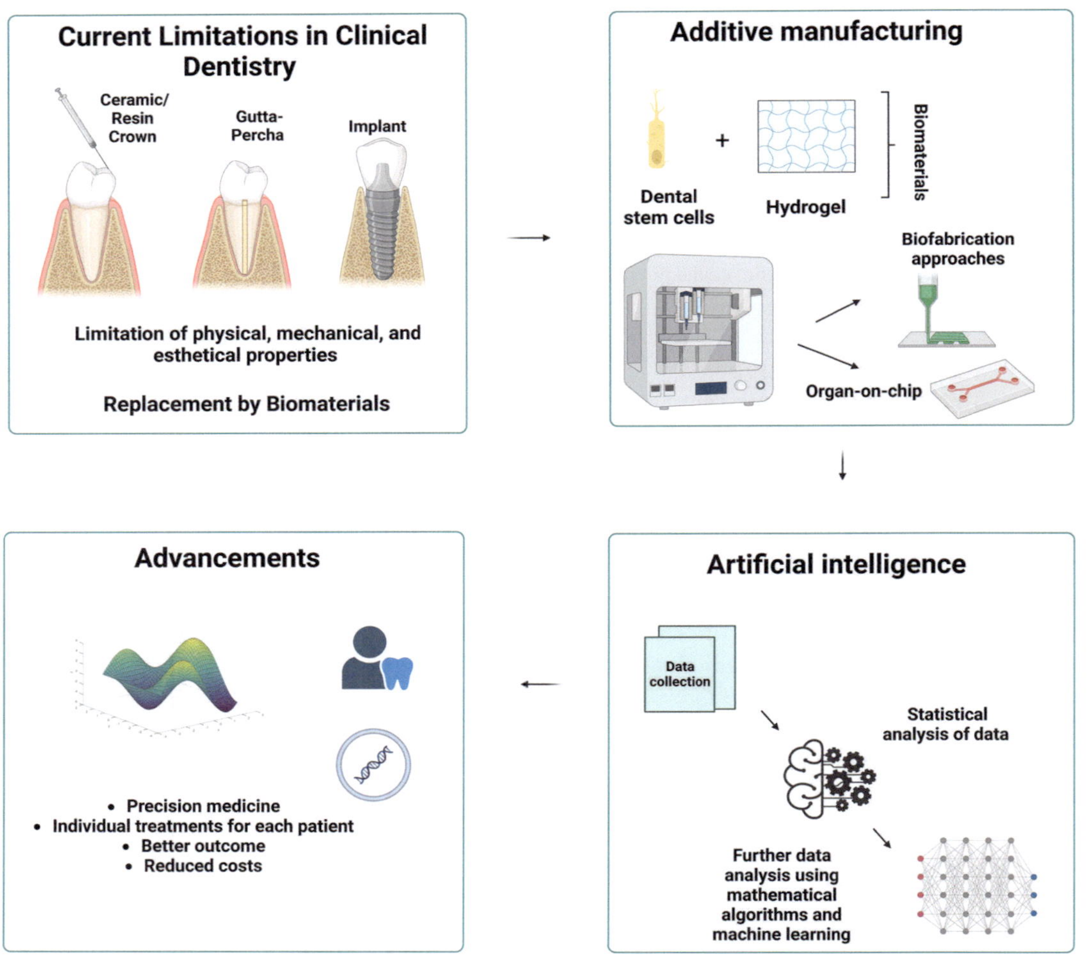

Fig. 16.2 Pipeline of workflow for dental tissue engineering in combination with artificial intelligence (AI) and machine learning (ML) toward personalized dentistry

16.6 Conclusions

Tissue engineering is directly associated to digital technologies. The signals of the microscopic world must be converted to digits to be translated into the macroscopic humanly interpreted language, while the human intervention must be elaborated to biological end physical components. The gap between the two worlds is bridged by highly advanced methodologies/software that are developed to serve this purpose. Apart from the fundamental methodologies, such as imaging, that are already conventionally used for many years in laboratories, new technologies are emerging that aim to fine-tune this translational process. The databases of biological data extraction and translation are continuously growing via new techniques, such as biosensors, high-throughput models, and lab-on-chips, making the relevant knowledge broader. The same applies to the designing, optimization, and manufacturing of engineered organs, through finite element analysis, computer-aided design and manufacturing, and 3D- and bioprinting. So far, digital applications are mainly focusing on serving human decision the best way possible, though there is much more to be gained. Digital twins and artificial intelligence through machine learning can lead to the next step of TERM/D, assisting the ultimate goal of personalized treatment.

References

1. Oshima M, Mizuno M, Imamura A, et al. Functional tooth regeneration using a bioengineered tooth unit as a mature organ replacement regenerative therapy. PLoS One. 2011;6:e21531. https://doi.org/10.1371/JOURNAL.PONE.0021531.
2. Oshima M, Tsuji T. Functional tooth regenerative therapy: tooth tissue regeneration and whole-tooth replacement. Odontology. 2014;102:123–36.
3. Ikeda E, Tsuji T. Growing bioengineered teeth from single cells: potential for dental regenerative medicine. Expert Opin Biol Ther. 2008;8:735–44.
4. Duailibi MT, Duailibi SE, Young CS, Bartlett JD, Vacanti JP, Yelick PC. Bioengineered teeth from cultured rat tooth bud cells. J Dent Res. 2004;83:523–8.
5. Stock UA, Vacanti JP. Tissue engineering: current state and prospects. Annu Rev Med. 2001;52:443–51.
6. Griffith LG, Naughton G. Tissue engineering—current challenges and expanding opportunities. Science. 2002;295:5557. https://doi.org/10.1126/SCIENCE.1069210.
7. Uygun BE, Soto-Gutierrez A, Yagi H, et al. Organ reengineering through development of a transplantable recellularized liver graft using decellularized liver matrix. Nat Med. 2010;16:814–20.
8. Abou Neel EA, Chrzanowski W, Salih VM, Kim HW, Knowles JC. Tissue engineering in dentistry. J Dent. 2014;42:915–28.
9. Langer R, Vacanti JP. Tissue engineering. Science. 1993;260:920–6.
10. Mandrycky C, Phong K, Zheng Y. Tissue engineering toward organ-specific regeneration and disease modeling. MRS Commun. 2017;7:332.
11. Pandya M, Diekwisch TGH. Enamel biomimetics—fiction or future of dentistry. Int J Oral Sci. 2019;11:1111–9.
12. Hashemi-Beni B, Khoroushi M, Foroughi MR, Karbasi S, Khademi AA. Tissue engineering: dentin—pulp complex regeneration approaches (a review). Tissue Cell. 2017;49:552–64.
13. Yang J, Yuan G, Chen Z. Pulp regeneration: current approaches and future challenges. Front Physiol. 2016;7:58.
14. Chen FM, Jin Y. Periodontal tissue engineering and regeneration: current approaches and expanding opportunities. Tissue Eng Part B Rev. 2010;16:219–55.
15. Liu J, Ruan J, Weir MD, Ren K, Schneider A, Wang P, Oates TW, Chang X, Xu HHK. Periodontal bone-ligament-cementum regeneration via scaffolds and stem cells. Cells. 2019;8:537.
16. Toma AI, Fuller JM, Willett NJ, Goudy SL. Oral wound healing models and emerging regenerative therapies. Transl Res. 2021;236:17–34.
17. Park JJ, Rochlin DH, Parsaei Y, Shetye PR, Witek L, Leucht P, Rabbani PS, Flores RL. Bone tissue engineering strategies for alveolar cleft: review of preclinical results and guidelines for future studies. Cleft Palate Craniofac J. 2022;60:1450. https://doi.org/10.1177/10556656221104954.
18. Wescoe KE, Schugar RC, Chu CR, Deasy BM. The role of the biochemical and biophysical environment in Chondrogenic stem cell differentiation assays and cartilage tissue engineering. Cell Biochem Biophys. 2008;52(2):85–102.
19. Ikeda E, Morita R, Nakao K, Ishida K, Nakamura T, Takano-Yamamoto T, Ogawa M, Mizuno M, Kasugai S, Tsuji T. Fully functional bioengineered tooth replacement as an organ replacement therapy. Proc Natl Acad Sci U S A. 2009;106:13475–80.
20. Gao ZH, Hu L, Liu GL, Wei FL, Liu Y, Liu ZH, Fan ZP, Zhang CM, Wang JS, Wang SL. Bio-root and implant-based restoration as a tooth replacement alternative. J Dent Res. 2016;95:642–9.
21. Geris L, Lambrechts T, Carlier A, Papantoniou I. The future is digital: in silico tissue engineering. Curr Opin Biomed Eng. 2018;6:92–8.
22. Tao F, Cheng J, Qi Q, Zhang M, Zhang H, Sui F. Digital twin-driven product design, manufacturing

and service with big data. Int J Adv Manuf Technol. 2018;94:3563–76.
23. Bassingthwaighte JB. Strategies for the physiome project. Ann Biomed Eng. 2000;28:1043–58.
24. Viceconti M, Clapworthy G, van Sint JS. The virtual physiological human—a European initiative for in silico human modelling. J Physiol Sci. 2008;58:441–6.
25. Möller J, Pörtner R. Digital twins for tissue culture techniques—concepts, expectations, and state of the art. Processes. 2021;9(3s):447.
26. Schneider CA, Rasband WS, Eliceiri KW. NIH image to ImageJ: 25 years of image analysis. Nat Methods. 2012;9:671–5.
27. Bunaciu AA, Hoang VD, Aboul-Enein HY. Vibrational micro-spectroscopy of human tissues analysis: review. Crit Rev Anal Chem. 2017;47:194–203.
28. McKinnon KM. Flow cytometry: an overview. Curr Protoc Immunol. 2018;120:511–5111.
29. Hornbeck PV. Enzyme-linked immunosorbent assays. Curr Protoc Immunol. 2015;110:211–2123.
30. Riss TL, Moravec RA, Niles AL, Duellman S, Benink HA, Worzella TJ, Minor L. Cell viability assays. In: Assay guidance manual. Bethesda, MD: Eli Lilly & Company and the National Center for Advancing Translational Sciences; 2004.
31. Bhalla N, Jolly P, Formisano N, Estrela P. Introduction to biosensors. Essays Biochem. 2016;60:1.
32. Mehrotra P. Biosensors and their applications—a review. J Oral Biol Craniofac Res. 2016;6:153–9.
33. Li YCE, Chi Lee I. The current trends of biosensors in tissue engineering. Biosensors (Basel). 2020;10:88. https://doi.org/10.3390/BIOS10080088.
34. Li Y-CE, Lee I-C. The current trends of biosensors in tissue engineering. Biosensors (Basel). 2020;10:88.
35. Entzeroth M, Flotow H, Condron P. Overview of high-throughput screening. Curr Protoc Pharmacol. 2009;44:Unit 9.4. https://doi.org/10.1002/0471141755.PH0904S44.
36. Seo J, Shin JY, Leijten J, Jeon O, Camci-Unal G, Dikina AD, Brinegar K, Ghaemmaghami AM, Alsberg E, Khademhosseini A. High-throughput approaches for screening and analysis of cell behaviors. Biomaterials. 2018;153:85–101.
37. Nam KH, Smith AST, Lone S, Kwon S, Kim DH. Biomimetic 3D tissue models for advanced high-throughput drug screening. SLAS Technol. 2015;20:201–15.
38. Peters A, Brey DM, Burdick JA. High-throughput and combinatorial technologies for tissue engineering applications. Tissue Eng Part B Rev. 2009;15:225–39. https://home.liebertpub.com/teb.
39. Yilmaz B, Yilmaz F. Lab-on-a-Chip Technology and its applications. In: Omics Technologies and bioengineering: towards improving quality of life, vol. 1. Cambridge, MA: Academic; 2018. p. 145–53.
40. Ertl P, Sticker D, Charwat V, Kasper C, Lepperdinger G. Lab-on-a-chip technologies for stem cell analysis. Trends Biotechnol. 2014;32:245–53.
41. Mobini S, Song YH, McCrary MW, Schmidt CE. Advances in ex vivo models and lab-on-a-chip devices for neural tissue engineering. Biomaterials. 2019;198:146.
42. Leung CM, de Haan P, Ronaldson-Bouchard K, et al. A guide to the organ-on-a-chip. Nat Rev Methods Primers. 2022;2:33.
43. Bhatia SN, Ingber DE. Microfluidic organs-on-chips. Nat Biotechnol. 2014;32:760–72.
44. Sackmann EK, Fulton AL, Beebe DJ. The present and future role of microfluidics in biomedical research. Nature. 2014;507:181–9.
45. Wu Q, Liu J, Wang X, Feng L, Wu J, Zhu X, Wen W, Gong X. Organ-on-a-chip: recent breakthroughs and future prospects. Biomed Eng Online. 2020;19:9. https://doi.org/10.1186/S12938-020-0752-0.
46. Sriram G, Alberti M, Dancik Y, Wu B, Wu R, Feng Z, Ramasamy S, Bigliardi PL, Bigliardi-Qi M, Wang Z. Full-thickness human skin-on-chip with enhanced epidermal morphogenesis and barrier function. Mater Today. 2018;21:326–40.
47. Vila Cuenca M, Cochrane A, van den Hil FE, de Vries AAF, Lesnik Oberstein SAJ, Mummery CL, Orlova VV. Engineered 3D vessel-on-chip using hiPSC-derived endothelial- and vascular smooth muscle cells. Stem Cell Rep. 2021;16:2159–68.
48. Hong N, Nam Y. Neurons-on-a-chip: in vitro NeuroTools. Mol Cells. 2022;45:76.
49. Hao S, Ha L, Cheng G, Wan Y, Xia Y, Sosnoski DM, Mastro AM, Zheng SY. A spontaneous 3D bone-on-a-Chip for bone metastasis study of breast cancer cells. Small. 2018;14:1702787.
50. Grosberg A, Nesmith AP, Goss JA, Brigham MD, McCain ML, Parker KK. Muscle on a chip: in vitro contractility assays for smooth and striated muscle. J Pharmacol Toxicol Methods. 2012;65:126–35.
51. França CM, Tahayeri A, Rodrigues NS, Ferdosian S, Puppin Rontani RM, Sereda G, Ferracane JL, Bertassoni LE. The tooth on-a-chip: a microphysiologic model system mimicking the biologic interface of the tooth with biomaterials. Lab Chip. 2020;20:405–13.
52. Driscoll M. The impact of the finite element method on medical device design. J Med Biol Eng. 2019;39:171–2.
53. Cebral JR, Lhner R. From medical images to anatomically accurate finite element grids. Int J Numer Methods Eng. 2001;51:985–1008.
54. Büchler P, Farron A. Benefits of an anatomical reconstruction of the humeral head during shoulder arthroplasty: a finite element analysis. Clin Biomech. 2004;19:16–23.
55. Taddei F, Schileo E, Helgason B, Cristofolini L, Viceconti M. The material mapping strategy influences the accuracy of CT-based finite element mod-

els of bones: an evaluation against experimental measurements. Med Eng Phys. 2007;29:973–9.
56. Freutel M, Schmidt H, Dürselen L, Ignatius A, Galbusera F. Finite element modeling of soft tissues: material models, tissue interaction and challenges. Clin Biomech. 2014;29:363–72.
57. Hou FJ, Lang SM, Hoshaw SJ, Reimann DA, Fyhrie DP. Human vertebral body apparent and hard tissue stiffness. J Biomech. 1998;31:1009–15.
58. Trivedi S. Finite element analysis: a boon to dentistry. J Oral Biol Craniofac Res. 2014;4:200.
59. Chen S, Lou H, Guo L, Rong Q, Liu Y, Xu TM. 3-D finite element modelling of facial soft tissue and preliminary application in orthodontics. Comput Methods Biomech Biomed Engin. 2012;15:255–61.
60. Zhang X, Tang Z, Liebschner MAK, et al. An eFace-template method for efficiently generating patient-specific anatomically-detailed facial soft tissue FE models for Craniomaxillofacial surgery simulation. Ann Biomed Eng. 2016;44:1656.
61. Knoops PGM, Borghi A, Ruggiero F, et al. A novel soft tissue prediction methodology for orthognathic surgery based on probabilistic finite element modelling. PLoS One. 2018;13:e0197209. https://doi.org/10.1371/JOURNAL.PONE.0197209.
62. Tian T, Yao HH, Wang W, Shi B, Zheng Q, Hao LC. Three-dimensional finite element analysis of the effect of alveolar cleft bone graft on the maxillofacial biomechanical stabilities of unilateral complete cleft lip and palate. Biomed Eng Online. 2022;21:1–20.
63. Rees JS, Hammadeh M. Undermining of enamel as a mechanism of abfraction lesion formation: a finite element study. Eur J Oral Sci. 2004;112:347–52.
64. Spears IR. A three-dimensional finite element model of prismatic enamel: a re-appraisal of the data on the young's modulus of Enamel. J Dent Res. 2016;76:1690–7. https://doi.org/10.1177/00220345970760101101.
65. Grzebieluch W, Bêdziñski R, Czapliñski T, Kaczmarek U. The mechanical properties of human dentin for 3-D finite element modeling: numerical and analytical evaluation. Adv Clin Exp Med. 2017;26:645–53.
66. Wang W, Roubier N, Puel G, Allain JM, Infante IC, Attal JP, Vennat E. A new method combining finite element analysis and digital image correlation to assess macroscopic mechanical properties of dentin. Materials. 2015;8:535–50.
67. Raj Vikram N, Senthil Kumar KS, Nagachandran KS, Mohamed Hashir Y. Apical stress distribution on maxillary central incisor during various orthodontic tooth movements by varying cemental and two different periodontal ligament thicknesses: a FEM study. Indian J Dent Res. 2012;23:213–20.
68. Moga RA, Cosgarea R, Buru SM, Chiorean CG. Finite element analysis of the dental pulp under orthodontic forces. Am J Orthod Dentofac Orthop. 2019;155:543–51.
69. Research O, Hemanth M, Deoli S, Raghuveer HP, Rani MS, Hegde C, Vedavathi B. Stress induced in the periodontal ligament under orthodontic loading (part I): a finite element method study using linear analysis. J Int Oral Health. 2015;7:129.
70. Toms SR, Dakin GJ, Lemons JE, Eberhardt AW. Quasi-linear viscoelastic behavior of the human periodontal ligament. J Biomech. 2002;35:1411–5.
71. Poiate IAVP, de Vasconcellos AB, de Santana RB, Poiate E. Three-dimensional stress distribution in the human periodontal ligament in masticatory, parafunctional, and trauma loads: finite element analysis. J Periodontol. 2009;80:1859–67.
72. Cattaneo PM, Dalstra M, Melsen B. The finite element method: a tool to study orthodontic tooth movement. J Dent Res. 2016;84:428–33. https://doi.org/10.1177/154405910508400506.
73. Chen YC, Tsai HH. Use of 3D finite element models to analyze the influence of alveolar bone height on tooth mobility and stress distribution. J Dent Sci. 2011;6:90–4.
74. Geramy A, Geramy AR, Fazli B. An expansion to the Nägerl's theory of proportionality in reduced alveolar bone height models: a 3D finite element analysis. BMC Oral Health. 2022;22:1–10.
75. Pérez del Palomar A, Doblaré M. Finite element analysis of the temporomandibular joint during lateral excursions of the mandible. J Biomech. 2006;39:2153–63.
76. Lai L, Huang C, Zhou F, Xia F, Xiong G. Finite elements analysis of the temporomandibular joint disc in patients with intra-articular disorders. BMC Oral Health. 2020;20:1–8.
77. Sagl B, Schmid-Schwap M, Piehslinger E, Kundi M, Stavness I. A dynamic jaw model with a finite-element temporomandibular joint. Front Physiol. 2019;10:1156.
78. Wakabayashi N, Suzuki T. Patient-specific finite element analysis of viscoelastic masticatory mucosa. J Dent Biomech. 2013;4:1–7.
79. Ramakrishnan AN, Röhrle O, Ludtka C, Varghese R, Koehler J, Kiesow A, Schwan S. Finite element evaluation of the effect of adhesive creams on the stress state of dentures and Oral mucosa. Appl Bionics Biomech. 2021;2021:1. https://doi.org/10.1155/2021/5533770.
80. Chen J, Ahmad R, Li W, Swain M, Li Q. Biomechanics of oral mucosa. J R Soc Interface. 2015;12:20150325. https://doi.org/10.1098/RSIF.2015.0325.
81. Garbin CA, Spazzin AO, Meira-Júnior AD, Loretto SC, Lyra AMVC, Braz R. Biomechanical behaviour of a fractured maxillary incisor restored with direct composite resin only or with different post systems. Int Endod J. 2010;43:1098–107.
82. Song HY, Huh YH, Park CJ, Cho LR. A two-short-implant-supported molar restoration in atrophic

posterior maxilla: a finite element analysis. J Adv Prosthodont. 2016;8:304–12.
83. Olivares AL, Marsal È, Planell JA, Lacroix D. Finite element study of scaffold architecture design and culture conditions for tissue engineering. Biomaterials. 2009;30:6142–9.
84. Ciocca L, de Crescenzio F, Fantini M, Scotti R. CAD/CAM and rapid prototyped scaffold construction for bone regenerative medicine and surgical transfer of virtual planning: a pilot study. Comput Med Imaging Graph. 2009;33:58–62.
85. Asaad F, Pagni G, Pilipchuk SP, Giannì AB, Giannobile WV, Rasperini G. 3D-printed scaffolds and biomaterials: review of alveolar bone augmentation and periodontal regeneration applications. Int J Dent. 2016;2016:1. https://doi.org/10.1155/2016/1239842.
86. Zhang S, Vijayavenkataraman S, Lu WF, Fuh JYH. A review on the use of computational methods to characterize, design, and optimize tissue engineering scaffolds, with a potential in 3D printing fabrication. J Biomed Mater Res B Appl Biomater. 2019;107:1329–51.
87. Matai I, Kaur G, Seyedsalehi A, McClinton A, Laurencin CT. Progress in 3D bioprinting technology for tissue/organ regenerative engineering. Biomaterials. 2020;226:119536. https://doi.org/10.1016/J.BIOMATERIALS.2019.119536.
88. Tamay DG, Usal TD, Alagoz AS, Yucel D, Hasirci N, Hasirci V. 3D and 4D printing of polymers for tissue engineering applications. Front Bioeng Biotechnol. 2019;7:164.
89. Zhu W, Ma X, Gou M, Mei D, Zhang K, Chen S. 3D printing of functional biomaterials for tissue engineering. Curr Opin Biotechnol. 2016;40:103–12.
90. Sufaru IG, Macovei G, Stoleriu S, Martu MA, Luchian I, Kappenberg-Nitescu DC, Solomon SM. 3D printed and bioprinted membranes and scaffolds for the periodontal tissue regeneration: a narrative review. Membranes (Basel). 2022;12:902. https://doi.org/10.3390/MEMBRANES12090902.
91. Roato I, Masante B, Putame G, Massai D, Mussano F. Challenges of periodontal tissue engineering: increasing biomimicry through 3D printing and controlled dynamic environment. Nanomaterials (Basel). 2022;12:3878.
92. Park CH, Rios HF, Jin Q, Bland ME, Flanagan CL, Hollister SJ, Giannobile W, v. Biomimetic hybrid scaffolds for engineering human tooth-ligament interfaces. Biomaterials. 2010;31:5945–52.
93. Park CH, Rios HF, Jin Q, Sugai JV, Padial-Molina M, Taut AD, Flanagan CL, Hollister SJ, Giannobile WV. Tissue engineering bone-ligament complexes using fiber-guiding scaffolds. Biomaterials. 2012;33:137–45.
94. Rasperini G, Pilipchuk SP, Flanagan CL, Park CH, Pagni G, Hollister SJ, Giannobile WV. 3D-Printed bioresorbable Scaffold for periodontal repair. J Dent Res. 2015;94:153S–7S. https://doi.org/10.1177/0022034515588303.
95. Lee CH, Hajibandeh J, Suzuki T, Fan A, Shang P, Mao JJ. Three-dimensional printed multiphase scaffolds for regeneration of periodontium complex. Tissue Eng Part A. 2014;20:1342–51.
96. Goh BT, Teh LY, Tan DBP, Zhang Z, Teoh SH. Novel 3D polycaprolactone scaffold for ridge preservation—a pilot randomised controlled clinical trial. Clin Oral Implants Res. 2015;26:271–7.
97. Mangano C, Barboni B, Valbonetti L, Berardinelli P, Martelli A, Muttini A, Bedini R, Tetè S, Piattelli A, Mattioli M. In vivo behavior of a custom-made 3D synthetic bone substitute in sinus augmentation procedures in sheep. J Oral Implantol. 2015;41:240–50.
98. Athirasala A, Tahayeri A, Thrivikraman G, Franca CM, Monteiro N, Tran V, Ferracane J, Bertassoni LE. A dentin-derived hydrogel bioink for 3D bioprinting of cell laden scaffolds for regenerative dentistry. Biofabrication. 2018;10:024101.
99. Nejad ZM, Zamanian A, Saeidifar M, Vanaei HR, Amoli MS. 3D Bioprinting of polycaprolactone-based Scaffolds for pulp-dentin regeneration: investigation of physicochemical and biological behavior. Polymers. 2021;13(13):4442.
100. Han J, Kim DS, Jang H, Kim HR, Kang HW. Bioprinting of three-dimensional dentin-pulp complex with local differentiation of human dental pulp stem cells. J Tissue Eng. 2019;10:204173141984584. https://doi.org/10.1177/2041731419845849.
101. Mohabatpour F, Duan X, Yazdanpanah Z, Tabil XL, Lobanova L, Zhu N, Papagerakis S, Chen X, Papagerakis P. Bioprinting of alginate-carboxymethyl chitosan scaffolds for enamel tissue engineering in vitro. Biofabrication. 2022;15:015022.
102. Mooney DJ, Powell C, Piana J, Rutherford B. Engineering dental pulp-like tissue in vitro. Biotechnol Prog. 1996;12:865–8.
103. Cordeiro MM, Dong Z, Kaneko T, Zhang Z, Miyazawa M, Shi S, Smith AJ, Nör JE. Dental pulp tissue engineering with stem cells from exfoliated deciduous teeth. J Endod. 2008;34:962–9.
104. Park S, Kim G, Jeon YC, Koh Y, Kim W. 3D polycaprolactone scaffolds with controlled pore structure using a rapid prototyping system. J Mater Sci Mater Med. 2009;20:229–34.
105. Lee W, Debasitis JC, Lee VK, Lee JH, Fischer K, Edminster K, Park JK, Yoo SS. Multi-layered culture of human skin fibroblasts and keratinocytes through three-dimensional freeform fabrication. Biomaterials. 2009;30:1587–95.
106. Cohen DL, Malone E, Lipson H, Bonassar LJ. Direct freeform fabrication of seeded hydrogels in arbitrary geometries. Tissue Eng. 2006;12:1325–35.
107. Schütz K, Placht AM, Paul B, Brüggemeier S, Gelinsky M, Lode A. Three-dimensional plotting of a cell-laden alginate/methylcellulose blend: towards biofabrication of tissue engineering constructs with clinically relevant dimensions. J Tissue Eng Regen Med. 2017;11:1574–87.

108. Derby B. Printing and prototyping of tissues and scaffolds. Science. 2012;338:921–6.
109. Hamet P, Tremblay J. Artificial intelligence in medicine. Metabolism. 2017;69:S36–40.
110. Agrawal P, Nikhade P. Artificial intelligence in dentistry: past, present, and future. Cureus. 2022;14(7):e27405. https://doi.org/10.7759/CUREUS.27405.
111. Deo RC. Machine learning in medicine. Circulation. 2015;132:1920–30.
112. Xu J, Ge H, Zhou X, Yang D. Tissue engineering scheming by artificial intelligence. Int J Artif Organs. 2018;28:74–8. https://doi.org/10.1177/039139880502800112.
113. Guo JL, Januszyk M, Longaker MT. Machine learning in tissue engineering. Tissue Eng Part A. 2022;29:2. https://doi.org/10.1089/TEN.TEA.2022.0128.
114. Barrera MDB, Franco-Martínez F, Lantada AD. Artificial intelligence aided design of tissue engineering scaffolds employing virtual tomography and 3D convolutional neural networks. Materials. 2021;14:5278.
115. Gao W, Wang C, Li Q, Zhang X, Yuan J, Li D, Sun Y, Chen Z, Gu Z. Application of medical imaging methods and artificial intelligence in tissue engineering and organ-on-a-chip. Front Bioeng Biotechnol. 2022;10:985692. https://doi.org/10.3389/FBIOE.2022.985692.
116. Mackay BS, Marshall K, Grant-Jacob JA, Kanczler J, Eason RW, Oreffo ROC, Mills B. The future of bone regeneration: integrating AI into tissue engineering. Biomed Phys Eng Express. 2021;7:052002.
117. Pillar N, Ozcan A. Virtual tissue staining in pathology using machine learning. 2022. https://doi.org/10.1080/1473715920222153040.
118. Wang MFZ, Fernandez-Gonzalez R. (Machine-) Learning to analyze in vivo microscopy: support vector machines. Biochim Biophys Acta Proteins Proteom. 2017;1865:1719–27.
119. Xu J, Ge H, Zhou X, Yan J, Chi Q, Zhang Z. Prediction of vascular tissue engineering results with artificial neural networks. J Biomed Inform. 2005;38:417–21.
120. Thomson H, Yang S. Cochran S (2022) machine learning-enabled quantitative ultrasound techniques for tissue differentiation. J Med Ultrason. 2001;49:517–28.
121. Knighton NJ, Cottle BK, Tiwari S, Mondal A, Kaza AK, Sachse FB, Hitchcock RW. Toward cardiac tissue characterization using machine learning and light-scattering spectroscopy. J Biomed Opt. 2021;26:116001. https://doi.org/10.1117/1.JBO.26.11.116001.
122. Arzani A, Wang JX, Sacks MS, Shadden SC. Machine learning for cardiovascular biomechanics modeling: challenges and beyond. Ann Biomed Eng. 2022;50(60):615–27.
123. Yun SSC, Peña Fernández M, Tozzi G, Buehler MJ. Deep learning approach to assess damage mechanics of bone tissue. J Mech Behav Biomed Mater. 2021;123:104761. https://doi.org/10.1016/J.JMBBM.2021.104761.
124. Gerazov B, Caligari Conti DA, Farina L, Farrugia L, Sammut CV, Schembri Wismayer P, Conceição RC. Application of machine learning to predict dielectric properties of in vivo biological tissue. Sensors (Basel). 2021;21:6935. https://doi.org/10.3390/S21206935.
125. Coronnello C, Francipane MG. Moving towards induced pluripotent stem cell-based therapies with artificial intelligence and machine learning. Stem Cell Rev Rep. 2022;18:559–69.
126. Shende P, Devlekar NP. A review on the role of artificial intelligence in stem cell therapy: an initiative for modern medicines. Curr Pharm Biotechnol. 2021;22:1156–63.
127. Varoquaux G, Cheplygina V. Machine learning for medical imaging: methodological failures and recommendations for the future. NPJ Digit Med. 2022;15:1–8.

Digital Storage Systems PACS Servers and Cloud Dentistry

17

Antigoni Delantoni and Kaan Orhan

PACS is defined as physical access control system and other terms used for it according to its acronyms are

Physical Access Control Systems and

Picture Archiving and Communication System and finally

Picture Archiving and Communication System(s).

Medical imaging is a critical component in the proper patient care that often helps with the diagnosis and treatment planning of the patient's care. There are various systems for data storage, but the system that provides for the acceptance, transfer, display, storage, and digital processing of medical images is known as the picture archiving communications system (PACS) and is nearly everywhere in healthcare environments.

Basically PACS can be defined as an imaging technology in medical environments, which provide economical storage and convenient access to images from multiple modalities, that are basically different source machine types. The digital or electronic images and their reports are transmitted digitally via PACS; eliminating the need to manually file, retrieve, or transport film or film jackets. The universal format for PACS image storage and transfer is DICOM (digital imaging and communications in medicine) [1].

PACS fits within a highly complex environment and may interface with a range of enterprise information technology systems and healthcare professionals both internal and external to the Healthcare Delivery Organization.

This complexity leads to cybersecurity challenges.

The challenge with PACS is securing disparate, interconnected systems. A medical imaging infrastructure offers a broad attack surface with equipment that may have varying vulnerabilities, configurations, and control implementations.

The healthcare professionals may reside in different departments and have components hosted and used across a wide geography. Some of the people involved with the date acquisition may be external to the HDO, interacting with sensitive information across the internet.

As threats to the operational environment increase, PACS and other healthcare systems may become increasingly vulnerable to:

- disruption of the system, leading to inability to render timely diagnosis and treatment,
- inability to access the system for standard use, including inability to schedule procedures,

A. Delantoni (✉)
Faculty of Dentistry, Aristotle University of Thessaloniki, Thessaloniki, Greece
e-mail: andelant@dent.auth.gr

K. Orhan
Faculty of Dentistry, Ankara University, Ankara, Turkey

Ankara University Medical Design Application and Research Center (MEDITAM), Ankara, Turkey

Department of Oral Diagnostics, Faculty of Dentistry, Semmelweis University, Budapest, Hungary

A. Delantoni, K. Orhan (eds.), *Digital Dentistry*, https://doi.org/10.1007/978-3-031-52826-2_17

- compromise of image data, leading to incorrect diagnosis and treatment,
- compromise of components, allowing malicious actors to use the components as pivot points to attack other parts of the HDO infrastructure.

Securing picture archiving and communication system (PACS) is the major concern that may lead to fraudulent or improper use of patient's data and can identity theft solution.

17.1 What Is a PACS Server?

PACS servers are an essential component of a type of clinical IT system called PACS as previously described.

The hardware and software components of PACS acquire digital images from PACS imaging modalities (such as ultrasound CT MRI and radiography) store them into the DICOM (digital imaging and communications in medicine) file format and transfer them to workstations where they can be accessed and reviewed (Fig. 17.1)

A PACS server provides storage for the database of these DICOM files [2–5]. DICOM also signifies the universal transmission protocol for PACS systems, enabling the archiving, retrieval, and distribution of these files (Fig. 17.2).

Given that PACS imaging is able to be integrated not only with Radiology Information Systems (RIS), but with Hospital Information Systems (HIS), Electronic Medical Records (EMR), and Practice Management Software

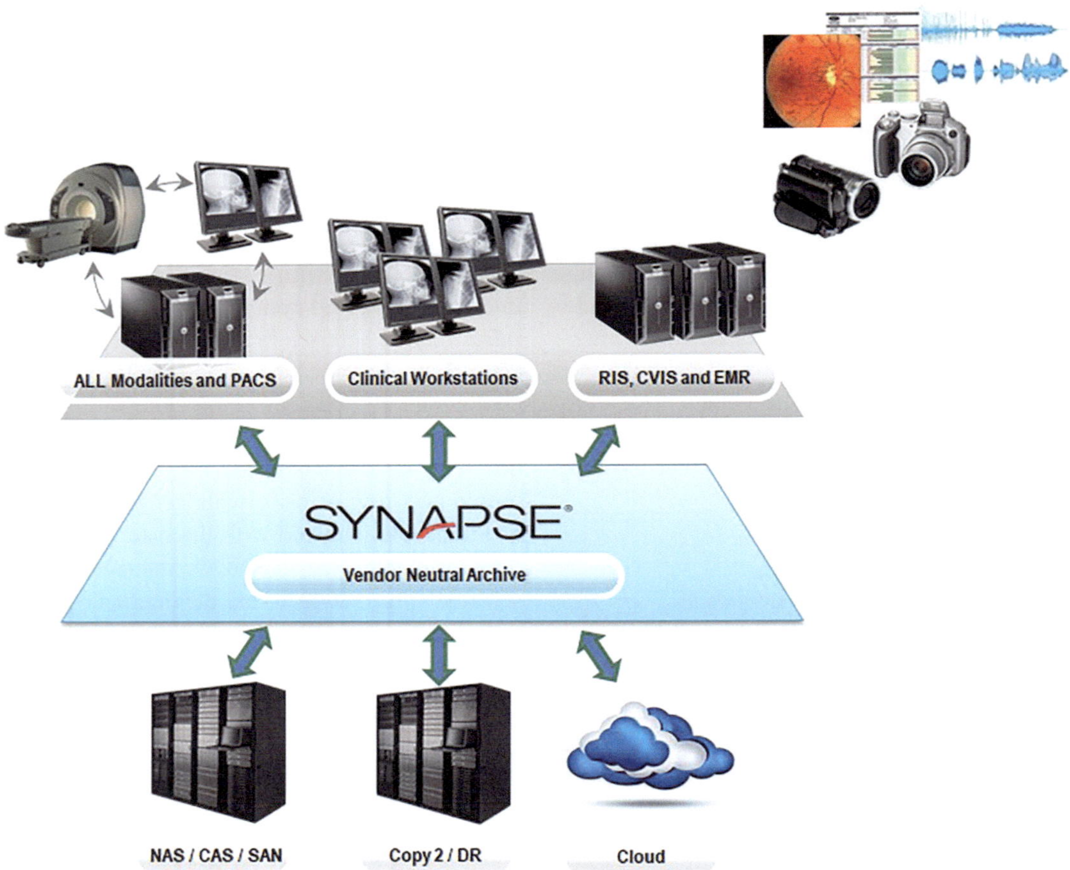

Fig. 17.1 A Typical workflow for Medical Informatics in a Routine hospital set-up. (Courtesy of FUJIFILM Turkey)

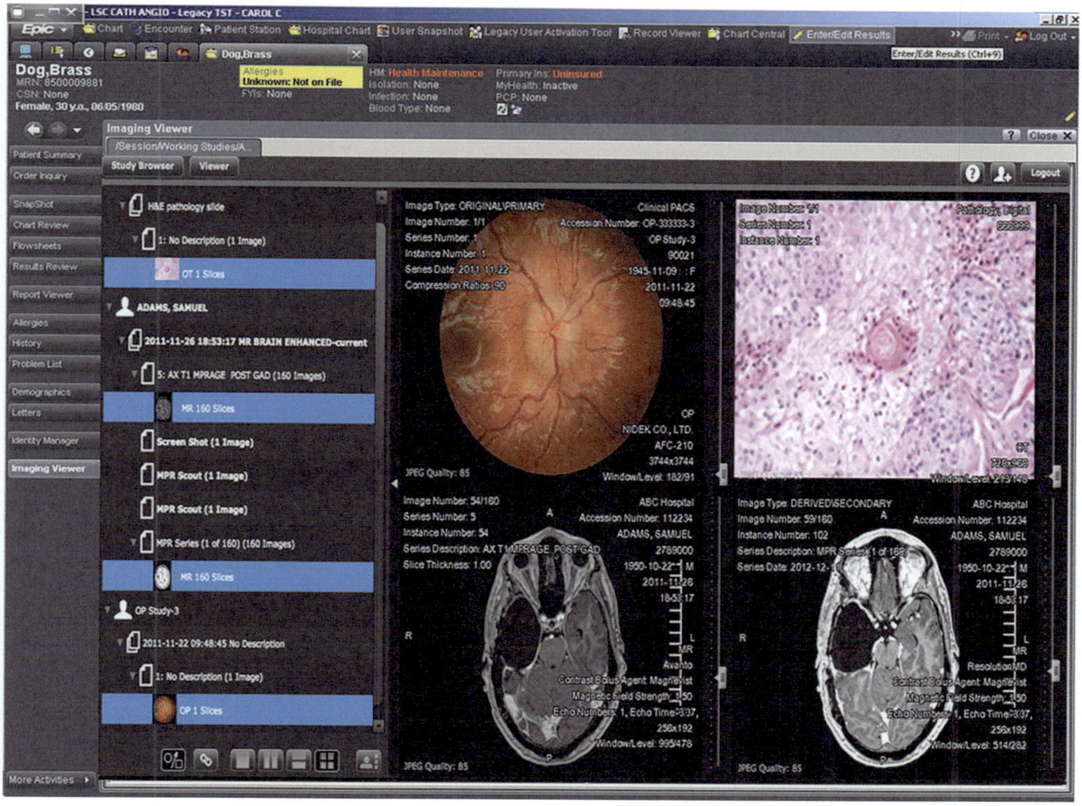

Fig. 17.2 A PACS server provides storage for the database of these DICOM files. (Courtesy of FUJIFILM Turkey)

(PMS), PACS in medical imaging is steadily becoming the norm as an increasing number of hospitals are beginning to implement it beyond their radiology departments.

17.2 PACS Systems or Servers Include

- A local server, which is the main hardware component of PACS systems, and is the part that provides storage for archiving images and related documents.
- Modalities—which are basically various radiographic techniques and modalities devices, such as Cone beam Competed tomography (CBCT) computed tomography (CT), magnetic resonance imaging (MRI), ultrasound (US), nuclear medicine, and positron emission tomography (PET).
- Workstations.
- A computer network that basically connects the system components (Fig. 17.3).

While PACS systems initially consisted of local PACS servers, recently there has been an increase of PACS systems with cloud-based PACS servers to enable distant storage of images. A prime example of this is PostDICOM, that optimizes the PACS system even further, with regard to archiving capacity, cost effectiveness, data security, and data accessibility, and eliminates the need for local PACS servers in all healthcare locations.

PostDICOM acts as a cloud-based PACS server, enabling DICOM files to be stored in the

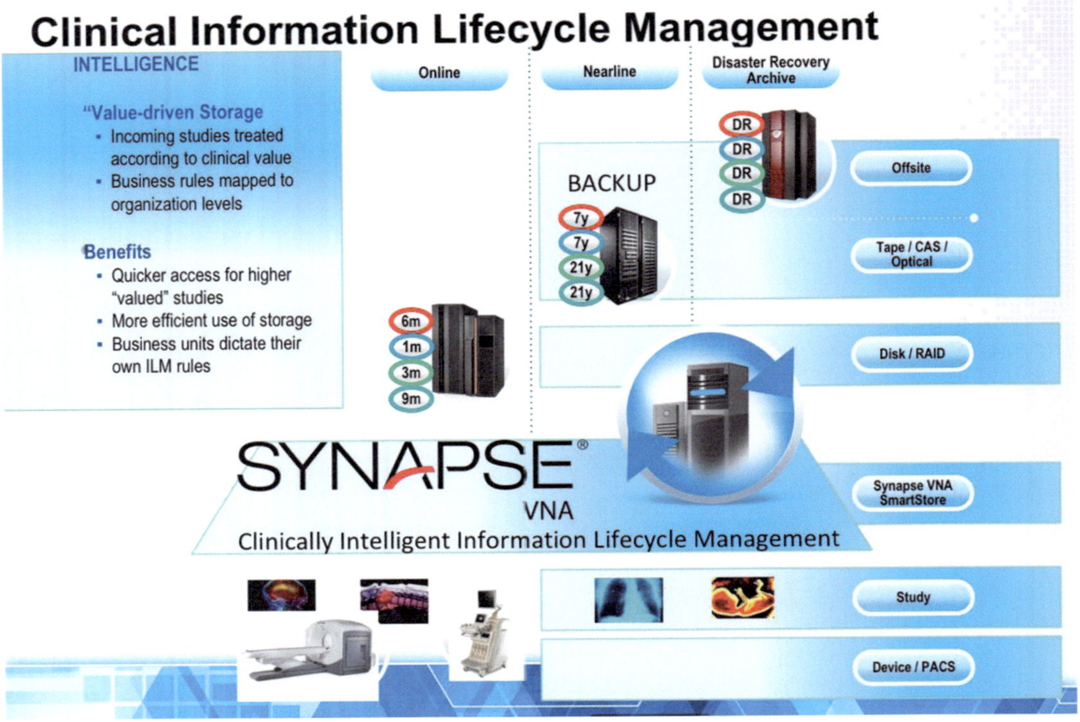

Fig. 17.3 Clinical Information Lifecycle management. (Courtesy of FUJIFILM Turkey)

cloud while preserving the functions of regular PACS systems relying on local servers. Basically it backs up to the cloud so that local servers can be used without any disruptions. Images obtained from any PACS radiology imaging method (e.g., ultrasound, MRI, CT, or radiography) are stored into the DICOM format with any related documents in PDF, JPG, BMP, and AVI within the cloud environment.

17.3 Who Uses PACS Servers?

PACS servers are used mostly by radiologists but also by other medical doctors in hospitals, research institutions, clinics, and increasingly in smaller practices. They are often used in conjunction with another type of clinical IT system—RIS (radiology information system)—as a convenient way of scheduling patients, tracking and interpreting examinations, and as an easy retrieval system.

Although the usage of PACS has been primarily within radiology its application has been steadily expanding to other medical fields such as dentistry radiotherapy cardiology oncology nuclear medicine neurology orthopedics ophthalmology pathology veterinary medicine and clinical research

Post-DICOM is used by medical professionals with diverse specializations—radiologists, cardiologists, nuclear imaging specialists, biomedical researchers, as well as professors, students, and patients who are looking for secure storage, retrieval, and exchange of medical imaging data.

PACS servers have become a part of radiology departments and practices globally mainly because of the system's ability to simplify and speed up the management of imaging files obtained. They also significantly improve workflow and are considered by many to increase the productivity compared to films and finally improving time efficiency of the work space. These advantages make PACS systems, a logical and needed in many cases upgrade for medical practices. Their use in radiology will continue to grow as the digitization of the field, in radiology as it is happening with many other specialties, becomes inevitable [3, 5–8].

PACS servers' benefits

- Reduced costs digital storage is significantly less expensive than storage needed for hard-copy films
- Faster workflow—PACS servers eliminate the need for manual filing, retrieval, and transport of folders.
- Faster image retrieval and the ability to access the images remotely help radiologists to work at a much quicker pace.
- *More organized and convenient management of patient data—All patient information can be reached through a single point of access*
- *Improved image analysis—Sophisticated diagnostic monitors with enhanced resolution and functions enable clearer visualization of images*

With the recent development of cloud-based PACS such as post DICOM, all of these benefits can be enhanced even further.

By transferring the system to the cloud, costs are lowered, and its maintenance is no longer required. Remote access is made available to anyone with an internet connection willing to set up an account, and communication between doctors and their peers is further facilitated.

The benefits of working with soft copy and viewing images on computer screens seem quite self-evident when opposed to relying on paper and film-based procedures and reading images on light boxes. As the adoption of filmless departments' gains further momentum, the digitization of medical imaging is likely to become ubiquitous, and the transfer to cloud-based systems likes Post DICOM the next logical step.

17.4 Security of PACS Servers

Securing Picture Archiving and Communication System (PACS) shows how biomedical engineers, networking engineers, security engineers, and IT professionals can help securely configure and deploy PACS within HDOs by using available, open-source tools and technologies that are consistent with cybersecurity standards.

The advantages include helping an organization:

- To improve strength and performance in the network infrastructure,
- To limit unauthorized movement within the HDO enterprise network, to address the potential risk of an "insider threat."
- To analyze behavior and detect malware throughout the ecosystem.
- To enable those organizations to limit the effects of a potential threat such as secure sensitive data (e.g., personally identifiable information or protected health information).

The approach used to develop the NCCoE reference solution include risk assessment and analysis, logical design, build development, test and evaluation, and security control mapping.

A large scale attempt by The National Cybersecurity Center for Excellence to explain and standardize PACS included a large number of scientists to develop the reference solution, the protocol, reviewed known vulnerabilities in PACS, the Digital Imaging and Communications in Medicine (DICOM) protocol and medical imaging process flow, leveraging use cases described by Integrating Health Enterprise (IHE). They examined how the architecture and component integration could be designed to increase the security of the device. The systems security engineering (SSE) framework discussed in NIST SP 800–160 Volume 1 was utilized to introduce a disciplined, structured, and standards-based set of SSE activities and tasks to the project.

Based on the PACS Project Description document, the scenarios of note are as follows:

Sample Radiology Practice Workflows;

Access to Aggregations and Collections of Different Types of Images; Accessing, Auditing, and Monitoring; Image Object Change Management; and Remote Access. This practice guide does not examine pervasive risks an HDO may face but focuses on the risks specific to the medical imaging ecosystem. The guide considers specific elements that may be required for safe and secure hosting of PACS. It addresses measures that would enhance the security posture for the overall PACS and medical imaging ecosystem, but there may be elements that HDOs should address beyond the recommendations offered in safeguarding PACS and the overall medical imaging ecosystem.

17.5 Cloud Computing in Dentistry

Cloud computing is the provision of computing digital resources via the internet (e.g., servers, apps, etc.) from central systems that are remote from the end user. The end user id provided with automated processes that result to easing and a flexibility of connection.

Basically, it is a system that helps data management over the web. Companies such as Cisco, Intel, Microsoft, Apple and Google are among those that have introduced the technology, the applications, and the platforms, that are known as cloud.

As a definition of the term, the National institute Of Standards and Technology (NIST) gives the following.

Cloud computing is a model for enabling ubiquitous, convenient, on-demand network access to a shared pool of configurable computing resources (e.g., networks, servers, storage, applications, and services) that can be rapidly provisioned and released with minimal management effort or service provider interaction. This cloud model is composed of five essential characteristics, three service models, and four deployment models.

The concept of Cloud Computing first appeared in the 1950s in educational institutes and companies, and its use was carried out by mainframe computers with large computing and storage capabilities [9]. Users accessed these computers through terminals, which had neither computing power nor storage capabilities. The term cloud computing became more widely known in the 1970s, when IBM and Google decided to collaborate in this technology field. Initially, IBM introduced the virtual machine operating system (VM operating system), which provided the ability to work multiple virtual machines (virtual machines) on the same machine. Each virtual machine is—was—a self-contained entity that runs its own operating system and provides computing resources such as—a central processing unit, memory, and I/O units [2].

In the 90s virtual private networks appeared, until their era the telecommunications companies, supported the data circuits, from point to point.

By 2000, IT giants such as Amazon, Microsoft, and Google were engaged in the development and provision of cloud computing services. What followed were some events that are widely regarded as milestones in the history of cloud computing.

In 2006, Amazon introduced Elastic Compute Cloud (EC2). A commercial service based on the World Wide Web, which provided the user with the ability to implement applications on leased-rented machines.

In 2008, eucalyptus, the first open-source platform for developing private clouds, was launched. In the same year, Google released Google App Engine, a platform that supported various cloud computing services.

Following developments in 2011, IBM introduced IBM SmartCloud while in 2012 Oracle Cloud was launched. Finally, Microsoft also announced that it will introduce cloud computing in the next major update of Dynamics ERP solutions and they will run through the Windows Azure platform [10–12].

Cloud computing architecture defines the components and sub-components required for cloud computing. In its simplest form, the foundations of cloud computing can be classified into two parts: front end and back end, which are connected to each other through a virtual network or the Internet. Cloud computing consists of the following key features and functions:

- front-end platform. The principles of cloud computing (the front-end platform) are also called clients or cloud clients. These clients are servers, tablets and mobile devices. These client platforms interact with cloud data storage through an application (middleware) and through a web browser or through a virtual session.
- back-end platforms (servers, storage), an electronic network storage, where data is stored and accessible to many clients.
- delivery based on cloud computing such as (IaaS—Infrastructure as a Service), platforms with a programming environment (PaaS—Platform as a Service) and software (SaaS—Software as a Service), and,

- a network (Internet, Intranet, and Intercloud). The development models are either private or public (internet) or a combination of the two (hybrid/intercloud).

A large number of universities, vendors, and even governments are investing money in research assessing cloud computing. IBM and Google have developed an academic cloud computing interactive which is partially applied in many universities. The evolution is such that numerous conferences and seminars on cloud computing take place daily.

So where is dentistry today with respect to cloud computing platforms?

The oldest web-based dental software is Denticon from Planet DDS. For storage of dental imaging systems, cloud computing is not as robust as the current client server software, and this is related to the problem of digital sensor integration.

Several other systems such as Dentisoft online, Denticon, DentalCollab, etc. are available with cloud capacity, many of them are dentists orientated and even supplied by dental products companies,

With respect to the storage of digital X-ray images mostly in DICOM format, companies using cloud platforms are limited, though many practices nowadays use cloud storage systems in their local network.

There are different types of networks in cloud computing and therefore, Cloud service deployment can be done in any of the following ways:

1. Public Cloud: It is available from a third-party service provider over the Internet and is very cost-effective for SMEs to develop IT solutions. For example, Google Apps.
2. Private Cloud: It is easy to use within an organization and suitable for large enterprises (managed within enterprises).
3. Community Cloud: It is used and controlled by a group of people who have common interests.
4. Hybrid cloud: It is a combination of public and private cloud.

So the major advantages from their use are:

- Cost of performance—Cloud computing is probably the most efficient method to use, maintain and upgrade to use, maintain and upgrade user information. A traditional desktop software costs a lot, in financing terms. Adding multi-user license fees can prove very expensive for such an installation. The cloud on the other hand, is available at a much cheaper price and hence, can significantly reduce IT expenses. Besides, there are many payment options, e.g., pay-as-you-go and other tiered options available.
- Almost unlimited storage—Storing information in the cloud gives you almost unlimited storage / capacity.
- Backup and Restore—Given that all data when stored in the cloud, backing up and restoring the same is relatively easier than storing the same on a physical device. In addition, most cloud service providers are usually capable of handling information retrieval. Hence, it makes the entire backup and recovery process much simpler than other traditional data storage methods.
- Automatic software integration—In the cloud, software integration is done automatically. This means that in the cloud, users don't need to put in extra effort to customize and integrate their apps to their liking. The app takes care of itself.
- Easy access to information—Once users register with Cloud Computing, they can access information from anywhere there is an Internet connection. This handy feature allows users to move beyond their time zone and geographic location.
- Fast deployment—When the user decides to use Cloud computing, the system is fully operational in minutes.
- Easier scale of services—It is easy for a provider to adapt to user requirements.
- Provision of new services—Makes it possible to accept new categories/requests/delivery of new services that are interactive in nature.

- There are, however, some limitations to cloud computing in dentistry as well as in other more technical applications:
- Technical issues—There are times when the system may have some temporary glitches.
- Cloud Security—As a user one should make sure that they choose the most reliable service provider for the security of their information.
- Vulnerability to attacks—Storing information in the cloud may make user data vulnerable to external hacker attacks and online threats.
- Potential downtime—This is where the reliability of the internet connection comes into play.
- Lack of support—According to user comments, the level of service for web applications is still not satisfactory for all websites.

To conclude the authors would like to propose the potential benefits of incorporating a PACS or Cloud storage. They include the following:

- Computers are a part of our daily routine, with the use of PACS, Cloud or other storage systems and applications there is reduced need for more processing power and memory on the current computer systems providing economy,
- Software update costs, and with those systems, the downtime from storage updating are reduced or even eliminated.
- Storage capacity expansion can be increased as needed.
- There is multisite access to patient info and data bases as well as imaging studies.
- There is security against equipment theft, office or equipment damage.
- Data is encrypted and secure with DICOM friendly systems.
- Finally for a large multisite practice, for group practice or dental schools, and even hospitals, there will be a significant reduction of cost, for server infrastructure and IT support (Fig. 17.4).

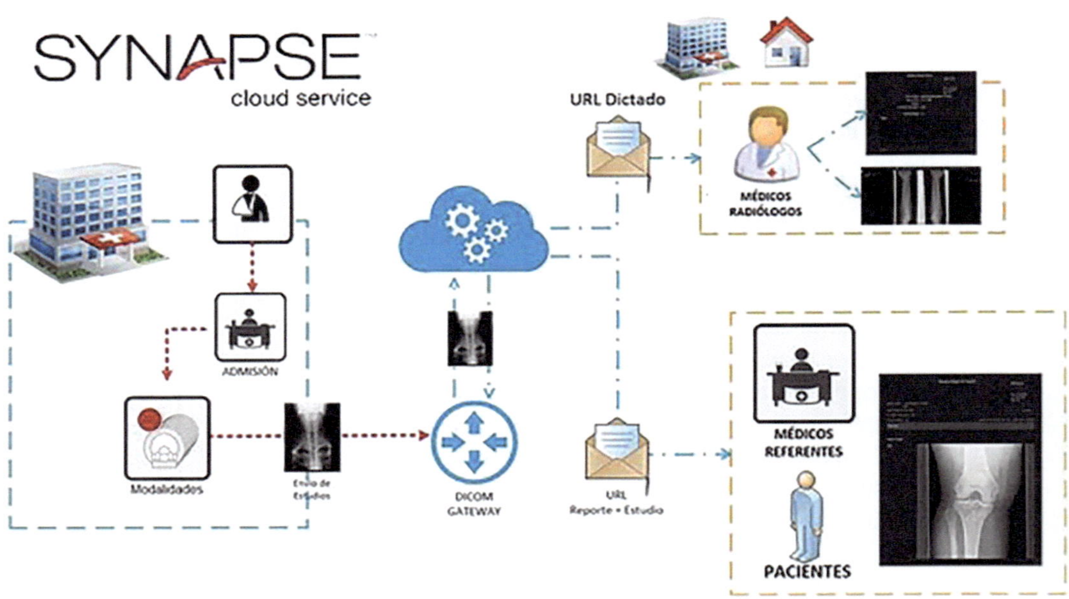

Fig. 17.4 Typical usage of Cloud system in combination of PACS. (Courtesy of FUJIFILM Turkey)

17.6 What Is a Vendor-Neutral Archive (VNA)?

Healthcare providers have always relied on clinical imaging when making diagnoses, compiling treatment plans, and analyzing treatment efficacy. While the majority of images have traditionally been handled by the radiology department, healthcare enterprises now obtain images from a variety of service lines. If a patient has a suspicious mole or a serious wound, for example, chances are a dermatologist or wound care specialist will take a picture to document a baseline and assist with their proposed care strategy. To keep pace with this proliferation of clinical imaging, healthcare organizations are starting to implement an enterprise imaging strategy to help manage all of the imaging content coming in from across the care continuum. That's where a vendor-neutral archive comes in.

A vendor-neutral archive, or VNA, was designed for imaging interoperability. Many solutions on the market, including Fujifilm's Best in KLAS Synapse® VNA, provide secure, easy-to-manage storage, and allow access to the complete patient imaging record. They also integrate with electronic health records (EHRs) and health information technology (HIT) systems to provide the complete picture health picture (Fig. 17.5).

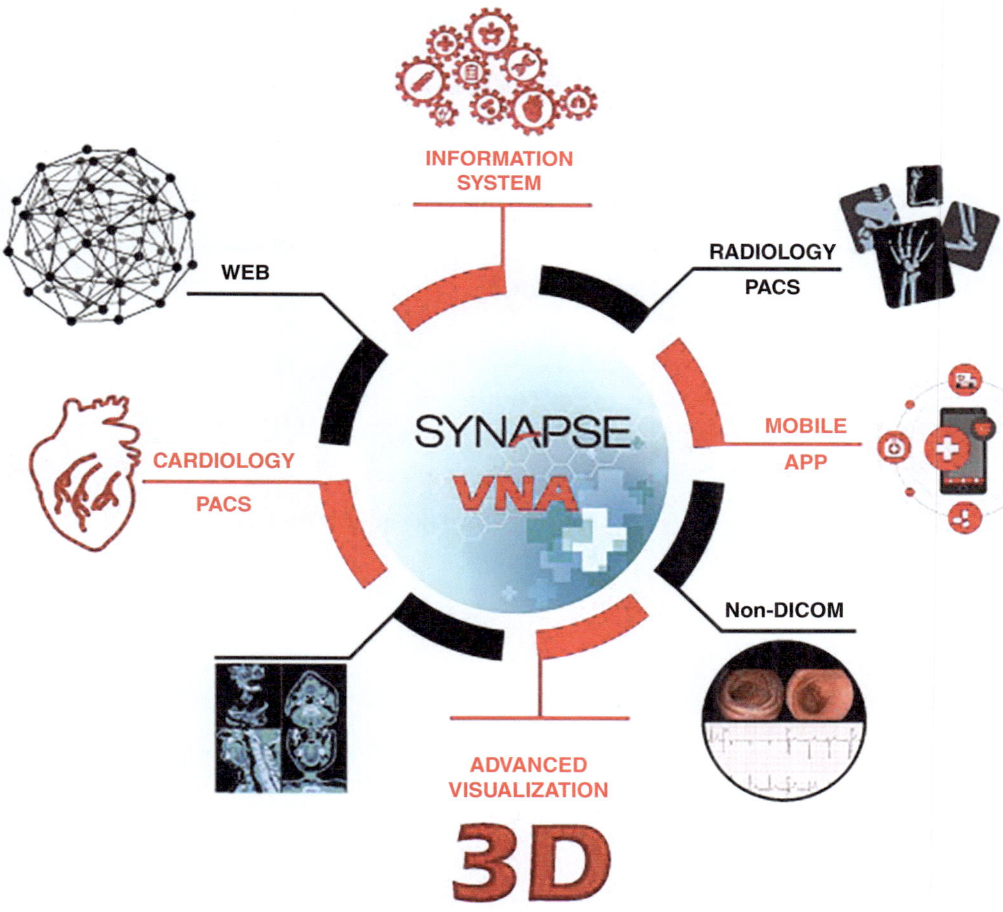

Fig. 17.5 Typical usage of VNA in combination of PACS. (Courtesy of FUJIFILM Turkey)

17.7 A Few Other Important Features of VNAs Include

Secures and enables control of all image data on the organization's preferred enterprise-class storage media or in the cloud.

Creates a single, patient-centric view across the entire continuum of care.

Manages all DICOM and specialty department (non-DICOM) clinical imaging content from across the enterprise.

Captures imaging content using VNA-inherent workflows for encounters-based service lines.

Facilitates image sharing and collaboration amongst a community of care providers (Fig. 17.6).

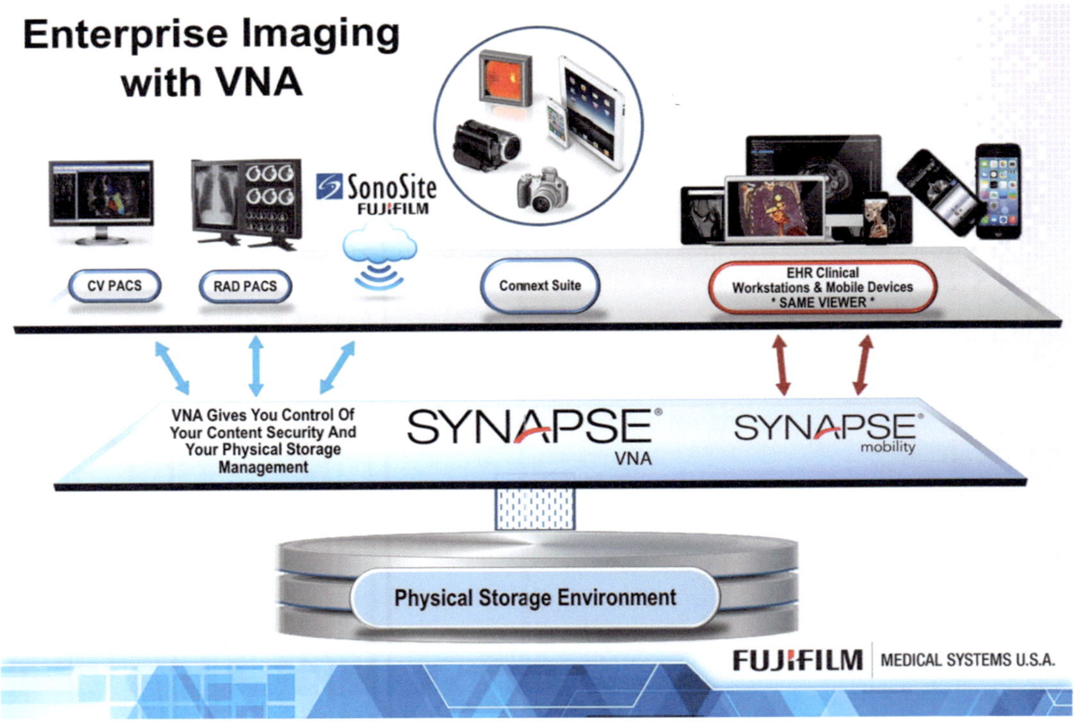

Fig. 17.6 An example of Overall Imaging in combination of VNA. Courtesy of FUJIFILM Turkey

17.8 Presents Patient Data Through Advanced Analytics and Configurable Dashboards

17.8.1 Why Do I Need a VNA?

Healthcare enterprises first realized the need for a VNA with the proliferation of picture archiving communication systems—or PACS. Radiology departments have used picture archiving PACS for more than 40 years, which primarily manage and archive DICOM images. However, as more vendors entered the market with their own variations of PACS technology and DICOM conformance, the ability to easily exchange and view images between PACS systems became challenging, causing demand for the VNA to grow. Add in the influx of specialty departments now curating images in a variety of non-DICOM formats – A/V, MPEG, WAV, JPG, PDF, to name a few—and you can see why the need for one, all-inclusive image archive solution becomes so critical.

17.8.2 So How Does It Work?

A VNA captures, stores, archives, manages, and distributes DICOM and non-DICOM images in one common archive, regardless of the imaging device, file format, or department. Some specific benefits of having a VNA as the core to your enterprise imaging strategy include:

Reduced storage and operational costs: Simplifying data storage with a VNA reduces storage costs and eliminates the need for costly future data migrations.

Secure patient data: A HIPAA-compliant VNA that provides data in accordance with your organization's access control policies helps keep patient information secure, with centralized data security across the healthcare enterprise.

Streamlined physician workflows: A VNA with EHR interoperability allows providers to access images and patient records through a single interface, streamlining workflows, and improving clinician satisfaction while allowing them to spend more time on patient care.

Improved patient care: Access to complete imaging data allows providers to see the whole patient, so they can treat the whole patient.

References

1. Silva E III, Breslau J, Liebscher LA, Bohl M, Hoffman T, Boland GWL, Sherry C, Kim W, Shah SS, Tilkin M. ACR white paper on teleradiology practice: a report from the task force on teleradiology practice. J Am Coll Radiol. 2013;10(8):575–85.
2. Rajaraman V. Cloud computing. Resonance. 2014;19:242–58.
3. Iwasaki H, Honda E, Nishitani H, Takahashi H, Yamamoto Y, Ooguro T, Tanaka K. Hanging protocol and viewers for a dental full picture [corrected] archiving and communication system (PACS) [corrected]. Dentomaxillofac Radiol. 2007;36(5):285–95.
4. Thodberg HH, Böttcher J, Lomholt J, Kreiborg S, Wolf G. Pfeil a.A new implementation of digital X-ray radiogrammetry and reference curves of four indices of cortical bone for healthy European adults. Arch Osteoporos. 2016;11:17.
5. Hirschorn D, Eber C, Samuels P, Gujrathi S, Baker SR. Filmless in New Jersey: the New Jersey Medical School PACS Project. J Digit Imaging. 2002;15(Suppl 1):7–12.
6. Chow F, Muftu A, Shorter R. Virtualization and cloud computing in dentistry. J Mass Dent Soc. 2014;63:14.
7. Goonasekera N, Mahmoud A, Chilton J, Afgan E. Galaxy cloud runner: enhancing scalable computing for Galaxy. Bioinformatics. 2021;37(12):1763–5.
8. Spangler HD, Simancas-Pallares MA, Ginnis J, Ferreira Zandoná AG, Roach J, Divaris K. A web-based rendering application for communicating dental conditions. Healthcare (Basel). 2021;9(8):960.
9. Decasena CN. Impact study of cloud computing on business development. Oper Res Appl Int J (ORAJ). 2014;1(1):1–17.
10. Lin CY, Peng KL, Chen J, Tsai JY, Tseng YC, Yang JR, Chen MH. Improvements in dental care using a new mobile app with cloud services. J Formos Med Assoc. 2014;113(10):742–9.
11. Johnson L, Callaghan C, Balasubramanian M, Haq H, Spallek HJ. Cost comparison of an on-premise IT solution with a cloud-based solution for electronic health records in a dental school clinic. Dent Educ. 2019;83(8):895–903.

12. Lightbody G, Haberland V, Browne F, Taggart L, Zheng H, Parkes E, Blayney JK. Review of applications of high-throughput sequencing in personalized medicine: barriers and facilitators of future progress in research and clinical application. Brief Bioinform. 2019;20(5):1795–811.
13. Estai M, Kanagasingam Y, Xiao D, Vignarajan J, Huang B, Kruger E, Tennant MJ. A proof-of-concept evaluation of a cloud-based store-and-forward telemedicine app for screening for oral diseases. Telemed Telecare. 2016;22(6):319–25.
14. Kaur PD. Chana I cloud based intelligent system for delivering health care as a service. Comput Methods Prog Biomed. 2014;113(1):346–59.
15. Spanakis EG, Santana S, Tsiknakis M, Marias K, Sakkalis V, Teixeira A, Janssen JH, de Jong H. Tziraki C technology-based innovations to Foster personalized healthy lifestyles and Well-being: a targeted review. J Med Internet Res. 2016;18(6):e128.

18 Artificial Intelligence in Dentistry

Kaan Orhan and Gürkan Ünsal

The scientific community has never fully grasped how to develop an exact model that duplicates the functioning of the human brain. Scientists have been slavishly advancing "artificial intelligence" for a long time (AI).

The progresses in AI initiated in 1943 but the term AI was created in 1956 at a conference in Dartmouth by John McCarthy with the definition of "computerized synthetic human cognitive function". During that time the term was called as machine learning (ML). Main objective of the AI is to utilize computer technology to reproduce critical thinking, decision-making, and intelligent behaviour that is operated by organic brain. When a computer mimics analytical skills that people usually connect with other human brains, such as "learning and problem-solving", the term "AI" is employed.

There has been a lot of experimentation with AI techniques as clinical trial tools, specifically to help in decision-making for prognosis and projection, as well as each phase of diagnosis and subsequent therapy, as a result of their excellent capabilities and capacities in recognizing significant data patterns. AI was created to address issues in certain fields by picking up different modes of perception and thought. This particular aptitude to solve problems lends itself to virtual use via the use of software-type techniques.

AI has been shown to improve precision, accuracy, and efficiency to the same level as doctors more rapidly and economically. It already has an influence on our everyday life because of different office and practice management software.

A few apps that have created intelligent conversational user interfaces for any device, application language, or environment utilizing artificial intelligence are Siri, Google Now, Cortana, Alexa, Google Assistant, and other voice command software.

It is crucial to distinguish AI or ML from conventional computing software. The basis of computing software is a logistical "IF" statement. The easiest way to explain this is that an input "A" is supplied, computed using a sequence of IF questions, and then an output "B" is provided. IF statements are non-variable logic tools. While doing highly helpful jobs for humanity, this only offers a little amount of availability for augmentation and adaption to unexplored datasets. AI operates in a unique way. Convolutional neural networks (CNNs), artificial neural networks (ANNs), deep learning (DL), which have different programme formats from this start to end

K. Orhan
Faculty of Dentistry, Ankara University, Ankara, Turkey

Ankara University Medical Design Application and Research Center (MEDITAM), Ankara, Turkey

Department of Oral Diagnostics, Faculty of Dentistry, Semmelweis University, Budapest, Hungary
e-mail: knorhan@dentistry.ankara.edu.tr

G. Ünsal (✉)
Department of Dentomaxillofacial Radiology, Faculty of Dentistry, Near East University, Nicosia, Cyprus

A. Delantoni, K. Orhan (eds.), *Digital Dentistry*, https://doi.org/10.1007/978-3-031-52826-2_18

IF-based procedure, make up the majority of this discipline. When creating an AI-based tool, you must supply both the input "A" and the necessary output "B". The AI technique will then fine-tune the tool to capitalize on the relationship between the two, which can then be used to previously unexplored comparable data.

Through data learning, machines are able to develop algorithms that enable them to tackle prediction-related tasks independently. Neural networks (NNs) use artificial neurons that are akin to human neural networks to simulate the human brain in a mathematical nonlinear model. NNs may imitate certain aspects of human cognition, such as decision-making and learning-based problem resolution and human reasoning. Input, hidden, and output layers are the three layers that make up simple neural networks. Information enters the system through the input layer, while data processing takes place in the hidden layer (where the system decides what to do). Given a collection of mathematical models, NNs may outline any input to an output. If sufficient data is provided, these NNs may be trained to represent the data's intrinsic statistical statistics.

Artificial neural networks (ANNs) replicate the biological neuron system with many connections between neurons that is employed in "learning" and uses it in its algorithm to understand the link between qualities and the truth.

Digital pictures are seen as analogues or as an ongoing stream of information by humans. However, a digital image is nothing more than the fusion of countless millions of little colour pixels. Thus, rather than representing a visual image, these pixel series may be thought of as strings of data that software can display as code. CNNs may be trained to recognize these strings, enabling them to search through new picture datasets for related patterns. CNNs need to go through a "training" phase before they can carry out this task. Humans define these data sets throughout the training process, instructing a CNN on what to search for. Picture analysis frequently requires on professionals labelling interesting image portions so that CNN can locate them later. For instance, humans would put a circle around the nodules on a photograph of a lung to indicate the right digital value of the code so that CNN could identify them. Through a process known as supervised learning, the CNN will get better at mimicking the transcribing process as more nodules are shown to it, eventually enabling it to do this work on its own.

AI has two phases: the first is "training" and the second is "testing". The training data determines the model set's parameters. The model employs data from earlier examples, such as patient data or data from data sets with different examples, retrospectively. The test sets are then subjected to these criteria.

Last but not least, DL has matched and enhanced human performance for extremely difficult tasks in disciplines like sound processing and picture processing like object detection, facial recognition, speech synthesis and processing.

The use of artificial intelligence (AI) has resulted in significant developments that have improved our daily lives and routine tasks in several ways (facial recognition, self-driving cars, and image classification, among others). The most significant cause for the most current wave of AI innovation is the dramatic growth of the data collecting in the past few decades. Data on its own, however, is insufficient. High-performance computing (HPC) advancements have made it possible for new, potent AI algorithms to extract knowledge from acquired data in a thorough and perceptive manner. ML, the data-driven component of AI, is what is commonly referred to as the information extraction process. Its goal is to enable machines (algorithms implemented on computer systems) to learn about a particular topic from a certain available dataset. Typically, supervised learning approaches are used for this sort of information extraction. These techniques have been quite successful in solving a wide range of issues.

Both virtual and physical, AI have applications in the healthcare sector. A growing number of industries stand to gain from the use of AI, including the surgical field (e.g., intelligent systems for assisted surgery, and video-surgery), automatic disease diagnosis (e.g., decision support diagnosis systems from images), and the recently developed personalized medicine, which provided the predisposition to diseases, diagnosis, and selection of the best treatment for a given patient. The primary domain of the virtual type is the mathematical equations for medicine dosage, diagnosis and prognosis, appointment scheduling, drug interactions, electronic health records, and imaging. Rehabilitation, telepresence, robotic assistance during surgery, and companion robots for senior care are all examples of the physical element.

While CNNs may sometimes accurately identify a picture, they are most frequently employed as supportive tools, allowing AI to highlight regions that are most likely to have the desired disease or image type. AI may be utilized in the development of more efficient treatments, prophylaxis, and the lowering of healthcare expenses. The majority of the medical fields that AI can help with include radiology, pathology, oncology (detection of malignant lesions), cardiology (ECG analysis), psychiatry, nuclear medicine, detection of anomalies in chest X-rays, lesions with the potential to become cancerous, and radiology (to detect specific types of retinopathies), and numerous other branches of medicine and dentistry.

However, it has been argued that some of the work in these disciplines may not be as precise as medical specialists or, in fact, robust enough to be fully generalizable to all clinical settings.

AI is being used more frequently in dentistry and medicine as a supporting tool, and it is increasingly seen as a need for delivering secure and efficient healthcare.

Large amounts of data may be analysed by DL networks to carry out particular tasks. These are typically utilized in the healthcare industries for image analysis, patient records analysation, and logistic regression.

In medicine, there has been progress in predicting Alzheimer's disease, depression, sepsis, and dementia using medical records of patients and metabolite data. The phrase "augmented intelligence" was used by the American Medical Association to describe the advancements in bit-based computer technology's data processing capabilities, namely in the fields of medicine and dentistry. This explains how AI is conceptualized in the context of healthcare, emphasizing how it may help doctors.

While there are some obvious advantages to using AI in healthcare, such as minimizing human error, aiding with diagnosis, simplifying data processing, and task performance, which might eventually result in more effective and affordable services, its adoption is not without challenges. These can specifically include a lack of hardware, data curation, code exchange, and readability. Additionally, there are problems that come with integrating any emerging innovations into a service, such as resistance to change, integrating new technology into existing facilities, and continuous maintenance costs. The existence of implicit biases in training datasets and their direct effects on AI performance have been the subject of more recent criticism.

According to epidemiological and demographic changes, significant increase in the cost of oral and dental problems is expected. The price and accessibility of oral and dental treatment are also threatened by the lack of skilled experts, which places further demand on already overloaded healthcare systems. AI has considerable promise, especially in the area of oral and dental care because of its potential for higher efficacy, safety, and efficiency, which permits the providing of better oral healthcare to a wider number of people.

AI is also becoming increasingly common in the dental industry as a result of technological advancements and the digitization of the profession. Nowadays, computers could offer a second opinion in a number of dental disciplines. Neural networks' precision, rapidity, and effectiveness can be used to enhance diagnosis.

Among the AI research in dentistry that have been published on PubMed Database in 2020, the incidence of caries lesions, periodontal attachment loss, periodontally compromised teeth, apical lesions, and diagnosis of odontogenic cysts are only a few.

Dentistry clinical utility favour more sophisticated AI technologies like 3D convolutional neural networks and cone beam computed tomography (CBCT). They are often utilized, even in interdisciplinary fields like forensic dentistry.

In terms of problem-solving capacity, the "strong" or "deep" artificial general intelligence is similar to a human. Physicians have the ability to think abstractly, plan in advance, and generate innovation, but even the most advanced AI systems currently fail at these skills. It will eventually be possible for artificial general intelligence to think extremely similarly to humanity. Artificial Super Intelligence will be able to learn and develop beyond the capabilities of humans, going beyond our current comprehension.

Although it might not appear that advances in AI have had much of an impact on dentistry, there have been significant advancements in areas like image-based automatic disease diagnosis and other diagnosis-support systems, image segmentation for automatic detection of oral lesions, and resolution enhancement of dental images.

In dentistry, the input data may be visual (experimental parameters), textual (medical or treatment records), or voice-based (handpiece noises) (spectral or radiographic images, photos). These input data are processed by the neural networks, who then provide an output.

The outcome might be a prognosis, diagnosis, course of therapy, or forecast of the condition. To make a diagnosis, it can decipher clinical clues, do cephalometric analysis, or identify lesions based on voxel differences. By identifying the typical structures, inducing and assessing the results, transforming the speech data, or connecting data capture and CAD/CAM, it foretells how the input will be treated. The AI software may use gene analysis, risk factor prioritization, or outcome prediction to predict the disease or its prognosis.

The diagnosis of carious lesions, the staging and grading of periodontal disease, the identification of apical pathology, or the evaluation of peri-implant health are common causes for acquiring dental radiographs. A dentist will often prescribe and provide feedback on these scans. Inter-rater and intra-rater agreement in the identification of dental caries and bone loss has been demonstrated to be low, facilitating CNN with this research.

A complete digital process shift is required for clinical AI applications for dentists. Currently, a number of examples of latest dental technology based on digital processes are available. Their objective is to improve the effectiveness and calibre of the services provided.

As December 30th 2022, most of the dental applications in AI include:

1. X-ray and other diagnostics, caries.
2. Implant dentistry.
3. Photography analysis.
4. Practice management, tele-dentistry.
5. Clinical predictions (maturation, growth, age).

AI can be utilized in every single aspect of the dentistry as follows:

1. Oral Diagnosis and Maxillofacial Radiology.
2. Oral and Maxillofacial Surgery.
3. Orthodontics.
4. Periodontology.
5. Endodontics.
6. Restorative Dentistry.
7. Prosthodontics.
8. Pedodontics.
9. Patient and Practice Management.
10. Forensic Odontology.
11. Dental Education.
12. Controversies.

18.1 Oral Diagnosis and Maxillofacial Radiology

Artificial intelligence may be used to diagnose and cure disorders of the oral cavity, as well as to identify and categorize suspiciously altered mucosa that has undergone premalignant and malignant modifications. Even tiny alterations at the single-pixel level that the human eye could overlook are detected. The genetic predisposition for oral cancer in a broad population may be appropriately identified by artificial intelligence. An AI-based machine learning system is a helpful tool for assessing the future of dental conditions in relation to the chosen treatment protocol. A comprehensive treatment plan must be thoroughly examined in order to assess a tooth's chances for long-term dental health and function.

As most of the AI applications that were mentioned before also included radiological techniques, in this part the radiomic applications of AI in Oral Diagnosis and Maxillofacial Radiology which was not mentioned in the previous chapters will be discussed.

On normal dental radiography interpretations, odontogenic lesions are frequently discovered by chance. Because these lesions are often cystic in appearance, it can be difficult for a non-specialist dentist to differentiate cysts from tumours on radiographs. Several research have created AI model, using OPGs for automatic diagnosis of lesions of the jaws, driven by the requirement for more rapid and accurate detection of maxillofacial cysts and tumours. Ameloblastoma, odontogenic keratocysts, dentigerous cysts, and radicular cysts were the lesions that received the majority of their attention. The suggested models achieved good diagnostic accuracy on level with oral-maxillofacial surgeons. On OPG and CBCT, Lee et al. built CNN models for the automated identification, segmentation, and classification of odontogenic keratocysts, dentigerous cysts, and radicular cysts. Unsurprisingly, the model that was trained using CBCT performed better than the model that was trained on OPGs given that 3D images can provide more detail without geometric limitations. CNN models were created by Bispo et al. and Chai et al. to differentiate between ameloblastoma and odontogenic keratocysts on computed tomography scans. The effectiveness of the model was evaluated with that of 7 senior and 30 junior oral-maxillofacial surgeons by Chai et al. The model had an accuracy of 85% and a quick execution time of just under 3 ms per interpretation, outperforming both seniors and juniors. These DL models may help practitioners recognize various jaw cysts and tumours on CBCT during routine dental care, enabling prompt referral to oral-maxillofacial specialists and, therefore, the start of therapy as soon as practical. The sixth most common kind of cancer in the world is oral squamous cell carcinoma (OSCC), which has a high incidence of lymph node metastases and invasiveness. One of the main diagnostic factors in OSCC patients that is directly associated with a worse overall survival rate is cervical lymph node metastases, according to research. Unseen lymph node metastases is a prevalent occurrence in clinical practice, hence patients with OSCC frequently have preventive neck dissection. The neck dissection, though, has the potential to cause serious motor and sensory issues that have a significant impact on the patients' standard of living. Due of the debate surrounding preventive neck dissection for OSCC patients, highly accurate non-invasive methods for detecting lymph node metastases are sought for. One of the most popular imaging methods for diagnosing lymph node metastases in OSCC patients is contrast-enhanced CT. The key characteristics for recognizing cervical lymph node metastases are size, necrosis, and extranodal extension. However, it is still difficult to identify every metastatic lymph node using CT scans and solely the visible nodal characteristics. The creation of a non-invasive method for precisely identifying the kind of cervical lymph nodes in individuals with OSCC appears to be supported by AI. In order to distinguish between the positive and negative cervical lymph nodes on trimmed contrast-enhanced CT images of OSCC patients, Ariji et al. initially created a deep learning model. With an AUC (area under the curve) of 0.80, the model's accuracy was satisfactory and on par with that of two seasoned radiologists (AUC of 0.83). On trimmed contrast-enhanced CT images of OSCC patients, Ariji et al. further suggested a CNN model to distinguish between metastatic lymph nodes both with and without extranodal expansion. The model surpassed four expert radiologists and attained better accuracy with an AUC of 0.82. (AUCs of 0.52–0.63). All cervical lymph nodes had to be manually identified and trimmed on several CT image slices since these algorithms could only use the trimmed pictures of individual lymph nodes to make choices. The application of these models for everyday clinical usage would undoubtedly be constrained by the time-consuming manual classification and trimming tasks. Ariji et al.

established CNN models for the automated identification and segmentation of metastatic and non-metastatic cervical lymph nodes on contrast-enhanced CT images in order to increase overall practical value. In terms of identifying cervical lymph nodes with metastatic disease, the most recent model fared better than two seasoned radiologists (AUC of 0.90), albeit segmentation accuracy might yet be enhanced. In order to generate prediction algorithms for undetected cervical lymph node metastases in patients with tongue cancer, Kubo et al. used a variety of classifiers from machine learning and CT-derived radiomic characteristics. With an AUC of 0.98, the model predicted regional lymph node metastases with an almost perfect accuracy. For patients with tongue cancer, Zhong et al. created prediction algorithms based on CT-derived radiomic characteristics and related clinical indicators for undetected cervical lymph node metastases. The model with radiomic characteristics and clinical lymph node condition (AUC of 0.94) outperformed the model with just radiomic features (AUC of 0.92). Morgan et al. created a number of algorithms based on radiomic characteristics acquired from CT and CBCT. The model with the best predictive accuracy, with an AUC of 0.87 for main cancer and 0.91 for nodal formations, was trained on both radiomic characteristics and clinical data.

Dentists' expertise and imaging techniques are very important in the diagnosis of disorders of the salivary glands. Due to MRI scans' advantages above other imaging modalities in visualizing soft tissues, DL models for the detection of disorders of the salivary gland have been primarily based on MRI images. Nonetheless, because MRI is not frequently used by dentists and practitioners, CT continues to play a crucial role in determining the presence and significance of neoplasms. To automatically spot the fatty degeneration of the salivary gland which is a decisive diagnostic feature for the diagnosis of Sjogren's syndrome, Kise et al. created a CNN algorithm using CT scans. The algorithm outscored three novice radiologists while performing comparably to three expert radiology specialists. To differentiate pleomorphic adenoma and malignant tumours of the parotid gland on CT scans, Yuan et al. created a CNN model that achieved a 90% classification accuracy. Likewise, Zhang et al. developed a number of CNN models to differentiate benign and malignant tumours of the parotid gland and those models achieved up to 98% classification accuracy. The same scientists also created a model to differentiate high-grade and low-grade mucoepidermoid carcinoma based on CT-derived radiomic characteristics and Xu et al. created a similar model to differentiate parotid gland's malignant and benign tumours. To differentiate between pleomorphic adenoma and Warthin tumours of the parotid glands, Liu et al. created two prediction models, one based on MRI and another based on CT-derived radiomic characteristics. The performance of the model on MRI had 0.91 AUC value, while the model on CT had 0.88 AUC value. These models might be used as supplemental instruments to help dentists recognize patients with malignant salivary gland tumours.

In order to prevent patients from receiving unnecessary tests and surgical procedures, correct identification of TMJ problems is challenging for general dentistry practitioners and necessitates significant clinical expertise. For these reasons, several research were conducted and published in the literature. Numerous research studies on TMJ disease have used CBCT scans, despite the fact they are unable to reveal the soft tissue components such ligaments, muscles, and the articular disc. In order to automatically segment the mandibular ramus and condyle using CBCT images, Lee et al. built a CNN model and Kim et al. developed a CNN model that can segment and measure the cortical thickness of the mandibular condyle. de Dumast et al.'s DL model achieved a high agreement in TMJ osteoarthritis classification (AUC 91%) with 2 radiology specialists. With the aid of this diagnostic model, screening individuals with early TMJ osteoarthritis seems possible. As TMJ disorders affect a significant number of the population, those developments can surely assist the dentists with their examinations.

Maxillary sinus has the biggest volume among all paranasal sinuses and may get damaged during oral and maxillofacial surgery and implant procedures. One of the most important aspects in assuring a reliable clinical outcome is the accurate diagnosis of maxillary sinus diseases before performing any surgical operations involving the sinus area. Yet, as general practitioners may feel less competent and confident to diagnose maxillary sinus disorders on radiographs, numerous DL models were developed by the researchers. The maxillary sinus and the mucosal changes of the sinus are can be segmented automatically on CT images using CNN models and to differentiate the mucosal thickening and mucous retention cysts of the maxillary sinus, Jung et al. created a CNN algorithm on CBCT which obtained a favourable segmentation performance. Hung et al. conducted another study on maxillary sinuses and they reported that their 3D CNN model showed outstanding efficiency in the detection, segmentation, and quantitative determination of mucosal thickening and mucous retention cysts of the sinus on both standard dose and low dose CBCT images. Their AUC value for the standard dose and low dose were 0.89–0.93 and 0.84–0.89, respectively.

The only mobile and most often fractured bone of the craniofacial region in trauma instances is the mandible. To automatically identify mandibular fractures on CT scans, a CNN model was created. The models initially produced an OPG that was synthesized from the CT imaging. The mandibular area was then straightened and separated into image patches with nine sub-areas in the reconstructed OPG image. In the end, the model identified if a fracture existed or not on the image patches of particular mandibular sub-areas. With AUC values ranging from 0.93 to 0.98 throughout the nine mandibular sub-areas, our model showed good fracture detection accuracy, which may be especially helpful for diagnosing hidden condylar fractures particularly for the inexperienced dentists.

18.2 Oral and Maxillofacial Surgery

The collected research suggests that NNs might even be extensively utilized in oral surgery. The aim of Chien-Hsun Lu et al. study's was to assess and enhance patient-specific postorthognathic surgery visual projections. NN simulations may allow surgeons, orthodontists, and patients to refine their therapeutic approaches. The study by Patcas et al. suggested that AI might become capable of determining how orthognathic surgery affects facial attractiveness and look of ageing. Orthognathic patients' before- and after-treatment photos were obtained, and CNNs were trained on more than 0.5 million pictures for age estimate and more than 17 million ratings for beauty. According to the algorithms, the 66.4% of patients' appearances improved with therapy, giving them a look that was almost a year younger.

In the study of Byung Su Kim et al., CNNs were utilized to determine if third molar extraction may result in nervus alveolaris inferiores damage. Prior to the extraction, OPGs were taken, and the CNN used the physical contact between the mandibular canal and tooth roots to foretell the occurrence of nerve paraesthesia. However, the scientists came to the conclusion that OPGs would produce more false positive and false negative findings, necessitating further study.

The identification of odontogenic lesions may benefit from DL. Ameloblastoma and odontogenic keratocyst are two predominant pathologies that can affect the jaws, particularly the mandibular ramus and mandibular posterior region. OPGs were utilized in Liu et al.'s study to identify these two pathologies since 2D radiographs cost less and are more widely available than CT or MR scans. In OPGs, it is challenging for the observer to do a differential diagnosis between them, hence a CNN was built using the transfer learning method. The histopathology analysis verified all of the lesions and in comparison, to the accuracy of three other NNs utilized in the same research, the CNN's accuracy score of 90.36% was higher.

Previous research suggests that NNs might be applied in implantology. AI algorithms may make it easier to design CBCT image-based dental implant therapy. CNNs can also be utilized to determine the stage of therapy and to recognize dental implant brands on OPGs. Using CNNs, the osteointegration's quality may be evaluated. The existence of a soft tissue layer (non-mineralized bone tissue) along the bone-implant contact, which may be seen during a sonography, may be the cause of the osteointegration problems. Finally, studies have using AI to quantify peri-implant bone loss.

NNs in oral surgery may be extensively utilized in a variety of procedures, from orthognathic operations to therapy for alterations in the bones or issues following extractions. Due to the requirement for extreme accuracy and precise management, implantology is a field that is evolving very quickly, and the use of NNs in daily practice may be quite beneficial. NNs may also assist in predicting and subsequently preventing many surgical intervention problems.

The major use of AI in oral surgery is the development of robotic surgery. Image-guided cranial surgical techniques that have proved effective in clinical situations include dental implants, the removal of tumours and foreign objects, biopsies, and TMJ surgery. Robotic surgery has often been associated with shorter operating times, more intraoperative precision, and safer manipulation around fragile tissues. With imaging guidance, a much more thorough surgical resection is achievable, simultaneously lowering the need for revision procedures. AI has revolutionized surgery, and there are currently a number of robotic surgeons that do semi-automated surgical operations under the guidance of a qualified surgeon with increasing efficiency.

Predicting outcomes and organizing orthognathic and craniofacial surgical operations using digital imaging, pictures, 3D photos, and intraoral scanning are other uses of AI in maxillofacial surgery. Since the data now accessible in the tissue-prediction area are a compilation of various measurements, 2D and 3D planning, and imaging, more pertinent 3D data and outputs are required. The industry is also making large expenditures in practical AI research and development for robotic surgery and digital orthodontics. All craniofacial surgeons have a duty to gather digital data and establish a productive relationship with the clinical usage of AI since it has the capacity to be an incredibly formidable tool in oral and maxillofacial surgery in the coming days.

18.3 Orthodontics

AI-powered individualized orthodontic treatment is the most discussed topic recent development. Nowadays, AI may be used for orthodontic diagnosis, planning, and treatment outcomes. For diagnostic and treatment planning, radiographs and visuals captured using intraoral scanners and cameras can be analysed. The results are frequently much more accurate than human understanding, and it eliminates the necessity for several lab tests as well as creating patient impressions. A customized treatment plan may easily be 3D printed for the aligners using precise 3D scans and virtual models. An algorithm that automatically decides under what amount of force and how patient teeth might be moved, as well as force sites particular to that tooth, is created as the massive volumes of information are analysed.

The aligners with AI support promise to speed up treatment times and optimize appointment scheduling as well as providing precise treatment delivery and progress tracking.

Lateral cephalometric evaluation is one of the fundamentals of the orthodontic treatment and combines computerized 3D cephalometric assessment based on cutting-edge 3D CNN models with the power of automated CBCT segmentations.

Currently, for better diagnosis accuracy and efficacy, AI automated facial surface analysis sourced from CBCT or any other face scanner may be used. Another specialization that is being replaced by AI models as they take over prediction and planning is facial development and ageing. Numerous businesses have spent the previous 10 years collecting enormous data on teeth movement brought on by aligner therapies. As a consequence, they now have the necessary groundwork for cutting-edge AI solutions that assist efficient tooth movement.

Some of them have even developed an effective AI-managed solution for the pre-treatment or retention stage of orthodontic therapy as specified by orthodontic professionals, which may be routinely assessed by AI using patient's personal video recordings.

Owing to predictive algorithms, AI models can assess the prevalence of cleft lip and palate and may detect genetic and environment-related risk indicators in diverse demographics.

While a cleft lip cannot be missed during a foetal ultrasonography, it can be challenging to diagnose a congenital defect early in pregnancy. The morphological pattern identification technique created by Jurek et al. might be one of the useful applications of AI. A DL algorithm developed by Kuwada et al. may also be used to detect and categorize unilateral cleft on OPGs postnatally.

In CLP patients, AI technology has also been used to detect lateral cephalometric landmarks, assess cephalometric analyses, forecast the requirement for orthognathic surgery following the completion of maturation, and predict soft tissue alterations following surgery. A customized technology known as "AID" may be used to do anthropometric assessment of face symmetry in images of CLP patients. This method has proven to be straightforward, quick, and trustworthy for this purpose. When panel ratings are conducted, dispersion-related problems may be eliminated by using AI to rate the face beauty of treated CLP patients after the conclusion of therapy. AI may be used to analyse speaking in patients with CLP, focusing primarily on the presence and degree of hypernasality.

In their research, Peilini et al. utilized an ANN to determine if or not participants' treatment plans required dental extractions before orthodontic treatment. They also took into account the anchoring patterns. The ANN correctly predicted the usage of maximal anchoring with a 92.8% accuracy rate and the effectiveness of the treatment plan with a 94.0% accuracy rate for extractions. These findings suggest that orthodontists can utilize ANN to create more exact treatment regimens.

A method based on ANNs was created by Auconi et al. to forecast the course of treatment for individuals in classes II and III. The study might identify reactive regions for a therapeutic strategy to misaligned teeth and perhaps predict the co-occurrence of auxological abnormalities throughout individual maxillofacial maturation.

According to the studies, NNs may be the most effective for diagnosing TMJ osteoarthritis. TMJ diseases, which afflict 5% to 12% of the population, are the second-most prevalent musculoskeletal problem, and the chronic impairment of TMJ osteoarthritis rises with ageing. The major objective is to identify TMJ dysfunction before anatomical deterioration has place. In the study by Bianchi et al., TMJ CBCT scans, blood testing, and saliva tests were performed to accomplish that purpose.

The cephalometric points were placed on the lateral cephalometric radiography in the study by Muraev et al. using ANN. The ANN's accuracy in placing cephalometric points was compared to that of three different dentist groups: experienced, average, and novice. The findings shown that ANN could design cephalometric points as accurately as a skilled dentist, and in certain instances, they could be far more accurate than brand-new medical professionals.

The estimation of the growth and development phases may also benefit from the use of ANN. In the study by Kök et al., children between the ages of 8 and 17 provided the cephalometric and hand-wrist radiographs. The cervical vertebrae were used to establish the gender, growth-development phases, and accuracy was found to be 94.27%.

Niño-Sandoval TC et al., Banumathi et al., Yu et al., Radwan et al. and Amasya et al. conducted studies to classify the maturation of the patients in lateral cephalograms with AI. An AI algorithm that classifies craniofacial categorization and does away with the landmark identification procedure was created using around 5900 lateral cephalometric radiographs. In this analysis, it was noted that AI demonstrated sensitivity and accuracy over 90.0% in the categorization of the vertical and sagittal skeletons. Additionally, it was discovered that vertical classification had a greater prediction performance than sagittal classification. On the CBCT images acquired, a programme was also created to automatically identify twenty cephalometric landmarks. In a different investigation, it was discovered that human measurements and findings were quite comparable to the automated cephalometric landmark recognition in CBCT and the established method.

An AI algorithm that automatically provides craniofacial classification and does away with the landmark identification procedure was created using around 5900 lateral cephalometric radiographs. In this analysis, it was noted that AI demonstrated sensitivity and accuracy over 90.0% in the categorization of the vertical and sagittal skeletons. Additionally, it was discovered that vertical classification had a greater prediction performance than sagittal classification. On the CBCT images collected, a programme was also created to automatically identify 20 cephalometric sites. In a different investigation, it was discovered that human measurements and findings were quite comparable to the automated cephalometric landmark recognition in CBCT images and the established method.

In orthodontic patients, congenital tooth abnormalities are frequent. Arranging orthodontic treatment becomes challenging when teeth that are abnormal in size, form, or location affect the length and occlusion of the upper and lower arches. Orthodontic treatments may involve filling up tooth arch cavities and creating openings for implants or prosthetic replacements. Sometimes the choice of orthodontic therapy can be selected for this reason. AI algorithms that can assist in making this choice have been created. The average accuracy was estimated to be approximately 80% in the Machine learning model, which was created to determine if the extraction procedure would be helpful in orthodontic patients aged between 11 and 15.

18.4 Periodontology

The integrity, aesthetics, and functionality of the teeth serve as an indicator for periodontal health as a component of the social life quality. Given the high incidence and the possibility that it could eventually result in the loss of all teeth, periodontitis is a serious public health concern.

Worldwide, periodontitis affects billions of individuals and, if left untreated, can result in tooth mobility and, in more severe situations, tooth loss. Early detection of periodontitis and efficient treatment are required to stop this from occurring. A thorough intraoral examination is necessary to provide a trustworthy diagnosis. Dental probing is done in order to assess clinical attachment loss and pocket depth. Because the effectiveness of periodontal examination varies depending on the particular clinician, Dental radiographs are a frequently utilized secondary examination wherein assessment also depends on the examiner's experience. NNs have been utilized by several researchers to reduce diagnostic inaccuracy.

Krois et al. utilized CNNs to analyse OPGs to diagnose periodontal bone loss as a proportion of the length of the tooth root. The outcomes were compared with the findings of six skilled clinicians' measurements. As opposed to dentists, who were effective in diagnosing periodontal bone loss in 80% of cases, CNN had higher precision and dependability as CNN was able to successfully diagnose bone loss in 83% of cases.

Periapical radiographs can identify peri-implant bone loss, although it can be challenging since the borders of the bone around the implants are sometimes ambiguous or might overlap. As a result, CNNs may evaluate the marginal bone level at different levels of the implants. The bone loss percentage was estimated and categorized using an AI model in the study by Jun-Young Cha et al. and they stated that clinicians can evaluate the severity of peri-implantitis using this technique.

In the study by Lee et al., radiographs were analysed to determine the radiographic bone loss for each tooth. Comparative measures between CNN's grading, probable diagnosis, and radiographic bone loss measurements were made. The NN's accuracy was 85%. Therefore, NNs may be helpful instruments in determining radiographic periodontal assessment and measuring radiographic bone loss.

Vadzyuk et al. exploited behavioural traits to detect the beginning of periodontitis. They got to the conclusion that the patients' levels of stress hormones and anxiety had an impact on their periodontitis.

In their research, Lin et al. stated that regions of automatic alveolar bone loss could be found in periapical films; and in a subsequent investigation, they created a model that could determine the extent of alveolar bone destruction.

Mason et al. utilized an AI algorithm in a study to determine whether ethnicity could be predicted from microflora observed in dental plaque and saliva samples. This study can help people of many ethnic backgrounds understand why their mouth regions have diverse bacteria.

It has been demonstrated that the AI model, developed by using fluorescent biomarkers and experts, is very precise at detecting the presence and position of dental plaque in intraoral images. In order to control plaque using intraoral images and detect early periodontal disease without the need of numerous plaque imaging techniques or specialists, researchers have created an AI model. An AI model developed in another study can identify both healthy and inflamed gingiva from fluorescence pictures taken using intraoral cameras. Gingivitis may be identified in intraoral photographs using the established model, helping to halt the development of more severe periodontitis.

Using salivary methyl mercaptan levels and oral microflora, Nakano et al. identified halitosis using ANN, albeit with only moderate success. The same research team found that when that situation was classified using DL, it was more accurate and sensitive than when it was done in the earlier trial.

18.5 Endodontics

The finest possible care will be given during endodontic therapy with the aim of keeping the tooth in its functioning state and avoiding any future issues. In endodontics, AI algorithms have shown a variety of uses, including examining the morphology of the root canal system, spotting periapical diseases and root fractures, measuring working lengths, forecasting the survivability of dental pulp stem cells, and foretelling the efficacy of retreatment treatments. The development of artificial intelligence for periapical lesion evaluation utilizing digital periapical radiographs, panoramic radiographs, and CBCT images has been the major emphasis of CAD.

For less experienced dentists and non-specialists, AI-based algorithms can be a significant assistant since they can be utilized in practical applications to determine the apical foramen and endodontic working length. The identification of periapical diseases using AI tools has shown decent results with high sensitivity and moderate specificity. Early detection of vertical root fractures is crucial to preventing harm to periodontal structures. In contrast to periapical radiographs, AI methods demonstrated exceptional efficacy in identifying vertical root fractures on CBCT images.

Identifying a diagnosis and a programme of therapy for teeth having periapical lesions and/or related manifestations can be challenging for dentists. Apical periodontitis, a common disease, is to blame for around 75% of cases with radiolucent lesions. Early diagnosis might improve the effectiveness of treatment, prevent the disease from spreading to other tissues, and lessen future difficulties.

The two 2D diagnostic imaging techniques that are most routinely utilized in routine clinical practice to identify apical osteitis are periapical radiography and OPGs. On radiographs, periapical lesions frequently appear as radiolucencies; however, the data obtained from these periapical radiographs is unreliable since the genuine 3-D anatomy is reduced into a 2-D picture with flaws. As a 3D imaging technology, CBCT imaging was created to precisely identify periapical lesions and evaluate their position and size. The accuracy ratings for the periapical lesions for CBCT, conventional periapical radiograph, and digital periapical radiograph were 0.96, 0.73, and 0.72, respectively, according to a meta-analysis. CBCT imaging performed less accurately in the diagnosis of apical periodontitis in teeth with root canal fillings.

The characteristics of periapical radiolucency and alveolar bone loss might be useful to AI algorithms for the detection of periapical pathology and periodontitis. Two models were proposed by Lin et al., one for diagnosing alveolar bone resorption and the other for assessing the degree of bone loss.

With the use of CNN, Ekert et al. examined OPGs for the presence of periapical lesions. They came to the conclusion that due to the radiographic image technique; different tooth morphologies are difficult to analyse on OPGs in various ways. In spite of the findings of periapical lesion detection by NN being excellent, the diagnosis may still be unsure and the sensitivity has to be increased. The CNN's sensitivity in molars was 87% and this sensitivity was higher than it was in other teeth, but its specificity was lower.

Lee et al. created a model based on a DL network of neurons to detect periodontally compromised molars and premolars and predict hopeless prognosis of molars and premolars depending on the degree of alveolar bone destruction. Models to classify the severity of periapical lesions in relation to the diagnosis of periapical disease were also developed by Mol et al. and Carmody et al. Endres et al. stated that a DL algorithm model is equally accurate at detecting periapical radiolucencies on OPGs as oral and maxillofacial surgeons.

In the research by Orhan et al., CNN was also utilized to identify periapical lesions on CBCT. 142 of 153 periapical lesions were successfully classified by the convolutional neural network with a 92.8% accuracy. The outcomes achieved by CNN were identical to those of a skilled dentist. DL was also used by Setzer et al. to detect periapical lesions on CBCT and the lesion detection performance was 93%. Furthermore, Flores et al. developed a way to distinguish periapical cysts from apical granulomas using CBCT scans; this method is highly valued in clinical care since it enables apical granulomas to heal following root canal therapy without the requirement for an enucleation for the cystic lesion.

Vertical root fractures, which account for 2% to 5% of crown/root fractures, are a significant consequence that may need root resection or tooth extraction. A vertical root fracture, which may be difficult to diagnose, is identified with the use of CBCT and 2D radiographs. Additionally, a delay in diagnosis may result in unnecessary surgery or tooth extraction. The low sensitivity and clinical manifestations of conventional radiography in the detection of vertical root fractures typically restrict a dentist's therapeutic choices.

CNN may be a helpful technique for spotting vertical root fractures in OPGs, according to research by Fukuda et al. In a separate study, a NN was built using CBCT and periapical radiographs to detect vertical root fractures in teeth. Researchers discovered that fracture detection of roots on CBCT is more accurate in terms of specificity, accuracy, and sensitivity compared to images from two dimensional radiographs.

The exact working length selection is critical for excellent root canal therapy success. 2D intraoral radiography is one technique used to evaluate working length and other techniques include CBCT imaging, electronic apex locators, digital tactile sensation, and the patient's response to a paper or file point inserted into the root canal system. Radiography and electronic apex locators are two routine procedures used in endodontic treatments. Digital radiograph's quality is crucial for a correct evaluation of the configuration of the root canal system. However, a number of other variables influence radiographic evaluation, which might result in misdiagnosis. As a result, AI solutions are required to deliver consistently accurate working lengths.

Saghiri et al. claim that using ANNs as a recommendation to find the radiographic apical foramen can improve the precision of working length measurement. In similar studies, Saghiri et al. evaluated the accuracy of working length measurement by an artificial neural network using a model of a human cadaver to simulate a clinical scenario. They found that there was no difference in the root length measurements when they compared an ANN with the actual measurement after extraction. In addition, they reported that the ANN performed much better than an endodontist when using periapical radiographs to identify anatomic narrowings. The accuracy of the ANN was 96% while the accuracy of the endodontists was 76%. An ANN can therefore be considered a precise method for calculating working length.

The efficiency of nonsurgical root canal treatment depends critically on an understanding of the various configurations of roots and root canal systems. This has frequently been accomplished using periapical radiography and CBCT. CBCT imaging has demonstrated to be more accurate in detecting the root and root canal morphologies when compared to radiography. However, due to issues related to ionizing radiation, this cannot be recommended in routine clinical practice.

Lahoud et al. created an automated, 3D teeth segmentation using the CNN approach. In a rapid, accurate, and effective clinical reference evaluation of 433 CBCT segmentations of teeth, the authors found that AI performed exactly as well as a human operator while working much faster.

Research by Bindal et al. evaluated the stem cells taken out of the tooth pulp in several regeneration therapies using the neurofuzzy inference approach. This method was able to forecast the outcome by monitoring the stem cells' survival after being treated with bacterial lipopolysaccharides in a representative clinical setting. The neurofuzzy inference system was proposed as a tool to predict cell survival following a variety of regeneration processes that are susceptible to microbial invasion. The cells were examined for vitality after being treated with lipopolysaccharide to cause an inflammatory response in pulp stem cells. The accuracy of the prediction made by using adaptive neurofuzzy interferences to anticipate these stem cells' survival after microbiological infiltration was then assessed by the researchers.

18.6 Restorative Dentistry

Since dental caries is the most prevalent dental condition, it is essential to disclose it as soon as possible. Dentists mostly utilize dental probes for the detection and diagnosis of dental caries, and they may tell if a tooth is healthy or not by looking at its texture and colouring. This approach is very individualized and depends on the dentist's expertise. The interproximal surfaces in particular might cause issues during a dental check-up.

Modern dentistry requires additional testing that can help diagnose carries, including dental radiography. Bitewing, periapical, and OPG radiological imaging are the most often utilized in caries detection.

AI is used in therapeutic dentistry for a variety of purposes, mostly for image-based disease detection and other diagnosis-support systems. A CNN system built on deep learning can be used to identify dental cavities in periapical radiographs. This may improve the identification and diagnosis of dental cavities in clinical dentistry practice.

AI can assist in the diagnosis of proximal caries on bitewings. Due to its better sensitivity in the diagnosis and arrest of early caries lesions, this could be cost-effective. The dentist can benefit from CNN-based AI algorithms as clinical decision support systems.

A deep CNN system may be used to automatically generate dental records and identify the teeth in bitewing radiographs, saving the practitioner time.

Neural networks may help in dental caries diagnosis on radiographic images, allowing for a quicker and more accurate assessment. The use of neural networks in conservative dentistry has grown significantly but is still not particularly common. Due to picture noise and poor contrast, algorithms can be used to distinguish between the edges of anatomical and pathological features, which may be quite similar to one another.

An ANN was used in a research by Geetha et al. to identify whether or not caries existed in the 105 radiographs. From the segmented picture, they retrieved 16 feature vectors, which served as the input layers. There were two output nodes made up of sound or carious teeth. The percentage of false positives was 2.8%, while the accuracy of caries detection was 97.1%. This study suggests that neural networks may identify tooth decay far more accurately than an intraoral examination.

AI may be used to identify and categorize dental restorations, as demonstrated in a 2020 study by Abdalla-Aslan et al. On 83 panoramic photos, the algorithms utilized in their research were able to identify 93.6% of dental restorations. In addition, restorations were divided into 11 groups based on the distribution and form of the grey values.

An artificial neural network was used in a study by Javed et al. to predict the post-Streptococcus mutans prior to the excavation of dental caries (ANN). A total of 45 primary molars with occlusal caries were used in the study. Pre- and post-Streptococcus mutans colony forming units were noted. The study shows that ANN can foresee which excavation technique is most suitable for a certain patient. The ANN's accuracy was 99.03%, and it had undergone microbiologic scrutiny. When post-Streptococcus mutans is predicted, pulpal trauma from the excavated cavity, re-examination of post-Streptococcus mutans, and re-excavation are all avoided.

According to Moutselos et al., they used the region-based convolutional neural network (R-CNN) model to identify occlusal tooth decay in pictures taken with the intraoral camera.

In this study, Lee et al. examined the convolutional neural network (CNN) model's ability to identify dental decay in periapical radiographies. They discovered that the accuracy rate for premolar teeth was 89.2%, for molar teeth it was 88.5%, and for combined premolar and molar teeth it was 82.3%. In other research, radiographic data was used to construct models that may identify dental decay in removed teeth.

When high-speed spinning dental instruments come into contact with teeth and restorative materials, they produce noises and Zakeri et al. evaluated/distinguished those different noises. Their study's goal was to assist dentists by reducing unintentional loss of substance from dental tissue during the removal of restorations. Amalgam and composite were employed as repair materials.

18.7 Prosthodontics

The development of neural networks has enabled dental laboratories to use AI to autonomously design cutting-edge dental restorations that adhere to the highest criteria for fit, function, and aesthetics.

Today, prosthodontics uses all facets of modern dentistry. Intraoral scans now begin workflows that formerly began with analogue impressions. Particularly in single-crown or smaller bridge restorations, intraoral scanners have shown to be precise enough for routine use. During the scanning procedure, artificial intelligence is employed to automatically eliminate extra soft tissues and substances.

In fixed prosthodontics, margin identification comes following intraoral scan capture; AI is utilized for this, and the suggested margins can be changed subsequently.

Dental restorations that are both fixed and removable can be created using CAD/CAM technology. In this method, machine learning may be used to generate the ideal crown design for certain circumstances using millions of real crowns.

It is never easy for the dental technician to adapt denture teeth in edentulous patients such that they fulfil both practical and cosmetic standards. By properly positioning the teeth, machine learning in CAD/CAM software can re-establish healthy intermaxillary connections.

AI can assist with accurate colour matching in challenging cosmetic scenarios that involve a single central incisor or several front teeth. Intraoral scanners can identify implant placements in implant prosthodontics and instantly input them into CAD software.

At the moment, "smile design" is an integral part of digital workflow that cuts across many different dental specializations. In order to virtualize patient morphology, the cornerstone of any treatment planning affecting the patient's smile, it makes use of the previously unheard-of simplicity of digital scanning, including 3D face scanning, and the availability of virtual fusions of 3D data, including segmented CBCT, intraoral scans, and face scans. Due to its benefits, a lot of companies offer software that automates the process of creating smiles.

Dental prosthetics are used to replace missing teeth, natural teeth that have lost their structure, and abnormalities in the oral and maxillofacial tissues. Mastication, phonation, aesthetics, and patient health are all intended to be corrected and maintained. Prosthetic restorations need high levels of accuracy throughout the preparatory steps, which can be completed using traditional or computerized technologies. AI in prosthetic treatments has risen along with the advancement of digital systems and the increasing usage of AI in dentistry.

The design and fabrication of prostheses in prosthetic therapies are significantly impacted by CAD/CAM technology. However, accessing these technologies might not always be simple. The resemblance of occlusal morphology between the reconstructions made by the AI model and the hand-made reconstructions finished by the dental laboratory technician was compared in the studies by Ender et al., Litzenburger et al., and Kollmus et al. Their findings demonstrated that AI model was as effective as the dental technician's reconstruction.

Removable dentures are still utilized as the main therapy since they are a more affordable alternative to implants, despite the popularity of implant applications growing. A clinical decision support model was created by Chen et al. to build removable prosthesis since there is a financial difference and they reported AI algorithms can successfully design removable dentures as well.

18.8 Pedodontics

Diagnoses that are made more quickly and accurately in paediatric dentistry allow for improved patient cooperation and a higher success rate. Paediatric patients are frequently diagnosed by dentists using periapical and OPGs. Recently, AI-based technologies have been created to improve the precision of radiological diagnosis and stop dentists from missing dental issues. Most of the studies were conducted in order to automatic detection/numbering of the deciduous teeth, detection of permanent dental germs, and detection of mesiodenses.

Kılıç et al. examined 421 OPGs of paediatric patients between the ages of 5 and 7 to assess the effectiveness of the deep learning approach in the automated detection and counting of the deciduous teeth. A similar study was conducted by Kaya et al. in 4518 OPGs of young patients between the ages of 5 and 12. They used the deep CNN algorithm YOLOv4 to detect permanent dental germs with the goal of making the proper diagnosis while minimizing process and human-induced mistakes. Çalışkan et al. found that the approach showed great accuracy for identifying impacted deciduous teeth in the OPGs of 74 paediatric patients aged 5–12 years.

Ahn et al. utilized four different deep learning techniques to identify mesiodens in OPGs from the deciduous and mixed dentition periods utilizing a total of 1100 pictures with and without 550 mesiodens. They stated that the Inception-ResNet-V2 and ResNet-101 models performed more effectively. In this study, it is hypothesized that AI-supported OPGs will aid physicians in the early detection of mesiodens, which will lessen potential dental problems in the future. The goal of Ha et al. was to create an AI model that can recognize mesiodens in OPGs from various dental eras. 612 OPGs were utilized for this, and a CNN model based on YOLOv3 was created to find mesiodens. The proposed approach has demonstrated good performance and holds promise for clinical use to identify mesiodens in OPGs from various dentition phases.

18.9 Patient Practice Management

AI-powered virtual dental assistants can do a variety of tasks in the dentist clinic with more accuracy and fewer errors while using less personnel as a result. It may assist with a variety of duties, including clinical diagnosis, treatment planning, appointment scheduling, insurance and paperwork management, and numerous others. Knowing the patient's medical background and any habits, such tobacco and alcohol, is very important for the dental professional. The patient might choose emergency teleassistance in emergencies, particularly if the clinician is not present.

18.10 Forensic Odontology

Artificial intelligence is a scientific advancement that has been heavily utilized in forensic medicine. It has shown to be quite useful in identifying the biological age and gender of healthy and sick people. It is also used to forecast mandibular morphology and analyse biting marks.

Some of the most exciting applications of AI are expected to assist dentistry. A key element of dental practices, the dental chair, saw a considerable transformation from physiologic, hydraulic pressure chairs with a manual pump to electronic chairs with many sensors connected. The most current development is a voice-activated dental chair that eliminates the need for the doctor to physically perform any actions.

All actions are conducted through voice instructions. Soon, dental chairs will be able to keep track of a patient's weight, vital signs, degree of anxiety, and the duration of the procedure while also reassuring the patient and alerting the operating doctors if any deviations are discovered, among other things. This is due to the persistent labour that all clever brains are putting towards AI.

Last but not least, one of the most inventive applications of artificial intelligence is in the field of "bioprinting", which enables the creation of organic material and even organs in a series of thin layers of cells. This technology might someday be used to replace the missing oral hard and soft tissues that were lost due to pathological or iatrogenic causes.

18.11 Dental Education

Since its inception in the 1980s, the field of intelligent tutoring systems has made major advancements. AI is commonly used in the field of dentistry education to create scenarios that mimic clinical work on patients and reduce all the risks associated with training on a live patient. As a consequence, the students' preclinical virtual patient feedback has improved dramatically. The interactive interphase produces high-quality learning environments by enabling students to evaluate their work and compare it to the ideal. Numerous evaluations of these systems' efficacy have demonstrated that, compared to traditional simulator units, these systems enable students to achieve competency-based skill levels more quickly.

18.12 Controversies

Various organizations are creating new standards and technologies to assure the safety, effectiveness, and reliability of AI solutions in order to ensure their safe use in healthcare, particularly in dentistry. A notable dilemma involving legal culpability for flaws in AI algorithm evaluation and potential erroneous medical action is one of the issues surrounding AI use. AI can be trained using any person's prejudices, as we all know.

Even though the provided AI models have shown promising outcomes, it is still required to confirm their generalizability and dependability utilizing relevant external data collected from recently enrolled patients or amassed from other dental facilities. Future goals of AI research in the dental field include not just improving AI model performance to expert levels but also spotting early lesions that are unseen to the human eye. Majority of the AI algorithms were developed and tested using a single centre's CT and OPG scans which may lead to an overfitting of the algorithm and can cause a bias. Some research claimed that when evaluated on data from an external institution, their models performed worse. There is a need for further testing that proactively gather additional datasets to evaluate the effectiveness of the algorithms. To ensure the model's genuine universal applicability, the performance should preferably be assessed using external image data that was collected using various scanners and radiography techniques from external institutions.

Even while deep learning approaches have outperformed people in a number of categories, they are nevertheless prone to mistakes that they are considerably less likely to make than humans, such as misclassifying hostile cases. The enormous achievements made possible by these approaches should not be diminished in any way, but fresh efforts should be directed towards robustness and interpretability. These issues are dealt with through collaboration between computational models and human specialists, and they perform better together than they would apart.

As local servers cannot be expanded to handle more data, data exchange gets challenging. That problem might be resolved by cloud storage, which have experienced a fast increase in both users and suppliers over the past decade. Because of the expense of sustaining and upgrading local servers and computing platforms once they become out of date, businesses have begun migrating their data platforms to cloud computing and storage services. When all of these sources of data were accessible, every individual could receive personalized medication. For example, the utilization of genetic data can help patients receive better diagnosis, effective monitoring, and more customized therapy. By doing so, the recovery time for patients would be shortened, and the effectiveness of the treatment would be increased. As dental data sharing grows, its integration with DL would improve the already outstanding findings that have been produced in coming years. The endeavours to collect additional data are a critical starting point for the improvement of the actual models since, as was already established, DL needs a lot of data to work at its best.

A significant portion of the dental community feared that AI would eliminate clinical employment in medicine and dentistry as early as the 1970s, but this has not happened. Science fiction will portray AI as an all-encompassing, comprehensive intellect, but this is not the case. It is crucial to emphasize that artificial intelligence (AI) assists, not replaces, the work of dental practitioners. An increasing number of dental clinics are using digital workflows and AI for planning diagnostic and treatment procedures. Even then, there are still relatively few "smart dentistry clinics", or dental offices, that fully integrate AI into their operating procedures.

Dental Education Tools in Digital Dentistry

19

Charis Beltes, Antigoni Delantoni, and Kaan Orhan

19.1 Introduction

The profession of dentistry is continuously improving and becoming more innovative in many aspects. The sheer breadth of the new digital technologies in the dental practice workflow positively impacts dental care quality and patient satisfaction. Revolutionary digital equipment has been introduced to the field of dentistry, including cone-beam computed tomography (CBCT), 3D intraoral and facial scanners, 3D printers, and integrated processing software, such as the computer-assisted design/computer-assisted-manufacturing (CAD/CAM) prosthetic software and dental implant planning software. The introductions of these recent techniques, together with the pivotal advances in dental materials, are transforming the entire field of dentistry. The digitization of the dental profession offers advantages that combine analog workflows with recent digital technologies. The main clinical advantage of their use is the enhancement of the perceived and measured quality of care. Digital dental applications can support dentists in making the most accurate diagnostic-based decisions. For example, intraoral scanners allow tooth preparations to be viewed in a high contrast magnified field on a computer monitor and often directly at the patient's sight. This permits real-time modifications and precise esthetic/functional-driven planning for the restoration and improves the quality of the provided dental treatments. The widespread adoption of electronic patient records that emanated from the use of intraoral scanners and contemporary digital imaging techniques brings many advantages to dentistry, including improved communication between the dentists, patients, dental laboratory technicians, as well as third-party stakeholders, more outstanding quality and data archiving, and improved patient experiences [1].

Programs have been introduced to enhance students' spatial ability, their interactivity, critical thinking, and clinical correlations with the integration of multiple dental disciplines. Augmented reality in 3D visualization allows insights in tooth morphology, and also facilitates treatment planning with fixed or removable partial denture programs [2]. Digital technologies also include the 3D printing of virtual teeth, which has been suggested to enhance transpar-

C. Beltes
Department of Endodontology, School of Dentistry, Aristotle University of Thessaloniki, Thessaloniki, Greece

A. Delantoni (✉)
Faculty of Dentistry, Aristotle University of Thessaloniki, Thessaloniki, Greece
e-mail: andelant@dent.auth.gr

K. Orhan
Faculty of Dentistry, Ankara University, Ankara, Turkey

Ankara University Medical Design Application and Research Center (MEDITAM), Ankara, Turkey

Department of Oral Diagnostics, Faculty of Dentistry, Semmelweis University, Budapest, Hungary
e-mail: knorhan@dentistry.ankara.edu.tr

A. Delantoni, K. Orhan (eds.), *Digital Dentistry*, https://doi.org/10.1007/978-3-031-52826-2_19

ency for all students due to the identical setups [3]. In communicating with dental professionals, medical doctors, dental technicians, and insurance providers, dental students have to be prepared to manage digitized data, ensure patient safety, and understand the benefits and limitations of conventional and digital processes.

Overall, digitalization seems to have had a major impact on dental education, addressing various aspects, such as e-learning and Web-based knowledge transfer, but also related to diagnostics using 3D imaging and digital radiography, and practically oriented trainings in terms of dental simulator motor skills including intraoral optical scanning (IOS) with 3D printing, prototyping, and digital surface mapping. Digital applications can provide additional opportunities to evaluate and improve education, implementing evidence-based surveys related to the penetration and acceptance of digital education. There is no disagreement that in order to produce qualified clinical doctors, it is necessary to conduct clinical education as much as possible. Currently, many clinical lectures engage medical students through various media, especially photographs and videos, and several educational methods that enhance immersion using recent technologies are also emerging [4].

19.2 Digital Trends in Medical Education. Teaching and Learning

19.2.1 Computer-Assisted Learning

This learning method has the advantage of being able to easily visualize complex procedures, and its principal advantage may be excellent accessibility. In particular, through the widespread use of the internet and various electronic devices, clinical education, which traditionally could only be conducted in the school setting, and especially in practice rooms, can now be carried out at home, on the road, and above all, repeatedly at the pace of learning until the students are fully acquainted with the corresponding material. Specific examples are digital libraries providing online videos and countless photographs derived from some of the most current technologies (CBCT and micro-CT) enabling researchers to even view the complexity of head and neck anatomy, dental tissues, and root canal system in three dimensions [3].

19.2.2 Virtual Patients

This is a form of education that has not been used by many medical schools after it was first proposed by Harless in 1971 [5]. The main reason for this is that it is expensive to build such a system, and maintaining it is also not straightforward. Nevertheless, an advantage of this type of education is that customized education is easily available and that students can easily engage in learning through this method without special preparation. The definition of a virtual patient proposed by the American Association for Medical Colleges is a special type of computer program capable of implementing a real patient clinical scenario; it is said that learners can imitate their role as healthcare providers by acquiring a patient's medical history, conducting a physical examination, and making diagnosis and treatment decisions.

19.2.3 Augmented Reality

The equipment called Hololens from Microsoft (Microsoft Corp., Redmond, WA, USA), in the form of augmented reality, provides the unique experience of seeing a real patient and acquiring related medical information, including images and charts. In a study by Pratt et al. [6] in 2018, images could be controlled by voice through the Hololens device, and a case of reconstructive surgery was reported using this technique. According to the results of a systematic review comparing the virtual patient education method with the existing traditional education method, it was found that the use of virtual patients was more effective in helping students to acquire clinical skills and knowledge compared to existing education methods [7].

19.2.4 Human Patient Simulation

This is the most traditional medical education format, and it provides an environment suitable for educational goals using mannikins or models, in which students receive training to cope with various situations models. Although this is a traditional educational method, it has recently become possible to produce a model of the same shape as the patient's organs using 3-dimensional (3D) imaging techniques and 3D printing, so it has begun to receive attention once again. Most of all, this simulation method enables repetitive practice of specific skills using only partial organs rather than the patient's entire body, so that immersion is excellent, active experiences are possible, and emotional and sensory learning can be maximized. In addition, it is an excellent learning method for transferring the content of basic medicine to clinical practice. However, in order to provide such equipment, there are problems of cost and space, and it has been pointed out that it may be difficult to provide equipment depending on the number of students [8, 9].

19.2.5 Web-Video Platforms

The biggest advantage of video platforms, such as YouTube, is that students can easily access on any device, and they are already fully comfortable with how to use the platform. The YouTube algorithm automatically selects similar content and provides suggested videos alongside. Students can make connections with the original video and acquire profound insights related to materials by watching similar videos from different viewpoints. In addition, by using the basic streaming function of YouTube, it is possible to provide real-time interactive classes to remote medical students. For instance, the teacher conducts live surgery remotely broadcasted using the YouTube live streaming feature to students. This is a very intriguing way to communicate the overall content of surgery to students and to induce interest, and above all, it is thought that using this technique can make the class more meaningful for students who are taking their first steps as clinicians. However, YouTube live streaming clearly has the disadvantage of being unable to evaluate students' reactions face to face, although students can at least communicate through comments in real time. Fortunately, this technical limitation can be easily over- come by using various types of video conferencing tools, especially Zoom or Google Meet.

19.3 Digital Trends in Medical Education. Assessment

Evaluation methods are the field showing the most changes in light of developments in educational technology. Most evaluation methods used in existing medical education are paper-written, oral, or practical tests, and the biggest problem pointed out regarding paper-written tests is that it is difficult to provide sufficient feedback to students due to the structural factor of the overwhelmingly small number of evaluators compared to the number of students. Many medical school professors experience difficulties simply in preparing exam questions, scoring them, and notifying students of their grades in time. In addition, as most tests involve checking a large amount of knowledge within a short time through simple memorization, short answer, and multiple-choice questions predominate. However, if there is a situation in which a virtual patient takes blood pressure pills regularly, exercises hard, and has recently adjusted his weight, but his blood pressure has not improved at all, that would be a real-world problem that would require the student to think about "why" such a problem arises and "how" to solve the problem, not "what" is the criterion for defining hypertension. Perhaps the true evaluation and preparation for the real world will be helping students to solve real-world situations based on "why" and "how," not just "what." On a similar note, the most suitable assessment of students will not be to test whether they know something, but to identify what they do not understand, which must be corrected during the assessment. However, this goal has not been easy to achieve in the traditional assessment format.

Dental students' acquisition of psychomotor skills is the core feature and main competency of pre-clinical operative dentistry and the area where the majority of pre-clinical teaching time is devoted. Globally, dental curricula allocate more time for practicing and enhancing psychomotor skills rather than didactic or theoretical teaching. The most widespread approach in teaching psychomotor skills is the traditional approach lecture/demonstration method. In these traditional methods, the teaching content is delivered as a package of information; the teacher tells the students and shows them how to do the task. The students practice the task in the lab then evaluate their work with the teacher according to a definite detailed criterion-referenced rubric. Therefore, clinically unacceptable errors may be encountered more frequently after they are made especially during the initial stage of psychomotor skills acquisition. The student relies on instructor feedback and availability, and may not readily develop skills of self-assessment and critical thinking [10].

19.4 Augmented Reality (AR) and Virtual Reality (VR)

Augmented reality (AR) and virtual reality (VR) have their use in a variety of specialties of dentistry, as presented in Fig. 19.1

AR/VR technologies have a promising role in the field of dentistry. The details of its application in oral health are described below.

19.4.1 Dental Education and Training

In the delivery of dental education and training, instructors can help students to achieve precision in pre-clinical/clinical skills, respectively, with 3D real-time digital simulations as well. Learning and retaining the anatomy of the head and neck is a crucial part of dental education. Lectures and 2D images from textbooks of anatomy have been used for teaching this subject to students. In this traditional mode of teaching, cadaveric skulls are commonly employed, and students are instructed

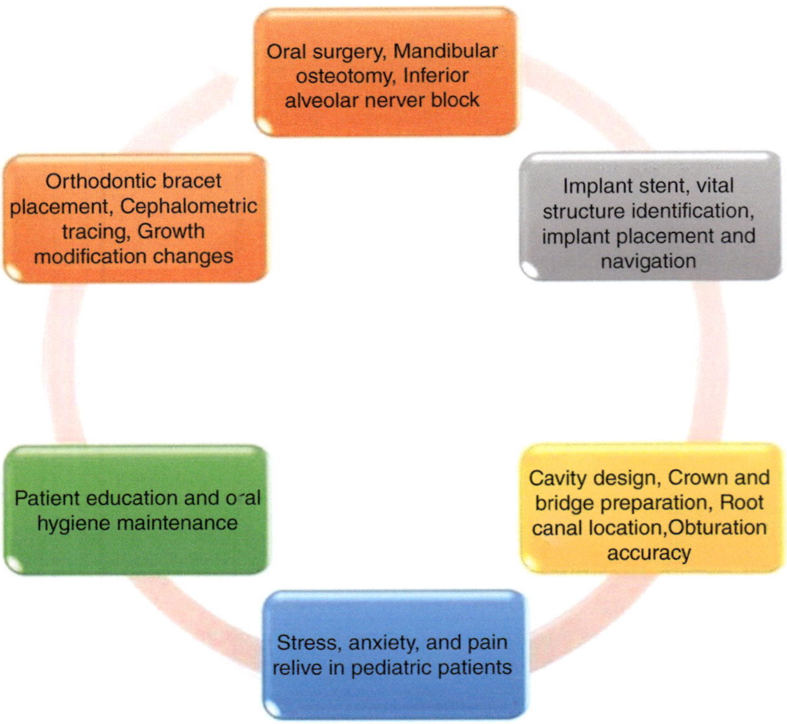

Fig. 19.1 AR/VR applications in dentistry (Fahim S. et al. 2022)

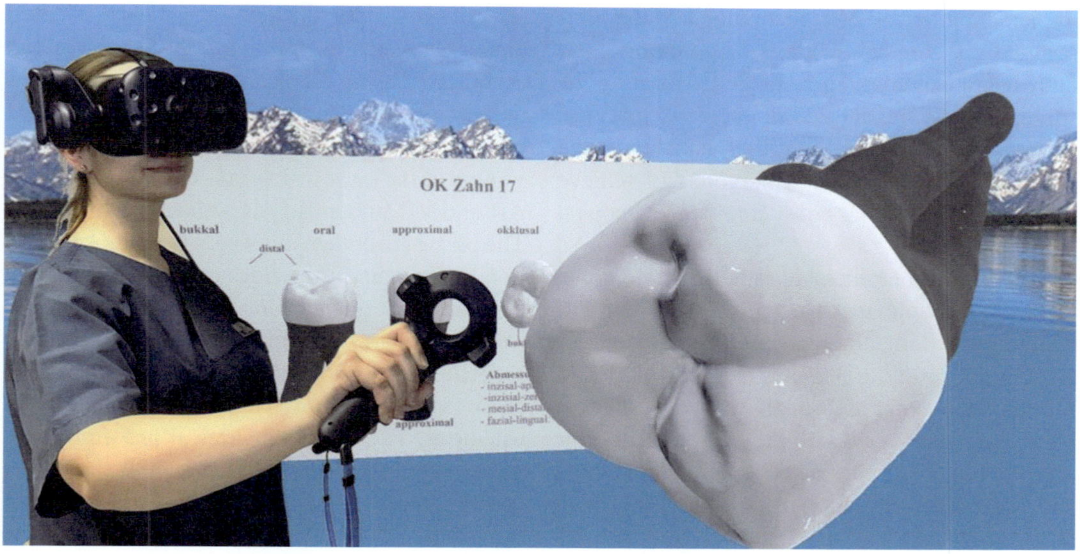

Fig. 19.2 VR education: Dental morphologies in a virtual teaching environment

through these. However, the visualization of all associated muscular, neural, vascular, and other structures is quite challenging for students and it is not fully effective either. In the midst of the COVID-19 pandemic, students suffered due to limited learning opportunities and the ability to enhance their pre-clinical skills as students could not train at their universities without the instructor's direct supervision. Therefore, helping these students to learn while controlling the spread of COVID-19 has been the most challenging aspect for the universities. Innovative techniques have been proposed to teach clinically relevant anatomy to students of dentistry and replace cadavers with dissected and sliced plastinated specimens. However, one recent study incorporated digital tools and a 3D augmented curriculum, which is an interactive 3D experience that combines the view of the actual world with elements generated by computers along with traditional teaching methods (lectures and cadavers). The study demonstrated improved understanding and a positive influence on the retention of anatomical knowledge in students as compared to the control group (taught via textbooks and 2D images) [11].

Learning, also, in the VR dental learning environment showed a high level of acceptance among all students and should be integrated as a fixed element in the dental curriculum, offering additional learning opportunity of dental morphologies [12] (Fig. 19.2)

19.4.2 Oral and Maxillofacial Surgery

In recent years, many technological advancements have taken place in the field of surgery such as the introduction of augmented and virtual reality. The application of AR and VR technology has been explored in many surgical fields of medical science, such as laparoscopic surgery, neurosurgery, and plastic surgery. In dentistry, the use of AR in oral and maxillofacial surgery has focused on the placement of dental implants, craniofacial surgery, and orthognathic surgery. The use of AR technology allows the users to combine information and images to bring them to reality.

The training period of surgical residents is a crucial phase where the residents learn and practice their surgical skills on different simulators before actually performing on patients. Pulijala et al. [13] evaluated the effectiveness of virtual reality in surgical training and found that many of the surgeons were not confident about performing the surgeries. With the introduction and implementation of VR technologies, this has resulted in surgical residents improving their knowledge and confidence while performing the surgeries. VR is an additional tool that has immense importance in further enhancing the skills already possessed by surgeons to achieve optimal outcomes that boost confidence amongst surgeons.

Inferior alveolar block anesthesia is one of the most fundamental anesthesia used in dentistry to operate on the mandibular teeth for procedures such as root canal treatment, extractions, dental fillings, and complex surgeries. Many factors have been associated with the failure of inferior alveolar block anesthesia such as poor technique, and anatomical variations. In a study by Won et al. [14], AR was used for inferior alveolar block anesthesia and it was concluded the use of AR in this block anesthesia can improve the effectiveness when block anesthesia is used alone. AR helps in improving the precision and accuracy of using block anesthesia as the images that are directly generated from the patient help in converting those images to reality (Figure 19.3).

One of the most widely studied applications of AR and VR in dentistry is orthognathic surgery. The prime advantage of using AR-guided navigation tools is that it provides real surgical images and virtual surgical plans to guide through the treatment plan. One of the important surgical procedures in orthognathic surgery is mandibular angle split osteotomy. Mandibular angle split osteotomy is a cosmetic surgical procedure that aims to improve the prominent mandibular angle, thereby improving the esthetics of the patient.In their study, Zhu et al. [15] used AR for mandibular angle split osteotomy and found that the use of AR enhances the translocation of the maxilla

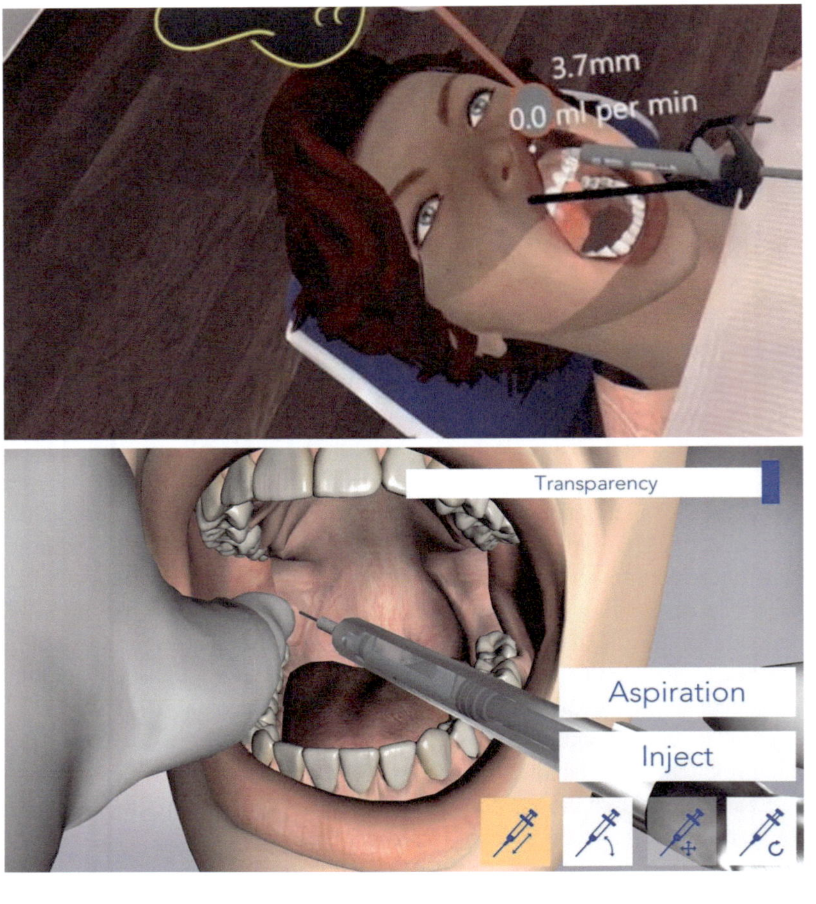

Fig. 19.3 VR education: Dental anesthesia

in orthognathic surgery. The use of such AR systems allows surgeons to operate real-time streaming video images that allow them to plan the surgery and study the anatomical structures of the patient, thus enhancing the accuracy of such orthognathic surgical procedures.

The use of AR has also been studied in distraction osteogenesis. In a study by Qu et al. [16], patients suffering from hemifacial microsomia were treated with an intraoral distractor using AR and it was found that AR was more accurate in proper positioning of the osteotomy planes as compared to the conventional methods. Additionally, one study explored the use of AR systems where images were overlaid, which allowed surgeons to observe and follow the virtual surgical plans to reposition the bones of the patient after performing maxillary osteotomies [17]. Additionally, to further enhance the surgical skills, VR technology replicated different functions such as drilling, place fixation, and bone sawing with the help of hepatic force feedback [18, 19].

So, the importance of VR and AR in oral and maxillofacial surgery can be appreciated given the improved accuracy of the surgery performed, the decrease in the chance of errors by the surgeons, and the unlimited number of training sessions available to surgeons. Therefore, VR and AR as an adjunct can prove to be more than beneficial tools for surgeons.

19.4.3 Pediatric Dentistry

Pediatric dentistry is one of the most challenging specialties of dentistry as the commonest factor determining the treatment outcomes in such patients is their compliance. To improve patient cooperation and compliance, different tools have been used ranging from the armamentarium of the dentist, such as behavior modification, and pharmacological interventions. Pediatric patients who are visiting the dental practice often present with tremendous amounts of anxiety as most of the time it is their first interaction with dentists. Managing the anxieties and behavior of children is one of the crucial factors in patient management.

To decrease the levels of anxiety and stress of such patients, virtual reality is one of the innovative tools that have been discussed in the literature, although to a limited extent. Different techniques to manage anxiety include in vivo exposure therapy (IVET) and virtual reality exposure therapy (VRET). IVET consists of the direct confrontation of patient's fear to reduce their anxiety levels and this method has been categorized as a gold standard method. VRET is a recent technique that consists of computer-generated images for patients where the simulation makes the patient experience their fears without facing them in reality, thereby helping them to reduce their anxiety [20]. One of the most important factors that determine the treatment outcomes in patients in this age group is the anxiety and stress associated with visiting the dental practice. Virtual reality can help to provide an artificial environment that is more relaxing for the patients, which can help them overcome their fears and should be taught in all dental universities.

19.4.4 Dental Implantology

Many advances have been made in dentistry in regard to the replacement of missing teeth or teeth in the mandibular and maxillary arches of patients such as removable dentures, fixed dental prostheses, and dental implants. Dental implants have emerged as a suitable and preferable choice for many patients because of their high success rate and the long-term benefits associated with them. The introduction of AR technology in dental implants has significantly improved many procedures associated with the placement of implants. Initially, the AR surgical navigation technology was used to place implants using the retinal imaging display as the surgeon keeps his visual on the operative area, avoiding the need for the surgeon to turn away [21].

In a study by Jiang et al. [17], it was found that the use of augmented reality resulted in higher accuracy and applicability for guided placement of dental implants as compared to the traditional two-dimensional navigational method. Such AR navigation systems help the surgeon to concentrate only on the site of the implant placement, thereby providing only useful information to the surgeon, which eventually reduces the cost and time of the procedure [22]. It is of prime importance that the location of the implants should be as accurate as possible because negligence in this step of implant placement could be one of the factors responsible for future implant failure.

Moreover, one study used augmented reality-based dental implant placement to evaluate the virtual placement of the implant as compared to the actual prepared implant site created [23]. It was found that the use of augmented reality resulted in a significantly decreased deviation in implant placement from the actual planned site. Since AR navigation-based systems help the surgeon to accurately locate and place the dental implants, the accuracy of such procedures thereby increases as compared to the traditional methods. The placement of the dental implant is a surgical procedure, so with the help of VR technology, patients have an opportunity to get a detailed explanation of the treatment and what they will experience while the treatment is being performed.

19.4.5 Restorative Dentistry and Endodontics

Restorative dentistry and endodontics are some of the most challenging and exhausting fields of general dentistry. Conventionally, students are first trained in the laboratory on a phantom head where the mannequin mimics the patient, which allows the students to work as if they are working on an actual patient as in a clinical setup [24]. Procedures such as cavity preparation are practiced on these mannequins by the students. In a study by Llena et al. [25], cavity preparation using AR technology was studied. It was found that the participants that used AR technology showed an improvement in their knowledge and skills. With the help of AR, realistic simulations can be delivered to the students in order to practice and improve their clinical skills without the need for live test subjects.

To overcome the chances of failure in endodontic treatments in patients, augmented reality has been used in endodontics for the reliable detection of root canals. In a study by Bruellmann et al. [26], augmented reality was used to detect root canals where it was found that overall higher sensitivity was noted in detecting root canals in molars and premolars [27]. In a preliminary study of Marras et al. [28] in 2008, a virtual tooth drilling model was introduced. The dental simulator described had the potential, 15 of being a very promising educational and research tool that allows the user to practice virtual tooth drilling for endodontic cavity preparation or other related procedures on high-detail teeth models placed within an adaptable and animated 3D face and oral cavity model (Fig. 19.4).

19.4.6 Dental Radiology

Currently, a novel virtual dental tool was established, called VIRED® , designed for advanced dental training in several treatments, such as implantology and radiology. All modules are based in real-life case studies and facilitate the teaching of new techniques, procedures, and product use in modern dental practice. Academic institutions, private dental companies, dental organizations, as well as individuals associated with the dental profession could greatly benefit from adopting VIRED virtual reality dental modules in their continuing education. In the field of radiology, virtual reality tool is intended to train dentists, dental students, and dental assistants in the techniques of X-ray taking, including all the necessary steps (proper handling of equipment, radiation safety) before and after the actual X-ray, in a realistic and customizable way. The trainee can be exposed to different X-ray taking procedures (different dental X-rays, variable in complexity) and his/her performance is recorded by means of completion certain pre-determined tasks (steps). At the end of the training process, a detailed report is issued where all the errors (critical and non-critical) are listed and analyzed (Fig. 19.5).

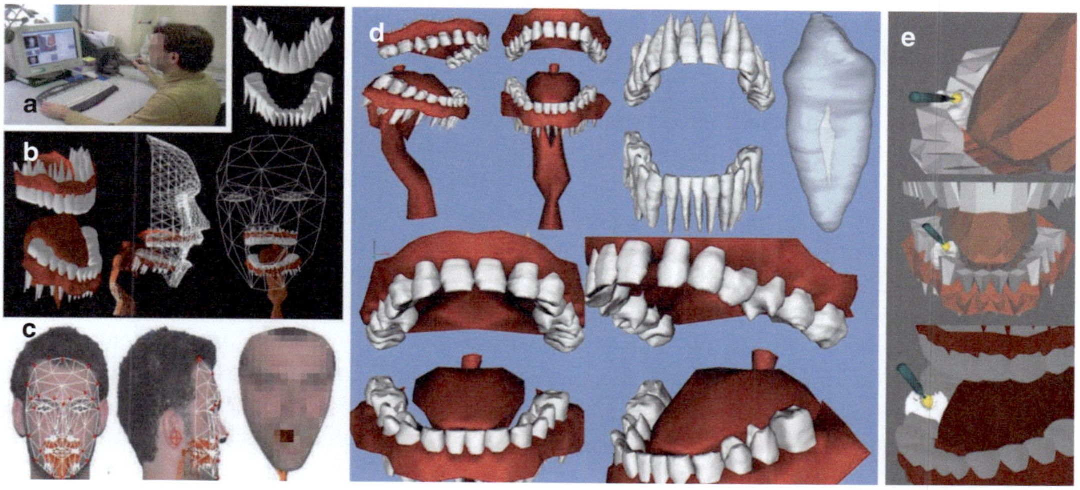

Fig. 19.4 (**a**) System hardware components, (**b**) A 3D model of the head and the oral cavity, including the prototype simple teeth models, with and without mesh subdivision, (**c**) Adaptation of the generic facial mesh model to the characteristics of a specific person, (**d**) The database of detailed surface teeth models used in V DP simulator, (**e**) Prototype tooth (with and without mesh subdivision) replacement with a detailed one for performing dental operations. (Marras et al., 2008)

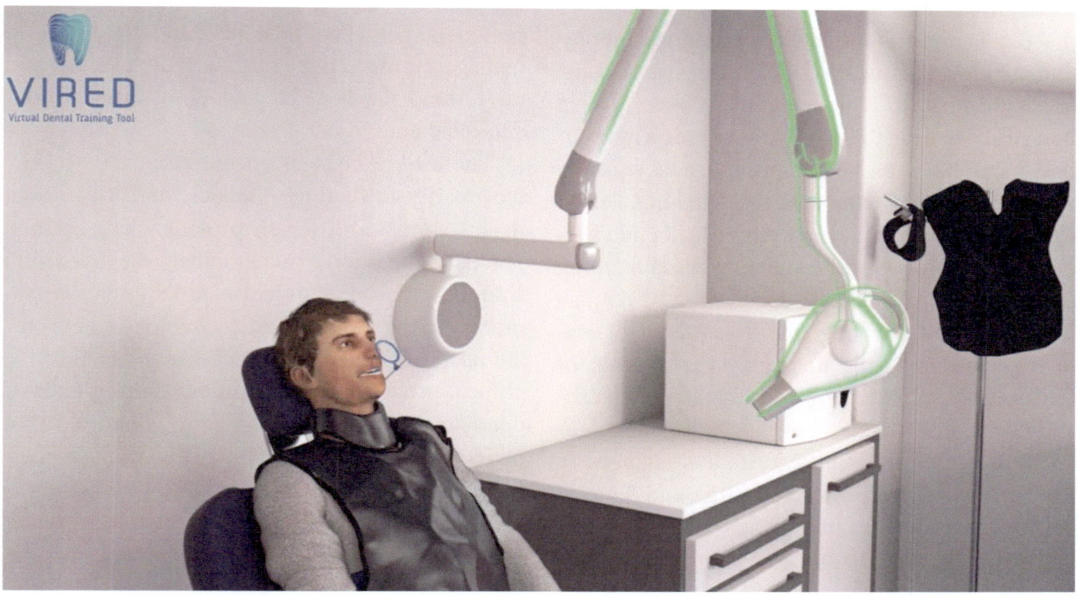

Fig. 19.5 A virtual reality tool customized to train dentists, dental students, and dental assistants in the techniques of intraoral radiology

19.5 Haptic Virtual Reality Simulators (HVRS)

Dental schools use the phantom head simulator for teaching psychomotor skills in pre-clinical operative dentistry using plastic teeth which is considered the mainstay simulation since its existence. Unfortunately, plastic teeth do not simulate enamel and dentine hardness. No pathosis, such as caries, exist in plastic teeth and it is difficult for the teacher to explain the real tactile sensation [29, 30]. In 1894, the first historic phantom head simulator was developed and designed by Oswald Fergus with the purpose of providing dental students with a training model that resembled a real patient scenario. This would subsequently help to facilitate their acquisition of essential restorative dentistry skills and resultantly prepare students for professional practice [31]. The phantom head simulator has extensively evolved from what started as a low-fidelity model to systems with high-fidelity status and to this day is the main effective training tool in pre-clinical dental education. For the last decade, simulation-based mannequins have been described as near to being "ergonomically accurate" and have proven to establish a learning environment that enhances the teaching, learning, and practice of certain motor skills and precision [32]. However, mannequin-based learning systems require constant supervision, which can impact faculty teaching, the assessment of student performance and managing the safe use of the simulators; for example, navigating "electrically driven handpieces" of phantom head simulators. This, paired with continuous changes in the curriculum, can introduce time and support constraints affecting the ability to effectively teach clinical skills to students to ensure they are up to qualifying standard [32, 33]. Moreover, the implementation of many new complex operative techniques into the pre-clinical training cannot be demonstrated with traditional clinical simulator systems. In effect, they do not allow the practice and judgment of some characteristics/skills which can be seen in complex patient cases or are crucial to accurately performing procedures, for example, hand-eye coordination. With the requirement to be competent in increasingly complex procedures, standalone phantom head simulators do not offer an effective solution and technological advances are required to address their limitations [33].

The application of augmented reality (AR) and virtual reality (VR) in dental medicine demonstrated that the use of AR/VR technologies for educational motor skill training and clinical testing of surgical protocols is increasing [34]. These digital technologies are valuable in dental undergraduate and postgraduate education, offering interactive learning concepts with 24/7 access and objective evaluation. A recent scoping review analyzed the application of VR in pre-clinical dental education and identified four educational thematic areas (simulation hardware, realism of simulation, scoring systems, and validation), highlighting the need for a better evidence base for the utility of VR in dental education [35]. In communicating with dental professionals, medical doctors, dental technicians, and insurance providers, dental students have to be prepared to manage digitized data, ensure patient safety, and understand the benefits and limitations of conventional and digital processes.

There have been recent developments in virtual reality technology, haptics, and robotics in dental simulation, which provide more optimal practice conditions to smoothen the transition from the traditional model-based simulation laboratory to the clinic. These technologies help create an environment in which users can practice clinical procedures in the different disciplines of dentistry [36]. For example in Japan, a robot patient was developed, which can provide real-life simulations such as coughing, shaking neck, tongue thrusting, and salivary secretion which was found to enhance dental skills and improve management of dental emergencies in a dental setting [37, 38]. Furthermore, virtual reality simulation offers the prospect of creating a digital environment for its users to perform various exercises, in the field of operative dentistry, such as cavity preparation, caries excavation, and light-curing techniques [39].

Most recently, combining haptic technology with virtual reality simulation introduced haptic virtual reality simulators (HVRS); a cutting-edge technology that revolutionized dental education globally [39]. Haptic virtual reality simulators provide a sense (haptic) of feedback through the device being held by the user in the form of sounds, pressure, and vibrations. The goal is to simulate an optimal and genuine sense of the clinical procedure, providing a learning experience that resembles reality [40]. This kind of haptic simulation in pre-clinical operative dentistry provides sensory feedback of preparation in enamel and dentine, as well as caries excavation [29]. In addition, it provides standardized cases, objective assessment, and interactivity. Furthermore, it stimulates the use of reflective forms of assessment that involve students in a self-assessment process to identify individual learning needs and self-directed learning [41]. It was claimed that adjunctive training in these simulators seems to enhance students' learning and psychomotor skill acquisition, provide unlimited access to practice clinical tasks, and reduce the required faculty supervision time [32, 42].

Despite the many benefits of the application of digital technologies, several factors influence their adoption in dentistry. The lack of knowledge and skills is one of the most important factors limiting technology's efficient integration and utilization in dentistry [43]. Therefore, many dental schools have started to incorporate the most recent digital technologies in their curricula to provide students with the knowledge and skills necessary to keep pace with the rapidly growing need for the implementation of digital techniques and workflows in dentistry [44–49].

The arrival of social media, mobile devices, personal computers, clinical technologies, and visual technologies have modified how and where education occurs. These technological resources allow students to access information easily, to re-use learning materials, to study at a distance, and simulate training environments [50, 51]. While limitations still exist, mainly because of the costs involved in the acquisition of this technology, dental education has now incorporated technology-based resources into its training and one key example is 3D technology [52]. Moreover, current curricular trends in dentistry consider simulation-based learning as an essential part of training [53].

Currently, many dental schools are suffering from limited educational circumstances in which students and teachers must keep social distance, due to the recent coronavirus disease 2019 (Covid-19) pandemic. As one of the countermeasures for the pandemic situation, the haptic 3Dvirtual reality dental training simulator has been drawn attention. In training using the device, trainees cut teeth on a 3D monitor using a special controller that imitates an air- turbine handpiece. In the combination with internet technology, such digital device would contribute to realize remote training to minimize the spread out the infection. Additionally, some studies have reported usefulness of the digital educational device from standpoints of objective assessment. Thus, the digital simulator would hold the promise of its great potential in dental education, however, it has not yet been widespread in dental schools in the world. Majority is still the conventional simulator training, in which trainees cut artificial teeth attached on phantom head and teachers perform visual inspection to make assessment and instruction. To introduce the novel device into conventional courses and make the best use, revealing difference between two instruction process is important [54].

The concept of VR (virtual reality) originates from the 1830s when the first stereoscope was invented and used to project an image using a set of mirrors, giving the user a feeling of depth and immersion. VR-like haptic features were later introduced in 1929 via a flight simulator used to train US air force pilots; this system was able to mimic air turbulence and plane movements [50]. In the early 1960s, Ivan Sutherland first introduced and set into motion "virtual reality" as we now know it, by creating the first head-mounted display [55]. In the 1970s, VR development was chiefly driven by NASA and military training needs through the creation of various vehicle simulators [56]. By the late 1980s and early 1990s, VR systems had become coupled with haptic gloves and computer systems, including part of NASA's astronaut training projects. Publicly available VR systems also gained huge popularity as video games, in the form of arcade machines, such us Virtuality, Sega VR and Virtual Boy by Nintendo. Since 2012, new VR systems, incorporating headsets, were introduced to the public and commercially released: Oculus, Project Morpheus, and HTC VIVE. These systems ignited a new wave of interest toward virtual reality and augmented reality (VR/AR) and use now extends outside of the gaming sphere into social networking, skills training and education, to name a few. VR is now used in many spheres, ranging from training pilots to military simulations and education. AR is also making its way into everyday life through mobile applications.

As VR/AR are emerging technologies definitions vary widely; the Oxford English Dictionary defines VR as "a computer-generated simulation of a lifelike environment that can be interacted with in a seemingly real or physical way..." and AR as "the addition of computer- generated output, such as images or sound, to a person's view or experience of his or her physical surroundings by means of any of various electronic devices." Broadly, VR can be thought of as immersion into a computer-generated environment. Contrastingly, AR can be thought of as superimposition of a computer-generated environment on reality.

The practice of dentistry encompasses a unique spectrum of skills; the teaching of which incorporates in-depth head and neck anatomy and physiology, complex technical skills (restorative, endodontic, periodontic, prosthodontic and surgical therapy), subtle clinical skills (from communication to clinical judgment), sound academic understanding and leadership skills, to name a few. The breadth of learning in dental education provides many areas where VR/AR may be exploited to aid teaching.

Generally, VR/AR technology systems are apparent as head- mounted devices with OLED screens, either with or without haptic controllers, which allow the user to interact with virtual models/features of applications. a novel s/w system aiming to disrupt the healthcare training industry with the first psychomotor virtual reality (VR) surgical training solution. We provide the means for performing surgical operations in VR, thereby facilitating training in a fail-safe environment that very accurately simulates reality and significantly reduces training costs, offering surgeons and the healthcare ecosystem a way to improve operation outcomes drastically [54].

A novel system (M.A.G.E.S. 3.0, OramaVR SA) in medicine aiming to disrupt the healthcare training industry with the first psychomotor virtual reality (VR) surgical training solution, was presented in 2018. The means for performing surgical operations in VR, thereby facilitating training in a fail-safe environment that very accurately simulates reality and significantly reduces training costs, offering surgeons and the healthcare ecosystem a way to improve operation outcomes drastically, was provided. The system generates a fail-safe, realistic environment for surgeons to master and extend their skills in an affordable and portable solution. Is an educational tool for orthopedic surgeries to enhance the learning procedure with gamification elements, advanced interactability, and cooperative features in an immersive VR operating theater? The presented system was focused on a completed total knee arthroplasty (TKA) virtual reality operating module, opening the way for making available a full suite of virtual reality operations in surgery. The methodology transforms medical training to a cost-effective and easily and broadly accessible process. The latter is accomplished by employing the latest VR, gamification, and tracking technologies for virtual character-based, interactive 3D medical simulation training. It requires standard h/w (PCs, laptops) irrelevant of the operating system. For optimal user experience, a commodity VR head-mounted display (HMD) should be employed along with motion or other hand-controller sensors. The open ovidVR architecture supports all current and forthcoming VR HMDs and standard 3D content generation. These technologies facilitate presence that is the feeling of "being there" and "acting there" in the virtual world, thereby offering the means for unprecedented training. The most current software is the MAGES 4.0, a novel Software Development Kit (SDK) to accelerate the creation of collaborative medical training scenarios in VR and AR. It offers a versatile authoring platform for developers to create medical simulations in a future-proof, low-code environment. Students can collaborate using virtual and augmented reality devices at the same medical scene [57, 58]. The platform incorporates the following novel advancements:

(a) 5G edge-cloud remote rendering and physics dissection,
(b) realistic real-time simulation of organic tissues as soft-bodies,
(c) a highly realistic cutting and tearing algorithm,
(d) neural network assessment for user profiling and,
(e) VR recorder to record and replay or resume the training simulation from any perspective. (Fig. 19.6).

In dentistry, professionally orientated systems, such as the Virteasy dental trainer simulator and Simodont dental trainer (VR system), often consist of 3D displays, which show a virtual tooth, jaw models and instruments, and usually include a "handpiece-replica" device, which provides haptic feel [24] (Fig. 19.7)

Those include absence of haptic feel but real computer-tracked handpiece and real plastic tooth models capable of augmenting the reality through presenting a virtual 3D model of the real-time preparation, giving instant feedback on-screen. PerioSim® and DentSim® (DenX Corp., Jerusalem, Israel) describes as the first dental simulators of VR and haptic technology, since 2006. In 2010, Moog Industrial Group of Amsterdam, built the dental homework trainer named Simodont® and at the same time the ACTA university in Amsterdam developed its courseware. Recently, dental trainer Simodont® has been acquired by Nissin Dental Product Inc, the Japanese manufacturer of digital dental training and simulation systems. Its manufacture has been extended to 571 units, distributed in 117 dental schools in Asia, Europe, America and Oceania.

Simodont Dental Trainers apply sophisticated haptic technology used in flight simulators, adapted and tailored for dental simulation, with a highly realistic haptic (force) feedback provided through a dental drill hand-piece and mirror Fig. 19.8.

The intention is that students develop psychomotor skills and confidence more rapidly so they spend less time in the traditional phantom head setting and transfer safely to patients sooner. Haptic trainers provide an opportunity to upload patient-specific dental information and images. This will allow students to practice a particular procedure on a particular tooth of their patient, virtually, before undertaking the same procedure on the actual patient. The result is a much more realistic training experience that allows students to see, by using 3-D glasses for depth perception and work on a virtual tooth, with different colors representing its layers (e.g., dentin is yellow and pulp is red), and to "feel" what makes each layer unique using virtual dental instruments. Most

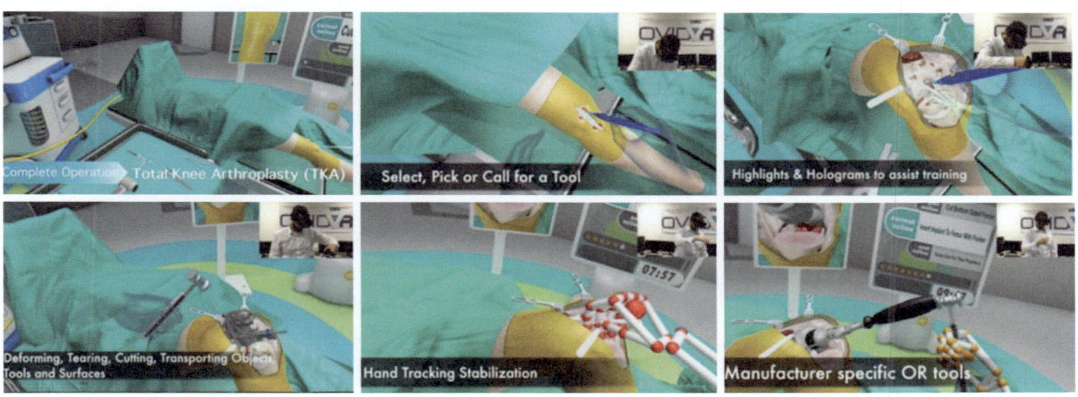

Fig. 19.6 The psychomotor virtual reality surgical training solution MAGES

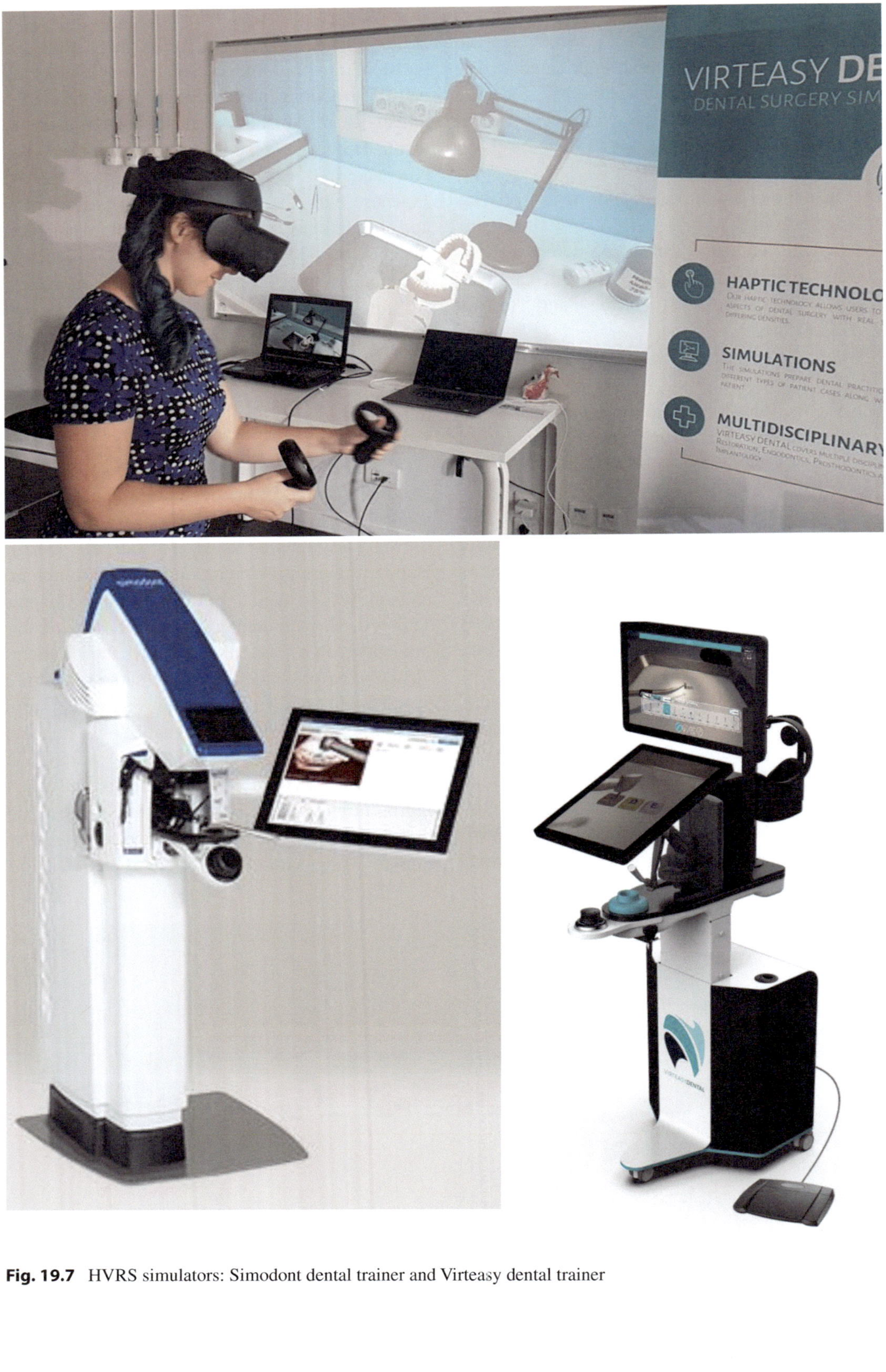

Fig. 19.7 HVRS simulators: Simodont dental trainer and Virteasy dental trainer

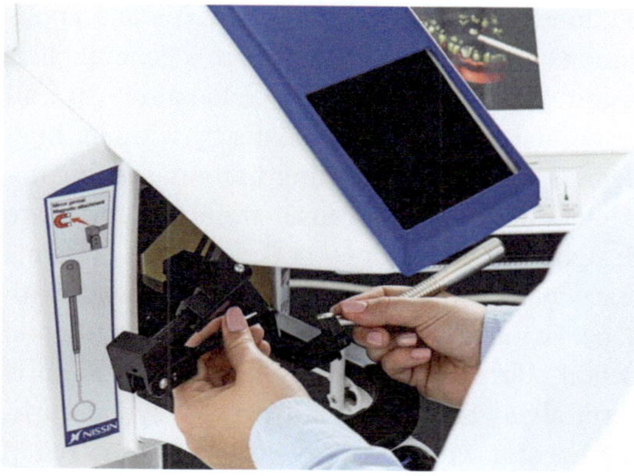

Fig. 19.8 The dental handpiece in Simodont provides highly precise force feedback and a dental mirror is available for indirect vision training

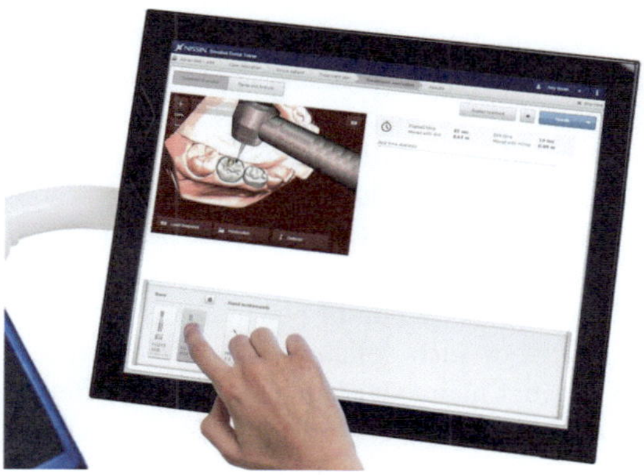

Fig. 19.9 The student navigates through the exercises with a touch screen in Simodont device. This interface is used to select cases, create treatment plans, select instruments, answer questions, read teacher feedback and more

users begin their training by practicing cutting out different shapes with the virtual drill, choosing a level of difficulty, and selecting the proper bur. When they have mastered the various levels of drilling skills, they graduate to working on a virtual tooth, which they select through a virtual case study, complete with patient photo, background, patient history, and treatment plan. They are tasked with selecting the proper virtual tools to drill or scoop out decayed tooth sections and fill the cavity (Fig. 19.9).

19.6 Digitalization in Dental Education

Digitalization in dental education is frequently used to enhance the accessibility and exchange of documents and to facilitate the collaboration and communication among students, teachers, and administrative staff. Digitalization enables cloud-based records, evaluation, and feedback, as well as the provision of e-learning modules [59]. Students today, particularly the Millennials, expect services instantly, expect to be able to download their grades, course schedules, and other information automatically, and to be able to get assistance 24/7. In order to satisfy these expectations, it is necessary to promote a change of mindset of the dental faculty and provide instructors with training in e-learning and e-teaching to enable theoretical and practical knowledge transfer [59]. The coronavirus disease (COVID-19) pandemic that started in 2019 caused dental schools around the world to close, and highlighted the need for alternative channels for education (e.g., Web-based learning platforms) [60]. Scheduled webinars can provide a structure for students' theoretical learning. Additional applications of digital features include educational videos illustrating clinical exams or therapeutic steps, interactive systems, adaptive systems that monitor students' ability and adjust teaching accordingly, online collaborative tools, etc. The use of pictograms instead of scripts in educational videos facilitates a language-independent application in several countries.

Especially in the field of motor skills training, digital software tools can be used to evaluate the manual abilities of potential candidates for the dental curriculum, to analyze students' pre-clinical preparations, to enable self-assessment, and to enhance the quality of education. The objective and exact nature of these digital evaluations helps to improve students' visualization, provides immediate feedback, and enhances instructor evaluation and student self-evaluation and self-correction [61, 62]. Students can learn to self-assess their work with self-reflection and faculty guidance in conjunction with a specially designed digital evaluation tool. IOS and digital impression techniques can be included early in the dental curriculum to help familiarize students with ongoing development in the computer-assisted technologies used in oral rehabilitation [63].

While undergraduate students today have to be prepared for digital dentistry, they still need to acquire the knowledge of conventional treatment strategies and processes. Growing up in the digital world, they will easily adapt to digital features. Digital dentistry offers several options for an objective standardized evaluation of students' performance, which should be used for quality enhancement. It is currently a "teaching transition time," and new standards have to be defined for dental education in general. Open questions remain, such as:

1. in which phase of the dental curricula should digital technologies be introduced as the routine tool;
2. which analog techniques can be omitted; and,
3. which digital content should be taught in which disciplines? [64].

Nevertheless, faculty should be aware of their responsibility in teaching young dentists, who are treating individuals with individual needs requiring empathy and an informed consent for any treatment decision. Digitalization cannot replace all educational lessons or courses, and the role-model function of faculty is important when supervising students during patient treatment in the clinical courses. It should be emphasized that there are still no uniform standards in dental education with regard to the digital tools applied. Such standards are essential to ensure uniformity in teaching, which is particularly important for an international exchange. Society as well as dentistry is currently undergoing a digital transformation. It is necessary to clarify learning contents, to what extent conventional workflows should still be taught, and what can be done digitally. While digital tools and applications in knowledge transfer are a general challenge for undergraduate education in all disciplines, the field of dentistry with its high degree of practical training units is specifically demanding. Just because training units are designed digitally does not mean that students learn on their own. Continuous training with supervision and feedback is still the key to good dental education. In this context, digitization is certainly a great opportunity to convey the learning content with more joy and newly awakened enthusiasm.

Following the rule, "you can only teach what you are able to perform yourself," a highly motivated faculty is needed that is willing to embrace the latest digital technologies. Besides personal motivation, the financial aspect of implementing the various digital tools and applications has to be managed at dental universities. Collaborations with industry would be helpful here. This is a classic "win–win situation"—the dental school would be equipped with the latest products and updates, and the industry would get access to the youngest target group of potential customers. In the event of such collaborations, it is vital that universities maintain their objectivity by offering a variety of products from diverse companies; otherwise, there is a risk of unduly influencing dental students and biasing them toward one particular technological option. The rapid pace of change in dental technology must also be considered. Dental technology companies are constantly introducing new products and workflows. While this provides exciting opportunities for dental research, to test and analyze those new developments, it complicates the implementation of digital workflows in dental education programs. New job descriptions are also necessary at dental schools in order to maintain the technical infrastructures required for these new technologies and to guarantee a smooth operation in clinical practice. In future, the best dental schools will be ranked according to their digital infrastructure combined with the level of innovation of the teaching faculty.

19.7 Conclusions

Digital tools and applications are now widespread in routine dental care. Therefore, this trend toward ongoing developments must be considered in dental curricula in order to prepare future dentists for their daily work-life. There is a need to establish generally accepted digital standards of education, at least among the different dental universities within individual countries. Digitalization offers the potential to revolutionize the entire field of dental education. More interactive and intuitive e-learning possibilities will arise that motivate students and provide a stimulating, enjoyable, and meaningful educational experience with convenient access 24/7.

At present, digital dental education encompasses several areas of teaching interests, including Web-based knowledge transfer and specific technologies such as digital surface mapping, dental simulator motor skills including IOS, and digital radiography. Furthermore, it is assumed that AR/VR technology will play a dominant role in the future development of dental education.

Given the increasing interest in technology mainly driven by industry, it is essential to explore whether dental students' knowledge and expectations of digital dentistry are current with the continually updated dental curricula. Understanding dental students' perception and awareness of digital dentistry are vital in influencing institutional admission processes and decision-making regarding resource investment. Moreover, an exploration of dental students' current knowledge and experiences in digital dentistry will significantly adjust pedagogical methods, research collaboration, and future dental practice. Undoubtedly, the direct exchange with the learning tool is a milestone for all in-depth knowledge of the technological genres. However, in the case of the teaching activity, anticipation and training background are necessary to make the most of practice time, technical and human resources, protect equipment and create a training culture in which the learner is the protagonist. The prevalence of traditional concepts such as dependence on the teacher and asking the teacher questions to solve setbacks, raise the need to look for more innovative training solutions. These training solutions must be supported by technology, teamwork, and the linking of face-to-face activities with e- learning resources in a dynamic way and with more powerful intrinsic and extrinsic motivations.

Both students and teachers considered that the technical domain (to operate the simulator at a basic level necessary to perform the exercise) was the one that prevailed the most, which speaks favorably of the intuitive and friendly interface of the simulators. However, this level of domain may not be enough for a correct use of the simulator.

There was a tendency for students not to value highly the prior technological preparation. The study of the didactic resources created in the study did not reach the desirable high levels. Both students and teachers considered that the best knowledge/learning strategy was the direct exchange with the simulator. However, in the teaching activities that concern us, anticipation and the training background are necessary to make the most of the practice times, human and technical resources, to protect the equipment and to create a training culture in which the student has the leading role.

References

1. Mangano F, Gandolfi A, Luongo G, Logozzo S. Intraoral scanners in den-tistry: a review of the current literature. BMC Oral Health. 2017;17(1):1–11.
2. Goodacre CJ. Digital learning resources for prosthodontic education: the perspectives of a long-term dental educator regarding 4 key factors. J Prosthodont. 2018;27:791–7.
3. De Boer IR, Wesselink PR, Vervoorn JM. The creation of virtual teeth with and without tooth pathology for a virtual learning environment in dental education. Eur J Dent Educ. 2013;17:191–7.
4. Prager MC, Liss H. Assessment of digital workflow in Predoctoral education and patient Care in North American Dental Schools. J Dent Educ. 2019;84:350.

5. Harless WG, Drennon GG, Marxer JJ, Root JA, Miller GE. CASE: a computer- aided simulation of the clinical encounter. J Med Educ. 1971;46:443–8.
6. Pratt P, Ives M, Lawton G, Simmons J, Radev N, Spyropoulou L, Amiras D. Through the HoloLens(TM) looking glass: aug- mented reality for extremity reconstruction surgery using 3D vascular models with perforating vessels. Eur Radiol Exp. 2018;2:2.
7. Kononowicz AA, Woodham LA, Edelbring S, Stathakarou N, Davies D, Saxena N, Tudor Car L, Carlstedt-Duke J, Car J, Zary N. Virtual patient simulations in health professions education: systematic review and meta-analysis by the digital health education collaboration. J Med Internet Res. 2019;21:e14676.
8. Tallarico M. Computerization and digital workflow in medicine: focus on digital dentistry, vol. 13. Basel: Multidisciplinary Digital Publishing Institute; 2020.
9. Shaikh F, Inayat F, Awan O, Santos MD, Choudhry AM, Wa-Heed A, Kajal D, Tuli S. Computer-assisted learning applications in health educational informatics: a review. Cureus. 2017;9:e1559.
10. Donkers K, Bednarek M, Downey P, Ennulat C. Implementation of simulation-based learning in a physician assistant curriculum. J Allied Health. 2015;44:5E–9E.
11. Lahti S, Suominen A, Freeman R, Lähteenoja T, Humphris G. Virtual reality relaxation to decrease dental anxiety: immediate effect randomized clinical trial. JDR Clin Transl Res. 2020;5:312–8.
12. Liebermann A, Seefelder J, Huth K, Erdelt K. Mobile virtual tooth morphology teaching environment for preclinical dental students. J Dent Educ. 2023;87(1):130–8.
13. Pulijala Y, Ma M, Pears M, Peebles D, Ayoub A. Effectiveness of immersive virtual reality in surgical training—a randomized control trial. J Oral Maxillofac Surg. 2018;76:1065–72.
14. Won YJ, Kang SH. Application of augmented reality for inferior alveolar nerve block anesthesia: a technical note. J Dent Anesth Pain Med. 2017;17:129.
15. Zhu M, Chai G, Zhang Y, Ma X, Gan J. Registration strategy using occlusal splint based on augmented reality for mandibular angle oblique Split osteotomy. J Craniofac Surg. 2011;22:1806–9.
16. Qu M, Hou Y, Xu Y, Shen C, Zhu M, Xie L, Wang H, Zhang Y, Chai G. Precise positioning of an intraoral distractor using augmented reality in patients with hemifacial microsomia. J Cranio-Maxillofac Surg. 2015;43:106–12.
17. Jiang W, Ma L, Zhang B, Fan Y, Qu X, Zhang X, Liao H. Evaluation of the 3D augmented reality–guided intraoperative positioning of dental implants in edentulous mandibular models. Int J Oral Maxillofac Implant. 2018;33:1219–28.
18. Jo Y-J, Choi J-S, Kim J, Kim H-J, Moon S-Y. Virtual reality (VR) simulation and augmented reality (AR) navigation in orthognathic surgery: A case report. Appl Sci. 2021;11:5673.
19. Arikatla VS, Tyagi M, Enquobahrie A, Nguyen T, Blakey GH, White R, Paniagua B. High fidelity virtual reality orthognathic surgery simulator. In: Medical imaging 2018: image-guided procedures, robotic interventions, and modeling, vol. 10576. Bellingham, WA: International Society for Optics and Photonics; 2018. p. 1057612.
20. Albakri G, Bouaziz R, Alharthi W, Kammoun S, Al-Sarem M, Saeed F, Hadwan M. Phobia exposure therapy using virtual and augmented reality: a systematic review. Appl Sci. 2022;12:1672.
21. Yamaguchi S, Ohtani T, Ono S, Yamanishi Y, Sohmura T, Yatani TSAH. Intuitive surgical navigation system for dental Implantology by using retinal imaging display. In: Implant dentistry—a rapidly evolving practice. London: InTech; 2011.
22. Durham M, Engel B, Ferrill T, Halford J, Singh TP, Gladwell M. Digitally augmented learning in implant dentistry. Oral Maxillofac Surg Clin N Am. 2019;31:387–98.
23. Lin Y-K, Yau H-T, Wang I-C, Zheng C, Chung K-H. A novel dental implant guided surgery based on integration of surgical template and augmented reality. Clin Implant Dent Relat Res. 2015;17:543–53.
24. Leung AL-S, Yeung C, Chu S, Wong AW-Y, Yu OY, Chu C-H. Use of computer simulation in dental training with special reference to Simodont. Dent J. 2021;9:125.
25. Llena C, Folguera S, Forner L, Rodríguez-Lozano FJ. Implementation of augmented reality in operative dentistry learning. Eur J Dent Educ. 2018;22:e122–30.
26. Bruellmann DD, Tjaden H, Schwanecke U, Barth P. An optimized video system for augmented reality in endodontics: a feasibility study. Clin Oral Investig. 2012;17:441–8.
27. Zafar S, Zachar JJ. Evaluation of HoloHuman augmented reality application as a novel educational tool in dentistry. Eur J Dent Educ. 2020;24:259–65.
28. Marras I, Nikolaidis N, Mikrogeorgis G, Lyroudia K, Pitas I. A virtual system for cavity preparation in endodontics. J Dent Educ. 2008;72(4):494–502.
29. Perry S, Bridges SM, Burrow MF. A review of the use of simulation in dental education. Simul Healthc. 2015;10:31–7.
30. Taylor CL, Grey N, Satterthwaite JD. Assessing the clinical skills of dental students: a review of the literature. J Educ Learn. 2013;2:20–31.
31. Wang D, Zhao S, Li T, Zhang Y, Wang X. Preliminary evaluation of a virtual reality dental simulation system on drilling operation. Biomed Mater Eng. 2015;26:S747–56.
32. Plessas A. Computerized virtual reality simulation in preclinical dentistry: can a computerized simulator replace the conventional phantom heads and human instruction? Simul Healthc. 2017;12:332–8.

33. Vincent M, Joseph D, Amory C, Paoli N, Ambrosini P, Mortier É, Tran N. Contribution of haptic simulation to analogic training environment in restorative dentistry. J Dent Educ. 2020;84:367–76.
34. Joda T, Gallucci GO, Wismeijer D, Zitzmann NU. Augmented and virtual reality in dental medicine: a systematic review. Comput Biol Med. 2019;108:93–100.
35. Towers A, Field J, Stokes C, Maddock S, Martin N. A scoping review of the use and application of virtual reality in pre-clinical dental education. Br Dent J. 2019;226:358–66.
36. Tavkar A, Pawar A. Simulation in dentistry. EC Dent Sci. 2017;12:115–21.
37. Tanzawa T, Futaki K, Tani C, Hasegawa T, Yamamoto M, Miyazaki T, Maki K. Introduction of a robot patient into dental education. Eur J Dent Educ. 2012;16:e195–9.
38. Tanzawa T, Futaki K, Kurabayashi H, Goto K, Yoshihama Y, Hasegawa T, Yamamoto M, Inoue M, Miyazaki T, Maki K. Medical emergency education using a robot patient in a dental setting. Eur J Dent Educ. 2013;17:e114–9.
39. Imran E, Adanir N, Khurshid Z. Significance of haptic and virtual reality simulation (VRS) in the dental education: a review of literature. Appl Sci. 2021;11:10196.
40. Gal GB, Weiss EI, Gafni N, Ziv A. Preliminary assessment of faculty and student perception of a haptic virtual reality simulator for training dental manual dexterity. J Dent Educ. 2011;75:496–504.
41. Dutã M, Amariei CI, Bogdan CM, Popovici DM, Ionescu N, Nuca CI. An overview of virtual and augmented reality in dental education. Oral Health Dent Manag. 2011;10:42–9.
42. Al-Saud LM, Mushtaq F, Allsop MJ, Culmer PC, Mirghani I, Yates E, Keeling A, Mon-Williams MA, Manogue M. Feedback and motor skill acquisition using a haptic dental simulator. Eur J Dent Educ. 2017;21:240–7.
43. Matthews D, McNeil K, Brillant M, Tax C, Maillet P, McCulloch C, Glogauer M. Factors influencing adoption of new technologies into dental practice: a qualitative study. JDR Clin Transl Res. 2016;1(1):77–85.
44. Gratton DG, Kwon SR, Blanchette D, Aquilino SA. Impact of digital tooth preparation evaluation technology on preclinical dental students' technical and self- evaluation skills. J Dent Educ. 2016;80(1):91–9.
45. Schlenz MA, Michel K, Wegner K, Schmidt A, Rehmann P, Wöstmann B. Undergraduate dental students' perspective on the implementation of digital dentistry in the preclinical curriculum: a questionnaire survey. BMC Oral Health. 2020;20(1):1–10.
46. Siegel SC, Kramer SB, Deranek KM. Lean methods applied to CAD/CAM pedagogy in the dental simulation laboratory. J Dent Educ. 2019;83(9):1081–91.
47. Afshari FS, Sukotjo C, Alfaro MF. Integration of digital dentistry into a predoctoral implant program: program description, rationale, and utilization trends. J Dent Educ. 2017;81(8):986–94.
48. Ishida Y, Kuwajima Y, Kobayashi T, et al. Current implementation of digital dentistry for removable prosthodontics in US Dental Schools. Int J Dent. 2022;2022:7331185.
49. Jurado CA, Tsujimoto A, Punj A, Aida N, Miyazaki M, Watanabe H. Successful development and implementation of a digital dentistry cur- riculum at a US dental school. J Oral Sci. 2021;63(4):358–60.
50. Virtual Reality Society. History of virtual reality—Virtual Reality Society. 2020. https://www.vrs.org.uk/.
51. Caudell TP, Mizell DW. Augmented reality: an application of heads-up display technology to manual manufacturing processes. Institute of Electrical and Electronics Engineers (IEEE). IEEE, IEEE Xplore; 2003:669.
52. Issenberg SB, McGaghie WC, Petrusa ER, Gordon DL, Scalese RJ. Features and uses of high-fidelity medical simulations that lead to effective learning: a BEME systematic review. Med Teach. 2005;27:10–28.
53. Seymour NE, Gallagher AG, Roman SA, et al. Virtual reality train- ing improves operating room performance results of a randomized, double-blinded study. Ann Surg. 2002;236:458–64.
54. Dzyuba N, Jandu J, Yates J, Kushnerev E. Virtual and augmented reality in dental education: the good, the bad and the better. Eur J Dent Educ. 2022;00:1–19.
55. Sutherland IE. A head-mounted three dimensional display. Proceedings of the December 9–11, 1968, Fall Joint Computer Conference, Part I on—AFIPS '68 (Fall, Part I). ACM Press; New York, NY 1968:764.
56. The Franklin Institute. History of Virtual Reality|The Franklin Institute. https://www.fi.edu/virtual-realit.y. Accessed July 2020
57. Papagiannakis G, Lydatakis N, Kateros S, Georgiou S, Zikas P. Transforming medical education and training with VR using M.A.G.E.S. New York, NY: SIGGRAPH Association for Computing Machinery; 2018. https://doi.org/10.1145/3283289.3283291.
58. Hooper J, Tsiridis E, Feng J, Schwarzkopf R, Waren D, Long W, Poultsides L, Macaulay W, Papagiannakis G, Kenanidis RE, Slover Egol Phillips D, Friedlander S, Collins M. Virtual reality simulation facilitates resident training in Total hip arthroplasty: a randomized controlled. Trial. 2019;34(10):2278–83.
59. Alves LS, de Oliveira RS, Nora AD, Cuozzo Lemos LF, Rodrigues JA, Zenkner JEA. Dental students' performance in detecting in vitro occlusal carious lesions using ICDAS with E-learning and digital learning strategies. J Dent Educ. 2018;82:1077–83.
60. Meng L, Hua F, Bian Z. Coronavirus disease 2019 (COVID-19): emerging and future challenges for dental and Oral medicine. J Dent Res. 2020;99:481.

61. Miyazono S, Shinozaki Y, Sato H, Isshi K, Yamashita J. Use of digital technology to improve objective and reliable assessment in dental student simulation laboratories. J Dent Educ. 2019;83:1224–32.
62. Greany TJ, Yassin A, Lewis KC. Developing an all-digital workflow for dental skills assessment: part II, surface analysis, benchmarking, and grading. J Dent Educ. 2019;83:1314–22.
63. Zitzmann NU, Kovaltschuk I, Lenherr P, Dedem P, Joda T. Dental students' perceptions of digital and conventional impression techniques: a randomized controlled trial. J Dent Educ. 2017;81:1227–32.
64. Zitzmann NU, Matthisson L, Ohla H, Joda T. Digital undergraduate education in dentistry: a systematic review. Int J Environ Res Public Health. 2020;17:3269.

Future Prospective 20

Kaan Orhan, Antigoni Delantoni, Dilan Kırmızı, and Umut Aksoy

20.1 Digital Radiography

The future of dental digital radiography is likely to involve continued advances in digital technologies and the further integration of digital radiography into dental practice. Newer digital X-ray sensors have higher resolution and better image quality, making it easier for dentists to identify small details and abnormalities in the X-ray images.

20.1.1 Improved Image Sensors and Phosphor Plate Scanners

Image sensors are an important part of digital radiography systems and are used in place of traditional film-based X-ray systems. Both CCD and CMOS sensors are used in dental digital radiography systems, and the choice of which type to use may depend on the specific needs and budget of the dental practice. They are used in dentistry to capture high-resolution images of the teeth and supporting structures, such as the jawbone. These images can be used to diagnose a wide range of dental issues, including cavities, periodontal disease, and jaw abnormalities. In the future, it is likely that digital X-ray image sensors will continue to be an important part of dentistry and may be used for even more applications. For example, the use of image sensors in conjunction with artificial intelligence (AI) algorithms for the automatic detection and diagnosis of dental issues is expected to increase, potentially improving the accuracy and efficiency of dental care.

20.1.2 Dual-Energy CBCT

Dual-energy computed tomography (DECT) is a quantitative imaging technique that uses two X-ray spectra to identify and quantify different materials. It has a wide range of clinical applications, including virtual monochromatic imaging, perfused blood volume, automated bone removal, and urinary stone characterization. The technique has gained widespread acceptance in the diagnostic radiology community and is also of increasing interest for use in radiotherapy [1].

Cone beam computed tomography (CBCT) is an imaging modality that uses a flat-panel detector and has been widely used in clinical

K. Orhan (✉)
Faculty of Dentistry, Ankara University, Ankara, Turkey

Ankara University Medical Design Application and Research Center (MEDITAM), Ankara, Turkey

Department of Oral Diagnostics, Faculty of Dentistry, Semmelweis University, Budapest, Hungary

A. Delantoni
Faculty of Dentistry, Aristotle University of Thessaloniki, Thessaloniki, Greece
e-mail: andelant@dent.auth.gr

D. Kırmızı · U. Aksoy
Faculty of Dentistry, Department of Endodontics, Near University, Nicosia, Cyprus

A. Delantoni, K. Orhan (eds.), *Digital Dentistry*, https://doi.org/10.1007/978-3-031-52826-2_20

practice, including in dentistry, radiotherapy, and interventions. However, image inhomogeneity caused by X-ray scattering and beam hardening can affect the visibility of soft tissues and the accuracy of CT numbers. One limitation of CBCT is the presence of strong metal artifacts, which are caused by the strong X-ray attenuation of metal objects such as dental restorations and implants. These artifacts can appear as streaks or halos in the reconstructed 3D images and can degrade the image quality and compromise the diagnostic accuracy of CBCT, particularly in the evaluation of the osseointegration of implants. One way to reduce metal artifacts is through the use of dual-energy CT (DECT), which synthesizes virtual monoenergetic images (VMIs) at high energies. Dual-energy CBCT (DE-CBCT) has the potential to improve soft tissue contrast and provide quantitative imaging, and it has been studied for use in a range of fields, including dentistry, interventions, and radiotherapy. While DE-CBCT has shown promise in preliminary studies, it has not yet become routine clinical practice. Researchers are exploring ways to address these limitations by developing a low-cost DECT system for use in dental CBCT by retrofitting a regular CBCT scanner with an X-ray tube and a pair of spectral filters. The newly proposed system is able to produce VMIs at two different energies and has the advantage of a lower equipment cost compared to other methods for dual-energy imaging. Preliminary results show that the system can effectively reduce metal artifacts [2].

20.2 Dental Magnetic Resonance Imaging (MRI)

New generation high-resolution MRI has a higher spatial resolution, which allows for more detailed images of small structures such as teeth and surrounding tissues. New MRI machines featuring more advanced gradient coils and stronger magnets have been developed, resulting in the ability to produce higher quality images more quickly. Coils specifically designed for imaging the teeth and jaw, known as dental MRI coils, have been developed to improve the accuracy and detail of the resulting images.

Continuing efforts to increase the spatial resolution of MRI could lead to even more detailed and accurate images of small structures such as teeth and surrounding tissues. Advances in hardware and software may allow MRI machines to acquire images more quickly, reducing the amount of time patients need to spend in the scanner. In addition, the development of smaller, more portable MRI machines could make it easier to bring MRI capabilities to underserved areas or to use it in settings outside of traditional hospitals or clinics [3].

3D printing technology has been used to create models of teeth and jaw structures based on MRI data, which can be used for surgical planning and training. A recent study suggests that dental MRI is reliable and accurate enough to be used for creating surgical guides, but further research is needed to make it more accurate for use in implant planning outside of clinical trials [4]. Moreover, certain dental procedures, such as root canal therapy, can be performed with the assistance of MRI guidance to enhance accuracy and precision.

MRI can be used to visualize root canal topography and dental anatomy for endodontic treatment. While MRI offers high visibility of tissue without exposing the patient to ionizing radiation, it requires longer scan times and higher resolutions than other methods such as computed tomography (CT) or cone beam CT (CBCT). MRI is most effective at the microscopic level, with resolutions better than 100 mm^3, and can be useful in evaluating the health of dental pulp and in identifying inflammation or edema. The main limitation of using MRI in endodontic treatment is the long imaging time required, although this is expected to improve with technological developments [5].

In the future, functional MRI, which measures changes in blood flow and oxygenation, could be utilized more frequently in dentistry to evaluate the function of the teeth and jaw. Additionally, MRI has the potential to guide procedures such as biopsies or extractions in real-time, enabling more precise and minimally invasive technique.

Maxillary sinus volume and Schneiderian membrane thickness, and for computer-assisted implant surgery can be measured using MRI, which can also be applied to computer-assisted implant surgery. MRI has the advantage of being able to visualize soft tissues, such as the alveolar inferior nerve, more effectively than cone beam CT (CBCT), and can be used to evaluate the health and vascularization of dental pulp, detect missing canals, cracks, and fractures, and follow the progression of periapical lesions without exposing the patient to ionizing radiation [5]. Artificial intelligence (AI) technology has been successful in various medical imaging fields and in some applications of robotic surgery. It can be useful in recognizing landmarks in MRI and optimizing images [6, 7]. In the future, it is expected that AI technology will be applied to magnetic resonance imaging (MRI) to improve its usefulness in dental clinical practice and make it more suitable for use without exposing patients to ionizing radiation.

Overall, the future prospects for MRI in dentistry are promising and could lead to significant advances in the diagnosis and treatment of dental conditions.

20.3 Artificial Intelligence (AI)

Artificial intelligence (AI) refers to the ability of a computer or machine to perform tasks that typically require human-like intelligence, such as learning, problem-solving, decision making, and language understanding. It has the potential to revolutionize many aspects of the field of dentistry. AI can be used to assist with a variety of tasks, including diagnosis and treatment planning, predictive analytics, surgical procedures, and lab work [8]. AI has the potential to improve the accuracy and efficiency of dental care, leading to better outcomes for patients.

20.3.1 Diagnosis and Treatment Planning

One of the key areas where AI has the potential to make a significant impact in dentistry is in the realm of diagnosis and treatment planning. By analyzing dental images, such as X-rays, AI algorithms can help dentists identify issues that might not be immediately apparent to the human eye. This could include identifying signs of tooth decay, detecting abnormalities in the jaw, or identifying other issues that may require treatment. Once a diagnosis has been made, AI algorithms can be used to help dentists develop a customized treatment plan for each patient. This could include determining the best course of action, identifying the most appropriate materials to use, and estimating the cost of treatment. AI can also analyze a patient's medical history and other relevant data to provide recommendations to dentists on the best course of treatment. For example, an AI system might recommend a particular type of filling material based on the patient's allergies, or suggest a specific type of toothbrush for a patient with sensitive teeth.

20.3.2 Predictive Analytics

Predictive analytics in dentistry involves using AI algorithms to analyze data from electronic health records and other sources to predict which patients are at risk for certain dental conditions. This can allow dentists to intervene early and prevent problems from developing. In dentistry, predictive analytics can be used to identify patients at risk for periodontal disease, perform predictive maintenance on dental equipment, and identify patients at risk for tooth loss.

Predictive analytics involves using AI to analyze data and make predictions about future events. One potential use of AI in this context is the early detection of oral cancer [9]. By analyzing data from electronic health records, including patient history, demographic information, and dental images, AI algorithms could identify patients who are at risk for developing oral cancer. This could allow dentists to intervene early and provide treatment, increasing the chances of a successful outcome.

Another potential use of AI in predictive analytics is predictive scheduling. By analyzing data from electronic health records, including patient history and treatment plans, AI algorithms could predict when patients are likely to need follow-up visits or specific procedures. This could allow dentists to schedule appointments more efficiently, reducing wait times and improving patient satisfaction.

Predictive treatment planning is another area where AI could be used in the field of dentistry. By analyzing data from electronic health records, including patient history and treatment plans, AI algorithms could predict the most effective treatment plan for each patient. This could allow dentists to provide personalized care and improve patient outcomes.

20.3.3 Dental Surgery

AI has the potential to transform the field of dental surgery by assisting dentists in performing complex procedures. One way that AI could be used in this context is through the development of robotic assistants. These AI-powered robots could be equipped with cameras, sensors, and other technology to provide a high-resolution view of the surgical site and assist the dentist in performing the procedure.

AI algorithms could also be used in surgical planning. By analyzing patient data, including medical history, imaging studies, and other information, these algorithms could help dentists plan surgical procedures. They could suggest the best course of action, identify potential risks, and recommend the most appropriate materials to use.

In addition, AI algorithms could be used to create virtual simulations of surgical procedures. This could allow dentists to practice and refine their technique before performing surgery on a real patient.

20.3.4 Dental Lab Work

AI has the potential to improve the accuracy and efficiency of dental lab work, particularly in the design and fabrication of dental restorations like crowns and bridges. One way that AI could be used in this context is through design assistance. AI algorithms could analyze data from dental images, such as X-rays and 3D scans, to help dental technicians design custom restorations that fit each patient's unique anatomy.

AI algorithms could also be used to recommend the most appropriate materials for use in dental restorations based on data from electronic health records, including patient allergies and medical history. This could help ensure that patients receive restorations that are safe and effective.

AI-powered robotic assistants could also assist dental technicians in the fabrication process, allowing them to produce restorations more efficiently and accurately. This could improve the overall accuracy and efficiency of dental lab work.

In summary, AI has the potential to enhance the accuracy and efficiency of dental treatment, resulting in improved patient outcomes. However, the need for regulatory and ethical considerations should be addressed before certain AI technologies can be fully implemented, such as dental imaging diagnostics and robot-assisted surgeries. There is a concern that machine learning algorithms could contain bias and exacerbate disparities in care [10].

20.3.4.1 Digital Intraoral Scanners

Digital intraoral scanners are a tool used in dentistry that allows for the creation of digital impressions of a patient's teeth and mouth. These digital impressions can be used to make dental restorations, such as crowns and bridges, and to plan orthodontic treatment.

One potential benefit of digital intraoral scanners is their ability to create highly accurate digital impressions. This can lead to better treatment outcomes and more precise dental restorations. Additionally, digital impressions can be created much faster than traditional impressions, which can save time for both the patient and the dental team.

Digital intraoral scanners may also provide a more comfortable experience for patients compared to traditional impression materials. As a result, the use of these scanners is likely to continue to grow in the future as more dentists adopt the technology and it becomes more widely available.

In oral implantology, digital intraoral scanners can be used to design and create single or multiple dental implants [11]. The process involves acquiring 3D data using an intraoral scanner and then transmitting it to CAD software for implant design and a CAM device for manufacturing. Intraoral scanners can also be used to create digital impressions of complete arch implant cases and assist with arch implantation. Intraoral scanners can also be used to create computer-assisted implant surgery guide rails and locate implants during surgery, making the procedure more reliable and safer. However, some studies have found that there is inaccuracy in implant placement guidance when using virtual surgical planning based on data from CBCT scans and an intraoral scanner.

In orthodontics, digital orthodontic systems can be used for diagnosis, treatment planning, and manufacturing aligners and other custom devices. In oral and maxillofacial surgery, intraoral scanners can be used in combination with CT and stereo cameras to capture and visualize surrounding anatomy and virtual implants. However, the use of scanning systems in this field has been slow due to high implementation costs and infrequent use. Overall, while intraoral and extraoral scanners have become widely used in dentistry, they still have limitations such as image distortion, operator skill, patient movement, and restricted space in the oral cavity [12].

There are several potential innovations that may be developed for intraoral scanners in the future. For example, researchers may work to improve the accuracy of these scanners, or expand their capabilities to include a wider range of tasks. It is also possible that intraoral scanners will become more widely available and more affordable, making them accessible to more dental practices and patients. Additionally, intraoral scanners may be integrated with other technologies such as 3D printing or virtual reality in order to enhance their capabilities and improve the efficiency of dental procedures. Intraoral scanners can be used to customize almost every treatment to fit the specific needs of each patient in the future. Overall, the field of intraoral scanners is expected to continue to evolve and improve as new technologies and techniques are developed [13].

20.3.4.2 Computer-Aided Design and Computer-Aided Manufacturing (CAD/CAM)

Computer-aided design and computer-aided manufacturing (CAD/CAM) technologies have already had a significant impact on dentistry and are expected to continue to play an important role in the field in the future. These technologies allow dental practitioners to design and fabricate dental restorations, such as crowns and bridges, more accurately and efficiently. They also enable practitioners to create digital models of patients' teeth and jaws, which can be used for treatment planning and surgical guidance.

20.4 Dynamic Navigation in Implant Placement

Dental implants are a common treatment for replacing missing teeth. The success of these implants depends on their precise placement, which can be improved through the use of surgical guidance techniques. Static surgical guidance, which has been used for several decades, has improved the accuracy of implant placement, but it has limitations due to its rigid adherence to the planned implant position. Dynamic navigation is a relatively new technology in dentistry that allows for real-time, three-dimensional guidance during implant surgery. It has the potential to greatly improve the accuracy and precision of implant placement, which can lead to better outcomes for patients. Dynamic real-time clinical guidance, such as robot-assisted implant placement, offers the potential for more accurate and flexible implant placement. This technology provides visual and haptic guidance during treatment planning, osteotomy preparation, and implant placement [14].

In the future, it is likely that dynamic navigation will become more widely adopted in dental practices, as it has already started to do. In addition, it is possible that the technology will continue to evolve and improve, leading to even better results for patients.

Dynamic computer-assisted implant surgery (dCAIS) is a technology that can be used to guide implant placement in the mouth during surgery. It allows for real-time visualization of the relationship between the drill and important anatomical structures, which can reduce the risk of poor implant positioning or other intraoperative issues. A systematic review and meta-analysis were conducted to assess the accuracy of dCAIS compared to other methods of implant placement [15]. Overall, the review suggests that dCAIS may be more accurate than other methods of implant placement, but further research is needed to confirm these findings.

20.5 Virtual Reality (VR) Systems in Dentistry

Virtual reality (VR) systems have the potential to significantly impact the field of dentistry by providing a range of benefits. One potential use for VR in dentistry is the ability to simulate procedures in a virtual environment before performing them on a patient. This can allow dentists to practice new techniques or procedures and can be particularly helpful for complex or risky procedures. In addition, VR can be used to train dental students by providing a realistic, interactive environment for them to practice procedures and learn anatomy. This can be more effective than traditional methods such as lectures and textbooks, as students can learn by doing in a simulated environment.

20.5.1 VR Haptic Simulators

Haptic training simulator (HTS) is an advanced computer-based simulation (CBS) technology especially in the field of teaching and learning operative dentistry where perceptions and physiological arousals can be felt in the virtual environment with haptic feedback to the Virtual Reality (VR) environment [16, 17]. These simulators allow the user to feel sound, pressure and vibration through the holding device, thus providing an optimal simulation of the clinical procedure with a lifelike learning experience [18].

Haptic simulators provide preclinical operative dentistry in clinical integrations. These simulations can provide sensory feedback in enamel, dentin tissue, and a carious tissue [19]; even standard cases are evaluated and treated. In this way, the preclinical psychomotor skills of the students improve and the time they spend for clinical observation decreases. It has also been reported that haptic simulators can be used more easily and effectively than phantom simulators for left-handed students, however, that they cannot replace clinical practice [20].

In addition to the models produced with a joystick and desktop screen; A more realistic 3D environment is created by using VR glasses and haptic dental tool in current devices. They developed for dental practice include tactile instruments and dental mirrors. In this way, a tactile device that mimics a hand-held dental instrument is held in one hand, and a tracking device that mimics a mirror in the other to perform two-handed treatments. The hand skill on the devices was first tried to be developed by creating a shape on virtual blocks; in the next stage, opportunities such as working on haptic teeth and even jaws and detecting caries are offered. As a further level of this, it provides a virtual patient and clinical scene as an exact replica of reality, with moving VR patients and virtually generated clinical scenarios. Moreover, by transferring radiographs of real patients into practice, it is possible to define caries and create special cases in order to take learning to the next level. Manufacturers also provide a full classroom setup with the assistant console in order to observe, score and control the work done by the practitioner students in the dental classrooms and to produce new scenarios. This amazing technology offers the opportunity for better preclinical treatment in dentistry (Fig. 20.1).

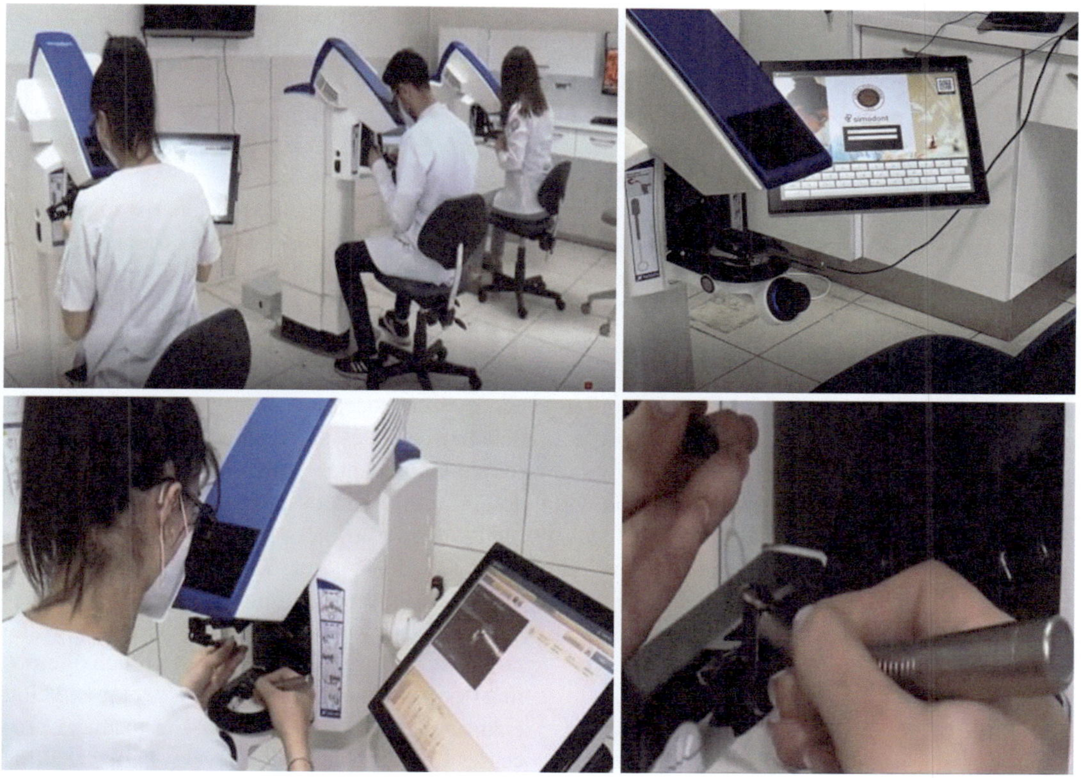

Fig. 20.1 Dental Haptic Simulators are used at Ankara University Faculty of Dentistry

20.5.2 Patient Education

VR can also be used to provide patient education, allowing patients to better understand their treatment options and procedures. By using VR, dentists can provide a more immersive and interactive experience, which can help patients feel more informed and involved in their own care. Additionally, VR can be used as a tool for pain management and anxiety reduction during dental procedures. By providing patients with a distraction in the form of a virtual reality experience, dentists may be able to reduce the perception of pain and discomfort during treatment.

In terms of communication, VR can be used to facilitate a more interactive and personalized experience between dentists and patients. For example, dentists could use VR to show patients 3D models of their teeth and explain treatment options in a more visual and interactive way.

Overall, the use of VR in dentistry has the potential to improve patient care, education, and training in the field, and may become an increasingly common tool in dental practice in the future.

20.6 Metaverse/Dentaverse

The metaverse is metadata store which called cyberspace. Metaverse provides a virtual forum for enhanced international engagement. After creating an avatar in a virtual reality environment using an application using a desktop or using virtual reality or augmented reality glasses, it is possible to interact with others, as well as entering conference rooms and developed for education in 3D [21]. The fact that dentistry education and applied courses are affected by the Pandemic COVID-19 outbreak has made the thought of distance learning and education in the metaverse even more important. It can enable virtual applications where fine motor movements such as wearing gloves, nerve blocking or suturing can be done [22].

A new platform has been created where access has been moved to the level of virtual help. Dentaverse is an online virtual reality portal aimed at providing virtual online 7/24 dental education services for dentistry students and post-graduated dentists. Dental students, professionals, and material suppliers can interact with each other, participate in many activities, VR conferences and exhibitions and even offer dental treatments and dental materials. The purchasable platform provides dental information and innovative technologies such as blockchain, web3 technology, Metaverse (VR) and education, which connects the dental community globally with the aim of increasing personal and professional development by connecting them in 3D and virtual reality.

Members have the opportunity to receive academic training through a dental VR link center that offers web3 tools and services. Using your VR headset and controllers, it is possible to work by creating an exact copy of the real environment in 3D. Also compatible with devices such as Windows PC, PlayStation 5, PlayStation 4, Xbox Series X, Xbox Series S, Xbox One, Nintendo Switch, Google Stadia, macOS, iOS, Android, ARKit, ARCore, OpenXR, SteamVR, Oculus, Linux, and SteamDeck.

Virtual interaction allows a dentist to simultaneously consult a specialist in a different country for a complex dental case procedure, simulate and perform the procedure and learn in detail the treatment process that should be applied by receiving feedback and guidance from colleagues about this procedure. Moreover, a web3-ready dental practice can be created in the virtual environment for dental professionals. Dentaverse is able to easily accept crypto payments by developing its own business-ready crypto platform.

The goal of the platform in 2023 is to make virtual reality applications that include intermediate dentistry skills available. Realizing the power of feedback and providing a touch of emotion in practitioners by virtual dental meeting environment. Its target in 2024 is to make processes that include high-level dentistry skills available. The creators of the platform consider Dentaverse to be an important milestone in the future of dentistry [23] (Fig. 20.1 and 20.2).

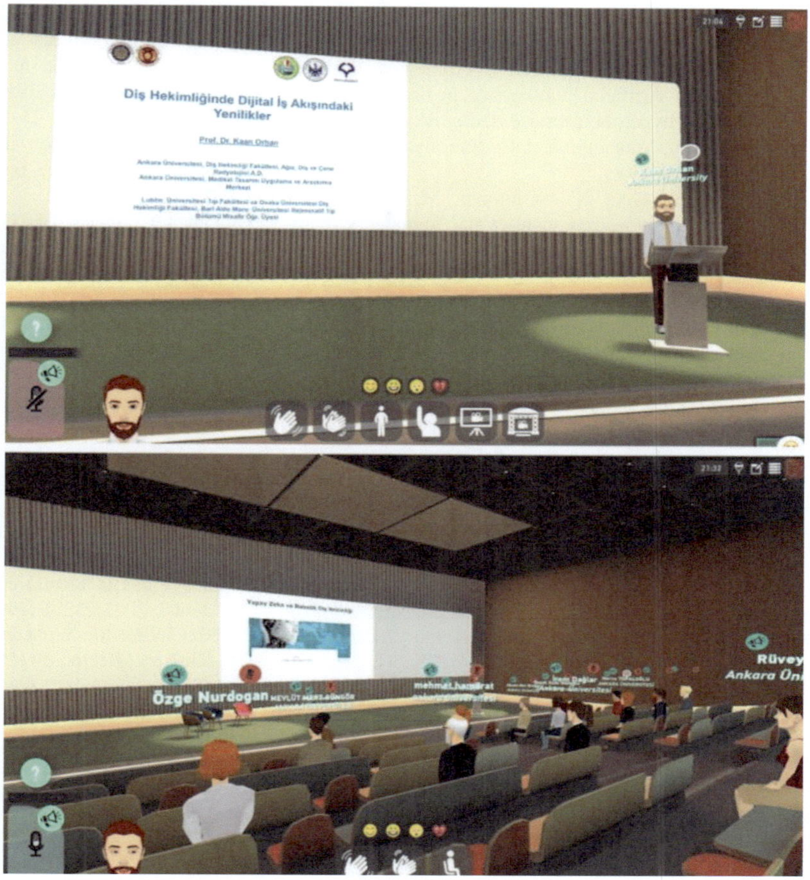

Fig. 20.1 and 20.2 Shows a virtual classroom in a Dentaverse platform set up. An avatar can be created in a virtual reality environment using a desktop application or VR/AR glasses, allowing for interaction with others and access to 3D conference rooms and educational spaces

References

1. Agostini A, Borgheresi A, Mari A, Floridi C, Bruno F, Carotti M, et al. Dual-energy CT: theoretical principles and clinical applications. Radiol Med. 2019;124(12):1281–95.
2. Li B, Spronk D, Luo Y, Puett C, Inscoe CR, Tyndall DA, et al. Feasibility of dual-energy CBCT by spectral filtration of a dual-focus CNT X-ray source. PLoS One. 2022;17(2):e02627.
3. Lang M, Rapalino O, Huang S, Lev MH, Conklin J, Wald LL. Emerging techniques and future directions. Magn Reson Imaging Clin N Am. 2022;30(3):565–82.
4. Hilgenfeld T, Juerchott A, Jende JM, Rammelsberg P, Heiland S, Bendszus M, et al. Use of dental MRI for radiation-free guided dental implant planning: a prospective, in vivo study of accuracy and reliability. Eur Radiol. 2020;30(12):6392–401.
5. Reda R, Zanza A, Mazzoni A, Cicconetti A, Testarelli L, Di Nardo D. An update of the possible applications of magnetic resonance imaging (MRI) in dentistry: a literature review. J Imaging. 2021;7(5):75.
6. Liu W, Wang Y, Jiang T, Chi Y, Zhang L, Hua XS. Landmarks detection with anatomical constraints for Total hip arthroplasty preoperative measurements. In: Martel AL, Abolmaesumi P, Stoyanov D, Mateus D, Zuluaga MA, Zhou SK, Racoceanu D, Joskowicz L, editors. Part I, proceedings of the medical image computing and computer assisted intervention—MICCAI 2020, Lima, Peru, 4–8 October 2020, vol. 12264. Cham: Springer; 2020.
7. Zhong Z, Li J, Zhang Z, Jiao Z, Gao X. An attention-guided deep regression model for landmark detection in Cephalograms. In: Proceedings of the languages and compilers for parallel computing, Shenzhen, China. Cham: Springer; 2019. p. 540–8.
8. Shan T, Tay FR, Gu L. Application of artificial intelligence in dentistry. J Dent Res. 2020;100(3):232–44.
9. García-Pola M, Pons-Fuster E, Suárez-Fernández C, Seoane-Romero J, Romero-Méndez A, López-Jornet P. Role of artificial intelligence in the early

diagnosis of oral cancer. A scoping review. Cancers. 2021;13(18):4600.
10. Matheny M, Thadaney Israni S, Ahmed M, Whicher D, editors. Artificial intelligence in health care: the Hope, the hype, the promise, the peril. NAM special publication. Washington, DC: National Academy of Medicine; 2019.
11. Yilmaz B, Guo X, Schimmel M, Abou-Ayash S. Effect of industrial scanner and framework material interaction on the marginal gaps of CAD-cam complete-arch implant frameworks. J Prosthet Dent. 2022;0022-3913(21):00586–2.
12. Mangano F, Gandolfi A, Luongo G, Logozzo S. Intraoral scanners in dentistry: a review of the current literature. BMC Oral Health. 2017;17(1):149.
13. Hou X, Xu X, Zhao M, Kong J, Wang M, Lee ES, et al. An overview of three-dimensional imaging devices in dentistry. J Esthet Restor Dent. 2022;34(8):1179–96.
14. Grischke J, Johannsmeier L, Eich L, Griga L, Haddadin S. Dentronics: towards robotics and artificial intelligence in dentistry. Dent Mater. 2020;36(6):765–78.
15. Afrashtehfar KI, Jurado CA, Moshaverinia A. Dynamic navigation may be used for most implant surgery scenarios due to its satisfactory accuracy. J Evid Based Dent Pract. 2022;22(4):101797.
16. Krogmeier C, Mousas C, Whittinghill D. Human–virtual character interaction: toward understanding the influence of haptic feedback. Computer Animation and Virtual Worlds. 2019;30(3–4):e1883.
17. Farag A, Hashem D. Impact of the haptic virtual reality simulator on dental students' psychomotor skills in preclinical operative dentistry. Clin Pract. 2021;12(1):17–26.
18. Gal GB, Weiss EI, Gafni N, Ziv A. Preliminary assessment of faculty and student perception of a haptic virtual reality simulator for training dental manual dexterity. J Dent Educ. 2011;75(4):496–504.
19. Perry S, Bridges SM, Burrow MF. A review of the use of simulation in dental education. Simul Healthc. 2015;10(1):31–7.
20. Wójcik A, Pakaszewski W, Smulewicz K, Ziomko B, Rusin B. Is simulation in dentistry able to replace clinical practice? Analysis of students' opinions. J Educ Health Sport. 2023;13(2):242–8.
21. Ravenscraft E. What is the metaverse, exactly? Wired. 2022. https://www.wired.com/story/what-is-the-metaverse.
22. Locurcio LL. Dental education in the metaverse. Br Dent J. 2022;232(4):191.
23. McClellan M. What is the metaverse—and how is dentistry affected by it? Dent Econ 2022;12(112).

Correction to: Digital Systems in Oral Pathology

Sofia Karachrysafi, Dimitrios Andreadis, and Athanasios Poulopoulos

Correction to:
Chapter 12 in: A. Delantoni, K. Orhan (eds.), *Digital Dentistry*, https://doi.org/10.1007/978-3-031-52826-2_12

The authors' names Karachrysafi Sofia, Andreadis Dimitrios, and Poulopoulos Athanasios were misspelled in this chapter. The authors' names have been changed to Sofia Karachrysafi, Dimitrios Andreadis, and Athanasios Poulopoulos.

The updated version of this chapter can be found at https://doi.org/10.1007/978-3-031-52826-2_12

A. Delantoni, K. Orhan (eds.), *Digital Dentistry*, https://doi.org/10.1007/978-3-031-52826-2_21

MIX
Papier aus verantwortungsvollen Quellen
Paper from responsible sources
FSC® C105338

If you have any concerns about our products,
you can contact us on
ProductSafety@springernature.com

In case Publisher is established outside the EU,
the EU authorized representative is:
Springer Nature Customer Service Center GmbH
Europaplatz 3, 69115 Heidelberg, Germany

Printed by Libri Plureos GmbH
in Hamburg, Germany